WITHDRAWN

AIDS
(Acquired Immune Deficiency Syndrome)
Bibliography

for 1981-86

AIDS
(Acquired Immune Deficiency Syndrome)
Bibliography

for 1981-86

Compiled by
Nancy C. Weissberg

The Whitston Publishing Company
Troy, New York
1988

TABLE OF CONTENTS

PREFACE

This is the first in a series of what will be an invaluable tool for research on the modern pandemic—AIDS. It is a complete bibliography of world-wide literature surrounding this central social and medical issue that has proven to be a persistent problem of alarming proportions.

This first volume covers the years 1981—the year of the first diagnosed case of AIDS in the United States—up to and including 1986. Hereafter, the *AIDS BIBLIOGRAPHY* will be updated annually. The Bibliography is divided into three sections: the first section is a list of books, government publications and monographs; the second section includes periodical literature alphabetically by title; the third section lists periodical literature by subject. The subject heads have been issued from the nature of the material indexed rather than being imposed from Library of Congress subject heads or other standard lists. A list of journals cited, a subject heading index, and an author index to the periodical literature all enhance the usefulness of this volume.

AIDS JOURNAL LIST

AAOHN JOURNAL
AANA JOURNAL
AARN NEWSLETTER: ALBERTA ASSOCIATION OF REGISTERED NURSES
    NEWSLETTER
ADAMHA NEWS
AGB REPORTS
AIDS RESEARCH
AJNR: AMERICAN JOURNAL OF NEURORADIOLOGY
AJR: AMERICAN JOURNAL OF ROENTGENOLOGY
AMB: REVISTA DA ASSOCIACAO MEDICA BRASILEIRA
ANNA JOURNAL: AMERICAN NEPHROLOGY NURSES ASSOCIATION
    JOURNAL
AORN JOURNAL: ASSOCIATION OF OPERATING ROOM NURSES
AUAA J: JOURNAL OF THE AMERICAN UROLOGICAL ASSOCIATION ALLIED
ACTA CLINICA BELGICA
ACTA CYTOLOGICA
ACTA DERMATO-VENEREOLOGICA
ACTA GASTROENTEROLOGICA BELGICA
ACTA HAEMATOLOGICA
ACTA HAEMATOLOGICA POLONICA
ACTA MEDICA PORTUGUESA
ACTA MEDICA SCANDINAVICA
ACTA NEUROLOGICA SCANDINAVICA
ACTA NEUROPATHOLOGICA
ACTA OPHTHALMOLOGICA
ACTA PATHOLOGICA, MICROBIOLOGICA, ET IMMUNOLOGICA SCANDI-
    NAVICA
ACTA UNIVERSITATIS PALACKIANAE OLOMUCENSIS FACULTATIS
    MEDICAE
L'ACTUALITE
ADVANCES IN ALCOHOL AND SUBSTANCE ABUSE
ADVANCES IN CANCER RESEARCH
ADVANCES IN EXPERIMENTAL MEDICINE AND BIOLOGY
ADVANCES IN INTERNAL MEDICINE
ADVANCES IN VETERINARY SCIENCE AND COMPARATIVE MEDICINE
ADVERTISING AGE
ADVOCATE
AFRICA
AGAINST THE CURRENT
AIR FORCE TIMES
ALABAMA JOURNAL OF MEDICAL SCIENCES
ALABAMA MEDICINE
ALBERTA REPORT

ALTERNATIVE MEDIA
AMERICA
AMERICAN ANNALS OF THE DEAF
AMERICAN BAR ASSOCIATION JOURNAL
AMERICAN BIOLOGY TEACHER
AMERICAN COLLEGE OF PHYSICIANS OBSERVER
AMERICAN FAMILY PHYSICIAN
AMERICAN HEALTH CARE ASSOCIATION JOURNAL
AMERICAN JOURNAL OF CARDIOLOGY
AMERICAN JOURNAL OF CLINICAL NUTRITION
AMERICAN JOURNAL OF CLINICAL PATHOLOGY
AMERICAN JOURNAL OF DISEASES OF CHILDREN
AMERICAN JOURNAL OF EMERGENCY MEDICINE
AMERICAN JOURNAL OF EPIDEMIOLOGY
AMERICAN JOURNAL OF FORENSIC MEDICINE AND PATHOLOGY
AMERICAN JOURNAL OF GASTROENTEROLOGY
AMERICAN JOURNAL OF HEMATOLOGY
AMERICAN JOURNAL OF HOSPICE CARE
AMERICAN JOURNAL OF INFECTION CONTROL
AMERICAN JOURNAL OF THE MEDICAL SCIENCES
AMERICAN JOURNAL OF MEDICAL TECHNOLOGY
AMERICAN JOURNAL OF MEDICINE
AMERICAN JOURNAL OF NURSING
AMERICAN JOURNAL OF OBSTETRICS AND GYNECOLOGY
AMERICAN JOURNAL OF OPHTHALMOLOGY
AMERICAN JOURNAL OF PATHOLOGY
AMERICAN JOURNAL OF PEDIATRIC HEMATOLOGY/ONCOLOGY
AMERICAN JOURNAL OF PSYCHIATRY
AMERICAN JOURNAL OF PUBLIC HEALTH
AMERICAN JOURNAL OF SURGICAL PATHOLOGY
AMERICAN JOURNAL OF TROPICAL MEDICINE AND HYGIENE
AMERICAN JOURNAL OF VETERINARY RESEARCH
AMERICAN LAUNDRY DIGEST
AMERICAN LIBRARIES
AMERICAN MEDICAL NEWS
AMERICAN NURSE
AMERICAN PHARMACY
AMERICAN PHOTOGRAPHER
AMERICAN PSYCHOLOGIST
AMERICAN REVIEW OF RESPIRATORY DISEASE
AMERICAN SCHOOL BOARD JOURNAL
AMERICAN SPECTATOR
ANALES ESPANOLES DE PEDIATRIA
ANALYTICAL AND QUANTITATIVE CYTOLOGY
ANALYTICAL CHEMISTRY
ANESTHESIA AND ANALGESIA
ANESTHESIOLOGY
ANNALES DE DERMATOLOGIE ET DE VENEREOLOGIE
ANNALES DE GASTROENTEROLOGIE ET D'HEPATOLOGIE
ANNALES D'OTOLARYNGOLOGIE ET DE CHIRURGIE CERVICO-FACIALE
ANNALES DE LA SOCIETE BELGE DE MEDECINE TROPICALE
ANNALES DE MEDECINE INTERNE
ANNALES FRANCAISES D'ANESTHESIE ET DE REANIMATION

ANNALS OF ALLERGY
ANNALS OF CLINICAL AND LABORATORY SCIENCE
ANNALS OF CLINICAL RESEARCH
ANNALS OF EMERGENCY MEDICINE
ANNALS OF INTERNAL MEDICINE
ANNALS OF NEUROLOGY
ANNALS OF THE NEW YORK ACADEMY OF SCIENCES
ANNALS OF OPHTHALMOLOGY
ANNALS OF PATHOLOGY
ANNALS OF SURGERY
ANNALS OF THORACIC SURGERY
ANNUAL REVIEW OF IMMUNOLOGY
ANNUAL REVIEW OF MEDICINE
ANTIBIOTICS AND CHEMOTHERAPY
ANTIMICROBIAL AGENTS AND CHEMOTHERAPY
APPLIED PATHOLOGY
APPLIED RADIOLOGY
ARCHIVES D'ANATOMIE ET DE CYTOLOGIE PATHOLOGIQUES
ARCHIVES OF DERMATOLOGICAL RESEARCH
ARCHIVES OF DERMATOLOGY
ARCHIVES OF DISEASE IN CHILDHOOD
ARCHIVES OF EMERGENCY MEDICINE
ARCHIVES OF GYNECOLOGY
ARCHIVES OF INTERNAL MEDICINE
ARCHIVES OF NEUROLOGY
ARCHIVES OF OPHTHALMOLOGY
ARCHIVES OF OTOLARYNGOLOGY
ARCHIVES OF OTO-RHINO-LARYNGOLQGY
ARCHIVES OF PATHOLOGY AND LABORATORY MEDICINE
ARCHIVES OF PHYSICAL MEDICINE AND REHABILITATION
ARCHIVES OF SURGERY
ARENA
ARIZONA NURSE
ARKANSAS TIMES
ARMY RESERVE NEWS
ARTFORUM
ASIAN AND PACIFIC JOURNAL OF ALLERGY AND IMMUNOLOGY
ATLANTIC INSIGHT
ATLANTIC MONTHLY
AUSTRALASIAN NURSES JOURNAL
AUSTRALIAN AND NEW ZEALAND JOURNAL OF MEDICINE
AUSTRALIAN AND NEW ZEALAND JOURNAL OF SURGERY
AUSTRALIAN DENTAL JOURNAL
AUSTRALIAN FAMILY PHYSICIAN
AUSTRALIAN JOURNAL OF EXPERIMENTAL BIOLOGY AND MEDICAL
    SCIENCE
AUSTRALIAN NURSES JOURNAL
BARRONS
BEST'S REVIEW
BIOMEDICINE AND PHARMACOTHERAPY
BIOSCIENCE
BLACK ENTERPRISE
BLOOD

BLUT
BODY POLITIC
BOLETIN-ASSOCIACION MEDICA DE PUERTO RICO
BOLLETTINO DELL INSTITUTO SIEROTERAPICO MILANESE
BORDERLINES
BOSTON
BRITISH DENTAL JOURNAL
BRITISH JOURNAL OF DERMATOLOGY
BRITISH JOURNAL OF DISEASES OF THE CHEST
BRITISH JOURNAL OF HAEMATOLOGY
BRITISH JOURNAL OF HOSPITAL MEDICINE
BRITISH JOURNAL OF INDUSTRIAL MEDICINE
BRITISH JOURNAL OF OPHTHALMOLOGY
BRITISH JOURNAL OF PSYCHIATRY
BRITISH JOURNAL OF SURGERY
BRITISH JOURNAL OF VENEREAL DISEASE
BRITISH MEDICAL JOURNAL
BULLETIN DE L'ACADEMIE NATIONALE DE MEDECINE
BULLETIN DE LA SOCIETE DE PATHOLOGIE ET DE SES FILIALES
BULLETIN DE LA SOCIETE DES SCIENCES MEDICALES DU GRAND-DUCHE
    DE LUXEMBOURG
BULLETIN DES SOCIETES D'OPHTHALMOLOGIE DE FRANCE
BULLETIN OF THE AMERICAN COLLEGE OF SURGEONS
BULLETIN OF THE WORLD HEALTH ORGANIZATION
BULLETIN ON NARCOTICS
BUSINESS AND HEALTH
BUSINESS HORIZONS
BUSINESS INSURANCE
BUSINESS WEEK
CRC CRITICAL REVIEWS IN IMMUNOLOGY
CRC CRITICAL REVIEWS ON CLINICAL LABORATORY SCIENCES
CALIFORNIA
CALIFORNIA NURSE
CALIFORNIA PRISONER
CANADA AND THE WORLD
CANADIAN ANAESTHETISTS SOCIETY JOURNAL
CANADIAN DENTAL ASSOCIATION JOURNAL
CANADIAN JOURNAL OF MEDICAL TECHNOLOGY
CANADIAN JOURNAL OF PSYCHIATRY
CANADIAN LIVING
CANADIAN MEDICAL ASSOCIATION JOURNAL
CANADIAN NURSE
CANCER
CANCER DETECTION AND PREVENTION
CANCER GENETICS AND CYTOGENETICS
CANCER IMMUNOLOGY AND IMMUNOTHERAPY
CANCER NURSING
CANCER RESEARCH
CANCER TREATMENT REPORTS
CARING
CASOPIS LEKARU CESKYCH
CATHOLIC WORKER
CELL

CELLULAR IMMUNOLOGY
CESKOSLOVENSKA PEDIATRIE
CHANGING MEN
CHANNELS OF COMMUNICATION
CHART
CHARTIST
CHATELAINE
CHEMICAL AND ENGINEERING NEWS
CHEMICAL INDUSTRY
CHEMICAL MARKETING REPORTER
CHEMICAL WEEK
CHEST
CHICAGO
CHILD WELFARE
CHIRURGIE
CHRISTIAN CENTURY
CHRISTIAN MINISTRY
CHRISTIANITY AND CRISIS
CHRISTIANITY TODAY
CHRONICLE OF HIGHER EDUCATION
CHUNG HUA CHIEH HO HU HSIHSI CHI PING TSA CHIH
CHUNG HUA LIU HSING PING HSUEH TSA CHIH
CHUNG HUA MIN KUO WEI SHENG WU CHI MIEN I HSUEH TSA CHIH
CHUNG HUA NEI KO TSA CHIH
CITY AND STATE HEALTH FINANCES
CIVIL LIBERTIES
CLEVELAND CLINIC QUARTERLY
CITIZEN AIRMAN
CLEVELAND MAGAZINE
CLINICA TERAPEUTICA
CLINICAL AND EXPERIMENTAL DERMATOLOGY
CLINICAL AND EXPERIMENTAL IMMUNOLOGY
CLINICAL AND LABORATORY MEDICINE
CLINICAL CHEMISTRY
CLINICAL ENGINEERING INFORMATION SERVICE
CLINICAL HAEMATOLOGY
CLINICAL IMMUNOLOGY AND IMMUNOPATHOLOGY
CLINICAL IMMUNOLOGY REVIEWS
CLINICAL NEPHROLOGY
CLINICAL NEUROLOGY AND NEUROSURGERY
CLINICAL NEUROPATHOLOGY
CLINICAL NEUROPHARMACOLOGY
CLINICAL NUCLEAR MEDICINE
CLINICAL PHARMACOLOGY AND THERAPEUTICS
CLINICAL PHARMACY
CLINICAL RADIOLOGY
CLINICAL RESEARCH
CLINICS IN HAEMATOLOGY
CLINICS IN LABORATORY MEDICINE
COLLEAGUE ON CALL
COLORADO MEDICINE
COLUMBIA JOURNALISM REVIEW
COMMENTARY

COMMONWEAL
COMMUNIQ'ELLES
COMMUNITY MEDICINE
COMPENSATION AND BENEFITS REVIEW
COMPREHENSIVE PSYCHIATRY
COMPREHENSIVE THERAPY
COMPTES RENDUS DE L'ACADEMIE DES SCIENCE. SERIE III: SCIENCES DE
    LA VIE
CONGRESSIONAL RESEARCH SERVICE REVIEW
CONNECTICUT MAGAZINE
CONNECTICUT MEDICINE
CONSERVATIVE DIGEST
CONSULTANT
CONSUMER'S RESEARCH MAGAZINE
CONTEMPORARY LONGTERM CARE
CONTEMPORARY REVIEW
CORPORATE SECURITY
CORRECTIONS DIGEST
CORRECTIONS TODAY
COSMOPOLITAN
CRIME CONTROL DIGEST
CRIME LABORATORY DIGEST
CRIMINAL JUSTICE NEWSLETTER
CRISIS
CRITICAL CARE MEDICINE
CRITICAL CARE NURSE
CRITICAL CARE UPDATE
CULTURAL SURVIVAL QUARTERLY
CURATIONIS
CURRENT DIGEST OF THE SOVIET PRESS
CURRENT PROBLEMS IN CANCER
CURRENT PROBLEMS IN DERMATOLOGY
CURRENT PROBLEMS IN PEDIATRICS
CURRENT REVIEWS FOR RECOVERY ROOM NURSES
CURRENT TOPICS IN MICROBIOLOGY AND IMMUNOLOGY
CUTIS
CYTOBIOS
D, THE MAGAZINE OF DALLAS
DANCE MAGAZINE
DEATH STUDIES
DEFENSE
DELAWARE ALTERNATIVE PRESS
DELAWARE MEDICAL JOURNAL
DEMOCRATIC LEFT
DERMATOLOGICA
DERMATOLOGISCHE MONATSSCHRIFT
DEUTSCHE MEDIZINISCHE WOCHENSCHRIFT
DEVELOPMENTAL MEDICINE AND CHILD NEUROLOGY
DIABETES EDUCATER
DIAGNOSTIC IMMUNOLOGY
DIAGNOSTIC MEDICINE
DIAGNOSTIC MICROBIOLOGY AND INFECTIOUS DISEASE
DIALOG

DIGESTIVE DISEASES AND SCIENCES
DIMENSIONS IN HEALTH SERVICES
DIMENSIONS OF CRITICAL CARE NURSING
DISABILITY RAG
DISCOVER
DISEASE-A MONTH
DRUG INTELLIGENCE AND CLINICAL PHARMACY
DRUGS
DUODECIM
ESA: ENGAGE/SOCIAL ACTION
EAR, NOSE, AND THROAT JOURNAL
EAST AFRICAN MEDICAL JOURNAL
EAST WEST JOURNAL
EBONY
THE ECONOMIST
EDITOR AND PUBLISHER: THE 4TH ESTATE
EDITORIAL RESEARCH REPORTS
EMERGENCY DEPARTMENT NEWS
EMERGENCY: JOURNAL OF EMERGENCY SERVICES
EMERGENCY MEDICAL SERVICES
EMERGENCY MEDICINE
EMERGENCY MEDICINE CLINICS OF NORTH AMERICA
EMMY
EMPIRE STATE REPORT
EMPLOYEE RELATIONS LAW JOURNAL
ENDOSCOPY
ENGINEERING NEWS-RECORD
EPIDEMIOLOGIC REVIEWS
EQUINOX
ESSENCE
ESQUIRE
ETUDES
EUROPEAN JOURNAL OF CANCER AND CLINICAL ONCOLOGY
EUROPEAN JOURNAL OF CLINICAL MICROBIOLOGY
EXECUTIVE EDUCATOR
EXECUTIVE HOUSEKEEPING TODAY
EXPERIENTIA
FDA CONSUMER
FDA DRUG BULLETIN
FAG RAG
FAMILY AND COMMUNITY HEALTH
FAMILY CIRCLE
FAMILY LAW REPORTER: COURT OPINIONS
FEDERAL REGISTER
FERTILITY AND STERILITY
FINANCIAL WORLD
FIRE COMMAND
FLASH-INFORMATIONS
FLORIDA NURSE
FOCUS ON CRITICAL CARE
FORBES
FORTSCHRITTE DER MEDIZIN
FORTUNE

FOUNDATION NEWS
FRONTIERS OF RADIATION THERAPY AND ONCOLOGY
FOUNDATION NEWS
FUNDAMENTALIST JOURNAL
FUTURIST
GAO REVIEW
GACETA MEDICA DE MEXICO
GALLUP REPORT
GAN TO KAGAKU RYOHO
GASTROENTEROLOGIE CLINIQUE ET BIOLOGIQUE
GASTROENTEROLOGY
GASTROINTESTINAL ENDOSCOPY
GAY COMMUNITY NEWS
GAY INFORMATION JOURNAL OF GAY STUDIES
GAZETTE OF THE INSTITUTE OF MEDICAL LABORATORY SCIENCES
GENERAL HOSPITAL PSYCHIATRY
GENITOURINARY MEDICINE
GIORNALE DI CLINICA MEDICA
GLAMOUR
GOOD HOUSEKEEPING
GROWTH
GUARDIAN
GUILD NOTES
GUT
HPN: HOSPITAL PURCHASING NEWS
HAMATOLOGIE UND BLUTTRANSFUSION
HAREFUAH
HARPERS
HARPER'S BAZAAR
HARVARD BUSINESS REVIEW
HARVARD LAW REVIEW
HASTINGS CENTER REPORT
HAUTARZT
HEALTH
HEALTH AND SOCIAL SERVICE JOURNAL
HEALTH BULLETIN
HEALTH CARE
HEALTH COST MANAGEMENT
HEALTH EDUCATION JOURNAL
HEALTH LAW VIGIL
HEALTH PAC BULLETIN
HEALTH POLICY
HEALTH PROGRESS
HEALTH VALUES
HEALTHRIGHT
HEALTHSHARING
HEALTHSPAN
HEMATOLOGICAL ONCOLOGY
HENRY FORD HOSPITAL MEDICAL JOURNAL
HEPATOLOGY
HERIZONS
HIGH TECHNOLOGY
HIROSHIMA JOURNAL OF MEDICAL SCIENCES

HISTOPATHOLOGY
HOME HEALTH JOURNAL
HOME HEALTHCARE NURSE
HOMEMAKERS' MAGAZINE
HOPPE-SEYLER'S ZEITSCHRIFT FUR PHYSIOLOGISCHE CHEMIE
HOSPICE JOURNAL
HOSPITAL AND COMMUNITY PSYCHIATRY
HOSPITAL EMPLOYEE HEALTH
HOSPITAL MANAGER
HOSPITAL MEDICINE
HOSPITAL PRACTICE
HOSPITAL PROGRESS
HOSPITAL SECURITY AND SAFETY MANAGEMENT
HOSPITAL TOPICS
HOSPITALS: JOURNAL OF THE AMERICAN HOSPITAL ASSOCIATION
HOUSTON CITY MAGAZINE
HUMAN DEVELOPMENT NEWS
HUMAN EVENTS
HUMAN IMMUNOLOGY
HUMAN ORGANIZATION
HUMAN PATHOLOGY
IARC SCIENTIFIC PUBLICATIONS
IMLS GAZETTE
INC
I KNOW YOU KNOW
ILLINOIS ISSUES
ILLINOIS MEDICAL JOURNAL
ILLUSTRATED LONDON NEWS
IMMUNITAT UND INFEKTION
IMMUNOBIOLOGY
IMMUNOLOGICAL INVESTIGATIONS
IMMUNOLOGICAL REVIEWS
IMPRINT
IN THESE TIMES
INDIANA MEDICINE
INDUSTRY WEEK
INFECTION
INFECTION AND IMMUNITY
INFECTION CONTROL
INFECTION CONTROL DIGEST
INFIRMIERE CANADIENNE
INTENSIVE CARE MEDICINE
INTERNATIONAL ARCHIVES OF ALLERGY AND APPLIED IMMUNOLOGY
INTERNATIONAL JOURNAL OF ANDROLOGY
INTERNATIONAL JOURNAL OF CANCER
INTERNATIONAL JOURNAL OF CLINICAL PHARMACOLOGICAL RESEARCH
INTERNATIONAL JOURNAL OF DERMATOLOGY
INTERNATIONAL JOURNAL OF IMMUNOPHARMACOLOGY
INTERNATIONAL JOURNAL OF LEPROSY AND OTHER MYCOBACTERIAL
    DISEASES
INTERNATIONAL JOURNAL OF ORAL SURGERY
INTERNATIONAL JOURNAL OF PSYCHIATRY IN MEDICINE
INTERNATIONAL NURSING REVIEW

INTERNATIONAL OPHTHAMOLOGY CLINICS
INTERNATIONAL REVIEW OF EXPERIMENTAL PATHOLOGY
INTERNIST
INTERNATIONAL SYMPOSIUM OF THE PRINCESS TAKAMATSU CANCER
    RESEARCH FUND
IOWA MEDICINE
IRISH JOURNAL OF MEDICAL SCIENCE
IRISH MEDICAL JOURNAL
ISRAEL JOURNAL OF MEDICAL SCIENCES
ISSUES IN COMPREHENSIVE PEDIATRIC NURSING
ISSUES IN RADICAL THERAPY
ISSUES IN SCIENCE AND TECHNOLOGY
JAMA: JOURNAL OF THE AMERICAN MEDICAL ASSOCIATION
JEN: JOURNAL OF EMERGENCY NURSING
JOGN NURSING: JOURNAL OF OBSTETRIC, GYNECOLOGIC AND NEONATAL
    NURSING
JNCI: JOURNAL OF THE NATIONAL CANCER INSTITUTE
JAPANESE JOURNAL OF NURSING
JET
JORDEMODERN
JOSANPU ZASSHI
JOURNAL OF THE AMERICAN ACADEMY OF DERMATOLOGY
JOURNAL OF AMERICAN COLLEGE HEALTH
JOURNAL OF THE AMERICAN COLLEGE OF CARDIOLOGY
JOURNAL OF THE AMERICAN DENTAL ASSOCIATION
JOURNAL OF THE AMERICAN DIETETIC ASSOCIATION
JOURNAL OF THE AMERICAN HEALTH CARE ASSOCIATION
JOURNAL OF THE AMERICAN OPTOMETRIC ASSOCIATION
JOURNAL OF THE AMERICAN OSTEOPATHIC ASSOCIATION
JOURNAL OF THE AMERICAN PODIATRIC MEDICAL ASSOCIATION
JOURNAL OF THE AMERICAN VETERINARY MEDICAL ASSOCIATION
JOURNAL OF ANTIMICROBIAL CHEMOTHERAPY
JOURNAL OF THE ARKANSAS MEDICAL SOCIETY
JOURNAL OF BIOLOGICAL CHEMISTRY
JOURNAL OF BIOLOGICAL RESPONSE MODIFIERS
JOURNAL OF CELLULAR BIOCHEMISTRY
JOURNAL OF CHRISTIAN NURSING
JOURNAL OF CHRONIC DISEASES
JOURNAL OF CLINICAL AND LABORATORY IMMUNOLOGY
JOURNAL OF CLINICAL APHERESIS
JOURNAL OF CLINICAL GASTROENTEROLOGY
JOURNAL OF CLINICAL IMMUNOLOGY
JOURNAL OF CLINICAL INVESTIGATION
JOURNAL OF CLINICAL MICROBIOLOGY
JOURNAL OF CLINICAL ONCOLOGY
JOURNAL OF CLINICAL PATHOLOGY
JOURNAL OF CLINICAL PHARMACOLOGY
JOURNAL OF CLINICAL PSYCHIATRY
JOURNAL OF CLINICAL TOMOGRAPHY
JOURNAL OF COMMUNITY HEALTH NURSING
JOURNAL OF COMPUTER ASSISTED TOMOGRAPHY
JOURNAL OF CONTINUING EDUCATION IN NURSING
JOURNAL OF COUNSELING AND DEVELOPMENT

JOURNAL OF CUTANEOUS PATHOLOGY
JOURNAL OF DERMATOLOGIC SURGERY AND ONCOLOGY
JOURNAL OF EMERGENCY MEDICAL SERVICES
JOURNAL OF EMERGENCY MEDICINE
JOURNAL FOR ENTEROSTOMAL THERAPY
JOURNAL OF EXPERIMENTAL MEDICINE
JOURNAL OF THE FLORIDA MEDICAL ASSOCIATION
JOURNAL OF FORENSIC SCIENCES
JOURNAL OF HEALTH POLITICS, POLICY AND LAW
JOURNAL OF HEPATOLOGY
JOURNAL OF HOMOSEXUALITY
JOURNAL OF HOSPITAL INFECTION
JOURNAL OF IMMUNOLOGY
JOURNAL OF INFECTION
JOURNAL OF INFECTIOUS DISEASES
JOURNAL OF INTERFERON RESEARCH
JOURNAL OF INVESTIGATIVE DERMATOLOGY
JOURNAL OF THE IOWA MEDICAL SOCIETY
JOURNAL OF THE KANSAS MEDICAL SOCIETY
JOURNAL OF THE KENTUCKY MEDICAL ASSOCIATION
JOURNAL OF LABORATORY AND CLINICAL MEDICINE
JOURNAL OF LAW AND EDUCATION
JOURNAL OF THE LOUISIANA STATE MEDICAL SOCIETY
JOURNAL OF THE MEDICAL ASSOCIATION OF GEORGIA
JOURNAL OF THE MEDICAL ASSOCIATION OF THAILAND
JOURNAL OF THE MEDICAL SOCIETY OF NEW JERSEY
JOURNAL OF MEDICAL TECHNOLOGY
JOURNAL OF MEDICAL VIROLOGY
JOURNAL OF MEDICINAL CHEMISTRY
JOURNAL OF THE NATIONAL CANCER INSTITUTE
JOURNAL OF THE NATIONAL MEDICAL ASSOCIATION
JOURNAL OF NEPHROLOGY NURSING
JOURNAL OF NEUROLOGY
JOURNAL OF NEUROPATHOLOGY AND EXPERIMENTAL NEUROLOGY
JOURNAL OF NEUROSCIENCE NURSING
JOURNAL OF NEUROSURGERY
JOURNAL OF NEUROSURGICAL NURSING
JOURNAL OF NURSE-MIDWIFERY
JOURNAL OF OBSTETRIC, GYNECOLOGIC AND NEONATAL NURSING
JOURNAL OF OCCUPATIONAL MEDICINE
JOURNAL OF THE OKLAHOMA STATE MEDICAL ASSOCIATION
JOURNAL OF OPHTHALMIC NURSING AND TECHNOLOGY
JOURNAL OF ORAL AND MAXILLOFACIAL SURGERY
JOURNAL OF THE PAKISTAN MEDICAL ASSOCIATION
JOURNAL OF PATHOLOGY
JOURNAL OF PEDIATRIC GASTROENTEROLOGY AND NUTRITION
JOURNAL OF PEDIATRICS
JOURNAL OF PRACTICAL NURSING
JOURNAL OF PROSTHETIC DENTISTRY
JOURNAL OF PROTOZOOLOGY
JOURNAL OF PSYCHOHISTORY
JOURNAL OF PSYCHOSOCIAL ONCOLOGY
JOURNAL OF RELIGION AND HEALTH

JOURNAL OF RHEUMATOLOGY
JOURNAL OF THE ROYAL NAVAL MEDICAL SERVICE
JOURNAL OF THE ROYAL SOCIETY OF HEALTH
JOURNAL OF THE ROYAL SOCIETY OF MEDICINE
JOURNAL OF SCHOOL HEALTH
JOURNAL OF THE SOUTH CAROLINA MEDICAL ASSOCIATION
JOURNAL OF STERILE SERVICE MANAGEMENT
JOURNAL OF SUBMICROSCOPIC CYTOLOGY
JOURNAL OF SUBSTANCE ABUSE AND TREATMENT
JOURNAL OF SURGERY AND ONCOLOGY
JOURNAL OF THORACIC AND CARDIOVASCULAR SURGERY
JOURNAL OF UROLOGY
JOURNAL OF VIROLOGICAL METHODS
JOURNAL OF VIROLOGY
JOURNAL OF VISUAL IMPAIRMENT AND BLINDNESS
JUVENILE JUSTICE DIGEST
KANGO
KANGO GIJUTSU
KANGOGAKU ZASSHI
KANSAS CITY MAGAZINE
KANSAS MEDICINE
KENTUCKY NURSE
KLINICHESKAIA MEDITSINA
KLINISCHE MONATSBLAETTER FUR AUGENHEILKUNDE
KLINISCHE WOCHENSCHRIFT
KRANKENPFLEGE
KRANKENPFLEGE JOURNAL
KRANKENPFLEGE SOINS INFIRMIERS
LABOR NOTES
LABORATORY ANIMAL SCIENCE
LABORATORY ANIMALS
LABORATORY INVESTIGATION
LADIES HOME JOURNAL
LAKARTIDNINGEN
LAMP
LANCET
LARYNGOLOGIE, RHINOLOGIE, OTOLOGIE
LARYNGOSCOPE
LAUNDRY NEWS
LAW AND ORDER
LAW ENFORCEMENT NEWS
LESBIAN CONTRADICTION
LESBIAN INSIDER INSIGHTER INCITER
LIFE
LIJECNICKI VJESNIK
LINACRE QUARTERLY
LISTENER
LONGEST REVOLUTION
LOS ANGELES
LUNG
LUTHERAN FORUM
LYMPHOKINE RESEARCH
LYMPHOLOGY

MCN: AMERICAN JOURNAL OF MATERNAL CHILD NURSING
MD
MLO: MEDICAL LABORATORY OBSERVER
MMWR: MORBIDITY AND MORTALITY WEEKLY REPORT
MS
MSRT JOURNAL
MCCALLS
MACLEAN'S
MADEMOISELLE
MAGISTRATE
MANAGEMENT REVIEW
MANAGEMENT WORLD
MARYLAND MEDICAL JOURNAL
MASSACHUSETTS NURSE
MEDECINE TROPICALE
MEDIAFILE
MEDICAL BULLETIN OF THE US ARMY, EUROPE
MEDICAL CLINICS OF NORTH AMERICA
MEDICAL HEALTH CARE
MEDICAL HYPOTHESES
MEDICAL JOURNAL OF AUSTRALIA
MEDICAL LABORATORY SCIENCES
MEDICAL LETTER ON DRUGS AND THERAPEUTICS
MEDICAL MICROBIOLOGY AND IMMUNOLOGY
MEDICAL PEDIATRICS AND ONCOLOGY
MEDICAL PRODUCTS SALES
MEDICAL SELF CARE
MEDICAL WORLD NEWS
MEDICINA
MEDICINA CLINICA
MEDICINE
MEDICINSKI PREGLED
MENTAL DISABILITY LAW REPORTER
MIAMI/SOUTH FLORIDA MAGAZINE
MICHIGAN HOSPITALS
MICHIGAN MEDICINE
MICROBIOLOGY AND IMMUNOLOGY
MIDWIFE, HEALTH VISITOR AND COMMUNITY NURSE
MIKROBIYOLOJI BULTENI
MILITANT
MILITARY MEDICINE
MINERVA MEDICA
MINERVA PEDIATRICA
MINERVA STOMATOLOGICA
MINNESOTA MEDICINE
MISSOURI MEDICINE
MODERN HEALTHCARE
MOLECULAR AND CELLULAR BIOCHEMISTRY
MOLECULAR BIOLOGY AND MEDICINE
MONEY
MONTH
MOSAIC
MOTHER JONES

MOUNT SINAI JOURNAL OF MEDICINE
MUENCHENER MEDIZINISCHE WOCHENSCRIFT
NAACOG NEWSLETTER: NURSES ASSOCIATION OF THE AMERICAN COL-
    LEGE OF OBSTETRICIANS AND GYNECOLOGISTS
NACLA'S REPORT ON THE AMERICS
NASSP BULLETIN
NIPH ANNALS
NITA: JOURNAL OF THE NATIONAL INTRAVENOUS THERAPY ASSOCIATION
NLM TECHNICAL BULLETIN
NARCOTICS CONTROL DIGEST
NATION
NATIONAL CATHOLIC REPORTER
NATIONAL GUARD
NATIONAL JOURNAL
NATIONAL NOW TIMES
NATIONAL PRISON PROJECT JOURNAL
NATIONAL REVIEW
NATIONAL SAFETY AND HEALTH NEWS
NATIONAL UNDERWRITER
NATURAL HISTORY
NATURE
NEBRASKA NURSE
NEDERLANDS TIJDSCHRIFT VOOR GENEESKUNDE
NERVENARZT
NETHERLANDS JOURNAL OF MEDICINE
NEUROLOGIC CLINICS
NEUROLOGY
NEURORADIOLOGY
NEUROSURGERY
NEW AGE
NEW ENGLAND JOURNAL OF MEDICINE
NEW JERSEY NURSE
NEW PHYSICIAN
NEW REPUBLIC
NEW SCIENTIST
NEW SOCIETY
NEW STATESMAN
NEW TIMES
NEW YORK
NEW YORK JOURNAL OF DENTISTRY
NEW YORK REVIEW OF BOOKS
NEW YORK STATE JOURNAL OF MEDICINE
NEW YORK TIMES MAGAZINE
NEW ZEALAND HOSPITAL
NEW ZEALAND MEDICAL JOURNAL
NEW ZEALAND NURSING FORUM
NEW ZEALAND NURSING JOURNAL
NEWS AND FEATURES FROM NIH
NEWSWEEK
NIPPON RINSHO
NO TO SHINKEI
NORDISK MEDICIN
NORTH CAROLINA MEDICAL JOURNAL

NORTHWEST PASSAGE
NOT MAN APART
NOUVELLE REVUE FRANCAISE D'HEMATOLOGIE
NUOVI ANNALI D'IGIENE E MICROBIOLOGIA
NURS RSA VERPLEGING
NURSE PRACTITIONER
NURSING
NURSING AND HEALTH CARE
NURSING CLINICS OF NORTH AMERICA
NURSING ECONOMICS
NURSING FORUM
NURSING HOMES
NURSING JOURNAL OF INDIA
NURSING LIFE
NURSING MANAGEMENT
NURSING MIRROR
NURSING STANDARD
NURSING TIMES
NUTRITION AND CANCER
NUTRITION REVIEWS
OR MANAGER
OBSERVER
OBSTETRICS AND GYNECOLOGY
OCCUPATIONAL HEALTH
OCCUPATIONAL HEALTH AND SAFETY
OCCUPATIONAL HEALTH NURSING
OFF OUR BACKS
OFFENTLICHE GESUNDHEITSWESEN
OHIO NURSES REVIEW
OHIO STATE MEDICAL JOURNAL
OMNI
ONCOLOGY NURSING FORUM
OPERA NEWS
OPHTHALMOLOGY
ORAL SURGERY
ORAL SURGERY, ORAL MEDICINE, ORAL PATHOLOGY
OREGON NURSE
ORIGINS
ORVOSI HETILAP
OSTERREICHISCHE KRANKENPFLEGEZEITSCHRIST
OTOLARYNGOLOGY AND HEAD AND NECK SURGERY
OUT
PARENTS
PASTORAL PSYCHOLOGY
PATHOLOGIST
PATHOLOGY
PATHOLOGY ANNUAL
PATHOLOGY, RESEARCH AND PRACTICE
PATIENT CARE
PATIENT EDUCATION AND COUNSELING
PATOLOGE
PATOLOGICHESAIA FIZIOLOGIIA I EKSPERIMENTALNAIA TERAPIIA
PEDIATRIC CLINICS OF NORTH AMERICA

PEDIATRIC INFECTIOUS DISEASE
PEDIATRIC NURSING
PEDIATRIC PATHOLOGY
PEDIATRICS
PEDIATRIE
PENNSYLVANIA MEDICINE
PENNSYLVANIA NURSE
PEOPLE
PERSONNEL
PERSONNEL JOURNAL
PHARMACOTHERAPY
PHI DELTA KAPPAN
PHOENIX
PHYSICIAN AND SPORTS MEDICINE
PHYSICIAN ASSISTANT
PHYSICIAN EXECUTIVE
PLASTIC AND RECONSTRUCTIVE SURGERY
PLASTIC SURGICAL NURSING
PLAYBOY
POINT OF VIEW
THE POLICE CHIEF
POLICE JOURNAL
POLICY OPTIONS/OPTIONS POLITIQUES
POLSKI TYGODNIK LEKARSKI
POSTGRADUATE MEDICINE
PRAIRIE ROSE
PRAXIS UND KLINIK DER PNEUMOLOGIE
PRESENT TENSE
PRESSE MEDICALE
PREVENTION
PREVENTIVE MEDICINE
PRIEST
PROCEEDINGS, ANNUAL MEETING OF THE MEDICAL SECTION OF THE
    AMERICAN COUNCIL OF LIFE INSURANCE
PROCEEDINGS OF THE NATIONAL ACADEMY OF SCIENCES OF THE UNITED
    STATES OF AMERICA
PROCEEDINGS OF THE SOCIETY FOR EXPERIMENTAL BIOLOGY AND MEDI-
    CINE
PROCESSED WORLD
PROFESSIONAL MEDICAL ASSISTANT
PROFESSIONAL SANITATION MANAGEMENT
PROGRESS IN ALLERGY
PROGRESS IN CLINICAL AND BIOLOGICAL RESEARCH
PROGRESS IN MEDICAL VIROLOGY
PROGRESSIVE
PROVIDER
PRZEGLAD DERMATOLOGICZNY
PSYCHIATRIC NEWS
PSYCHOLOGICAL REPORTS
PSYCHOLOGY TODAY
PSYCHOSOMATICS
PUBLIC HEALTH REPORTS
PUBLIC OPINION

REVUE MEDICALE DE LIEGE
REVUE MEDICALE DE LA SUISSE ROMANDE
REVUE NEUROLOGIQUE
RINSHO BYORI
RISK MANAGEMENT
ROLLING STONE
SGA JOURNAL
ST LUKE'S JOURNAL OF THEOLOGY
SAN FRANCISCO
SANGRE
SATURDAY EVENING POST
SAVINGS INSTITUTIONS
SCNDINAVIAN JOURNAL OF GASTROENTEROLOGY
SCANDINAVIAN JOURNAL OF HAEMATOLOGY
SCANDINAVIAN JOURNAL OF IMMUNOLOGY
SCANDINAVIAN JOURNAL OF INFECTIOUS DISEASES
SCHWEIZERISCHE MEDIZINISCHE WOCHENSCHRIFT
SCHWEIZERISCHE MONATSSCHRIFT FUR ZAHNMEDIZIN
SCHWEIZERISCHE RUNDSCHAU FUR MEDIZIN PRAXIS
SCIENCE
SCIENCE DIGEST
SCIENCE FOR THE PEOPLE
SCIENCE NEWS
THE SCIENCES
SCIENTIFIC AMERICAN
SCOTTISH MEDICAL JOURNAL
SECURITY LETTER
SEMINARS IN ONCOLOGY
SEMINARS IN THROMBOSIS AND HEMOSTASIS
SERVIR
SEVENTEEN
SEXUALLY TRANSMITTED DISEASES
SOCIAL CASEWORK
SOCIAL POLICY
SOCIAL RESEARCH
SOCIAL SCIENCE AND MEDICINE
SOCIAL WORK
SOCIAL WORK IN HEALTH CARE
SOCIALIST REVIEW
SOCIALIST WORKER
SOINS
SOINS. GYNECOLOGIE, OBSTETRIQUE, PUERICULTURE, PEDIATRIE
SOJOURNERS
SOLDIERS
SOUTH AFRICAN MEDICAL JOURNAL
SOVIET MEDICINE
SPARE RIB
SPECTATOR
SRPSKI ARHIV ZA CELOKUPNO LEKARSTVO
STATE GOVERNMENT NEWS
STATE NURSING LEGISLATION QUARTERLY
SUNDAY TIMES
SURGERY ANNUAL

SURGICAL NEUROLOGY
SURGICAL TECHNOLOGIST
SURVEY AND SYNTHETICS OF PATHOLOGY RESEARCH
SURVEY OF IMMUNOLOGICAL RESEARCH
SWEDEN NOW
SYGEPLEJERSKEN
SYKEPLEIEN
TV GUIDE
TABLET
TANPAKUSHITSU KAKUSAN KOSO PROTEIN, NUCLEIC ACID, ENZYME
TECHNOLOGY REVIEW
TERAPEVTICHESKII ARKHIV
TEXAS HOSPITALS
TEXAS MEDICINE
TEXAS NURSING
THERAPEUTISCHE UMSCHAU
THORAX
THROMBOSIS AND HAEMOSTASIS
TIDSSKRIFT FOR DEN NORSKE LAEGEFORENING
TIJDSCHRIFT VOOR ALCOHOL, DRUGS EN ANDERE PSYCHOTROPE STOF-
      FEN
TIJDSCHRIFT VOOR ZIEKENVERPLEGING
TIME
TIMES
TIMES EDUCATIONAL SUPPLEMENT
TIMES HIGHER EDUCATION SUPPLEMENT
TIMES LITERARY SUPPLEMENT
TODAY'S OR NURSE
TOPICS IN CLINICAL NURSING
TRAINING
TRAINING AIDS DIGEST
TRANSACTIONS AND STUDIES OF THE COLLEGE OF PHYSICIANS OF
      PHILADELPHIA
TRANSACTIONS OF THE AMERICAN CLINICAL AND CLIMATOLOGICAL AS-
      SOCIATION
TRANSACTIONS OF THE AMERICAN OPHTHALMOLOGICAL SOCIETY
TRANSACTIONS OF THE ASSOCIATION OF AMERICAN PHYSICIANS
TRANSACTIONS OF THE OPHTHALMOLOGICAL SOCIETIES OF THE UNITED
      KINGDOM
TRANSACTIONS OF THE ROYAL SOCIETY OF TROPICAL MEDICINE AND HY-
      GIENE
TRANSFUSION
TRIAL
TROPICAL DOCTOR
US
US MEDICINE
US NEWS & WORLD REPORT
USA TODAY
UTNE READER
ULTRASTRUCTURAL PATHOLOGY
UNION MEDICALE DU CANADA
URBAN ANTHROPOLOGY
UROLOGIC CLINICS OF NORTH AMERICA

VACCINE
VARDFACKET
VASA
VENTURE
VERHANDLUNGEN DES DEUTSCHEN GESELLSCHAFT FUR INNERE MED-
    IZIN
VETERINARY IMMUNOLOGY AND IMMUNOPATHOLOGY
VETERINARY PATHOLOGY
VETERINARY RECORD
VILLAGE VOICE
VIRCHOWS ARCHIV. A. PATHOLOGIAL ANATOMY AND HISTOPATHOLOGY
VIROLOGY
VNITRNI LEKARSTVI
VOGUE
VOJNOSANITETSKI PREGLED
VOPROSY VIRUSOLOGII
VOX SANGUINIS
VRACHEBNOE DELO
VUTRESHNI BOLESTI
WALL STREET JOURNAL
WASHBURN LAW JOURNAL
WASHINGTON MONTHLY
WASHINGTON NURSE
WASHINGTON REPORT ON MEDICINE AND HEALTH
WASHINGTONIAN
WASTE AGE
WEST INDIAN MEDICAL JOURNAL
WEST VIRGINIA MEDICAL JOURNAL
WESTERN JOURNAL OF MEDICINE
WHOLE EARTH REVIEW
WIADOMOSCI LEKARSKIE
WIENER KLINISCHE WOCHENSCHRIFT
WISCONSIN MEDICAL JOURNAL
WITNESS
WOMANEWS
WOMAN'S DAY
WOMEN'S PRESS
WORLD HEALTH
WORLD OF IRISH NURSING
WORSHIP
YALE JOURNL OF BIOLOGY AND MEDICINE
ZFA. ZEITSCHRIFT FUR ALTERNSFORSCHUNG
ZEITSCHRIFT FUR AERZTLICHE FORTBILDUNG
ZEITSCHRIFT FUR HAUTKRANKHEITEN
ZEITSCHRIFT FUR GASTROENTEROLOGIE
ZEITSCHRIFT FUR RECHS MEDIZIN

SUBJECT INDEX

BOOKS, MONOGRAPHS AND PAMPHLETS

Altman, Dennis. AIDS IN THE MIND OF AMERICA. Anchor Press, 1986. viii + 228 pages. $16.95.

Alumbaugh, M. J. Social support, coping and auto immune deficiency syndrome (AIDS): an exploratory study. California School of Professional Psychology, Berkeley, 1985 (Ph.D. dissertation).

American Management Associations Membership Publications Division. AIDS: THE WORKPLACE ISSUE. New York: The Association, 1985. 81 pages. $7.50.

Baker, J. A.I.D.S. San Francisco: R & E Research Associates, 1983. $7.95 (paper).

Barker, C. S. A molecular characterization of the genome of Mason-Pfizer monkey virus. University of Alabama in Birmingham, 1985. (Ph.D. dissertation).

Berg, T. A. A WAY TO SURVIVE THE AIDS EPIDEMIC. Palm Publications, 1983. $4.95.

Cahill, Kevin M., editor. THE AIDS EPIDEMIC. New York: St. Martin's Press, 1983. $12.95 (hard); $7.95 (paper).

Cantwell, A., Jr. AIDS: THE MYSTERY AND THE SOLUTION. Los Angeles: Aries Rising Press, 1984. $14.95 (hard); $9.95 (paper).

Charles, K. A. Factors in the primary prevention of AIDS in gay and bisexual men. California School of Professional Psychology, Berkeley, 1985. (Ph.D. dissertation.

DeRose, J. A. A study of AIDS-related complex patients. United States International University, 1986. (Ph.D. dissertation).

Ebbeson, Peter, Robert J. Biggar and Mads Melbye, editors. AIDS: A BASIC GUIDE FOR CLINICIANS. Philadelphia: Saunders (Munksgaard), 1984. 313 pages. $45.00.

Feldman, Douglas A. and Thomas M. Johnson, editors. THE SOCIAL DIMENSIONS OF AIDS: METHOD AND THEORY. New York: Praeger Publishers, 1986. viii + 274 pages. $37.95.

Fettner, Ann Guidici and William A. Check, with a foreword by Bijan Safai. THE TRUTH ABOUT AIDS: EVOLUTION OF AN EPIDEMIC. New York: Holt, Rinehart and Winston, 1984. xiii + 288 pages. $15.95.

1

Friedman-Kien, Alvin E. and Linda J. Laubenstein, editors. AIDS: THE EPIDEMIC OF KAPOSI'S SARCOMA AND OPPORTUNISTIC INFECTIONS. New York: Masson Publishing USA, 1984. 351 pages.

Garoogian, Rhoda. AIDS, 1981-1983; AN ANNOTATED BIBLIOGRAPHY. Brooklyn: Vantage Information Consultants, 1984. 92 pages. $15.00 (paper).

Gottlieb, Michael S. and Jerome E. Groopman, editors. ACQUIRED IMMUNE DEFI-CIENCY SYNDROME; PROCEEDINGS OF A SCHERING CORPORATION-UCLA SYMPOSIUM HELD IN PARK CITY, UTAH, FEBRUARY 5-10, 1984. New York: Alan R. Liss, 1984. xxi, 438 pages.

GUIDELINES ON AIDS IN EUROPE, 1st revised edition. Copenhagen: WHO Regional Office for Europe, 1985.

Hirsch, D. A. Psychological aspects of the acquired immune deficiency syndrome. Yeshiva University, 1985. (Ph.D. dissertation).

Irwin, Michael H. K. AIDS: FEARS AND FACTS. Washington: Public Affairs Press, 1986. 28 pages. $1.00.

Kagan, L. S. L. Baccalaureate nursing students' attitudes toward patients with acquired immunodeficiency syndrome (AIDS). Columbia University Teachers College, 1986. (Ph.D. dissertation).

Kaisch, K. B. The psychological and social consequences of HTLV-III infection: homosexuals in Orange County, California. Utah State University, 1986. (Ph.D. dissertation).

Kassler, J. GAY MEN'S HEALTH. New York: Harper & Row, 1983. $12.95 (hard); $7.95 (paper).

Legrand, Edmund K. Monocyte function in rhesus monkeys with simian acquired immune deficiency syndrome. University of California, Davis, 1985. (Ph.D. dissertation).

Llewellyn-Jones, D. HERPES, AIDS, AND OTHER SEXUALLY TRANSMITTED DISEASES. London: Faber & Faber, 1985. $6.95 (paper).

Ma, Pearl and Donald Armstrong, editors. THE ACQUIRED IMMUNE DEFICIENCY SYNDROME AND INFECTIONS OF HOMOSEXUAL MEN. Yorke Medical Books, 1984. 442 pages.

Moulton, J. M. Adjustment to a diagnosis of acquired immune deficiency syndrome and related conditions: a cognitive and behavioral perspective. California School of Professional Psychology, Berkeley, 1985. (Ph.D. dissertation).

New Jersey. Department of Health. AIDS: A SPECIAL REPORT ON ACQUIRED IMMUNODEFICIENCY SYNDROME. Trenton: The Department, 1986. iv + 25 pages.

New York. Department of Health. AIDS: 100 QUESTIONS AND ANSWERS. Albany: The Department, 1985. 19 pages. Free.

PSYCHIATRIC IMPLICATIONS OF ACQUIRED IMMUNE DEFICIENCY SYNDROME. American Psychiatric Press, 1984. $12.00 (paper).

2

Scappaticcio, J. S. Aids risk as psychological threat: the experience of anxiety in gay men at risk for aids as a function of anxiety proneness, defense mechanisms, and self-assessment of AIDS risk. Columbia University, 1985. (Ph.D. dissertation).

Seirup, J. F. Dreams as the mirror-image of AIDS: a study of dream symbols in male homosexuals at risk for AIDS. The Wright Institute, Berkeley, 1986. (Ph.D. dissertation).

Siegal, F. P. AIDS, THE MEDICAL MYSTERY. New York: Grove Press, 1983.

Tyckoson, D. A. AIDS (ACQUIRED IMMUNE DEFICIENCY SYNDROME). Phoenix: Oryx Press, 1985. 60 pages. $12.50 (paper).

UNDERSTANDING AIDS. New Brunswick: Rutgers University press, 1985. $20 (hard); $9.95 (paper).

United States. Centers for Disease Control. RECOMMENDATIONS AND GUIDE-LINES CONCERNING AIDS. Atlanta: The Centers for Disease Control, 1986. 50 pages.

—. Congress. Office of Technical Assessment. REVIEW OF THE PUBLIC HEALTH SERVICE'S RESPONSE TO AIDS: A TECHNICAL MEMORANDUM. Washington: GPO, 1985. viii + 158 pages. $5.50 (paper).

—. House. Committee on Energy and Commerce. Subcommittee on Health and the Environment. ACQUIRED IMMUNE DEFICIENCY SYNDROME (AIDS): HEARING, SEPTEMBER 17, 1984. Washington: GPO, 1985. iii + 138 pages.

—. —. —. —. KAPOSI'S SARCOMA AND RELATED OPPORTUNISTIC INFEC-TIONS: HEARING APRIL 13, 1982. Washington: GPO, 1982. iii + 54 pages.

—. —. Committee on Government Operations. THE FEDERAL RESPONSE TO AIDS: TWENTY-NINTH REPORT, NOVEMBER 30, 1983. Washington: GPO, 1984. v + 36 pages.

—. —. —. Intergovernmental Relations and Human Resources Subcommittee. FEDERAL AND LOCAL GOVERNMENTS' RESPONSE TO THE AIDS EPI-DEMIC: HEARINGS, JULY 3-DECEMBER 2, 1985. Washington: GPO, 1986. v + 848 pages.

—. —. —. —. FEDERAL RESPONSE TO AIDS: HEARING, AUGUST 1-2, 1983. Washington, GPO, 1983. iv + 643 pages.

—. —. OFFICE OF TECHNOLOGY ASSESSMENT'S FINDINGS ON THE PUBLIC HEALTH SERVICE'S RESPONSE TO AIDS: JOINT HEARING, FEBRUARY 21, 1985, BEFORE A SUBCOMMITTEE OF THE COMMITTEE ON GOVERNMENT OPERATIONS AND THE COMMITTEE ON ENERGY AND COMMERCE. Washington: GPO, 1985. 79 pages.

Woods, W. J. A comparison study of the psychological status of AIDS-associated Kaposi's sarcoma patients, acute leukemia patients, and healthy gay and hetero-sexual men. Ohio State University, 1985. (Ph.D. dissertation).

PERIODICAL LITERATURE

TITLE INDEX

ABC of sexually transmitted diseases. Acquired immune deficiency syndrome, by I. Weller. BRITISH MEDICAL JOURNAL 288(6411):136-137, January 14, 1984.

Abdominal CT findings of disseminated Mycobacterium avium-intracellulare in AIDS, by D. A. Nyberg, et al. AJR 145(2):297-299, August 1985.

Abdominal CT in acquired immunodeficiency syndrome by R. B. Jeffrey, Jr., et al. AJR 146(1):7-13, January 1986.

Aberrations in chromosomes of peripheral lymphocytes of male homosexuals predisposed to acquired immune deficiency syndrome, by G. Manolov, et al. AIDS RESEARCH 1(3):157-162, 1983-1984.

Abetting the hysteria of AIDS, by E. E. Bartlett. PATIENT EDUCATION AND COUNSELING 8(2):111-113, June 1986.

Abnormal in vitro proliferation and differentiation of T colony forming cells in AIDS patients and clinically normal male homosexuals, by Y. Lunardi-Iskandar, et al. CLINICAL AND EXPERIMENTAL IMMUNOLOGY 60(2):285-293, May 1985.

Abnormal lymphocyte response to exogenous interleukin-2 in homosexuals with acquired immune deficiency syndrome (AIDS) and AIDS related complex (ARC), by J. L. Murray, et al. CLINICAL AND EXPERIMENTAL IMMUNOLOGY 60(1):25-30, April 1985.

Abnormal T-lymphocyte subpopulations associated with transfusion of blood-derived products [letter], by C. M. Kessler, et al. LANCET 1(8331):991-992, April 30, 1983.

Abnormalities of B-cell activation and immunoregulation in patients with the acquired immunodeficiency syndrome, by H. C. Lane, et al. NEW ENGLAND JOURNAL OF MEDICINE 309(8):453-458, August 25, 1983.

Abnormalities of circulating lymphocyte subsets in haemophiliacs in an AIDS-free population, by R. Carr, et al. LANCET 1(8392):1431-1434, June 30, 1984.

Abnormally high concentrations of beta 2 microglobulin in acquired immunodeficiency syndrome (AIDS) patients [letter], by R. B. Bhalla, et al. CLINICAL CHEMISTRY 29(8):1560, August 1983.

Abolishing the myths about AIDS, by P. Holmes. NURSING TIMES 80(49):19, December 5-11, 1984.

4

Absence of AIDS in haemophiliacs in Australia treated from an entirely voluntary blood donor system [letter], by K. A. Rickard, et al. LANCET 2(8340):50-51, July 2, 1983.

Absence of antibodies against prostaglandins in sera of AIDS patients, by R. A. Knazek, et al. AIDS RESEARCH 2(2):73-76, Spring 1986.

Absence of antibodies to HTLV-III in health workers after hepatitis B vaccination, by J. L. Dienstag, et al. JAMA 254:1064-1066, August 23-30, 1985.

Absence of detectable IgM antibody during cytomegalovirus disease in patients with AIDS [letter], by J. Dylewski, et al. NEW ENGLAND JOURNAL OF MEDICINE 309(8):493, August 25, 1983.

Absence of immunosuppression in healthy subjects from eastern Zaire who are positive for HTLV-III antibody, by L. Kestens, et al. NEW ENGLAND JOURNAL OF MEDICINE 312:1517-1518, June 6, 1985.

Absence of Kaposi's sarcoma in hemophiliacs with the acquired immunodeficiency syndrome [letter], by D. I. Cohn, et al. ANNALS OF INTERNAL MEDICINE 101(3): 401, September 1984.

Acalculous cholecystitis and cytomegalovirus infection in the acquired immuno-deficiency syndrome, by H. Kavin, et al. ANNALS OF INTERNAL MEDICINE 104(1):53-54, January 1986.

Accusations and a new drug, by N. Fain. ADVOCATE 416:22, March 19, 1985.

Acid-fast bacilli on buffy coat smears in the acquired immunodeficiency syndrome: a lesson from Hansen's bacillus, by B. S. Graham, et al. SOUTHERN MEDICAL JOURNAL 77(2):246-248, February 1984.

Acid-labile alpha interferon [letter]. NEW ENGLAND JOURNAL OF MEDICINE 310(14):922-924, April 5, 1984.

Acid-labile alpha interferon. A possible immunodeficiency syndrome in hemophilia, by M. E. Eyster, et al. NEW ENGLAND JOURNAL OF MEDICINE 309(10):583-586, September 8, 1983.

Acquired cellular immunodeficiency syndrome [editorial], by F. Andreu-Kern, et al. MEDICINA CLINICA 80(12):532-534, April 9, 1983.

Acquired cellular immunodeficiency syndrome: 3 observations in hemophiliacs, by M. L. Miranda, et al. MEDICINA CLINICA 81(1):24-26, June 11, 1983.

Acquired ichthyosis in the acquired immunodeficiency syndrome [letter], by C. Bories, et al. PRESSE MEDICALE 13(25):1573, June 16, 1984.

Acquired immune deficiency disease after three years. The unsolved riddle, by H. L. Ioachim. LABORATORY INVESTIGATION 51(1):1-6, July 1984.

Acquired immune deficiency in Haitians: opportunistic infections in previously healthy Haitian immigrants, by J. Vieira, et al. NEW ENGLAND JOURNAL OF MEDICINE 308(3):125-129, January 20, 1983.

Acquired immune deficiency syndrome. ANNALS OF THE NEW YORK ACADEMY OF SCIENCES 437:1-622, 1984.

— [letter]. BRITISH MEDICAL JOURNAL 288(6417):650, February 25, 1984.

—. JAMA 252:2037-2043, October 19, 1984.

—. MEDICAL JOURNAL OF AUSTRALIA 2(8):363, October 15, 1983.

—. NEDERLANDS TIJDSCHRIFT VOOR GENEESKUNDE 127(50):2308-2309, December 10, 1983.

—. NEDERLANDS TIJDSCHRIFT VOOR GENEESKUNDE 128(12):591, March 24, 1984.

—. NEDERLANDS TIJDSCHRIFT VOOR GENEESKUNDE 128(32):1546-1547, August 11, 1984.

—, by A. C. Collier, et al. UROLOGIC CLINICS OF NORTH AMERICA 11(1):187-197, February 1984.

—, by A. C. Parris, et al. HOSPITAL MEDICINE 20(9):141-142+, September 1984.

— [letter], by A. G. Lawrence. BRITISH MEDICAL JOURNAL 286(6370):1059-1060, March 26, 1983.

—, by A. J. Pinching. CLINICAL AND EXPERIMENTAL IMMUNOLOGY 56(1):1-13, April 1984.

—, by A. J. Pinching. MIDWIFE, HEALTH VISITOR AND COMMUNITY NURSE 22(5):142-145+, May 1986.

—, by A. M. Macher. AMERICAN FAMILY PHYSICIAN 30(6):131-144, December 1984.

—, by A. M. Macher. JOURNAL OF CLINICAL APHERESIS 2(4):410-422, 1985.

—, by A. P. Waterson. BRITISH MEDICAL JOURNAL 286(6367):743-746, March 5, 1983.

—, by A. R. Miller. JOURNAL OF THE ROYAL NAVAL MEDICAL SERVICE 71(2):70-75, Summer 1985.

—, by B. Christenson, et al. BOLETIN—ASOCIACION MEDICA DE PUERTO RICO 75(9):408-412, September 1983.

— [letter], by B. H. O'Connor, et al. BRITISH MEDICAL JOURNAL 286(6374):1354, April 23, 1983.

—, by B. Polsky, et al. SURGERY ANNUAL 18:280-295, 1986.

—, by C. Cernescu. REVISTA DE IGIENA, BACTERIOLOGIE, VIRUSOLOGIE, PARAZITOLOGIE, EPIDEMIOLOGIE, PNEUMOFTIZIOLOGIE, BACTERI-OLOGIA, VIRUSOLOGIA, PARAZITOLOGIA, EPIDEMIOLOGIA 29(2):111-121, April-June 1984.

—, by C. Taafee. WORLD OF IRISH NURSING 15(2):7-8, March-April 1986.

—, by D. J. LaCamera, et al. NURSING CLINICS OF NORTH AMERICA 20(1):241-256, March 1985.

—, by D. Land. MSRT JOURNAL 18:9-12, Summer 1984.

—, by D. Seger. JOURNAL OF EMERGENCY MEDICINE 2(2):117-128, 1984.

—, by D. T. Durack. ADVANCES IN INTERNAL MEDICINE 30:29-51, 1984.

—, by E. Kazimierska. WIADOMOSCI LEKARSKIE 38(3):203-206, February 1, 1985.

—, by H. Glenister. NURSING TIMES 80(28):43-45, July 11-17, 1984.

—, by H. Masur. DISEASE-A-MONTH 30(1):1-48, October 1983.

—, by H. Minkoff. JOURNAL OF NURSE-MIDWIFERY 31(4):189-193, July-August 1986.

—, by J. Hrúzik. CASOPIS LEKARU CESKYCH 123(38-39):1175-1177, September 28, 1984.

— [letter], by J. M. McLean, et al. BRITISH MEDICAL JOURNAL 286(6378):16751, May 21, 1983.

—, by J. Ulewicz-Filipowicz, et al. POLSKI TYGODNIK LEKARSKI 39(36):1211-1213, September 3, 1984.

—, by K. Crossley. MINNESOTA MEDICINE 69(4):211-213, April 1986.

— [editorial], by K. Mutton, et al. MEDICAL JOURNAL OF AUSTRALIA 1(12,:540-541, June 11, 1983.

—, by Kh. Odiseev. VUTRESHNI BOLESTI 24(2):1-7, 1985.

— [letter], by L. G. Scot. BRITISH DENTAL JOURNAL 154(12):392, June 25, 1983.

—, by M. C. Chang, et al. CHUNG-HUA MIN KUO WEI SHENG WU CHI MIEN I HSUEH TSA CHIH16(4):318-327, November 1983.

—, by M. Duca. REVISTA MEDICO-CHIRURGICALA A SOCIETATII DE MEDICI SI NATURALISTI DIN IASI 88(1):125-129, January-March 1984.

—, by M. L. Levin. MARYLAND STATE MEDICAL JOURNAL 32(9):692-694, September 1983.

— [letter], by M. R. Farrell, et al. BRITISH MEDICAL JOURNAL 286(6371):1143, April 2, 1983.

—, by M. S. Balaian. KLINICHESKAIA MEDITSINA 62(9):8-15, September 1984.

—, by M. S. Gottlieb, et al. ANNALS OF INTERNAL MEDICINE 99(2):208-220, August 1983.

— by M. Seligmann. NOUVELLE REVUE FRANCAISE D'HEMATOLOGIE 26(5):283-286, 1984.

—, by N. A. Farber. VOPROSY VIRUSOLOGII 30(1):9-15, January-February 1985.

—, by N. Ikegami. RINSHO BYORI 33(11):1230-1241, November 1985.

— [editorial], by N. M. Newman. AMERICAN JOURNAL OF OPHTHALMOLOGY 97(2):240-241, February 1984.

—, by P. Ungvarski. NURSING MIRROR 157(13):17-20, September 28, 1983.

— [letter], by P. R. Casner. ARCHIVES OF INTERNAL MEDICINE 144(8):1697, August 1984.

—, by P. W. Mansell, et al. PROGRESS IN CLINICAL AND BIOLOGICAL RESEARCH 130:217-235, 1983.

—, by R. Neuwirthová, et al. CASOPIS LEKARU CESKYCH 122(23):725-727, June 10, 1983.

—, by R. M. Khaitov. PATOLOGICHESKAIA FIZIOLOGIIA I EKSPERIMENTALNAIA TERAPIIA 1:77-84, January-February 1986.

—, by R. S. Hansen, et al. EMERGENCY MEDICINE CLINICS OF NORTH AMERICA 3(1):3-23, February 1985.

—, by R. S. Micic. SRPSKI ARHIV ZA CELOKUPNO LEKARSTVO 11(8):1169-1178, August 1983.

—,by V. Farga. REVISTA MEDICA DE CHILE 111(12):1300-1306, December 1983.

— [letter], by V. C. Amerena. AUSTRALIAN DENTAL JOURNAL 29(2):133, April 1984.

—, by W. Budzynski, et al. WIADOMOSCI LEKARSKIE 37(14):1097-1103, July 15, 1984.

—, by W. T. Speck. JOURNAL OF PEDIATRICS 103(1):161-163, July 1983.

—, by X. L. Ji. CHUNG-HUA NEI KO TSA CHIH 23(10):637-639, October 1984.

—, by Y. D. Chen. CHUNG HUA LIU HSING PING HSUEH TSA CHIH 5(6):367-369, December 1984.

—, by Z. Malcolm, et al. PHYSICIAN ASSISTANT 7(10):31-32+, October 1983.

—. AIDS: the widening gyre [news] by J. E. Groopman, et al. NATURE 303(5918):575-576, June 16-22, 1983.

—. Ascites disclosing necrotizing enterocolitis [letter], by E. Rene, et al. PRESSE MEDICALE 13(4):227, February 4, 1984.

—. Clinical data and immunologic studies on 9 patients examined in Mexico, by C. Abud-Mendoza, et al. REVISTA DE INVESTIGACION CLINICA 36(4):311-319, October-December 1984.

— Clinicopathologic study of 56 autopsies, by G. W. Niedt, et al. ARCHIVES OF PATHOLOGY AND LABORATORY MEDICINE 109(8):727-734, August 1985.

—. Commentary. Council on Scientific Affairs. JAMA 252(15):2037-2043, October 19, 1984.

—. A contemporary overview, by K. Crossley. MINNESOTA MEDICINE 69(1):29-30, January 1986.

—. A deadly new disease, by F. A. Khan, et al. POSTGRADUATE MEDICINE 74(2):180-185+, August 1983.

—. Distinctive features of bone marrow biopsies, by S. A. Geller, et al. ARCHIVES OF PATHOLOGY AND LABORATORY MEDICINE 109(2):138-141, February 1985.

—. A dynamic clinico-biological situation, by X. Estivill, et al. SANGRE 28(6):753-769, 1983.

—. Epidemiologic update, by J. N. Kuritsky, et al. MINNESOTA MEDICINE 67(1):37-41, January 1984.

—. The ever-broadening clinical spectrum [editorial], by A. S. Fauci. JAMA 249(17): 2375-2376, May 6, 1983.

— The first cases in Finland, by S. L. Valle, et al. ANNALS OF CLINICAL RESEARCH 15(5-6):203-205, 1983.

—. First confirmed case in Panamá, by M. M. de Ycaza, et al. REVISTA MEDICA DE PANAMA 10(1):66-73, January 1985.

—. Health and Public Policy Committee, American College of Physicians; and The Infectious Diseases Society of America. ANNALS OF INTERNAL MEDICINE 104(4):575-581, April 1986.

—. Implications for the practicing physician, by B. Varkey. POSTGRADUATE MEDICINE 73(5):138+, May 1983.

—. Infection control and public health law, by M. Mills, et al. NEW ENGLAND JOURNAL OF MEDICINE 314(14):931-936, April 3, 1986.

—. Introduction, by J. E. Groopman. SEMINARS IN ONCOLOGY 11(1):3, March 1984.

—. Measures to be taken in blood transfusion establishments in order to protect the personnel], by J. Y. Muller. REVUE FRANCAISE DE TRANSFUSION ET IMMUNO-HEMATOLOGIE 27(4):567-570, September 1984.

—. A new disease of infectious origin? PRESSE MEDICALE 12(39):2453-2456, November 5, 1983.

—. No evidence of the presence of cyclosporine, by H. F. Schran, et al. AMERICAN JOURNAL OF MEDICINE 77(5):797-804, November 1984.

—. Ophthalmic manifestations in ambulatory patients, by P. R. Rosenberg, et al. OPHTHALMOLOGY 90(8):874-878, August 1983.

—. Pathogenic mechanisms of ocular disease, by J. S. Pepose, et al. OPHTHAL-MOLOGY 92(4):472-484, April 1985.

—. A perspective for the medical practitioner, by R. J. Sherertz. MEDICAL CLINICS OF NORTH AMERICA 69(4):637-655, July 1985.

—. A proderomal form, by A. G. Dalgleish, et al. MEDICAL JOURNAL OF AUSTRALIA 1(12):558-560, June 11, 1983.

—. Recommendations to prevent transmission for hospitals and health care workers, by K. Crossley. MINNESOTA MEDICINE 69(4):211-213, April 1986.

—. A report of 2 South African cases, by G. J. Ras, et al. SOUTH AFRICAN MEDICAL JOURNAL 64(4):140-142, July 23, 1983.

—. Review of the literature. Apropos of a pre-AIDS case in a heroin addict, by F. Valentini, et al. MINERVA MEDICA 77(1-2): 7-11, January 14, 1986.

— A status report. The statement of a World Health Organization meeting. SERVIR 33(5):259-269, September-October 1985.

9

—. A surgical perspective, by J. M. Davis, et al. ARCHIVES OF SURGERY 119(1):90-95, January 1984.

Acquired immune deficiency syndrome abroad, by J. L. Marx. SCIENCE 222:998-999, December 2, 1983.

Acquired immune deficiency syndrome (AIDS). TOPICS IN CLINICAL NURSING 6(2): vi-vii+, July 1984.

—, by C. Scully, et al. BRITISH DENTAL JOURNAL 155(7):221-225, October 8, 1983.

— [editorial], by D. Michaeli. HAREFUAH 104(7):301-303, April 1, 1983.

— by D. J. Jeffries. MEDICAL LABORATORY SCIENCES 42(3):237-244, July 1985.

—, by D. T. Purtilo, et al. CLINICAL AND LABORATORY MEDICINE 6(1):3-26, March 1986.

—, by E. J. Fisher. MICHIGAN MEDICINE 83(24):229-230+, May 1984.

—, by I. Bojic. VOJNOSANITETSKI PREGLED 42(5):372-379, September-October 1985.

—, by J. D. Wilson. NEW ZEALAND MEDICAL JOURNAL 97(747):9-11, January 11, 1984.

—, by J. V. Wells, et al. AUSTRALIAN AND NEW ZEALAND JOURNAL OF MEDICINE 14(2):191-194, April 1984.

—, by W. L. Bayer, et al. MISSOURI MEDICINE 80(12):756-758, December 1983.

—. From the AIDS committee—Quebec. UNION MEDICALE DU CANADA 112(7):604-606+, July 1983.

—. Hypotheses on the etiology, by T. A. Kelly. MEDICAL HYPOTHESES 14(4):347-351, August 1984.

—. Light microscopic, ultrastructural and immunocytochemical studies of one case, by S. R. Allegra, et al. JOURNAL OF SUBMICROSCOPIC CYTOLOGY 16(3):561-568, July 1984.

—. Medical challenge of the 80's, by C. B. Daul, et al. POSTGRADUATE MEDICINE 76(1):167-174+, July 1984.

—. Report of the NHMRC Working Party. MEDICAL JOURNAL OF AUSTRALIA 141(9):561-568, October 27, 1984.

—. A review, by S. H. Landesman, et al. ARCHIVES OF INTERNAL MEDICINE 143(12):2307-2309, December 1983.

—. An update 1984, by S. R. Porter, et al. BRITISH DENTAL JOURNAL 157(11):387-391, December 8, 1984.

Acquired immune deficiency syndrome (AIDS) and consultation-liaison psychiatry, by D. L. Wolcott, et al. GENERAL HOSPITAL PSYCHIATRY 7(4):280-293, October 1985.

Acquired immune deficiency syndrome (AIDS) . . . critical care crossword, by A. L. Gilmour. CRITICAL CARE NURSE 4(5):134-135+, September-October 1984.

Acquired immune deficiency syndrome (AIDS): current status and implications for respiratory care practitioners, by T. J. Witek, Jr., et al. RESPIRATORY CARE 29(1):35-45, January 1984.

Acquired immune deficiency syndrome (AIDS): disease characteristics and oral manifestations, by D. T. Wofford, et al. JOURNAL OF THE AMERICAN DENTAL ASSOCIATION 111(2):258-261, August 1985.

Acquired immune deficiency syndrome (AIDS) HTLV-III/LAV; the causal agent and modes of transmission, by A. Smithies. HEALTH BULLETIN 44(4):234-238, July 1986.

Acquired immune deficiency syndrome (AIDS) in Europe. EUROPEAN JOURNAL OF CLINICAL MICROBIOLOGY 3(1):53-84, February 1984.

Acquired immune deficiency syndrome (AIDS) in hemophiliacs: a hypothesis, by T. V. Shankey, et al. AIDS RESEARCH 1(1):83-90, 1983-1984.

Acquired immune deficiency syndrome (AIDS) in a Jamaican, by C. Charles, et al. WEST INDIAN MEDICAL JOURNAL 33(2):130-133, June 1984.

Acquired immune deficiency syndrome (AIDS) manifesting as anogenital herpes zoster eruption: demonstration of virus-like particles in lymphosytes, by P. Thune, et al. ACTA DERMATO-VENEREOLOGICA. SUPPLEMENTUM 63(6):540-543, 1983.

Acquired immune deficiency syndrome (AIDS)—a multidisciplinary enigma [clinical conference]. WESTERN JOURNAL OF MEDICINE 140(1);66-81, January 1984.

Acquired immune deficiency syndrome (AIDS): number one priority, by E. D. Glover. HEALTH VALUES 8(2):3-12, March-April 1984.

Acquired immune deficiency syndrome (AIDS): of concern to us all [editorial], by D. N. Lawrence. JOURNAL OF THE FLORIDA MEDICAL ASSOCIATION 70(2):101-102, February 1983.

Acquired immune deficiency syndrome (AIDS): precautions for clinical and laboratory staffs. EMERGENCY MEDICAL SERVICES 12(5):69, September-October 1983.

—. MMWR 31(43):577-580, November 5, 1982.

Acquired immune deficiency syndrome (AIDS): precautions for clinical staff. CHART 83(5):7, May-June 1986.

Acquired immune deficiency syndrome (AIDS): speculations about its etiology and comparative immunology, by J. G. Sinkovics, et al. REVIEWS OF INFECTIOUS DISEASES 6(5):745-760, September-October 1984.

Acquired immune deficiency syndrome (AIDS) trends in the United States, 1978-1982, by R. M. Selik, et al. AMERICAN JOURNAL OF MEDICINE 76(3):493-500, March 1984.

Acquired immune deficiency syndrome (AIDS): an update for nurses, by N. P. Guarda, et al. FLORIDA NURSE 34(10):1+, November 1985.

11

Acquired immune deficiency syndrome, altered T cell subset ratios, and cytomegalo-virus infections among male homosexuals in The Netherlands, by J. Goudsmit, et al. ANTIOBIOTIC CHEMOTHERAPY 32:138-146, 1983.

Acquired immune deficiency syndrome and epidemic of infection with human immu-nodeficiency virus: costs of care and prevention in an inner London district, by A. M. Johnson, et al. BRITISH MEDICAL JOURNAL 293(6545):489-492, August 23, 1986.

Acquired immune deficiency syndrome and the fertility clinic, by G. D. Ball. FERTIL-ITY AND STERILITY 45(2):172-174, February 1986.

Acquired immune deficiency syndrome and the management of associated oppor-tunistic infections, by N. Dozier, et al. DRUG INTELLIGENCE AND CLINICAL PHARMACY 17(11):798-807, November 1983.

Acquired immune deficiency syndrome and multiple tract degeneration in a homosex-ual man, by D. S. Horoupian, et al. ANNALS OF NEUROLOGY 15(5);502-505, May 1984.

Acquired immune deficiency syndrome and pancytopenia, by J. L. Spivak, et al. JAMA 250(22):3084-3087, December 9, 1983.

Acquired immune deficiency syndrome and related complex. A report of 2 confirmed cases in Cape Town with comments on human T-cell lymphotropic virus type III in-fections, by F. H. Spracklen, et al. SOUTH AFRICAN MEDICAL JOURNAL 68(3): 139-143, August 3, 1985.

Acquired immune deficiency syndrome: a brief review and anesthetic implications, by J. Layon. CURRENT REVIEWS FOR RECOVERY ROOM NURSES 8(9):67-72, 1986.

Acquired immune deficiency syndrome: the causative agent and the evolving per-spective, by P. J. Fischinger. CURRENT PROBLEMS IN CANCER 9(1):1-39, January 1985.

Acquired immune deficiency syndrome: current status. Position of the German Association for the Control of Virus Diseases and the Virology Section of the German Society for Hygiene and Microbiology, by F. Deinhardt, et al. DEUTSCHE MEDIZINISCHE WOCHENSCHRIFT 110(7):274-276, February 15, 1985.

Acquired immune deficiency syndrome: dental considerations, by B. E. Evans. NEW YORK STATE DENTAL JOURNAL 49(9):649-652, November 1983.

Acquired immune deficiency syndrome—epidemiology and etiology, by I. Ahmed. JOURNAL OF THE PAKISTAN MEDICAL ASSOCIATION 35(9):269-271, Sep-tember 1985.

Acquired immune deficiency syndrome: the facts, by D. G. Penington, et al. QUEENSLAND NURSE 4(1):17-24, January-February 1985.

Acquired immune deficiency syndrome . . . impact of heredity and East Indian sexual practices, by S. Khanna. NURSING JOURNAL OF INDIA 76(4):91-93, April 1985.

Acquired immune deficiency syndrome: implications and directions, by W. A. Andes. AUAA JOURNAL 5(3):8-10, January-March 1985.

Acquired immune deficiency syndrome in Belgium, by N. Clumeck. EUROPEAN JOURNAL OF CLINICAL MICROBIOLOGY 3(1):59-60, February 1984.

Acquired immune deficiency syndrome in Belgium and its relation to Central Africa, by N. Clumeck, et al. ANNALS OF THE NEW YORK ACADEMY OF SCIENCES 437: 264-269, 1984.

Acquired immune deficiency syndrome in Black Africans [letter], by N. Clumeck, et al. LANCET 1(8325):642, March 19, 1983.

Acquired immune deficiency syndrome in Britain, August 1983. BRITISH MEDICAL JOURNAL 287(6400):1205, October 22, 1983.

Acquired immune deficiency syndrome in childhood, by K. M. Shannon, et al. JOURNAL OF PEDIATRICS 106(2):332-342, February 1985.

Acquired immune deficiency syndrome in children, by J. M. Oleske, et al. PEDIATRIC INFECTIOUS DISEASE 2(2):85-86, March-April 1983.

Acquired immune deficiency syndrome in the Federal Republic of Germany, by J. L'age-Stehr. EUROPEAN JOURNAL OF CLINICAL MICROBIOLOGY 3(1):61, February 1984.

Acquired immune deficiency syndrome in France, by J. B. Brunet. EUROPEAN JOURNAL OF CLINICAL MICROBIOLOGY 3(1):66, February 1984.

Acquired immune deficiency syndrome in infants and children, by S. W. Thompson, et al. PEDIATRIC NURSING 11(4):278-280+, July-August 1985.

Acquired immune deficiency syndrome in infants born of Haitian mothers [letter], by J. H. Joncas, et al. NEW ENGLAND JOURNAL OF MEDICINE 308(14):842, April 7, 1983.

Acquired immune deficiency syndrome in Kentucky, by J. M. Felser, et al. JOURNAL OF THE KENTUCKY MEDICAL ASSOCIATION 81(9):703-706, September 1983.

Acquired immune deficiency syndrome in low-risk patient. Evidence for possible transmission by an asymptomatic carrier, by A. E. Pitchenik, et al. JAMA 250(10): 1310-1312, September 9, 1983.

Acquired immune deficiency syndrome in the Middle East from imported blood, by M. E. Kingston, et al. TRANSFUSION 25(4):317-318, July-August 1985.

Acquired immune deficiency syndrome in a patient with prior sarcoidosis: case report with monocyte function studies, by S. Kalter, et al. TEXAS MEDICINE 81(9):44-46, September 1985.

Acquired immune deficiency syndrome in Scandinavia, by H. Repo, et al. EUROPEAN JOURNAL OF CLINICAL MICROBIOLOGY 3(1):65, February 1984.

Acquired immune deficiency syndrome in Switzerland, by B. Somaini. EUROPEAN JOURNAL OF CLINICAL MICROBIOLOGY 3(1):67, February 1984.

Acquired immune deficiency syndrome in Thailand, by H. Wilde, et al. ASIAN AND PACIFIC JOURNAL OF ALLERGY AND IMMUNOLOGY 3(1):104-107, June 1985.

Acquired immune deficiency syndrome in Thailand. A report of two cases, by A. Limsuwan, et al. JOURNAL OF THE MEDICAL ASSOCIATION OF THAILAND 69(3): 164-169, March 1986.

Acquired immune deficiency syndrome in The Netherlands, by C. M. Vanden-broucke-Grauls, et al. EUROPEAN JOURNAL OF CLINICAL MICROBIOLOGY 3(1):62, February 1984.

Acquired immune deficiency syndrome in 3 patients from Zaire, by H. Taelman, et al. ANNALES DE LA SOCIETE BELGE DE MEDECINE TROPICALE 63(1):73-74, March 1983.

Acquired immune deficiency syndrome in Trinidad. A report on two cases, by C. Bartholomew, et al. WEST INDIAN MEDICAL JOURNAL 32(3):177-180, September 1983.

Acquired immune deficiency syndrome in the United Kingdom, by M. McEvoy. EUROPEAN JOURNAL OF CLINICAL MICROBIOLOGY 3(1):63-64, February 1984.

Acquired immune deficiency syndrome in the United States: the first 1,000 cases, by H. W. Jaffe, et al. JOURNAL OF INFECTIOUS DISEASES 286(6374):1354, April 23, 1983.

Acquired immune deficiency syndrome in West Virginia: an 'imported' disease, by J. M. Bernstein, et al. WEST VIRGINIA MEDICAL JOURNAL 80(8):153-156, August 1984.

Acquired immune deficiency syndrome: an international health problem of increasing importance, by C. B. Oofsy, et al. KLINISCHE WOCHENSCHRIFT 62(11):512-522, June 1, 1984.

Acquired immune deficiency syndrome: is disseminated aspergillosis predictive of underlying cellular immune deficiency?, by A. Schaffner. JOURNAL OF INFECTIOUS DISEASES 149(5):828-829, May 1984.

Acquired immune deficiency syndrome: laboratory findings, clinical features, and leading hypotheses, by W. El-Sadr, et al. DIAGNOSTIC IMMUNOLOGY 2(2):73-85, 1984.

Acquired immune deficiency syndrome, leading to opportunistic infections, Kaposi's sarcoma, and other malignancies, by P. W. Mansell. CRITICAL REVIEWS IN CLINICAL LABORATORY SCIENCES 20(3):191-204, 1984.

Acquired immune deficiency syndrome: a new challenge for nursing, by C. Carneiro. MASSACHUSETTS NURSE 52(6):1+, June 1983.

Acquired immune deficiency syndrome: a new epidemic, by J. P. Griffin. CRITICAL CARE NURSE 3(2):21-24+, April-May 1983.

—. HOME HEALTHCARE NURSE 1(1):17-18+, September-October 1983.

Acquired immune deficiency syndrome—a new, thus far unexplained syndrome with a severe course, by J. Sejda, et al. VNITRNI LEKARSTVI 29(11):1107-1113, November 1983.

Acquired immune deficiency syndrome of macaque monkeys, by N. L. Letkin, et al. ANNALS OF THE NEW YORK ACADEMY OF SCIENCES 437:121-130, 1984.

Acquired immune deficiency syndrome, opportunistic infections and Kaposi's sarcoma: epidemic of a new disease, by P. Francioli, et al. SCHWEIZERISCHE MEDIZINISCHE WOCHENSCHRIFT 113(26):938-942, July 2, 1983.

Acquired immune deficiency syndrome—an overview, by J. A. Gracie, et al. SCOTTISH MEDICAL JOURNAL 30(1):1-7, January 1985.

Acquired immune deficiency syndrome part 1, by A. J. Pinching. MIDWIFE, HEALTH VISITOR AND COMMUNITY NURSE 22(5):142-146+, May 1986.

Acquired immune deficiency syndrome: the past as prologue, by J. W. Curran, et al. ANNALS OF INTERNAL MEDICINE 98(3):401-403, March 1983.

Acquired immune deficiency syndrome possibly related to transfusion in an adult without known disease-risk factors, by S. M. Gordon, et al. JOURNAL OF INFECTIOUS DISEASES 149(6):1030-1032, June 1984.

Acquired immune deficiency syndrome: postmortem findings, by L. A. Guarda, et al. AMERICAN JOURNAL OF CLINICAL PATHOLOGY 81(5):549-557, May 1984.

Acquired immune deficiency syndrome presenting as oral pharyngeal and cutaneous Kaposi's sarcoma, by B. L. NaPier, et al. LARYNGOSCOPE 93(11, Part 1):1466-1469, November 1983.

Acquired immune deficiency syndrome presenting as recalcitrant Candida, by A. Babajews, et al. BRITISH DENTAL JOURNAL 159(4):106-108, August 24, 1985.

Acquired immune deficiency syndrome—recommendations of the working party [letter]. JOURNAL OF HOSPITAL INFECTION 7(3):295-296, May 1986.

—, by R. E. Warren, et al. JOURNAL OF HOSPITAL INFECTION 7(3):306-307, May 1986.

Acquired immune deficiency syndrome—related lymphadenopathies presenting in the salivary gland lymph nodes, by J. R. Ryan, et al. ARCHIVES OF OTOLARYNGOLOGY 111(8):554-556, August 1985.

Acquired immune deficiency syndrome retinpathy, pneumocystis, and cotton-wool spots [editorial], by W. R. Freeman, et al. AMERICAN JOURNAL OF OPHTHALMOLOGY 9892):235-237, August 15, 1984.

Acquired immune deficiency syndrome: review, by C. Scully, et al. BRITISH DENTAL JOURNAL 161(2):53-60, July 19, 1986.

Acquired immune deficiency syndrome: a review, by K. C. Davis. RESPIRATORY THERAPY 14(5):15-16+, September-October 1984.

Acquired immune deficiency syndrome: specific aspects of the disease in Haiti, by J. M. Guerin, et al. ANNALS OF THE NEW YORK ACADEMY OF SCIENCES 437: 254-263, 1984.

Acquired immune deficiency syndrome: a study on impact of heredity, by S. Khanna. NURSING JOURNAL OF INDIA 76(4):91-93, April 1985.

Acquired immune deficiency syndrome—update, by A. Hasner, et al. HAREFUAH 108(9):448-453, May 1, 1985.

Acquired immune deficiency syndrome—an update, by D. M. Heebink. RESPIRATORY CARE 29(1):54-58, January 1984.

Acquired immune deficiency syndrome—update [editorial], by Z. Bentwich, et al. HAREFUAH 108(9):464-467, May 1, 1985.

Acquired immune deficiency syndrome: an update and interpretation, by C. B. Daul, et al. ANNALS OF ALLERGY 51(3):351-361, September 1983.

Acquired immune deficiency syndrome: a venereal disease? by P. A. Poulsen, et al. UGESKRIFT FOR LAEGER 146(5):355-356, JANUARY 30, 1984.

Acquired immune deficiency syndrome: viral infections and etiology, by D. Armstrong. PROGRESS IN MEDICAL VIROLOGY 30:1-13, 1984.

Acquired immune dysfunction in homosexual men: immunologic profiles, by A. J. Ammann, et al. CLINICAL IMMUNOLOGY AND IMMUNOPATHOLOGY 27(3):315-325, June 1983.

Acquired immunodeficiency, by A. González-Angulo, et al. GACETA MEDICA DE MEXICO 121(1-2):1-17, January-February 1985.

Acquired immunodeficiency, by O. A. Strand. TIDSSKRIFT FOR DEN NORSKE LAEGEFORENING 103(11):895-897, April 20, 1983.

Acquired immunodeficiency (AIDS), by H. G. Thiele. IMMUNITAT UND INFEKTION 11(5):177-180, September 1983.

Acquired immunodeficiency (AIDS) in pregnancy, by L. P. Jensene, et al. AMERICAN JOURNAL OF OBSTETRICS AND GYNECOLOGY 148(8):1145-1146, April 15, 1984.

Acquired immunodeficiency and the "one donor-one patient" principle, by A. I. Vorob'ev, et al. TERAPEVTICHESKII ARKHIV 57(7):3-6, 1985.

Acquired immunodeficiency and related syndromes, by J. Debold. PATHOLOGY, RESEARCH AND PRACTICE 179(1):124-126, September 1984.

Acquired immunodeficiency in haemophilia [editorial]. LANCET 1(8327):75, April 2, 1983.

Acquired immunodeficiency in Haitians [letter], by M. Boncy, et al. NEW ENGLAND JOURNAL OF MEDICINE 308(23):1419-1420, June 9, 1983.

Acquired immunodeficiency in homosexual men, by H. H. Handsfield. AJR139(4): 832- 833, October 1982.

Acquired immunodeficiency in an infant: possible transmission by means of blood products, by A. J. Ammann, et al. LANCET 1(8331):956-958, April 30, 1983.

'Acquired immunodeficiency 'of blood stored overnight [letter], by B. J. Weiblen, et al. NEW ENGLAND JOURNAL OF MEDICINE 809(13):793, September 29, 1983.

Acquired immunodeficiency syndrome [letter]. ANNALS OF INTERNAL MEDICINE 99(5):734-736, November 1983.

— [editorial]. LANCET 1(8317):162-164, January 22, 1938.

—, by D. J. LaCamera, et al. NURSING CLINICS OF NORTH AMERICA 20(1):241-256, March 1985.

—, by H. Minkoff. JOURNAL OF NURSE-MIDWIFERY 31(4):189-193, July-August 1986.

—, by J. M. Orenstein. HUMAN PATHOLOGY 16(12):1285-1286, December 1985.

—, by J. Racouchot. PRESSE MEDICALE 14(5):287, February 9, 1985.

—, by K. Crossley. MINNESOTA MEDICINE 69(4):211-213, April 1986.

Acquired immunodeficiency syndrome (AIDS). REVISTA DE ENFERMERIA 8(81): 55-59, April 1985.

—, by C. Bogdan, et al. FORTSCHRITTE DER MEDIZEN 103(35):817-821, September 19, 1985.

— (a review of the literature), by E. N. Sidorenko. VRACHEBNOE DELO 10:104-110, October 1985.

—, by F. Cambazard. SOINS. GYNECOLOGIE, OBSTETRIQUE, PUERICULTURE, PEDIATRIE 56:21-26, January 1986.

—, by F. S. Rosen. JOURNAL OF CLINICAL INVESTIGATION 75(1):1-3, January 1985.

—, by G. Levi. AMB 31(9-10):173-187, September-October 1985.

—, by H. Masur. PROGRESS IN CLINICAL AND BIOLOGICAL RESEARCH 182:271-276, 1985.

—, by J. Besner, et al. AARN NEWSLETTER 42(2):25-27, February 1986.

—, by J. Frottier. SOINS 930:53-56, May 1984.

—, by M. Dicato. BULLETIN DE LA SOCIETE DES SCIENCES MEDICALES DU GRAND-DUCHE DE LUXEMBOURG 121(2):5-6, 1984.

— [editorial], by M. S. Hutt. TROPICAL DOCTOR 15(1):1, January 1985.

—, by O. W. van Assendelft. NEDERLANDS TIJDSCHRIFT VOOR GENEESKUNDE 127(19):826-30, May 7, 1983.

—, by P. Jansa. ACTA UNIVERSITATIS PALACKIANAE OLOMUCENSIS FACULTATIS MEDICAE 108:193-195, 1985.

—, by S. A. Danner, et al. NEDERLANDS TIJDSCHRIFT VOOR GENEESKUNDE 127(19):830-832, May 7, 1983.

—, by V. Gong. AMERICAN JOURNAL OF EMERGENCY MEDICINE 2(4):336-346, July 1984.

—, by V. Suvakovic. SRPSKI ARHIV ZA CELOKUPNO LEKARSTVO 112(11-12):1205-1215, November-December 1984.

—, by Y. Ueda. NIPPON RINSHO 41(9):2185-2190, September 1983.

Acquired immunodeficiency syndrome (AIDS). Case reports and diagnosis, by O. Braun-Falco, et al. MUENCHENER MEDIZINISCHE WOCHENSCHRIFT 125(48): 1135-1139, December 2, 1983.

Acquired immunodeficiency syndrome (AIDS). Clinical, immunological, pathological, and microbiological studies of the first case diagnosed in Norway, by S. S. Froland, et al. SCANDINAVIAN JOURNAL OF GASTROENTEROLOGY 107:82-93, 1985.

Acquired immunodeficiency syndrome (AIDS). A 2-year review, by M. Vogt, et al. DEUTSCHE MEDIZINISCHE WOCHENSCHRIFT 108(50):1927-1933, December 16, 1983.

Acquired immunodeficiency syndrome (AIDS). An Update after 4 years, by M. Vogt, et al. SCHWEIZERISCHE MEDIZINISCHE WOCHENSCHRIFT 115(19):665-671, May 11, 1985.

Acquired immunodeficiency syndrome among patients with hemophilia. JAMA 250(24):3277-3278, December 23-30, 1983.

Acquired immunodeficiency syndrome (AIDS) and blood products, by R. D. Miller, et al. ANESTHESIOLOGY 58(6):493-494, June 1983.

Acquired immunodeficiency syndrome (AIDS) and Kaposi's sarcoma, by J. Martin. INTERNATIONAL JOURNAL OF DERMATOLOGY 23(7):482-486, September 1984.

Acquired immunodeficiency syndrome (AIDS)—apheresis and operative risks, by D. D. Kiprov, et al. JOURNAL OF CLINICAL APHERESIS 2(4):427-440, 1985.

Acquired immunodeficiency syndrome (AIDS) associated with transfusions by J. W. Curran, et al. NEW ENGLAND JOURNAL OF MEDICINE 310(2):69-75, January 12, 1984.

Acquired immunodeficiency syndrome (AIDS)—Canada. MMWR 32(48):635-636, December 9, 1983.

Acquired immunodeficiency syndrome (AIDS)—clinical course and prevention, by E. Sandström, et al. LAKARTIDNINGEN 80(7):529-530, February 16, 1983.

Acquired immunodeficiency syndrome (AIDS)—a current or future problem?, by Z. Kuratowska. POLSKI TYGODNIK LEKARSKI 39(36):1189-1192, September 3, 1984.

Acquired immunodeficiency syndrome (AIDS): the disease and its ocular manifestations, by J. A. Mines, et al. INTERNATIONAL OPHTHALMOLOGY CLINICS 26(2):73-115, Summer 1986.

Acquired immunodeficiency syndrome (AIDS): an epidemiologic and clinical overview, by K. G. Castro, et al. JOURNAL OF THE MEDICAL ASSOCIATION OF GEORGIA 78(8):537-542, August 1984.

Acquired immunodeficiency syndrome (AIDS)—Europe. JAMA 250(24):3278, December 23-30, 1983. Also in: MMWR 32(46):610-611, November 25, 1983.

Acquired immunodeficiency syndrome (AIDS): experience in the Puerto Rico Medical Center, by C. Climent, et al. BOLETIN—ASOCIACION MEDICA DE PUERTO RICO 77(2):50-55, February 1985.

Acquired immunodeficiency syndrome (AIDS) in Africa. A review, by R. Colebunders, et al. TROPICAL DOCTOR 15(1):9-12, January 1985.

Acquired immunodeficiency syndrome (AIDS) in Africans, by C. Katlama, et al. ANNALES DE LA SOCIETE BELGE DE MEDECINE TROPICALE 64(4):379-389, 1984.

Acquired immunodeficiency syndrome (AIDS) in Denmark. A report from the Copenhagen study group of AIDS on the first 20 Danish patients, by J. Gerstoft, et al. ACTA MEDICA SCANDINAVICA 217(2):213-224, 1985.

Acquired immunodeficiency syndrome (AIDS) in an economically disadvantaged population, by S. Maayan, et al. ARCHIVES OF INTERNAL MEDICINE 145(9):1607-1612, September 1985.

Acquired immunodeficiency syndrome (AIDS) in hemophilia, by B. L. Evatt, et al. CLINICS IN LABORATORY MEDICINE 4(2):333-344, June 1984.

Acquired immunodeficiency syndrome (AIDS) in hemophiliacs, by J. M. Jason, et al. SCANDINAVIAN JOURNAL OF HAEMATOLOGY. SUPPLEMENTUM 40:349-356, 1984.

Acquired immunodeficiency syndrome (AIDS) in hemophiliacs. Clinical course and post-mortem examination of the first cases described in Spain by M. A. Díaz-Torres, et al. MEDICINA CLINICA 82(19):866-867, May 19, 1984.

Acquired immunodeficiency syndrome (AIDS) in home care: maximizing helpfulness and minimizing hysteria, by J. Lillard, et al. HOME HEALTHCARE NURSE 2(5): 11-14+, November-December 1984.

Acquired immunodeficiency syndrome (AIDS) in a homosexual male with tuberculosis and medullary hyperplasia [letter], by T. Martín Jiménez, et al. MEDICINA CLINICA 85(1):39-40, June 1, 1985.

Acquired immunodeficiency syndrome (AIDS) in homosexual men—a new public health concern, by O. A. Strand. NIPH ANNALS 5(2):41-49, December 1982.

Acquired immunodeficiency syndrome (AIDS) in Kinshasa, Zaire: clinical and epidemi-ological observations, by W. Odio, et al. ANNALES DE LA SOCIETE BELGE DE MEDECINE TROPICALE 65(4):357-361, 1985.

Acquired immunodeficiency syndrome (AIDS) in male homosexuals in Frankfurt am Main, by E. B. Helm, et al. MUENCHENER MEDIZINISCHE WOCHENSCHRIFT 125(48):1129-1134, December 2, 1983.

Acquired immunodeficiency syndrome (AIDS) in persons with hemophilia. JAMA 252:2679-2680, November 16, 1984.

Acquired immunodeficiency syndrome (AIDS) in Spain [letter], by J. M. Arnau de Bolós, et al. MEDICINA CLINICA 82(18):827, May 12, 1984.

Acquired immunodeficiency syndrome (AIDS) in 2 homosexuals in Belgium, by J. Unger, et al. ACTA CLINICA BELGICA 38(6):401-405, 1983.

Acquired immunodeficiency syndrome (AIDS): is vaccination against hepatitis B a prevention for the risk?, by D. Vuitton, et al. GASTROENTEROLOGIE CLINIQUE ET BIOLOGIQUE 8(1):37-41, January 1984.

Acquired immunodeficiency syndrome 'AIDS': limits of the unknown, by W. Rozen-baum. ANNALES DE MEDECINE INTERNE 135(1):3-6, 1984.

Acquired immunodeficiency syndrome (AIDS) manifested as severe genital herpes. Apropos of 2 cases, by J. De Maubeuge, et al. DERMATOLOGICA 168(3):105-111, 1984.

Acquired immunodeficiency syndrome (AIDS)—a new pathology involving the res-piratory system, by F. Mihaltan. REVISTA DE IGIENA BACTERIOLOGIE, VIRUSOLOGIE, PARAZITOLOGIE, EPIDEMIOLOGIE, PNEUMOFITIZIOLOGIE, PNEUMOFTIZIOLOGIA 34(4):313-317, October-December 1985.

Acquired immunodeficiency syndrome (AIDS): new reports, by W. Mazurkiewicz. PRZEGLAD DERMATOLOGICZNY 71(5):423-429, September-October 1984.

Acquired immunodeficiency syndrome (AIDS): precautions for health-care workers and allied professionals. MMWR 32(34):450-451, September 2, 1983.

Acquired immunodeficiency syndrome (AIDS): report of the 1st autochthnous case in Brazil and immunological study, by V. Amato Neto, et al. REVISTA PAULISTA DE MEDICINA 101(4):165-168, July-August 1983.

Acquired immunodeficiency syndrome (AIDS): an update, by A. S. Fauci, et al. INTERNATIONAL ARCHIVES OF ALLERGY AND APPLIED IMMUNOLOGY 77(1-2):81-88, 1985.

Acquired immunodeficiency syndrome (AIDS)—an update, by L. Robinson. CRITI-CAL CARE NURSE 4(5):75-83, September-October 1984.

—. NEW ZEALAND NURSING FORUM 13(2):7-14, August-September 1985.

Acquired immunodeficiency syndrome (AIDS) update—United States. JAMA 250(3):335-336, July 15, 1983. Also in: MMWR 32(24):309-311, June 24, 1983.

Acquired immunodeficiency syndrome (AIDS) with Kaposi's sarcoma in homosexuals in Argentina [letter], by M. E. Estevez, et al. MEDICINA 43(4):477, 1983.

Acquired immunodeficiency syndrome among Haitians: an update, by M. A. Fischl, et al. ANNALS OF THE NEW YORK ACADEMY OF SCIENCES 437:325-333, 1984.

Acquired immunodeficiency syndrome among patients attending hemophilia treat-ment centers and mortality experience of hemophiliacs in the United States, by R. E. Johson, et al. AMERICAN JOURNAL OF EPIDEMIOLOGY 121(6):797-810, June 1985.

Acquired immunodeficiency syndrome: anatomo-pathological report of 2 necropsy cases,by V. L. Delmonte, et al. REVISTA DO INSTITUTO DE MEDICINA TROPI-CAL DE SAO PAULO 26(4):222-227, July-August 1984.

Acquired immunodeficiency syndrome and the emergency physician, by W. F. Skeen. ANNALS OF EMERGENCY MEDICINE 14(3):267-273, March 1985.

Acquired immunodeficiency syndrome and female sexual partners of bisexual men [letter], by C. L. Soskolne. ANNALS OF INTERNAL MEDICINE 100(2):312, Feb-ruary 1984.

Acquired immunodeficiency syndrome and homozygote sickle cell anemia. Apropos of a Zairian case, by K. W. Izzia, et al. ANNALES DE LA SOCIETE BELGE DE MEDECINE TROPICALE 64(4):391-396, 1984.

Acquired immunodeficiency syndrome and infection with hepatitis viruses in individ-uals abusing drugs by injection, by D. M. Novick, et al. BULLETIN ON NARCOT-ICS 38(1-2):15-25, January-June 1986.

Acquired immunodeficiency syndrome and Kaposi's sarcoma, by M. F. Muhlemann, et al. JOURNAL OF THE ROYAL SOCIETY OF MEDICINE 78(20:158-189, Feb-ruary 1985.

Acquired immunodeficiency syndrome and lupus anticoagulant [letter], by W. D. Haire. ANNALS OF INTERNAL MEDICINE 105(2):301-302, August 1986.

Acquired immunodeficiency syndrome and Mycobacterium avium-intracellulare bac-teremia in a patient with hemophilia, by J. L. Elliott, et al. ANNALS OF INTERNAL MEDICINE 98(3):290-293, March 1983.

Acquired immunodeficiency syndrome and nonmenstrual toxic shock syndrome [letter], by J. Sparano, et al. ANNALS OF INTERNAL MEDICINE 105(2):300-301, August 1986.

Acquired immunodeficiency syndrome and opportunistic infections [editorial], by R. de J. Pedro. REVISTA PAULISTA DE MEDICINA 101(4):123, July-August 1983.

Acquired immunodeficiency syndrome and opportunistic infections in a female, by E. Thornston, et al. SCHWEIZERISCHE MEDIZINISCHE WOCHENSCHRIFT 113(1):28-30, January 8, 1983.

Acquired immunodeficiency syndrome and other possible immunological disorders in European haemophiliacs, by A. L. Bloom. LANCET 1(8392):1452-1455, June 30, 1984.

Acquired immunodeficiency syndrome and related syndromes. Critical analysis of biological tests of cell-mediated immunity, by J. C. Gluckman, et al. PRESSE MEDICALE 13(32):1937-1941, September 22, 1984.

Acquired immunodeficiency syndrome and related syndromes in hemophiliacs: status throughout the world, by Y. Laurian, et al. REVUE FRANCAISE DE TRANSFUSION ET IMMUN0-HEMATOLOGIE 27(4):493-496, September 1984.

Acquired immunodeficiency syndrome and the transfusion service, by M. Hrubisko. VNITRNI LEKARSTVI 30(2):147-151, February 1984.

Acquired immunodeficiency syndrome and the treatment of hemophilia [letter], by V. Vicente, et al. MEDICINA CLINICA 81(5):231-232, July 16, 1983.

Acquired immunodeficiency syndrome and a trimethoprim-sulfamethoxazole adverse reaction [letter], by D. L. Cohn, et al. ANNALS OF INTERNAL MEDICINE 100(2): 311, February 1984.

Acquired immunodeficiency syndrome—another blood-transmitted disease?, by H. Seyfriedowa. ACTA HAEMATOLOGICA POLONICA 15(1-2):79-82, January-June 1984.

Acquired immunodeficiency syndrome: apropos of a case in an intravenous heroin user [letter], by A. Pintor Escobar, et al. MEDICINA CLINICA 82(1):42, January 14, 1984.

Acquired immunodeficiency syndrome—an assessment of the present situation in the world: memorandum from a WHO meeting. BULLETIN OF THE WORLD HEALTH ORGANIZATION 62(3):419-432, 1984.

Acquired immunodeficiency syndrome associated with Acanthamoeba infection and other opportunistic organisms, by M. M. Gonzalez, et al. ARCHIVES OF PATHOLOGY AND LABORATORY MEDICINE 110(8):749-751, August 1986.

Acquired immunodeficiency syndrome associated with blood-product transfusions, by J. R. Jett, et al. ANNALS OF INTERNAL MEDICINE 99(5):621-624, November 1983.

Acquired immunodeficiency syndrome associated with transfusions: the evolving perspective, by J. W. Curran, et al. ANNALS OF INTERNAL MEDICINE 100(2): 298-300, February 1984.

Acquired immunodeficiency syndrome: cerebral computed tomographic manifestations, by M. A. Whelan, et al. RADIOLOGY 149(2):477-484, November 1983.

Acquired immunodeficiency syndrome, chronic coccidiosis and Salmonella typhimurium septicemia in a couple from Zaire. Immunological functions and attempt at immunostimulation by thymopentin, by R. C. Martin-Du Pan, et al. SCHWEIZER-ISCHE MEDIZINISCHE WOCHENSCHRIFT 114(46):1645-1650, November 17, 1984.

Acquired immunodeficiency syndrome: current and future trends, by W. M. Morgan, et al. PUBLIC HEALTH REPORTS 101(5):459-465, September-October 1986.

Acquired immunodeficiency syndrome: current perspectives and future directions, by J. R. Minor. DRUG INTELLIGENCE AND CLINICAL PHARMACY 20(2):153-154, February 1986.

Acquired immunodeficiency syndrome: current status, by V. Quagliarello. YALE JOURNAL OF BIOLOGY AND MEDICINE 55(5-6):443-452, September-December 1982.

Acquired immunodeficiency syndrome: a discussion of etiologic hypotheses, by J. A. Sonnabend, et al. AIDS RESEARCH 1(2):107-120, 1983-1984.

Acquired immunodeficiency syndrome: epidemiological data in France and throughout the world, by J. B. Brunet, et al. BULLETIN DE L'ACADEMIE NATIONALE DE MEDECINE 168(1-2):278-281, January-February 1984.; also in REVUE FRANCAISE DE TRANSFUSION ET IMMUNO-HEMATOLOGIE 27(4):437-443, September 1984.

Acquired immunodeficiency syndrome: epidemiology, virology, and immunology, by A. Weiss, et al. ANNUAL REVIEW OF MEDICINE 36:545-562, 1985.

Acquired immuno-deficiency syndrome: a fatal but preventable disease, by N. Clumeck. ACTA CLINICA BELGICA 38(3):145-147, 1983.

Acquired immunodeficiency syndrome: guidelines for the control of infections in the ambulatory patient and in the hospitalized patient, by C. H. Ramírez-Ronda. BOLETIN—ASOCIACION MEDICA DE PUERTO RICO 77(4):143-150, April 1985.

Acquired immunodeficiency syndrome, hepatitis, and haemophilia [editorial], by P. Jones. BRITISH MEDICAL JOURNAL 287(6407):1737-1738, December 10, 1983.

Acquired immunodeficiency syndrome: highlights on the diagnosis and management of opportunistic infections, by C. E. Lopez. JOURNAL OF THE MEDICAL ASSOCIATION OF GEORGIA 73(8):525-533, August 1984.

Acquired immunodeficiency syndrome: impact and implication for neurological system, by M. M. Beckham, et al. JOURNAL OF NEUROSCIENCE NURSING 18(1):5-10, February 1986.

Acquired immunodeficiency syndrome in the adult. Its value in tropical medicine, by J. P. Coulaud, et al. MEDECINE TROPICALE 44(1):9-15, January-March 1984.

Acquired immunodeficiency syndrome in an African, by A. O. Obel, et al. EAST AFRICAN MEDICAL JOURNAL 61(9):724-726, September 1984.

Acquired immunodeficiency syndrome in African patients, by N. Clumeck, et al. NEW ENGLAND JOURNAL OF MEDICINE 310(8):492-497, February 23, 1984.

Acquired immunodeficiency syndrome in a child (preliminary report), by F. Iwanczak, et al. POLSKI TYGODNIK LEKARSKI 40(9):259-262, March 4, 1985.

Acquired immunodeficiency syndrome in the child of a haemophiliac, by M. V. Ragni, et al. LANCET 1(8421):133-135, January 19, 1985.

Acquired immunodeficiency syndrome in children [editorial], by B. Garty, et al. HARE-FUAH 107(9):262-263, November 1, 1984.

Acquired immunodeficiency syndrome in children, by F. Iwanczak, et al. POLSKI TYGODNIK LEKARSKI 40(9):245-248, March 4, 1985.

Acquired immunodeficiency syndrome in a cohort of homosexual men. A six-year follow-up study, by H. W. Jaffe, et al. ANNALS OF INTERNAL MEDICINE 103(2): 210-214, August 1985.

Acquired immunodeficiency syndrome in a colony of macaque monkeys, by N. L. Letvin, et al. PROCEEDINGS OF THE NATIONAL ACADEMY OF SCIENCES USA 80(9):2718-2722, May 1983.

Acquired immunodeficiency syndrome in correctional facilities: a report of the National Institute of Justice and the American Correctional Association. MMWR 35(12): 195-199, March 28, 1986.

Acquired immunodeficiency syndrome in a couple from Zaire, by P. Le Bras, et al. REVISTA DE MEDICINA INTERNA 5(3):225-227, September 1984.

Acquired immunodeficiency syndrome in a drug addict with Kaposi's sarcoma and chronic hepatitis B [letter], by A. García Díez, et al. MEDICINA CLINICA 83(12): 518, October 20, 1984.

Acquired immunodeficiency syndrome in Florida—a review, by C. L. MacLeod, et al. JOURNAL OF THE FLORIDA MEDICAL ASSOCIATION 71(9):712-717, September 1984.

Acquired immunodeficiency syndrome in four homosexuals, by W. Rozenbaum, et al. PRESSE MEDICALE 12(18):1149-1154, April 23, 1983.

Acquired immunodeficiency syndrome in France [letter], by J. B. Brunet, et al. LANCET 1(8326, Part 1):700-701, March 26, 1983.

Acquired immunodeficiency syndrome in gay men, by H. W. Jaffe, et al. ANNALS OF INTERNAL MEDICINE 103(5):662-664, November 1985.

Acquired immunodeficiency syndrome in Haiti, by J. W. Pape, et al. ANNALS OF INTERNAL MEDICINE 103(5):674-678, November 1985.

Acquired immunodeficiency syndrome in a heterosexual population in Zaire, by P. Piot, et al. LANCET 2(8394):65-69, July 14, 1984.

Acquired immunodeficiency syndrome in infants, by A. Rubinstein. AMERICAN JOURNAL OF DISEASES OF CHILDREN 137(9):825-827, September 1983.

Acquired immunodeficiency syndrome in infants, by G. B. Scott, et al. NEW ENGLAND JOURNAL OF MEDICINE 310(2):76-81, January 12, 1984.

Acquired immunodeficiency syndrome in infants and children, by A. J. Ammann. ANNALS OF INTERNAL MEDICINE 103(5):734-737, November 1985.

—, by L. J. Bernstein, et al. PROGRESS IN ALLERGY 37:194-206, 1986.

Acquired immunodeficiency syndrome in male prisoners. New insights into an emerging syndrome, by G. P. Wormser, et al. ANNALS OF INTERNAL MEDICINE 98(3):297-303 March 1983.

Acquired immunodeficiency syndrome in a male residing in Barcelona [letter], by R. Estruch, et al. MEDICINA CLINICA 81(14):645, November 5, 1983.

Acquired immunodeficiency syndrome in Mexico [letter], by G. J. Ruiz-Argüelles, et al. REVISTA DE INVESTIGACION CLINICA 35(4):265-266, October-December 1983.

Acquired immunodeficiency syndrome in New York City: evaluation of an active surveillance system, by M. E. Chamberland, et al. JAMA 254:383-387, July 19, 1985.

Acquired immunodeficiency syndrome in older children, by P. Baudoux, et al. PEDIATRIE 40(3):213-218, April-May 1985.

Acquired immunodeficiency syndrome in a patient with hemophilia, by K. C. Davis, et al. ANNALS OF INTERNAL MEDICINE 98(3):284-286, March 1983.

Acquired immunodeficiency syndrome in a patient with multiple risk factors, by S. B. Kalish, et al. ARCHIVES OF INTERNAL MEDICINE 143(12):2310-2311, December 1983.

Acquired immunodeficiency syndrome in a patient with no known risk factors: a pathological study, by A. D. Burt, et al. JOURNAL OF CLINICAL PATHOLOGY 37(4): 471-474, April 1984.

Acquired immunodeficiency syndrome in patients with hemophilia, by B. L. Evatt, et al. ANNALS OF INTERNAL MEDICINE 100(4):499-504, April 1984.

Acquired immunodeficiency syndrome in persons with hemophilia, by P. H. Levine. ANNALS OF INTERNAL MEDICINE 103(5):723-726, November 1985.

Acquired immunodeficiency syndrome in the prodromal phase in a drug addict [letter], by F. Cardellach, et al. MEDICINA CLINICA 81(14):645-646, November 5, 1983.

Acquired immunodeficiency syndrome in Rwanda, by P. Van de Pere, et al. LANCET 2(8394):62-65, July 14, 1984.

Acquired immunodeficiency syndrome in Saudi Arabia. The American-Saudi connection, by H. A. Harfi, et al. JAMA 255:383-384, January 17, 1986.

Acquired immunodeficiency syndrome in a small community, by S. S. Lee, et al. IOWA MEDICINE 75(8):351-352, August 1985.

Acquired immunodeficiency syndrome in a thalassemic child, by R. Paul, et al. PEDIATRIC INFECTIOUS DISEASE 5(2):274-276, March-April 1986.

Acquired immunodeficiency syndrome in The Netherlands, by H. Bijkerk. NEDERLANDS TIJDSCHRIFT VOOR GENEESKUNDE 127(19):856, May 7, 1983.

Acquired immunodeficiency syndrome in The Netherlands and United States. NEDERLANDS TIJDSCHRIFT VOOR GENEESKUNDE 127(31):1414-1415, July 30, 1983.

Acquired immunodeficiency syndrome in the United States: an analysis of cases outside high-incidence groups, by M. E. Chamberland, et al. ANNALS OF INTERNAL MEDICINE 101(5):617-623, November 1984.

Acquired immunodeficiency syndrome in the United States: a selective review, by J. Layon, et al. CRITICAL CARE MEDICINE 14(9):819-827, September 1986.

Acquired immunodeficiency syndrome in the wife of a hemophiliac, by A. E. Pitchenik, et al. ANNALS OF INTERNAL MEDICINE 100(1):62-65, January 1984.

Acquired immunodeficiency syndrome: infection control guidelines for the G.I suite, by R. L. Messner. SGA JOURNAL 8(2):37-38, Fall 1985.

Acquired immunodeficiency syndrome is an opportunistic infection and Kaposi's sarcoma results from secondary immune stimulation, by J. A. Levy, et al. LANCET 2(8341):78-81, July , 1983.

Acquired immunodeficiency syndrome, Kaposi's disease and cerebral toxoplasmosis in a young man. Review of the literature apropos of a case, by M. Janier, et al. ANNALES DE DERMATOLOGIE ET DE VENEREOLOGIE 111(1):11-23, 1984.

Acquired immunodeficiency syndrome: legal issues in the department, by L. D. Moskowitz, et al. JEN 12(5):297-300, September-October 1986.

Acquired immunodeficiency syndrome manifested as disseminated cryptococcosis, by G. Pittard, et al. JOURNAL OF EMERGENCY MEDICINE 3(4):275-279, 1985.

Acquired immunodeficiency syndrome; neuroradiologic findings, by W. M. Kelly, et al. RADIOLOGY 149(2):485-491, November 1983.

Acquired immunodeficiency syndrome—a new virus infection? VOPROSY VIRUSOLOGII 28(4):124-126, July-August 1983.

Acquired immunodeficiency syndrome, opportunistic infections, and malignancies in male homosexuals. A hypothesis of etiologic factors in pathogenesis, by J. Sonnabend, et al. JAMA 249(17):2370-2374, May 6, 1983.

Acquired immunodeficiency syndrome: an overview, by R. L. Baker, et al. INDIANA MEDICINE 78(6):459-465, June 1985.

Acquired immunodeficiency syndrome: an overview for anesthesiologists, by E. R. Greene, Jr. ANESTHESIA AND ANALGESIA 65(10):1054-1058, October 1986.

Acquired immunodeficiency syndrome possibly arthropod-borne [letter], by M. J. Blaser. ANNALS OF INTERNAL MEDICINE 99(6):877, December 1983.

Acquired immunodeficiency syndrome: report of a case in Chile, by F. Figueroa, et al. REVISTA MEDICA DE CHILE 112(10):1057-1059, October 1984.

Acquired immunodeficiency syndrome: rules for pestilential contagion revisited, by L. L. Rosendorf, et al. AMERICAN JOURNAL OF INFECTION CONTROL 12(1):31-33, February 1984.

Acquired immunodeficiency syndrome: a San Francisco perspective, by J. M. Luce, et al. INTENSIVE CARE MEDICINE 11(4):172-173, 1985.

Acquired immunodeficiency syndrome: state of immunological dysfunction in focus [editorial], by M. L. Santaella. BOLETIN-ASOCIACION MEDICA DE PUERTO RICO 75(9):391-392, September 1983.

Acquired immunodeficiency syndrome: an ultrastructural study, by G. S. Sidhu, et al. HUMAN PATHOLOGY 16(4):377-386, April 1985.

Acquired immunodeficiency syndrome: an update, by M. W. Moon. JEN 12(5):291-296, September-October 1986.

Acquired immunodeficiency syndrome: an update, by W. A. Stein, et al. PHYSICIAN ASSISTANT 10(1):23-24+, January 1986.

Acquired immunodeficiency syndrome with Kaposi's sarcoma in Ireland, by F. N. O'Keeffe, et al. IRISH JOURNAL OF MEDICAL SCIENCE 152(9):353-356, September 1983.

Acquired immunodeficiency syndrome with Pneumocystis carinii pneumonia and Mycobacterium avium-intracellulare infection in a previously healthy patient with classic hemophilia. Clinical, immunologic, and virologic findings, by M. C. Poon, et al. ANNALS OF INTERNAL MEDICINE 98(3):287-290, March 1983.

Acquired immunodeficiency syndrome with progressive multifocal leukoencephalopathy and monoclonal B-cell proliferaion, by J. L. Ho, et al. ANNALS OF INTERNAL MEDICINE 100(5):693-696, May 1984.

Acquired immunodeficiency syndrome with severe gastrointestinal manifestation in Haiti, by R. Malebranche, et al. LANCET 2(8355):873-878, October 15, 1983.

Acquired immunologic deficiency syndrome. Recommendations of group of French physicians and hemophilia specialists. REVUE FRANCAISE DE TRANSFUSION ET IMMUNO-HAEMATOLOGIE 28(3):273-274, June 1985.

Acquired immunosuppression syndrome associated with severe anguilluliasis [letter], by G. Pialoux, et al. PRESSE MEDICALE 13(32):1960, September 22, 1984.

Acquired neutrophil dysfunction in male homosexuals with the acquired immunodeficiency syndrome [letter], by G. J. Ras, et al. SOUTH AFRICAN MEDICAL JOURNAL 65(22):873-874, June 2, 1984.

Acquired-cell immune deficiency syndrome, by J. F. Heidelman, et al. ORAL SURGERY 55(5):452-453, May 1983.

Acquired-immunodeficiency-like syndrome in two haemophiliacs, by M. V. Ragni, et al. LANCET 1(8318):213-214, January 29, 1983.

Act of God—AIDS—fear of death, by J. Rule. BODY POLITIC 95:39, July 1983.

Actinomycetales infection in the acquired immunodeficiency syndrome, by H. A. Holtz, et al. ANNALS OF INTERNAL MEDICINE 102(2):203-205, February 1985.

Activation of the AIDS retrovirus promoter by the cellular transcription factor, Sp1, by K. A. Jones, et al. SCIENCE 232:755-759, May 9, 1986.

Activation of monocyte-mediated tumoricidal activity in patients with acquired immunodeficiency syndrome, by E. S. Kleinerman, et al. JOURNAL OF CLINICAL ONCOLOGY 3(7):1005-1012, July 1985.

Activation of a novel KpnI transcript by downstream integration of a human T-lymphotropic virus type I provirus, by T. Okamoto, et al. JOURNAL OF BIOLOGICAL CHEMISTRY 261:4615-4619, April 5, 1986.

Activation of tissue macrophages from AIDS patients: in vitro response of AIDS alveolar macrophages to lymphokines and interferon-gamma, by H. W. Murray, et al. JOURNAL OF IMMUNOLOGY 135(4):2374-2377, October 1985.

Activist urges unified plan on AIDS test, by P. Freiberg. ADVOCATE 4(8):12, November 27, 1984.

Activists campaign to fight AIDS initiative, by P. Freiberg. ADVOCATE 456:14, September 30, 1986.

Activists charge PBS AIDS show "unethical", by B. M. Gelbert. GAY COMMUNITY NEWS 13(36):2, March 29, 1986.

Activists, FDA clash over HTLV-III test, by B. Nelson. GAY COMMUNITY NEWS 12(34):1, March 16, 1985.

Acts of humor, acts of courage, by M. Bronski. GAY COMMUNITY NEWS 12(49):10, June 29, 1985.

Acute AIDS retrovirus infection. Definition of a clinical illness associated with seroconversion, by D. A. Cooper, et al. LANCET 1(8428):537-540, March 9, 1985.

Acute Cryptosporidium enteritis without immunologic weakness [letter], by U. Laukamm-Josten, et al. DEUTSCHE MEDIZINISCHE WOCHENSCHRIFT 110(25):1014-1015, June 21, 1985.

Acute encephalopathy coincident with seroconversion for anti-HTLV-III, by C. A. Carne, et al. LANCET 2(8466):1206-1208, November 30, 1985.

Acute HTLV III infection [letter], by K. R. Romeril. NEW ZEALAND MEDICAL JOURNAL 98(779):401, May 22, 1985.

Acute illnesses associated with HTLV-III seroconversion [letter], by C. Farthing, et al. LANCET 1(8434):935-936, April 20, 1985.

Acute myelofibrosis and infection with the lymphadenopathy-associated virus/human T-lymphotropic virus type III [letter], by C. Darne, et al. ANNALS OF INTERNAL MEDICINE 104(1):130-131, January 1986.

Adaptation of lymphadenopathy associated virus (LAV) to replication in EBV-transformed B lymphoblastoid cell lines, by L. Montagnier, et al. SCIENCE 225:63-66, July 6, 1984.

Add coccidioidomycosis to AIDS. EMERGENCY MEDICINE 16(16):43+, September 30, 1984.

Additional findings on the acquired deficiency syndrome, particularly in children, by J. Holy. CASOPIS LEKARU CESKYCH 122(45):1402, November 11, 1982.

Additional recommendations to reduce sexual and drug abuse-related transmission of human T-lymphotropic virus type III/lymphadenopathy-associated virus. JAMA 255(14):1843-1844+, April 11, 1986; also in: MMWR 35(10):152-155, March 14, 1986.

Addressing the AIDS crisis, by D. Collum. SOJOURNERS 15(2):6, February 1986.

Addressing the AIDS threat [interview with C. E. Koop]. CHRISTIANITY TODAY 29(7):52, November 22, 1985.

Addressing an epidemic: pending federal legislation on AIDS, by M. A. Kadzielski. REVIEW OF THE FEDERATION OF AMERICAN HEALTH SYSTEMS 19(3):48-49, May-June 1986.

Adenosquamous carcinoma of the lung and the acquired immunodeficiency syndrome [letter], by L. E. Irwin, et al. ANNALS OF INTERNAL MEDICINE 100(1): 158, January 1984.

Adenovirus and acquired immunodeficiency syndrome/Kaposi sarcoma [letter], by D. Ingrand, et al. PRESSE MEDICALE 12(46):2949, December 17, 1983.

Adenovirus isolates from urine of patients with acquired immunodeficiency syndrome, by P. J. deJong, et al. LANCET 1(8337):1293-1296, June 11, 1983.

Adequate precautions and extreme care: AIDS from inside the hospital, by R. Dobbins. VILLAGE VOICE 30:30-31, July 30, 1985.

Administration asks additional 45 million: AIDS, by D. Walter. ADVOCATE 428:10, September 3, 1985.

Administration of 3'-azido-3'-deoxythymidine, an inhibitor of HTLV-III/LAV replication, to patients with AIDS or AIDS-related complex, by R. Yarchoan, et al. LANCET 1(8481):575-580, March 15, 1986.

Administrative perspectives on care of patients with AIDS . . . the nurse administrator on the unit level, by D. Calliari. TOPICS IN CLINICAL NURSING 6(2):72-75, July 1984.

Admitting AIDS patients, by L. Raffel. CONTEMPORARY LONGTERM CARE 8(12): 54, December 1985.

Adrenal insufficiency as a complication of the acquired immunodeficiency syndrome, by L. W. Greene, et al. ANNALS OF INTERNAL MEDICINE 101(4):497-498, Oc--tober 1984.

Adrenal necrosis in the acquired immunodeficiency syndrome, by M. L. Tapper, et al. ANNALS OF INTERNAL MEDICINE 100(2):239-241, February 1984.

Adrenocortical function in the acquired immunodeficiency syndrome [letter], by R. S. Klein, et al. ANNALS OF INTERNAL MEDICINE 99(4):566, October 1983.

Advance against AIDS, by A. Steacy. MACLEAN'S 99:36, June 16, 1986.

Advances in the isolation of HTLV-III from patients with AIDS and AIDS-related complex and from donors at risk, by P. D. Markham, et al. CANCER RESEARCH 45(Suppl. 9):4588s-4591s, September 1985.

Advances in research on AIDS, by C. H. Gu. CHUNG-HUA NEI KO TSA CHIH 24(10): 627-629, October 1985.

Adverse effects of interferon in virus infections, autoimmune diseases, and acquired immunodeficiency, by J. Vilcek. PROGRESS IN MEDICAL VIROLOGY 30:62-77, 1984.

Adverse reactions associated wih pyrimethamine-sulfadoxine prophylaxis for Pneumocystis carinii infections in AIDS [letter], by T. R. Navin, et al. LANCET 1(8441): 1332, June 8, 1985.

Adverse reactions to pyrimethamine-sulfadoxine in context of AIDS [letter], by M. S. Gottlieb, et al. LANCET 1(8442):1389, June 15, 1985.

Adverse reactions to trimethoprim-sulfamethoxazole in patients with the acquired immunodeficiency syndrome, by F. M. Gordin, et al. ANNALS OF INTERNAL MEDICINE 100(4):495-499, April 1984.

Advocates for better health care, by P. Freiberg. ADVOCATE 3(72):13, July 21, 1983.

Aetiology of AIDS—antibodies to human T-cell leukaemia virus (type III) in haemophiliacs, by L. W. Kitchen, et al. NATURE 312(5992):367-369, November 22-28, 1984.

AF gearing up for AIDS testing in March, by L. Famiglietti. AIR FORCE TIMES 46:7, November 25, 1985.

AF to begin use of AIDS drug when approved. AIR FORCE TIMES 47:6, October 6, 1986.

AFL/CIO supports gay rights—AIDS. GUARDIAN 36(4):4, October 26, 1983.

AFRAIDS. THE NEW REPUBLIC 193:7-8+, Octoebr 14, 1985.

Africa and the origin of AIDS [news], by C. Norman. SCIENCE 230(4730):1141, December 6, 1985.

Africa's latest torment: AIDS. U.S. NEWS & WORLD REPORT 99:8, December 23, 1985.

African AIDS points to heterosexual link, by O. Sattaur. NEW SCIENTIST 106:10-11, April 25, 1985.

African 'eosinophilic bodies' in vivo in two American men with Kaposi's sarcoma and AIDS, by A. . Cantwell, Jr., et al. JOURNAL OF DERMATOLOGIC SURGERY AND ONCOLOGY 11(4):408-412, April 1985.

African form of the acquired immunodeficiency syndrome. Epidemiological reflections [letter], by D. Vittecoq, et al. PRESSE MEDICALE 13(42):2584, November 24, 1984.

African Kaposi's sarcoma and AIDS, by R. G. Downing, et al. LANCET 1(8375):478-480, March 3, 1984.

African swine fever and AIDS [letter], by C. V. Martins, et al. LANCET 1(8496):1504-1505, June 28, 1986.

African swine fever virus and AIDS [letter], by J. Beldekas, et al. LANCET 1(8480): 564-565, March 8, 1986.

African swine fever virus antibody not found in AIDS patients [letter], by J. Colaert, et al. LANCET 1(83333):1098, May 14, 1983.

After AIDS: a walk on the mild side, by N. Meredith. PSYCHOLOGY TODAY 18:60-61, January 1984.

After Amerika, AIDS, by A. Cockburn. IN THESE TIMES 10(31):17, August 6, 1986.

Aftercare instruction: AIDS brochure, by M. M. Hughes. JEN 9(6):340-342, November-December 1983.

Age of AIDS: a great time for defensive living (editorial], by G. D. Lundberg. JAMA 253(23):3440-3441, June 21, 1985.

Agglutination test for diagnosis of toxoplasmosis in AIDS [letter], by R. E. McCabe, et al. LANCET 2(8351)680, September 17, 1983.

AHA says feat of AIDS goes too far. RN 47:13, March 1984.

Aid to A.I.D.S. [editorial], by B. W. Otridge. IRISH MEDICAL JOURNAL 76(9):373-374, September 1983.

Aiding AIDS sufferers, by D. Miller. NEW ZEALAND NURSING JOURNAL 79(9):34, September 1986.

AIDophobia [letter], by E. Freed. MEDICAL JOURNAL OF AUSTRALIA 2(10):479, November 12, 1983.

AIDS [editorial]. AMERICAN FAMILY PHYSICIAN 28(1):111, July 1983.

—. LANCET 2(8497):51, July 5, 1986.

— [letter]. MEDICAL JOURNAL OF AUSTRALIA 2(12):601-602, December 10-24, 1983.

— [letter]. NATURE 319(6056):716, February 27-March 5, 1986.

— [special section]. NEWSWEEK 106:20-24+, August 12, 1985.

—. RIVISTA DELL INFERMIERE 3(1):51-53, March 1984.

—. SCIENCE NEWS 127:328, May 25, 1985.

—, by A. Rosser. POLICE JOURNAL 49(3):258-262, 1986.

—, by B. Dixon. WORLD HEALTH August 1983, p. 10-13.

—, by B. Hanczyk. PROFESSIONAL MEDICAL ASSISTANT 17(4):14-15, July-August 1984.

—, by B. Ott. AMERICAN LIBRARIES 16:681, November 1985.

—, by B. Ridgway. LAMP 42(2):7-9, March 1985.

—, by B. Stoller. JOURNAL OF PRACTICAL NURSING 35(4):26-31, December 1985.

—, by C. Dunphy. WASHINGTON NURSE 14(6):9, September 1984.

— [special section], by J. Langone. DISCOVER 6:28-33+, December 1985.

—[letter], by J. P. Krajeski. NORTH CAROLINA MEDICAL JOURNAL 44(8):525, August 1983.

—, by M. F. Silverman. EMERGENCY: JOURNAL OF EMERGENCY SERVICES 18(5):44-46, May 1986.

—, by M. Morichau-Beauchant. GASTROENTEROLOGIE CLINIQUE ET BIOLO-GIQUE 9(4):323-326, April 1985.

—, by R. A. Kiel. CORRECTIONS TODAY 48:68-70, February 1986.

—, by R. Augusta. JOURNAL OF PRACTICAL NURSING 33(8):48-51, September-October 1983.

—, by R. Wells, et al. INTERNATIONAL NURSING REVIEW 32(3):76-79, May-June 1985.

—, by T. Lizuka. KANGO 35(11):92-93, October 1983.

—, by W. F. Batchelor. AMERICAN PSYCHOLOGIST 39(11):1277-1278, November 1984.

AIDS: academy looks for strategy, by J. Palca. NATURE 319:441, February 6, 1986.

AIDS: acquired immune deficiency syndrome, by A. Ramirez. NEW ZEALAND NURSING JOURNAL 78(7):July 1985.

—, by J. A. Johson. CONGRESSIONAL RESEARCH SERVICE REVIEW 4(10):19-21, November 1983.

—, by J. Cohen. IMPRINT 31(4):50, November 1984.

—, by P. A. Miles. JEN 9(5):254-258, September-October 1983.

—. Epidemic or Hysteria? by S. Gesenhues. ZFA 59(33):1865-1869, November 30, 1983.

AIDS: acquired immunodeficiency syndrome. FLASH-INFORMATIONS 3:6-8, May-June 1985.

—, by G. Altay. MIKROBIYOLOJI BULTENI 19(4):238-251, October 1985.

—, by J. P. Soulier. REVUE FRANCAISE DE TRANSFUSION ET IMMUNO-HEMATOLOGIE 26(5):437-445, November 1983.

—, by K. O. Habermehl. INTERNIST 26(2):113-120, February 1985.

—, by M. Spoljar, et al. LIJECNICKI VJESNIK 106(1):21-24, January 1984.

—, by N. J. Gilmore, et al. CANADIAN MEDICAL ASSOCIATION JOURNAL 128(11):1281-1284, June 1, 1983.

—, by R. Piffer. RIVISTA DELL INFERMIERE 4(4):207-217, December 1985.

—, by W. Dowdle. SERVIR 34(3):151-157, May-June 1986.

AIDS, acquired immunodeficiency syndrome and its possible link to human T-cell leukemia-lymphoma virus, the retrovirus inducer of T-cell leukemia in the adult, by C. Dosne Pasqualini, et al. MEDICINA 43(4):472-474, 1983.

AIDS—acquired immunodeficiency syndrome, its importance for the dentist, by B. Maeglin. SCHWEIZERISCHE MONATSSCHRIFT FUR ZAHNMEDIZIN 95(8):697-699, August 1985.

AIDS: act now, don't pay later [editorial]. BRITISH MEDICAL JOURNAL 293(6543):348, August 9, 1986.

AIDS action line. BOSTON MAGAZINE 77:33, December 1985.

AIDS action: a policy of gestures. BODY POLITIC 96:21, September 1983.

AIDS activism against all odds, by S. Ault. GUARDIAN 38(26):10, April 2, 1986.

AIDS activist gets state job, by C. Guilfoy. GAY COMMUNITY NEWS 13(3):3, July 27, 1985.

31

AIDS activists—confidentiality issue, by C. Guilfoy. GAY COMMUNITY NEWS 12(5):1, August 11, 1984.

AIDS activists demand legislative action, by S. Connor. GAY COMMUNITY NEWS13(17):1, November 9, 1985.

AIDS: administrators fear the fear itself, by E. LeBourdais. HEALTH CARE 28(3):14-16, April 1986.

AIDS: African connection [editorial], by I. Braveny. EUROPEAN JOURNAL OF CLINICAL MICROBIOLOGY 2(6):521-522, December 1983.

AIDS: the African connection [letter], by P. Jenkins, et al. BRITISH MEDICAL JOURNAL 290(6477):1284-1285, April 27, 1985.

—, by P. Jones. BRITISH MEDICAL JOURNAL 291(6489):216, July 20, 1985.

AIDS—an African disease?, by K. M. De Cock. ADVANCES IN EXPERIMENTAL MEDICINE AND BIOLOGY 187:1-12, 1985.

AIDS' African genesis argued at symposium, by M. Helquist. ADVOCATE 437:20, January 7, 1986.

AIDS after coronary bypass surgery [letter], by G. Delpre, et al. LANCET 1(8368): 103, January 14, 1984.

AIDS aid, by S. Moorsom. NEW SOCIETY August 8, 1986, p. 12-13.

AIDS alarm, by F. Orr. ALBERTA REPORT 12:35, May 20, 1985.

AIDS alert. CORRECTIONS DIGEST 17(4):3, February 12, 1986.

AIDS alert [letter], by S. Ashman, et al. JOURNAL OF THE AMERICAN DENTAL ASSOCIATION 111(5):712, November 1985.

AIDS: allocating resources for research and patient care, by P. R. Lee. ISSUES IN SCIENCE AND TECHNOLOGY 2:66-73, Winter 1986.

AIDS also poses legal and political problems, by Phyllis Schlafly. HUMAN EVENTS 43:18, September 10, 1983.

AIDS amendment angers cancer institute [news] by B. J. Culiton. SCIENCE 226(4678):1056, November 30, 1984.

AIDS: the American nightmare, by D. Thompson. TIMES August 12, 1985, p. 8.

AIDS and the accident and emergency department [letter], by W. G. Tennant, et al. ARCHIVES OF EMERGENCY MEDICINE 2(1):47-49, March 1985.

AIDS and accuracy: Is TV testing positive?, by Jim Fiske. EMMY 8:38+, May-June 1986.

AIDS and African swine fever [letter], by E. Arnoux, et al. LANCET 2(8341):110, July 9, 1983.

—, by R. K. St John. LANCET 1(8337):1335, June 11, 1983.

AIDS and AIDS-related conditions: screening for populations at risk, by G. S. Carr, et al. NURSE PRACTITIONER 11(10):25-26+, October 1986.

AIDS and AIDS-related diseases—clinical manifestations and therapy, by A. Sönnerborg, et al. LAKARTIDNINGEN 82(20):1877-1880, May 15, 1985.

AIDS and the AIDS virus (HIV): facts and implications for magistrates, by A. J. Pinching. MAGISTRATE 42(12):192-198, 1986.

AIDS and all of us, by J. Zeh. GUARDIAN 38(31):20, May 7, 1986.

AIDS and the anaesthetist, by A. s. Cordero, et al. CANADIAN ANAESTHETISTS SOCIETY JOURNAL 32(1):45-48, January 1985.

AIDS and ARC: a theological reflection on the Church's ministry, by J. Hanvey. MONTH 19:326-331, December 1986.

AIDS and artificial insemination by donor [editorial], by a. Galvao-Teles. ACTA MEDICA PORTUGUESA 7(1):3-4, January-February 1986.

AIDS and associated syndromes: clinical manifestations, by C. Mayaud, et al. REVUE FRANCAISE DE TRANSFUSION ET IMMUNOHEMATOLOGIE 27(4):411-421, September 1984.

AIDS and the baths, by Freiberg, et al. ADVOCATE 3(75):20, September 1, 1983.

AIDS and the blood, by L. Goldsmith. GAY COMMUNITY NEWS 10(27):3, January 29, 1983.

AIDS and the blood bank, by H. F. Polesky. CLINICAL ENGINEERING INFORMATION SERVICE 7(5):152-153, September-October 1983.

AIDS and the blood bankers, by R. D. Eckert. REGULATION 10:15-24+, September-October 1986.

AIDS and blood donors [editorial], by A. I. Adams. MEDICAL JOURNAL OF AUSTRALIA 141(9):558, October 27, 1984.

AIDS and blood donors in Brazil [letter], by S. N. Wendel, et al. LANCET 2(8453): 506, August 31, 1985.

AIDS and blood products, by G. F. Rolland. BULLETIN DE LA SOCIETE DES SCIENCES MEDICALES DU GRAND-DUCHE DE LUXEMBOURG 121(2):7-12, 1984.

AIDS and the blood supply. KANSAS MEDICINE 87(3):76, March 1986.

AIDS and the blood supply, by R. D. Eckert. CONSUMERS' RESEARCH MAGAZINE 68:20-25, October 1985.

AIDS and blood transfusion in New Zealand [letter], by S. G. Whyte, et al. NEW ZEALAND MEDICAL JOURNAL 97(770):905, December 26, 1984.

AIDS and blood transfusions. NORTH CAROLINA MEDICAL JOURNAL 45(2):109-110, February 1984.

AIDS and the caregiver, by J. Lieberman. CALIFORNIA NURSE 82(4):3, May 1986.

AIDS and the church, by E. E. Shelp, et al. CHRISTIAN CENTURY 102(27):797-800, September 11-18,1985.

AIDS and the churches: belated, growing response, by B. J. Stiles. CHRISTIANITY AND CRISIS 45(22):534-536, January 13, 1986.

AIDS and civil rights, by A. Press, et al. NEWSWEEK 106(21):86+, November 18, 1985.

AIDS and clinical ethics: honoring patients' dignity, by D. J. Roy, et al. DIMENSIONS IN HEALTH SERVICE 63(7):32-33, October 1986.

AIDS and the common cup, by F. C. Senn. DIALOG 25(1):4-5, Winter 1986.

AIDS and communion. CHRISTIAN CENTURY 102:888, October 9, 1985.

AIDS and community health issues, by S. Cowell. JOURNAL OF AMERICAN COLLEGE HEALTH 33(6):253-258, June 1985.

AIDS and community supportive services. Understanding and management of psychological needs, by T. Goulden, et al. MEDICAL JOURNAL OF AUSTRALIA 141(9):582-586, October 27, 1984.

AIDS and confidentiality [letter], by W. H. Foege. NATURE 306(5938):10, November 3-9, 1983.

AIDS and the control of cell growth, by O. Sattaur. NEW SCIENTIST 102:20, May 10, 1984.

AIDS and the current significance of serological studies for the presence of antibodies against LAV/HTLV III, by W. J. van Gestel. NEDERLANDS TIJDSCHRIFT VOOR GENEESKUNDE 129(5):233-234, February 2, 1985.

AIDS and cryptococcosis (Zaire, 1977) [letter], by J. Vandepitte, et al. LANCET 1(8330):925-926, April 23, 1983.

AIDS and dentists in Australia [news], by C. H. Wall. BRITISH DENTAL JOURNAL 158(10):380, May 25, 1985.

AIDS and the disabiliy rights movement, by M. Owen. DISABILITY 7(2):14, March 1986.

AIDS and drug use. An overview of the epidemiology, virus, symptoms, and the relationship with intravenous drug use, by J. H. Moerkerk, et al. TIJDSCHRIFT VOOR ALCOHOL, DRUGS EN ANDERE PSYCHOTROPE STOFFEN 11(1):41+, 1985.

AIDS and ecology/wellfounded fears, by R. Summerbell. BODY POLITIC 94:6, June 1983.

AIDS and the electromyographer, by D. B. Karam. ARCHIVES OF PHYSICAL MEDICINE AND REHABILITATION 67(7):491, July 1986.

AIDS and employment issues, by C. A. Klein. NURSE PRACTITIONER 11(5):87-88+, May 1986.

AIDS and ethics, by A. R. Jonsen, et al. ISSUES IN SCIENCE AND TECHNOLOGY 2:56-65, Winter 1986.

AIDS and the executive directo. Perspectives in crisis management, by A. P. Brownstein. SCANDINAVIAN JOURNAL OF HAEMATOLOGY. SUPPLEMENTUM 40: 561-565, 1984.

AIDS and fungal infections, by K. Holmberg, et al. LAKARTIDNINGEN 83(19):1753-1759, May 7, 1986.

AIDS and gastroenterology, by A. Gelb, et al. AMERICAN JOURNAL OF GASTRO-
ENTEROLOGY 81(8):619-622, August 1986.

AIDS and the gay community: between the specter and the promise of medicine, by
R. Bayer. SOCIAL RESEARCH 52:581-606, Fall 1985.

AIDS and the gay community: the doctor's role in counseling [editorial], by G. Leach,
et al. BRITISH MEDICAL JOURNAL 290(6468):583, February 23, 1985.

AIDS and the gay man [letter], by N. R. Schram. NEW ENGLAND JOURNAL OF MED-
ICINE 310(19):1266-1267, May 10, 1984.

AIDS and gay rights collide in closings, by Helquist, et al. IN THESE TIMES 8(41):1,
October 31, 1984.

AIDS and the general population, by M. F. Silverman. FRONTIERS OF RADIATION
THERAPY AND ONCOLOGY 19:168-171, 1985.

AIDS and the gut, by I. V. Weller. SCANDINAVIAN JOURNAL OF GASTROENTER-
OLOGY 114:77-89, 1985.

AIDS and haemophilia, by A. L. Bloom. BIOMEDICINE AND PHARMACOTHERAPY
39(7):355-365, 1985.

AIDS and haemophilia: morbidity and morality in a well defined population, by P.
Jones, et al. BRITISH MEDICAL JOURNAL 291(6497):695-699, September 14,
1985.

AIDS and health care in the laboratory, by N. Gilmore. CANADIAN JOURNAL OF
MEDICAL TECHNOLOGY 47(4):267-268, December 1985.

AIDS and health education, by N. Freudenberg. HEALTH PAC BULLETIN 16(4):29,
July 1985.

AIDS and the health professions [editorial]. BRITISH MEDICAL JOURNAL 290
(6468):583-584, February 23, 1985.

—[letter]. BRITISH MEDICAL JOURNAL 290(6471):852-854, March 16, 1985.

AIDS and heat, by G. Weissmann. HOSPITAL PRACTICE 18(10):136-137+, October
1983.

AIDS and hemophilia [letter], by R. J. Ablin, et al. AUSTRALIAN AND NEW ZEALAND
JOURNAL OF MEDICINE 15(2):265-267, April 1985.

AIDS and hepatitis B [letter], by K. S. Froebel, et al. LANCET 1(8377):632, March 17,
1984.

AIDS and hepatitis B cannot be venereal diseases [letter], by J. R. Seale. CANADIAN
MEDICAL ASSOCIATION JOURNAL 130(9):1109-1110, May 1, 1984.

AIDS and herpes carry weighty policy implications for your Board, by K. McCormick.
AMERICAN SCHOOL BOARD JOURNAL 172(10):37-38, October 1985.

AIDS and Hodgkin's disease, by S. L. Schoeppel, et al. FRONTIERS OF RADIATION
THERAPY AND ONCOLOGY 19:66-73, 1985.

AIDS and the home health care industry—Part II, by D. Borfitz. HOME HEALTH
JOURNAL 4(12):27, December 1983.

AIDS and homologous blood transfusion [letter], by S. Flecknoe-Brown. MEDICAL JOURNAL OF AUSTRALIA 143(2):89, July 22, 1985.

AIDS and homosexual panic [letter], by M. Rapaport, et al. AMERICAN JOURNAL OF PSYCHIATRY 142(12):1516, December 1985.

AIDS and the hospital employer, by K. B. Stickler. HEALTH LAW VIGIL 8(26):1-4, December 27, 1985.

AIDS and hospital workers [letter], by M. B. McEvoy, et al. LANCET 1(8388):1245, June 2, 1984.

AIDS and HTLV-III in West Germany: the status February 1985, by R. Hehlmann, et al. KLINISCHE WOCHENSCHRIFT 63(9):385-388, May 2, 1985.

AIDS and HTLV-III infection, by H. M. Glenister. NURSING 3(6):229-231, June 1986.

AIDS and the human services. Agencies face a whole range of problems, by J. J. O'Hara, et al. PUBLIC WELFARE 44(3):7-13, Summer 1986.

AIDS and human T-cell leukemia/lymphoma virus III in Denmark, by G. Lange Wantzin. UGESKRIFT FOR LAEGER 147(5):389-391, January 28, 1985.

AIDS and hysterria a problem of health education, by N. J. Flumara. HEALTH VALUES 7(6):3, November-December 1983.

AIDS and immunologic abnormalities in European and American hemophiliacs, by D. Green. SCANDINAVIAN JOURNAL OF HAEMATOLOGY. SUPPLEMENTUM 40:367-369, 1984.

AIDS and the importance of donated blood, by L. K. Altman. THE NEW YORK TIMES MAGAZINE November 18, 1984, p. 136-137+.

AIDS and infection control, by S. R. Perdew. CARING 5(6):22-26, June 1986.

AIDS and its association with human tumors and viruses. A viral and/or immunogenetic cause?, by G. Mathé. BIOMEDICINE AND PHARMACOTHERAPY 37(4):153-159, 1983.

AIDS and its early-stage clinical signs, by S. L. Valle, et al. DUODECIM 102(7):405-412, 1986.

AIDS and its relation to a virus infection, by H. Bauer. DEUTSCHE MEDIZINISCHE WOCHENSCHRIFT 110(12):443-444, March 22, 1985.

AIDS and its significance to dentistry, by J. Hardie. CANADIAN DENTAL ASSOCIATION JOURNAL 49(8):565-569, August 1983.

AIDS and Kaposi's sarcoma, by M. A. Conant. CURRENT PROBLEMS IN DERMATOLOGY 13:92-108, 1985.

AIDS and the lab: infection control guidelines, by W. M. Valenti. MLO 18(2):53-56, February 1986.

AIDS and the laboratory worker [editorial], by A. Kellner. AMERICAN JOURNAL OF MEDICAL TECHNOLOGY 49(5):290, May 1983.

AIDS and lymphadenopathy [editorial], by M. J. Godley. BRITISH JOURNAL OF SURGERY 73(3):170-171, March 1986.

AIDS and Medicaid. The role of Medicaid in treating those with AIDS, by J. Luehrs, et al. PUBLIC WELFARE 44(3):20-28, Summer 1986.

AIDS and the mind, by N. Fain. ADVOCATE 3(79):22, October 27, 1983.

AIDS and moral issues, by T. Johson. ADVOCATE 3(79):24, October 27, 1983.

AIDS and the mythmakers, by B. Kochis. PROGRESSIVE 50(9):16, September 1986.

AIDS and the needle. NEW SCIENTIST 112:15, October 2, 1986.

AIDS and a new gay generation, by D. Sadownick. ADVOCATE 432:8, October 29, 1985.

AIDS and the new morality, by M. Godwin. GAY COMMUNITY NEWS 11(5):6, August 13, 1983.

AIDS and the nurse. Part 1, by H. Goble, et al. AUSTRALIAN NURSES JOURNAL 15(7):37-41+, February 1986.

—. Part 2, by P. Kerr, et al. AUSTRALIAN NURSES JOURNAL 15(7):42+, February 1986.

—. Part 3, by M. Fine. AUSTRALIAN NURSES JOURNAL 15(7):43-44, February 1986.

AIDS and oncogenesis, by J. L. Ziegler. FRONTIERS OF RADIATION THERAPY AND ONCOLOGY 19:99-104, 1985.

AIDS and organ transplantation [letter], by R. R. Bailey, et al. NEW ZEALAND MEDICAL JOURNAL 98(779):402-403, May 22, 1985.

AIDS and the paid donor [letter], by D. J. Gury. LANCET 2(8349):575, September 3, 1983.

AIDS and parasitic infections, including Pneumocystis carinii and cryptosporidiosis, by C. D. Berkowitz. PEDIATRIC CLINICS OF NORTH AMERICA 32(4):933-952, August 1985.

AIDS and parasitism [letter], by R. B. Pearce, et al. LANCET 1(8391):1411, June 23, 1984.

AIDS and the physician, by C. P. Erwin. WISCONSIN MEDICAL JOURNAL 82(10):5, October 1983.

AIDS and the physician's fear of contagion, by E. H. Loewy. CHEST 89(3):325-326, March 1986.

AIDS and a plague mentality, by R. Fisher. NEW SOCIETY 71(1157):322-325, February 28, 1985.

AIDS and the police: a loaded gun?, by P. M. Wright. LAW AND ORDER 34(1):38, January 1986.

AIDS and politics, by J. Foster. CALIFORNIA NURSE 82(4):9, May 1986.

AIDS and politics of despair, by M. Pally. ADVOCATE 436:8, December 24, 1985.

AIDS and preventive treatment in hemophilia [editorial], by J. F. Desforges. NEW ENGLAND JOURNAL OF MEDICINE 308(2):94-95, January 13, 1983.

AIDS and the professional ethic, by C. Healy. AUSTRALIAN NURSES JOURNAL 14(7):10, February 1985.

AIDS and promiscuity, by R. Royal. GAY COMMUNITY NEWS 11(5):6, August 13, 1983.

AIDS and prostitutes [letter], by D. A. Cooper, et al. MEDICAL JOURNAL OF AUS-TRALIA 145(1):55, July 7, 1986.

AIDS and public policy. NATIONAL REVIEW 35:796, July 8, 1983.

AIDS and related conditions. One year's experience in St. Vincent's Hospital, Syd-ney, by A. B. Hill, et al. MEDICAL JOURNAL OF AUSTRALIA 141(9):573-578, October 27, 1984.

AIDS and related conditions—infection control. Guidelines for health care workers in-volved in patient management and investigation, by R. Sher. SOUTH AFRICAN MEDICAL JOURNAL 68(12):843-848, December 7, 1985.

AIDS and the reluctant surgeon, by H. A. Dudley. MEDICAL JOURNAL OF AUS-TRALIA 142(12):651-652, June 10, 1985.

AIDS and the right to know, by J. Alter, et al. NEWSWEEK 108(7):46-47, August 18, 1986.

AIDS and the rights of the well, by B. Amiel. MACLEAN'S 98:11, September 30, 1985.

AIDS and the safety and adequacy of the Canadian blood supply [editorial], by J. B. Derrick. CANADIAN ANAESTHETISTS SOCIETY JOURNAL 33(2):117-122, March 1986.

AIDS and SCBA: a threat to the fire service?, by W. D. Kipp. FIRE COMMAND 53:17, January 1986.

AIDS and sexual behavior reported by gay men in San Francisco, by L. McKusick, et al. AMERICAN JOURNAL OF PUBLIC HEALTH 75(5):493-496, May 1985.

AIDS and 'slow viruses,' by R. W. Smith. ANNALS OF THE NEW YORK ACADEMY OF SCIENCES 437:576-607, 1984.

AIDS and social change, by D. A. Feldman. HUMAN ORGANIZATION 44:343-348, Winter 1985.

AIDS and the spectrum of HTLV-III/LAV infection, by A. J. Pinching, et al. INTERNA-TIONAL REVIEW OF EXPERIMENTAL PATHOLOGY 28:1-44, 1986.

AIDS (and STD) prophylaxis: urgent need for an effective genital antiseptic [letter], by A. Comfort. JOURNAL OF THE ROYAL SOCIETY OF MEDICINE 79(5):311-312, May 1986.

AIDS and the substance abuse treatment clinician [editorial], by J. Imhof, et al. JOUR-NAL OF SUBSTANCE ABUSE AND TREATMENT 2(3):137, 1985.

AIDS and succour, by N. Dickson. NURSING TIMES 80(41):18-19, October 9-15, 1985.

AIDS and sudden death [letter], by C. H. Sherlock, et al. CANADIAN MEDICAL ASSOCIATION JOURNAL 129(10):1079, November 15, 1983.

AIDS and surgery [editorial], by J. Ludbrook. AUSTRALIA AND NEW ZEALAND JOURNAL OF SURGERY 56(2):97-98, February 1986.

— [letter], by E. Owen. MEDICAL JOURNAL OF AUSTRALIA 142(2):164, January 21, 1985.

AIDS and taurolin [letter], by P. Bayardelle. CANADIAN MEDICAL ASSOCIATION JOURNAL 134(5):476, March 1, 1986.

AIDS and the threat to public health, by M. F. Silverman, et al. HASTINGS CENTER REPORT 15(Suppl. 19-22), August 1985.

AIDS and the treatment of hemophilia. MICHIGAN MEDICINE 84(1):62-63, January 1985.

AIDS and us, by E. Ropes. GAY COMMUNITY NEWS 10(47):5, June 18, 1983.

AIDS and the use of blood components and derivatives: the Canadian perspective [editorial], by J. B. Derrick. CANADIAN MEDICAL ASSOCIATION JOURNAL 131(1):20-22 July 1, 1984.

AIDS and women, by E. Cameron. CHATELAINE 59:56+, February 1986.

AIDS and zinc deficiency [letter], by R. G. Weiner. JAMA 252(11):1409-1410, September 21, 1984.

AIDS animal model. AMERICAN FAMILY PHYSICIAN 27:247, May 1983.

AIDS announcement raises questions, by J. Silberner. SCIENCE NEWS 128:293, November 9, 1985.

AIDS antibody in two health care workers. AMERICAN JOURNAL OF NURSING 85:1224-1225, November 1985.

AIDS antibody screening test: controversy surrounds a new ELISA assay designed to prevent the spread of AIDS through blood transfusions. ANALYTICAL CHEMISTRY 57:773A-4A+, June 1985.

AIDS: the antibody test, by S. Anderson. PROFESSIONAL MEDICAL ASSISTANT 19(2):22-25, March-April 1986.

AIDS antibody testing and counseling [letter], by G. H. Hall. BRITISH MEDICAL JOURNAL 29(6506):1424, November 16, 1985.

AIDS antibody tests effectively screen blood supply. AMERICAN FAMILY PHYSICIAN 32:274-275, October 1985.

AIDS anxiety. TIME 124:59, December 24, 1984.

—, by M. Daly. NEW YORK 16:24-29, June 20, 1983.

AIDS: are laboratorians at risk? MLO 17(4):9, April 1985.

AIDS, arms control, and the future, by A. Hammond. ISSUES IN SCIENCE AND TECHNOLOGY 2:2, Winter 1986.

AIDS as crisis and opportunity, by K. L. Vaux. CHRISTIAN CENTURY 102:910-911, October 16, 1985.

AIDS as a handicapping condition. MENTAL DISABILITY LAW REPORTER 9(6):402-406, November-December 1985.

AIDS as metaphor, by B. Teixiea. BODY POLITIC 96:40, September 1983.

AIDS as a sexually transmissible disease, by B. Donovan, et al. AUSTRALIAN FAMILY PHYSICIAN 15(5):620-633, May 1986.

AIDS—aspects of infection control part 2, by E. A. Jenner. MIDWIFE, HEALTH VISITOR AND COMMUNITY NURSE 22(6):181-182+, June 1986.

AIDS, associated disorders pose complex therapeutic challenges [news], by H. Cole. JAMA 252(15):1987-1988, October 19, 1984.

AIDS associated Kaposi's sarcoma in Afric [letter], by K. H. Marquart. BRITISH MEDICAL JOURNAL 292(6518):484, February 15, 1986.

AIDS-associated retroviruses (ARV) can productively infect other cells besides human T helper cells, by J. A. Levy, et al. VIROLOGY 147:442-448, December 1985.

AIDS-associated syndrome. Conference summation, by R. A. Good. ADVANCES IN EXPERIMENTAL MEDICINE AND BIOLOGY 187:163-172, 1985.

AIDS-associated syndromes. Proceedings of the International Conference on AIDS-Associated Syndromes. December 8-9, 1984, Irvine, California. ADVANCES IN EXPERIMENTAL MEDICINE AND BIOLOGY 187:1-181, 1985.

AIDS-associated ultrastructural changes [letter], by Z. Schaff, et al. LANCET 1(8337):1336, June 11, 1983.

AIDS-associated virus yields data to intensifying scientific study, by C. Marwick. JAMA 254:2865-2868+, November 22-29, 1985.

AIDS, athletes, and fears about contact, by M. M. Gauthier. PHYSICIAN SPORTS-MEDICINE 14:41, January 1986.

AIDS: attacking the problem, by D. Steele. SOLDIERS 41(1):6-11, January 1986.

AIDS autopsy precautions, by A. E. Mass. PATHOLOGIST 39(11):20-21, November 1985.

AIDS awareness in the emergency department, by N. M. Holloway. CRITICAL CARE NURSE 6(2):90-93, March-April 1986.

AIDS awareness month, by D. Morris. GAY COMMUNITY NEWS 10(27):2, January 29, 1983.

AIDS babies: walls around children?, by L. Gentry. HUMAN DEVELOPMENT NEWS Fall 1985, p. 11-12.

AIDS baby in Miami, Fla. finally gets foster home. JET 65:5, January 16, 1984.

AIDS: bad news, good news. NATURE 311:206, September 20, 1984. GENERAL

AIDS: a balance of sorrows, by L. L. Curtin. NURSING MANAGEMENT 17(3):7-8, March 1986.

AIDS: be informed. WORLD HEALTH November 1985, p. 6.

AIDS becoming an issue in pre-employment screening, other ways. SECURITY LETTER 16(16):1, August 15, 1986.

AIDS behind anti-gay scare campaign, by F. Feldman. MILITANT 47(25):6, July 8, 1983.

AIDS behind bars: lies and manipulation, by T. Schrieber. GAY COMMUNITY NEWS 13(35):3, March 22, 1986.

AIDS beyond the hospital. 1. A home care plan for AIDS, by H. Schietinger. AMERI-CAN JOURNAL OF NURSING 86(9):1021-1028, September 1986.

—. 1. What we know about AIDS, by J. A. Bennett. AMERICAN JOURNAL OF NURSING 86(9):1015-1021, September 1986.

AIDS bias ruling spurs debate, by D. B. Moskowitz, et al. ENGINEERING NEWS-RECORD 217:84, July 3, 1986.

AIDS bibliography, by J. P. Martin. CALIFORNIA NURSE 82(4):17, May 1986.

AIDS bill denounced. REGISTER 62:2, October 5, 1986.

AIDS bills hit legislature, by J. A. Smith. CALIFORNIA NURSE 82(4):8, May 1986.

AIDS: the blood-bank scare, by M. Clark, et al. NEWSWEEK 105(4):62, January 28, 1985.

AIDS: blood donor studies and screening programs, by H. S. Kaplan, et al. PRO-GRESS IN CLINICAL AND BIOLOGICAL RESEARCH 182:297-308, 1985.

AIDS blood screen approved, by J. Silberner. SCIENCE NEWS 127:148, March 9, 1985.

AIDS blood test: qualified success [ELISA test], by J. Silberner. SCIENCE NEWS 128:84, August 10, 1985.

AIDS: blood test trials inconclusive, by S. Budiansky. NATURE 316:96, July 11, 1985.

AIDS: boys and girls come out to play?, by C. Clementson. NURSING TIMES 82(7): 19-20, February 12-18, 1986.

AIDS—Brazil: official concern and cruising, by T. Stroll. BODY POLITIC 1(6):21, August 1984.

AIDS breakthrough, by D. Silburt. MACLEAN'S 97:56, May 7, 1984.

—, by Kate Nolan. PLAYBOY 31:59+, May 1984.

—, by M. Clark, et al. NEWSWEEK 106(20):88, November 11, 1985.

—: cause of disease probably identified. CHEMICAL & ENGINEERING NEWS 62:6-7, April 30, 1984.

AIDS brochure for distribution to patients, by M. M. Hughes. JEN 9(6):340-342, November-December 1983.

AIDS budget doubled, by S. Hyde. GAY COMMUNITY NEWS 11(7):1, September 3, 1983.

AIDS business: drug firms anticipate big market in products for immune disorder, by M. Chase. WALL STREET JOURNAL 207:1+, June 26, 1986.

AIDS: California publishes booklet providing helpful info. CORRECTIONS DIGEST 14(16):4-6, July 27, 1983.

—. CRIME CONTROL DIGEST 17(30):4-6, July 29, 1983.

—. NARCOTICS CONTROL DIGEST 13(16):3-5, August 3, 1983.

—. TRAINING AIDS DIGEST 8(8):5-7, August 1983.

AIDS care in the community, by H. Schietinger. AUSTRALIAN NURSES JOURNAL 15(7):50-51, February 1986.

AIDS: caring for your patient at home, by P. Jackson, et al. CANADIAN NURSE 82(3): 18-22, March 1986.

AIDS carrier arraigned on murder charges for spitting. CRIME CONTROL DIGEST 19(50):8-9, December 16, 1985.

AIDS case dismissed on legal technicality [news], by D. M. Barnes. SCIENCE 233(4762):414, July 25, 1986.

AIDS cases expected to triple. SCIENCE DIGEST 94:9, May 1986.

AIDS cases found concentrated in few prisons, study finds. CRIMINAL JUSTICE NEWSLETTER 17(5):4-5, March 3, 1986.

AIDS cases low in U.S. heartland, by R. J. Donahue. NATIONAL UNDERWRITER 90:4, March 29, 1986.

AIDS cases surpass 15,000. CHRISTIANITY TODAY 29(16):66, November 8, 1985.

AIDS cases top 7000; 5244 are gay men, by E. Guilfoy. GAY COMMUNITY NEWS 12(23):3, December 22, 1984.

AIDS casts a longer shadow [news], by J. Maddox. NATURE 312(5990):97, November 8-14, 1984.

AIDS: casual contact exonerated, by J. Silberner. SCIENCE NEWS 128:213, October 5, 1985.

AIDS: a challenge for contemporary nursing, Part 1, by J. G. Turner, et al. FOCUS ON CRITICAL CARE 13(3):53-61, June 1986.

—, Part 2, by J. G. Turner, et al. FOCUS ON CRITICAL CARE 13(4):41-50, August 1986.

AIDS: a challenge for the public health, by E. D. Acheson. LANCET 1(8482):662-666, March 22, 1986.

AIDS—challenge nurses cannot fail to meet, by R. Wells. NURSING STANDARD 448: 1, May 22, 1986.

AIDS: the challenge nurses have to face. NURSING JOURNAL OF INDIA 77(7):177, July 1986.

AIDS: the challenge to science and medicine, by M. Krim. HASTINGS CENTER REPORT 15(Suppl. 2-7), August 1985.

—, by M. Krim. QRB 12(8):278-283, August 1986.

AIDS: a Christian response. AMERICA 153:77, August 17-24, 1985. RELIGION

AIDS circular. NEW SCIENTIST 99:393, August 11, 1983.

AIDS cited as major administrative concern [interview], by V. Glesnes-Anderson. HOSPITALS 57(15):45-46, August 1, 1983.

AIDS: clarifying values to close in on ethical questions, by S. M. Steele. NURSING AND HEALTH CARE 7(5):246-248, May 1986.

AIDS—clinical research criteria [letter], by G. Yales. HOSPITAL PRACTICE 20(8):17, August 15, 1985.

AIDS: a clinical diagnosis, hence one with pitfalls, by S. A. Danner. NEDERLANDS TIJDSCHRIFT VOOR GENEESKUNDE 129(11):481-483, Mach 16, 1985.

AIDS comes to Halifax, by S. MacPhee. ATLANTIC INSIGHT 7:6, November 1985.

AIDS: a commentary . . . school health, by P. R. Nader. JOURNAL OF SCHOOL HEALTH 56(3):107-108, March 1986.

AIDS—complex challenge of the 80s: nurses are in a good position to offer help, by C. Dunphy. WASHINGTON NURSE 15(2):1+, February 1985.

AIDS, a complex syndrome, by A. Locke. MASSACHUSETTS NURSE 54(7):1+, August 1985.

AIDS concern grows in policing, by J. Nislow. LAW ENFORCEMENT NEWS 12(1): 1+, January 6, 1986.

AIDS concerns in Iowa: an interview with Laverne Wintermeyer. IOWA MEDICINE 75(8):346-347, August 1985.

AIDS, condoms, and gay abandon [letter], by C. J. Mitchell. MEDICAL JOURNAL OF AUSTRALIA 142(11):617, May 27, 1985.

AIDS, condoms and squeamish media, by R. Dorfman. QUILL 73:6-7, October 1985.

AIDS conference looks at the personal side, by C. Guilfoy. GAY COMMUNITY NEWS 12(37):3, April 6, 1985.

AIDS conference ponders the ethics of research, by C. Guilfoy. GAY COMMUNITY NEWS 12(42):1, May 11, 1985.

AIDS conference yields new warnings, by S. Burke. OUT 3(7):1, May 1985.

AIDS conflict, by J. Adler, et al. NEWSWEEK 106(13):18-24, September 23, 1985.

AIDS connection, by G. Kolata. SCIENCE 226:958, November 23,1 984.

AIDS contact [letter]. NATURE 304(5928):678, August 25-31, 1983.

AIDS contaminates world's blood, by S. Connor. NEW SCIENTIST 104:5, November 22, 1984.

AIDS (continued). SCIENCE NEWS 127:328, May 25, 1985.

AIDS control: problems of new blood test [news], by S. Budiansky. NATURE 309(5964):106, May 10-16, 1984.

AIDS controversies: scientists bicker while their search for a vaccine continues, by S. Gilbert. SCIENCE DIGEST 93:28, September 1985.

AIDS-conversation with a victim. SAN FRANCISCO 27:66+, April 1985.

AIDS: coping with the unknown. EMERGENCY MEDICINE 15(18):165-168+, October 30, 1983.

AIDS: the corporate response, by A. Halcrow. PERSONNEL JOURNAL 65(8):123-127, August 1986.

AIDS costs: employers and insurers have reasons to fear expensive epidemic. WALL STREET JOURNAL 206:1+, October 18, 1985.

AIDS could cause new havoc in starving Africa. NEW SCIENTIST 111:24, July 3, 1986.

AIDS could plague the world, or not. NEW SCIENTIST 105:5, February 14, 1985.

AIDS: could you be at risk, by D. Apuzzo-Berger. RN 46:67-68+, February 1983.

AIDS: counting the bodies and the antibodies. NEW SCIENTIST 108:20, October 3, 1985.

AIDS court case raises many serious right of privacy questions, by H. R. Halper. BUSINESS AND HEALTH 3(6):51-52, May 1986.

AIDS crisis action. CHRISTIAN CENTURY 102:1056, November 20, 1985.

AIDS crisis update. ADVOCATE 443:20, April 1, 1986; also in volumes 444, 445, 447, 448, 450, 452, 455.

AIDS crisis/what the ACLU must do, by T. Stoddard. CIVIL LIBERTIES 355:1, Fall 1985.

AIDS: the culprit found? DISCOVER 5:10-11, June 1984.

AIDS: current achievement, future problems [editorial], by L. H. Calabrese. CLEVE-LAND CLINIC QUARTERLY 52(2):217-218, Summer 1985.

AIDS—current concepts and implications for blood transfusion services and nursing staff, by C. J. Burrell, et al. AUSTRALIAN NURSES JOURNAL 14(7):45-47, February 1985.

AIDS: current status and present-day knowledge, by M. Vogt, et al. THERAPEUT-ISCHE UMSCHAU 42(11):798-804, November 1985.

AIDS data-sharing: help sought to combat bias, by C. Frank. AMERICAN BAR AS-SOCIATION JOURNAL 76:22, January 1, 1986.

AIDS: a deadly silence in Africa, by A. Stewart. TIMES November 8, 1985, p. 14.

AIDS debate: must we wait until all answers are at hand?, by S. B. Roll. SYKEPLEIEN 73(12):20+, July 4, 1986.

AIDS declared public enemy no. 1. AMERICAN JOURNAL OF NURSING 83:988, July 1983.

AIDS: definition and guidelines for the health professional, by M. J. Healey, Jr. RAD-IOLOGIC TECHNOLOGY 57(3):233-235, January-February 1986.

AIDS dementia complex: I. Clinical features, by B. A. Navia, et al. ANNALS OF NEU-ROLOGY 19(6):517-524, June 1986.

—: II. Neuropathology, by B. A. Navia, et al. ANNALS OF NEUROLOGY 19(6):525-535, June 1986.

AIDS development: NIH to license HTLV [news], by S. Budiansky. NATURE 309(5969):577, June 14-20, 1984.

AIDS diagnosis uncertain, by S. Yanchinski. NEW SCIENTIST 105:24, February 7, 1985.

AIDS diagnostic tests. CHEMICAL MARKETING REPORTER 228:5, August 5, 1985.

AIDS dilemma. TIME 122:54, October 24,1 983.

AIDS dilemma: recent court decisions place a burden of persuasion on public schools, by J. Beckham. NAASP BULLETIN 70(489):91-95, April 1986.

AIDS: dilemmas for the psychiatric patient [letter], by D. Summerfield. LANCET 2(8498):112, July 12, 1986.

AIDS: dilemmas for the psychiatrist [letter], by A. J. Pinching. LANCET 1(8479):496-497, March 1, 1986.

AIDS—discounting promiscuity theory, by B. Lewis. BODY POLITIC 92:11, April 1983.

AIDS discovery may unlock cancer secrets. NEW SCIENTIST 102:4, May 10, 1984.

AIDS: discrimination issues, by G. Tillet. LAMP 42(8):25+, October 1985.

AIDS: a disease of ancient Egypt? [letter], by R. J. Ablin, et al. NEW YORK STATE JOURNAL OF MEDICINE 85(5):200-201, May 1985.

AIDS: disease, research efforts advance, by J. Silberner. SCIENCE NEWS 127:260-261, April 27, 1985.

AIDS: does the control gene pX poison the lymphocytes?, by G. Miketta. FORT-SCHRITTE DER MEDIZIN 102(47-48):64-65, December 20, 1984.

AIDS: double exposure, by E. Jackson. BODY POLITIC 121:15, December 1985.

AIDS, drug abuse, and mental health [editorial], by H. A. Pincus. PUBLIC HEALTH REPORTS 99(2):106-108, March-April 1984.

AIDS drug shows promise in preliminary clinical trial [news], by J. L. Marx. SCIENCE 231(4745):1504-1505, March 28, 1986.

AIDS drugs: some relief, but adverse side effects, by S. Siwolop. DISCOVER 6:38-42+, December 1985.

AIDS education: the city's closet case, by P. Byron. VILLAGE VOICE 30:33, May 28, 1985.

AIDS education for staff, by H. Schietinger. JOURNAL OF CONTINUING EDUCA-TION IN NURSING 17(1)3-4, January-February 1986.

AIDS education need; conference highlight, by H. W. Jaffe. CORRECTIONS TODAY 48:49-50+, April 1986.

AIDS: an 80's epidemic, by L. David, et al. HEALTH 15:62+, May 1983. EPIDEMIOLOGY

AIDS elephant, by R. D. Smith. THE SCIENCES 24:8+, March-April 1984.

AIDS . . . emergency care personnel, by M. F. Silverman. EMERGENCY: JOURNAL OF EMERGENCY SERVICES 18(5):44-46, May 1986.

AIDS: the emerging ethical dilemmas. HASTINGS CENTER REPORT 15(Suppl. 32): August 1985.

AIDS: an employer's dilemma, by R. S. Letchinger. PERSONNEL JOURNAL 63(2): 58-63, February 1986.

AIDS encephalopathy, by R. W. Price, et al. NEUROLOGIC CLINICS 4(1):285-301, February 1986.

AIDS—the end of permissive society?, by J. Clements. NEW ZEALAND NURSING JOURNAL 78(7):12-13, July 1985.

AIDS enters the brain, by M. Small. SCIENCE DIGEST 94:18, April 1986.

AIDS epidemic. US NEWS AND WORLD REPORT 94:56, June 6, 1983.

—, by J. Seligmann. NEWSWEEK 101:74-79, April 18, 1983.

—, by S. H. Landesman, et al. NEW ENGLAND JOURNAL OF MEDICINE 312(8): 521-525, February 21, 1985.

—, by S. L. Hellman. AAOHN JOURNAL 34(6):285-290, June 1986.

AIDS epidemic and the communion cup, by O. N. Griese. LINACRE QUARTERLY 53:15-25, May 1986.

AIDS epidemic and gay bathhouses: a constitutional analysis, by J. A. Rabin. JOURNAL OF HEALTH POLITICS, POLICY AND LAW 10(4):729-747, Winter 1986.

AIDS epidemic: continental drift [news], by J. E. Groopman, et al. NATURE 307(5948):211-212, January 19-25, 1984.

AIDS epidemic continues, moving beyond high-risk groups, by R. M. Baum. CHEMI- CAL AND ENGINEERING NEWS 63:19-22+, April 1, 1985.

AIDS epidemic creates educational, product demands, by E. Beck. MEDICAL PRODUCTS SALES 16(12):1+, December 1985.

AIDS epidemic: dilemmas facing nurse managers . . . how the University of California San Diego Medical Center has responded, by M. M. Jackson, et al. NURSING ECONOMICS 4(3):109-116, May-June 1986.

AIDS epidemic: multidisciplinary trouble, by J. E. Osborn. NEW ENGLAND JOURNAL OF MEDICINE 314(12):779-782, March 20, 1986.

AIDS—the epidemic of the decade and the medical mystery of the century, by D. E. Stover. RESPIRATORY CARE 29(1):19-20, January 1984.

AIDS—an epidemic of hysteria, by Ardill. SPARE RIB 153:13, April 1985.

AIDS epidemic: an overview of the science, by J. E. Osborn. ISSUES IN SCIENCE AND TECHNOLOGY 2:40-55, Winter 1986.

AIDS epidemic: the price of promiscuity. HUMAN EVENTS 43:5+, June 18, 1983.

AIDS epidemic: risk containment for home health care providers, by J. G. Turner, et al. FAMILY AND COMMUNITY HEALTH 8(3):25-37, November 1985.

AIDS: epidemiology and potential for nosocomial transmission, by D. K. Henderson. TOPICS IN CLINICAL NURSING 6(2):1-11, July 1984.

AIDS: epidemiology update, by J. A. Bennett. AMERICAN JOURNAL OF NURSING 85(9):968-972, September 1984.

AIDS: an ethical challenge for our time, by C. Levine. QRB 12(8):273-277, August 1986.

AIDS: ethical duties of nurses, by S. J. Smith. CALIFORNIA NURSE 79(3):4, September 1983.

AIDS, ethics, and the blood supply. A report of a conference of the American Blood Commission and the Hastings Center, Institute of Society, Ethics and the Life Sciences, January 29 and 30, 1985, by W. V. Miller, et al. TRANSFUSION 25(2): 174-175, March-April 1985.

AIDS—etiology, pathogenesis and epidemiology, by A. Vaheri, et al. DUODECIM 102(7):396-403, 1986.

AIDS: evidence of the growing burden of ethical dilemmas in health care, by M. K. Mitchell. NURSING AND HEALTH CARE 7(5):229, May 1986.

AIDS exacerbates psoriasis, by T. M. Johnson, et al. NEW ENGLAND JOURNAL OF MEDICINE 313:1415, November 28, 1985.

AIDS exiles in Paris, by M. Clark, et al. NEWSWEEK 106(6):71, August 5, 1985.

AIDS exorcism—suck toes, by J. McNiel. FAG RAG 40:1, 1983.

AIDS exposure in health care workers, by R. D. Danielsen, et al. PHYSICIAN ASSISTANT 10(5):37-38+, May 1986.

AIDS: express train to death, by R. Wells. NURSING MIRROR 160(7):16-18, February 13, 1985.

AIDS extra. Fighting bigotry as well as an epidemic, by A. Veitch. GUARDIAN November 5, 1985, p. 11.

—. A model for the world's struggle, by A. Brummer. GUARDIAN November 6, 1985, p. 23.

AIDS fact book, by E. Mabrey. DELAWARE ALTERNATIVE PRESS 6(2):17, January 1984.

AIDS—facts and fiction, by M. Karlovac. MEDICINSKI PREGLED 38(9-10):429-433, 1985.

AIDS: facts and myths [interview with A. Pinching], by H. Wilce. THE TIMES EDUCATIONAL SUPPLEMENT 3613:10, September 27, 1985.

AIDS: the facts behind the fears [interview with B Starrett], by J. Kluger. MCCALL'S 111:66, April 1984.

AIDS: the facts, the fears, the future, by D. Fallowell. TIMES March 6, 1985, p. 10.

AIDS: facts not fear, by C. Weinstein. CALIFORNIA PRISONER 14(3):12, April 1985.

AIDS: the facts of life, by S. Ault. GUARDIAN 38(25):1, March 26, 1986.

AIDS: fatal, incurable and spreading. PEOPLE WEEKLY 23:42-49, June 17, 1985.

AIDS fatalities in Hamburg (status: February 1985)—legal medicine aspects, by K. Püschel, et al. ZEITSCHRIFT FUR RECHTSMEDIZIN 95(2):113-121, 1985.

AIDS fear affects first UK school [Hampshire, England], by S. Bayliss. THE TIMES EDUCATIONAL SUPPLEMENT 3612:3, September 20, 1985.

AIDS: fear and loathing. EMERGENCY MEDICINE 15(18):157-161, October 30, 1983.

AIDS fear cited in Atlanta bathhouse bust, by S. Poggi. GAY COMMUNITY NEWS 12(31):1, February 23, 1985.

AIDS fear is leading to safer sex, expert says [views of Dr. L. Edwards]. JET 68:5, September 2, 1985.

AIDS fear may cause less kissing under the mistletoe. JET 69:25, December 23, 1985.

AIDS fear poses crisis for some, market for others, by P. Winters. ADVERTISING AGE 57:1+, February 3, 1986.

AIDS fear prompts recall of blood products, by S. Connor. NEW SCIENTIST 111:19, July 17, 1986.

AIDS fear puts panic in open-mouth kissing for actors, actresses. JET 69:59, November 18, 1985.

AIDS fears. CHRISTIAN CENTURY 103(10):290, March 19-26, 1986.

AIDS fears spark row over vaccine [news], by D. Dickson. SCIENCE 221(4609):437, July 29, 1983.

AIDS figures mount as researchers seek answers to the puzzle. AMERICAN FAMILY PHYSICIAN 28:331+, September 1983.

AIDS film honored, by C. Guilfoy. GAY COMMUNITY NEWS 13(3):12, July 27, 1985.

AIDS: financial implications for Michigan, by D. W. Benfer, et al. MICHIGAN HOSPITALS 22(8):13-16, August 1986.

AIDS—the first cases in Finland, by H. Repo, et al. DUODECIM 100(11):656-657, 1984.

AIDS 1st leak cited on TV, by B. Gelbert. GAY COMMUNITY NEWS 13(39):1, April 19, 1986.

AIDS: Footdragging on public health, by M. Stanton Evans. HUMAN EVENTS 45:7, September 21, 1985.

Aids for AIDS, by P. David. NATURE 303:743, June 30, 1983.

AIDS for all by the year 2000? [letter], by M. McEvoy, et al. BRITISH MEDICAL JOURNAL 290(6466):463, February 9, 1985.

AIDS forum—it hasn't gone away, by M. Perigard. GAY COMMUNITY NEWS 11(36):3, March 31, 1984.

AIDS forum: politics & science collide, by C. Guilfoy. GAY COMMUNITY NEWS 12(31):3, February 23, 1985.

AIDS found in female prostitute. RN 46:15, April 1983.

AIDS: France to screen blood donors, by R. Walgate. NATURE 315:705, June 27, 1 1985.

AIDS: French sue over who was first, by C. Joyce, et al. NEW SCIENTIST 108:3, December 19-26, 1985.

AIDS: a fresh lead. THE ECONOMIST 287:94-95, May 28, 1983.

AIDS—from the clinical viewpoint, by H. D. Pohle. OFFENTLICHE GESUNDHEIT-SWESEN 47(8):349-352, August 1985.

AIDS: from fear to fightback, by K. Kelley. GUARDIAN 37(31):1, May 8, 1985.

AIDS from west to east?, by M. Khurana. NURSING JOURNAL OF INDIA 77(8):207+, August 1986.

AIDS from women to men. NEW SCIENTIST 108:27, November 7, 1985.

AIDS funding and research hiked; Haitians' risk debated. AMERICAN FAMILY PHYSICIAN 28:17-18, September 1983.

AIDS funding decisions lack consensus opinion, by J. Firshei. HOSPITALS 60(1):35, January 5, 1986.

AIDS funding jeopardized by veto, by D. Nelson. GAY COMMUNITY NEWS 10(48):3, June 25, 1983.

AIDS funds approved. BODY POLITIC 91:19, March 1983.

AIDS—a further development, by T. Aoki, et al. GAN TO KAGAKU RYOHO 13(5): 1791-1797, May 1986.

AIDS: the gay epidemic, by F. Fisher. NEW SCIENTIST 96:713-715, December 16, 1982.

AIDS, gay men and the insurance industry, by R. Mohr. GAY COMMUNITY NEWS 14(10):5, September 21, 1986.

AIDS gay mens health crisis, by P. Byron. GAY COMMUNITY NEWS 11(3):8, July 30, 1983.

AIDS—general characteristics and new clues in the studies of etiopathogenesis of the syndrome—the role of HTLV, by K. Jonderko. WIADOMOSCI LEKARSKIE 38(15):1061-1066, August 1, 1985.

AIDS: getting the facts, by M. L. Stein. EDITOR AND PUBLISHER, THE FOURTH ESTATE 118:16-17, November 2, 1985.

AIDS: getting past the diagnosis and on to discharge planning, by P. H. Wolff, et al. CRITICAL CARE NURSE 6(4):76-81, July-August 1986.

AIDS goes hetero, by M. Castleman. MEDICAL SELF CARE 30:18, September 1985.

AIDS goes straight, by N. Fain. VILLAGE VOICE 30:30-31, May 14, 1985.

AIDS: the good news. SCIENTIFIC AMERICAN 255:55, November 1986.

AIDS grant. ADAMHA NEWS 9(20):1, November 18, 1983.

AIDS group doubts study, by K. Popert. BODY POLITIC 124:15, March 1986.

AIDS group urges monitoring,by C. Guilfoy. GAY COMMUNITY NEWS 12(9):6, September 15, 1983.

AIDS: a growing cause of blindness, by L. P. Wahl. JOURNAL OF VISUAL IMPAIRMENT AND BLINDNESS 80:544, January 1986.

AIDS: a growing 'pandemic'?, by M. Clark. NEWSWEEK 105:71, April 29, 1985.

AIDS: a growing threat, by C. Wallis, et al. TIME 126(6):40-45+, August 12, 1985.

AIDS guidance for heads [Great Britain], by J. Meikle. THE TIMES EDUCATIONAL SUPPLEMENT 3639:10, March 28, 1986.

AIDS guide offsets hysteria [Australia], by L. Garcia. THE TIMES EDUCATIONAL SUPPLEMENT 3609:11, August 30, 1985.

AIDS guidelines can reduce legal risks for hospitals, by D. L. Wing. HOSPITAL MANAGER 16(4):1-3, July-August 1986.

AIDS: guidelines for caring for AIDs patients, by C. Field. LAMP 42(1):21-21, February 1985.

AIDS guidelines too stringent [letter], by A. J. Pinching, et al. BRITISH MEDICAL JOURNAL 290(6469):709-710, March 2, 1985.

—, by S. McKechnie. BRITISH MEDICAL JOURNAL 290(6473):1006, March 30, 1985.

AIDS guidelines urge common-sense care, by S. B. Young, et al. AIR FORCE TIMES 46:34, November 25, 1985.

AIDS: the Haitian connection, by H. M. Smith. MD 27(12):46-52, December 1983.

AIDS: The Haitian Factor, by Alfredo S. Lanier. CHICAGO 33:120+, August 1984.

AIDS has both sexes running scared, by E. Cantarow. MADEMOISELLE 90:158-159+, February 1984.

AIDS health care American style, by D. Altman. DEMOCRATIC LEFT 14(3):3, May 1986.

AIDS: the health crisis of the 80's, by P. Alexander. NATIONAL NOW TIMES 18(8):4, February 1986.

AIDS—a health education approach in West Glamorgan, by C. Griffiths, et al. HEALTH EDUCATION JOURNAL 44(4):172-173, 1985.

AIDS—a health education challenge, by Z. Kurtz. HEALTH EDUCATION JOURNAL 44(4):169-171, 1985.

AIDS—health—politics, by D. Feinberg. GAY COMMUNITY NEWS 11(19):8, November 26, 1983.

AIDS, hepatitis, and the national blood policy. REGULATION 9(4):5-7, July-August 1985.

AIDS, hepatitis B and the problems of confidentiality [letter], by R. C. Hitchcock. BRITISH DENTAL JOURNAL 159(8):243, October 19, 1985.

AIDS: here's how health experts and the legal community have viewed the disease: how some progressive businesses are working to enlighten their employees and peers; and what AIDS has meant to those living—and dying— with it. PERSONNEL JOURNAL 65:112-127, August 1986.

AIDS: the heterosexual connection. NEW SCIENTIST 100:644, December 1, 1983.

AIDS: histopathological aspects, by P. R. Millard. JOURNAL OF PATHOLOGY 143(4): 223-239, August 1984.

AIDS hits heterosexuals. SCIENCE NEWS 123:341, May 28, 1983.

AIDS hits second tier cities, by M. Helquist. ADVOCATE 430:23, October 1, 1985.

AIDS: Hollywood jitters, by E. Salholz. NEWSWEEK 106:73, August 26, 1985.

AIDS home care and hospice program. A multidisciplinary approach to caring for persons with AIDS, by J. P. Martin. AMERICAN JOURNAL OF HOSPICE CARE 3(2): 35-37, March-April 1986.

AIDS: homosexual plague, by M. Stanton Evans. HUMAN EVENTS 43:15, August 6, 1983.

AIDS horror story worsens, by M. Stanton Evans. HUMAN EVENTS 45:7, November 30, 1985.

AIDS: hospital guidelines, clinical clues. AHA panel hits exaggerated precautions, by D. Lefton. AMERICAN MEDICAL NEWS 26(48):1+, December 23-30, 1983.

AIDS: how do we continue in the interim?, by J. Huisman. NEDERLANDS TIJD-SCHRIFT VOOR GENEESKUNDE 129(31):1459-1462, August 3, 1985.

AIDS: how the immune system works. CALIFORNIA NURSE 82(4):11, May 1986.

AIDS: how a problem became a priority, by B. J. Stiles. FOUNDATION NEWS 27(2): 48-56, March-April 1986.

AIDS: how real is the risk for women? GLAMOUR 83:308+, November 1985.

AIDS: how we kept the kids in school and averted a panic, by P. J. Hagerty, et al. EXECUTIVE EDUCATOR 8(1):28-30, January 1986.

AIDS: the human element, by J. Aberth. PERSONNEL JOURNAL 65(8):119-123, August 1986.

AIDS hunt homes in on Haitian pigs, by O. Sattaur. NEW SCIENTIST 98:199, April 28, 1983.

AIDS hunt: precaution or privacy violation? NEWSWEEK 106:27, September 2, 1985.

AIDS hygiene: practices and precautions, by D. Bille. ADVOCATE 421:34, May 28, 1985.

AIDS hysteria. NEWSWEEK 101:42, May 30, 1983.

AIDS hysteria [letter], by J. C. Katz. CANADIAN MEDICAL ASSOCIATION JOURNAL 134(6):573+, March 15, 1986.

AIDS hysteria and the common cup: take and drink, by R. W. Hovda. WORSHIP 60(1):67-73, January 1986.

AIDS hysteria: a contagious side effect, by M. Korcok. CANADIAN MEDICAL AS-SOCIATION JOURNAL 133(12):1241-1248, December 15, 1985.

AIDS hysteria: a housekeeper's nightmare, by M. Polito. EXECUTIVE HOUSEKEEPING TODAY 7(3):10, March 1986.

AIDS hysteria: how it began and what nurses can do [editorial], by P. N. Palmer. AORN JOURNAL 43(2):418+, February 1986.

AIDS hysteria strikes New York City, by P. Freiberg. ADVOCATE 431:13, October 15, 1985.

AIDS IDs: protection or hysteria?, by J. Shevach. NEW AGE May 1986, p. 12.

AIDS an illness with many questionmarks, by N. Albrecht-van Lent, et al. TIJD-SCHRIFT VOOR ZIEKENVERPLEGING 36(21):666-668, October 18, 1983.

AIDS—an immunologic reevaluation, by M. Seligmann, et al. NEW ENGLAND JOUR-NAL OF MEDICINE 311(20):1286-1292, November 15, 1984.

AIDS immunopathologic network a tangled web [news]. HOSPITAL PRACTICE 19(1):39-40+, January 1984.

AIDS: the impact on the health care worker, by G. I. Lusby. FRONTIERS OF RADIA-TION THERAPY AND ONCOLOGY 19:165-167, 1985.

AIDS' impact on hemophiliacs, by M. Helquist. ADVOCATE 451:23, July 22, 1986.

AIDS impairs mental function. ADAMHA NEWS 11(8):1, August 1985.

AIDS: the impending quarantine, by R. Cohen. HEALTH PAC BULLETIN 16(4):9, July 1985.

AIDS: the implications for home care, by M. G. Boland, et al. MCN 11(6):404-411, November-December 1986.

AIDS: implications for South African nurses I, by M. C. Herbst. CURATIONIS 8(3):13-14+, September 1985.

— II, by M. C. Herbst. CURATIONIS 8(4):18-20, December 1985.

AIDS: an imported disease?, by B. Somaini. SCHWEIZERISCHE MEDIZINISCHE WOCHENSCHRIFT 116(24):818-821, June 14, 1986.

AIDS in Africa. NEW SCIENTIST 108:14, November 28, 1985.

AIDS in Africa: a heterosexuals' disease, by O. Sattaur. NEW SCIENTIST 104:9, October 18, 1984.

AIDS in an apparently risk-free woman [letter], by J. Cabane, et al. LANCET 2(8394):105, July 14, 1984.

AIDS in Arabia. NEW SCIENTIST 109:23, January 30, 1986.

AIDS in association with malignant melanoma and Hodgkin's disease [letter], by G. E. Moore, et al. JOURNAL OF CLINICAL ONCOLOGY 3(10):1437, October 1985.

AIDS in Australia, by S. Hyde. GAY COMMUNITY NEWS 12(22):2, December 15, 1984.

AIDS in the bathhouse, by T. Allen-Mills. SPECTATOR March 9, 1985, p. 7-8.

AIDS in the black community, by D. Walter. ADVOCATE 454:10, September 2, 1986.

AIDS in a black Malian [letter], by D. Vittecoq, et al. LANCET 2(8357):1023, October 29, 1983.

AIDS: in the blood. SCIENTIFIC AMERICAN 251:89+, September 1984.

AIDS in a bodybuilder using anabolic steroids [letter], by H. M. Sklarek, et al. NEW ENGLAND JOURNAL OF MEDICINE 311(26):1701, December 27, 1984.

AIDS in a Canadian woman who had helped prostitutes in Port-au-Prince [letter], by D. B. Rose, et al. LANCET 2(8351):680-681, September 17, 1983.

AIDS in a child 5 1/2 years after a transfusion [letter], by M. J. Maloney, et al. NEW ENGLAND JOURNAL OF MEDICINE 312(19):1256, May 9, 1985.

AIDS in children, by G. Fontán. ANNALES ESPANOLES DE PEDIATRIA 23(3):157-162, September 1985.

AIDS in children: a review of the clinical, epidemiologic and public health aspects, by M. F. Rogers. PEDIATRIC INFECTIOUS DISEASE 4(3):230-236, May-June 1985.

AIDS in Colorado: rumor and reality. COLORADO MEDICINE 30(11):314-317, November 1983.

AIDS in a Danish surgeon (Zaire, 1976) [letter], by I. C. Bygbjerg. LANCET 1(8330): 925, April 23, 1983.

AIDS in Denmark and immunological parameters among homosexual Danish men with special reference to the prognosis of patients with low H/S rations. A report from the CAID, by J. Gerstoft, et al. ANTIBIOTIC CHEMOTHERAPY 32:127-137, 1983.

AIDS in the east: now it's official. NEW SCIENTIST 109:25, March 6, 1986.

AIDS in the emergency room, by V. Svesko. NEW YORK 18:36-37, September 23, 1985.

AIDS in Europe [letter], by J. Green, et al. BRITISH MEDICAL JOURNAL 287(6506): 1715-1716, December 3, 1983.

AIDS in Europe, by P. Ebbesen, et al. BRITISH MEDICAL JOURNAL 287(6402): 1324-1326, November 5, 1983.

AIDS in the family, by M. Blackwell. ESSENCE 16:54-56+, August 1985.

AIDS in the family [case of L. Nassaney], by S. Haller. PEOPLE 24:136-138+, November 18, 1985.

AIDS in the female, by W. Stille, et al. ARCHIVES OF GYNECOLOGY 238(1-4):825-832, 1985.

AIDS in French prisons, by I. Porras. CORRECTIONS TODAY 48:128, August 1986.

AIDS in the 'gay' areas of San Francisco [letter], by A. R. Moss, et al. LANCET 1(8330):923-924, Apri 23, 1983.

AIDS in Germany: a failed challenge, by H. Fiedler. DEUTSCHE MEDIZINISCHE WOCHENSCHRIFT 110(47):1830-1831, November 22, 1985.

AIDS in haemophilia patients in Spain [letter], by E. Lissen, et al. LANCET 1(8331): 992-993, April 30, 1983.

AIDS in haemophiliacs in Spain [letter], by M. Leal, et al. LANCET 1(8423):275, February 2, 1985.

—, by O. Tello. LANCET 2(8417-8418):1472, December 22, 1985.

AIDS in Haitian-Americans: a reassessment, by E. Frank, et al. CANCER RESEARCH 45(Supplement 9):4619s-4620s, September 1985.

AIDS in a Haitian couple in Paris [letter], by E. Dournon, et al. LANCET 1(8332):1040-1041, May 7, 1983.

AIDS in Haitian immigrants [letter], by R. A. Fralick. CANADIAN MEDICAL ASSOCIA-TION JOURNAL 130(10):1266, May 15, 1984.

AIDS in Haitian immigrants and in a Caucasian woman closely associated with Haitians, by M. Laverdière, et al. CANADIAN MEDICAL ASSOCIATION JOURNAL 129(11):1209, 1212, December 1, 1983.

AIDS in a Haitian woman with cardiac Kaposi's sarcoma and Whipple's disease [letter], by B. Autram, et al. LANCET 1(8327):767-768, April 2, 1983.

AIDS in hemophilia, by M. W. Hilgartner, et al. ANNALS OF THE NEW YORK ACADEMY OF SCIENCES 437:466-471, 1984.

AIDS in hemophiliacs. AMERICAN FAMILY PHYSICIAN 32:222, July 1985.

AIDS in a heterosexual population. AMERICAN FAMILY PHYSICIAN 31:292, February 1985.

AIDS in homosexual men—the first cases in Sweden, by P. Pehrson, et al. LAKAR-TIDNINGEN 80(7):545-548, February 16, 1983.

AIDS in a hospital worker [letter], by A. Belani, et al. LANCET 1(8378):676, March 24, 1984.

AIDS in Houston, by P. I. Evans, et al. HOUSTON CITY MAGAZINE 9:56+, October 1985.

AIDS in the human brain, by C. H. Fox, et al. NATURE 319:8, January 2, 1986.

AIDS in the infant, by E. Vilmer, et al. REVUE FRANCAISE DE TRANSFUSION ET IMMUNO-HEMATOLOGIE 27(4):423-426, September 1984.

AIDS in infants, by S. Eliot. HEALTHSHARING 7(1):6, Winter 1985.

AIDS in Italy [letter], by G. Rezza, et al. LANCET 2(8403):642, September 15, 1984.

AIDS in Japan. No screening of blood donors [news], by D. Swinbanks. NATURE 318(6044):306, November 28-December 4, 1985.

AIDS in Johannesburg [letter], by R. Sher. SOUTH AFRICAN MEDICAL JOURNAL 68(3):137-138, August 3, 1985.

AIDS in Michigan. The public health approach, by R. Pope. MICHIGAN HOSPITALS 22(8):6-11, August 1986.

AIDS in the mind of America, by G. Keenan. SCIENCE FOR THE PEOPLE 18(2):31, March 1986.

AIDS in monkeys. AMERICAN FAMILY PHYSICIAN 33:372, February 1986.

AIDS in monkeys and men [letter]. LANCET 1(8333):1097-1098, May 14, 1983.

AIDS in New York City with particular reference to the psycho-social aspects, by N. Deuchar. BRITISH JOURNAL OF PSYCHIATRY 145:612-619, December 1984.

AIDS in New Zealand [letter], by S. D. Somerfield. NEW ZEALAND MEDICAL JOURNAL 98(774):160-161, March 13, 1985.

AIDS in 1949? [letter], by G. Williams, et al. LANCET 2(8359):1136, November 12, 1983.

AIDS in 1968 [letter], by M. H. Witte, et al. JAMA 251(20):2657, May 25, 1984.

AIDS in Ohio. How the state is handling the problem, by K. S. Edwards. OHIO STATE MEDICAL JOURNAL 81(10):695-699+, October 1985.

AIDS in one city. An interview with Mervyn Silverman, Director of Health, San Francisco [interview by Stephen F. Morin], by M. Silverman. AMERICAN PSYCHOLOGIST 39(11):1294-1296, November 1984.

AIDS in a patient with Crohn's disease, by J. M. Dhar, et al. BRITISH MEDICAL JOURNAL 288(6433):1802-1803, June 16, 1984.

AIDS in a patient with hemophilia receiving mainly cryoprecipitate, by H. C. Gerstein, et al. CANADIAN MEDICAL ASSOCIATION JOURNAL 131(1):45-47, July 1, 1984.

AIDS in perspective. CANADIAN NURSE 80:16, May 1984.

—, by N. Fain. ADVOCATE 3(98):20, July 10, 1984.

—, by A. Nichols. JOURNAL OF NEPHROLOGY NURSING 2(3):101-104, May-June 1985.

AIDS in pregnancy, by A. Loveman, et al. JOGN NURSING15(2):91-93, March-April 1986.

AIDS in pregnancy, donors and tears. SCIENCE NEWS 128:187, September 21, 1985.

AIDS in the prison system: some suggestions on how to prevent new outbreaks, by T. Bassinger. CORRECTIONS DIGEST 14(16):3-4, July 27, 1983.

AIDS in schoolchildren [letter], by P. M. Shah, et al. DEUTSCHE MEDIZINISCHE WOCHENSCHRIFT 110(42):1631, October 18, 1985.

AIDS in the schools: a special report, by S. Reed. PHI DELTA KAPPAN 67:494-498, March 1986.

AIDS in South Carolina [editorial], by C. S. Bryan. JOURNAL OF THE SOUTH CAROLINA MEDICAL ASSOCIATION 79(8):452-453, August 1983.

AIDS in a surgeon [letter], by J. J. Sacks. NEW ENGLAND JOURNAL OF MEDICINE 313(16):1017-1018, October 17, 1985.

AIDS in 'sweeps' time, by V. Russo. CHANNELS OF COMMUNICATIONS 5:6+, September-October 1985.

AIDS in Switzerland, by B. Somaini. SCHWEIZERISCHE MEDIZINISCHE WOCHENSCHRIFT 114(16):538-544, April 21, 1984.

AIDS in The Netherlands. Clinical and microbiological data on 36 cases, by S. A. Danner, et al. NETHERLAND JOURNAL OF MEDICINE 28(10):487-497, 1985.

AIDS in tropical areas: Haitian and African foci, by H. Taelman et al. ANNALES DE LA SOCIETE BELGE DE MEDECINE TROPICALE 64(4):331-334, 1984.

AIDS in the USA and the RSA—an update [letter], by M. Malan. SOUTH AFRICAN MEDICAL JOURNAL 70(2):119, July 1986.

AIDS in West Germany [letter], by J. L'age-Stehr, et al. LANCET 2(8363):1370-1371, December 10, 1983.

AIDS in a woman in England [letter],by C. L. Smith, et al. LANCET 2(8354):846, October 8, 1983.

AIDS in the workplace. AAOHN JOURNAL 34(7):347-348, July 1986.

—. TRIAL 22(1):82-83, January 1986.

—, by A. Buzy. WASHINGTON NURSE 16(7):21, July-August 1986.

—, by A. Halcrow. PERSONNEL JOURNAL 64:10-11, October 1985.

—, by B. S. Murphy, et al. PERSONNEL JOURNAL 64:20+, December 1985.

—, by H. Z. Levine. PERSONNEL JOURNAL 63(3):56-64, March 1986.

—, by J. Aberth. MANAGEMENT REVIEW 74(12):49-51, December 1985.

—, by L. T. Duffie. CONTEMPORARY LONGTERM CARE 9(4):21-22, April 1986.

—, by M. Clark, et al. NEWSWEEK 108(1):62-63, July 7, 1986.

—, by P. G. Engel. INDUSTRY WEEK 228:28-30, February 3, 1986.

—, by W. L. Kandel. EMPLOYEE RELATIONS LAW JOURNAL 11(4):678-690, Spring 1986.

—: an epidemic fear. NATIONAL SAFETY AND HEALTH NEWS 133:34-39, January 1986.

—: the ethical ramifications, by R. Bayer, et al. BUSINESS AND HEALTH 3(3):30-34, January-February 1986.

—: facing the legal issues. CORPORATE SECURITY December 1985, pp. 2-3.

—. How to prevent the transmission of the infection. INTERNATIONAL NURSES REVIEW 33(4/268):117-122+, July-August 1986.

—. How to reach out to those among us, by C. Ryan. PUBLIC WELFARE 44(3): 29-33, Summer 1986.

AIDS in the workplace: facing the legal issues. CORPORATE SECURITY December 1985, pp. 2-3.

AIDS incidence higher in older recruits, by P. Smith. AIR FORCE TIMES 46:3, April 14, 1986.

AIDS incidence increases as experts continue investigations. AMERICAN FAMILY PHYSICIAN 33:328-329, March 1986.

AIDS-induced decline of the incidence of syphilis in Denmark, by A. Poulsen, et al. ACTA DERMATO-VENEREOLOGICA 65(6):567-569, 1985.

AIDS-infected chimps. AMERICAN FAMILY PHYSICIAN 30:343, October 1984.

AIDS-infected members limited to ConUS duty, by L. Famiglietti. AIR FORCE TIMES 46:6, July 28, 1986.

AIDS infection control precautions, by M. A. Johnson. FRONTIERS OF RADIATION THERAPY AND ONCOLOGY 19:160-163, 1985.

AIDS, infectivity, and health care workers, by P. B. Kernoff. BRITISH JOURNAL OF HAEMATOLOGY 60(2):207-211, June 1985.

AIDS: information for dentists. New York State Department of Health. NEW YORK JOURNAL OF DENTISTRY 54(6):256, September-October 1984.

AIDS: an information perspective, by L. Kabbash, et al. BIBLIOTHECA MEDICA CAN-ADIANA 8(2):71-78, 1986.

AIDS insurance and health bills slated for votes, by K. Westheimer. GAY COM-MUNITY NEWS 13(36):1, March 29, 1986.

AIDS-insurance investigation slated by NAIC, by J. Diamond. NATIONAL UNDER-WRITER 89:8, December 27, 1985.

AIDS investigators identify secnd retrovirus [news], by J. Maurice. JAMA 250(8): 1010-1011+, August 26, 1983.

AIDS investigators want input on prevention of disease. AMERICAN FAMILY PHYSICIAN 29:18, June 1984.

AIDS is all of us, by J. Carpenter. NORTHWEST PASSAGE 24(4):6, November 1983.

AIDS is getting to us, by J. Adams. LESBIAN CONTRADICTION 16:20, Summer 1986.

AIDS is here, by D. Fallowell. TIMES July 27, 1983, p. 8.

AIDS: is it the body turned against itself?, by M. Helquist. ADVOCATE 435:23, December 10, 1985.

AIDS: is it a major threat to blacks?, by T. Martin. EBONY 40:91-92+, October 1985.

AIDS is less transmissible than hepatitis, say guidelines. AMERICAN JOURNAL OF NURSING 86:201, February 1986.

AIDS is no work environment risk with the correct protective measures, by I. Lernevall. VARDFACKET 9(7):22-23, April 4, 1985.

AIDS is not for men only, by C. Norwood. MADEMOISELLE 91:198-199+, September 1985.

AIDS: is Retrovirus HTLV-III the causative agent?, by H. G. Thiele. IMMUNITAT UND INFEKTION 12(5):256-258, October 1984.

AIDS is running rampant through Africa. NEW SCIENTIST 110:26, June 26, 1986.

AIDS is top priority for U.S. Public Health Service. FLORIDA NURSE 31(10):7+, November 1983.

AIDS: 'isolate the disease, not the patient,' by P. Holmes. NURSING TIMES 81(6):15-16, February 6-12, 1985.

AIDS issue hits the schools, by E. McGrath. TIME 126:61, September 9, 1985.

AIDS—issues in Rights Bill hearing, by L. Goldsmith. GAY COMMUNITY NEWS 11(36):1, March 31, 1984.

AIDS: it can be avoided, by J. H. Tanne. READER'S DIGEST 128:94-98, February 1986.

AIDS—its implications for South African homosexuals and the mediating role of the medical practitioner, by G. Isaacs, et al. SOUTH AFRICAN MEDICAL JOURNAL 68(5):327-330, August 31, 1985.

AIDS: 'it's just a matter of time,' by R. Streitmatter. QUILL 72:22-25+, May 1984.

AIDS: Its victims are this century's lepers, by B. Kenkelen. NATIONAL CATHOLIC REPORTER 20:6-7, July 6, 1984.

AIDS IV: a recovery, by K. Hale-Wehmann. GAY COMMUNITY NEWS 14(2):7, July 20, 1986.

AIDS: Japan screens donated blood, by D. Swinbanks. NATURE 319:610, February 20, 1986.

AIDS journal, by M. Helquist. ADVOCATE 3(79):26, October 27, 1983.

AIDS: journalism in a plague year, by David Nimmons. PLAYBOY 30:35+, October 1983.

AIDS, Kaposi's sarcoma and the dermatologist [editorial], by N. P. Smith. JOURNAL OF THE ROYAL SOCIETY OF MEDICINE 78(2):97-99, February 1958.

AIDS kids: the education of parents, by A. Mayo. VILLAGE VOICE 30:20, September 24, 1985.

AIDS: a killer confined, by L. A. Engelhard, et al. TODAY'S OR NURSE 5(10):26-30+, December 1983.

AIDS kills Virginia inmate. CORRECTIONS DIGEST 16(10):6, May 8, 1985.

AIDS: the latest facts, by B. Weinhouse. LADIES' HOME JOURNAL 100:100+, November 1983.

AIDS: legacy of the '60s?, by J. G. Fuller. SCIENCE DIGEST 91:84-86+, December 1983.

AIDS: the legal debate, by D. L. Wing. PERSONNEL JOURNAL 65(8):114-119, August 1986.

AIDS: a legal, medical, and social problem, by C. J. Postell. TRIAL 22(8):76-78, August 1986.

AIDS: a legal perspective on employer costs, by G. P. Cunningham. HEALTH COST MANAGEMENT 3(1):1-6, January-February 1986.

AIDS: a lethal mystery story, by M. Clark. NEWSWEEK 100:63-64, December 27, 1982.

AIDS-like immunologic alterations in clinically unaffected drug users, by G. Fiorini, et al. AMERICAN JOURNAL OF CLINICAL PATHOLOGY 84(3):354-357, September 1985.

AIDS likely to spread unless causes can be identified, by P. L. Polakoff. OCCUPATIONAL HEALTH AND SAFETY February 1984, p. 44-45.

AIDS: a link with poverty? [Belle Glade, Florida], by J. Conant. NEWSWEEK 105:37, June 24, 1985.

AIDS linked to gamma interferon deficiency. CHEMICAL AND ENGINEERING NEWS 62:7, April 9, 1984.

AIDS: a living nightmare: psychosocial intervention by the GIA, by S. Lewis, et al. SGA JOURNAL 7(4):16-21, Spring 1985.

AIDS lobby and educ proj proposed, by D. Slaw. GAY COMMUNITY NEWS 10(50):3, July 9, 1983.

AIDS: London scare ends [news], by M. Chown. NATURE 310(5979):614, August 23-29, 1984.

AIDS: London's last chance, by K. Conlon, et al. ILLUSTRATED LONDON NEWS 2 74:26-30, December 1986.

AIDS: looking for the cure, by E. Dobson. FUNDAMENTALIST JOURNAL 4(9):14, October 1985.

AIDS: majority would permit children to attend school with AIDS victim. GALLUP REPORT pp. 19-22, April 1986.

AIDS management: the federal role, by J. S. Oliver. JOURNAL OF MEDICAL TECHNOLOGY 3(3):159-166, March 1986.

AIDS material called "porno", by M. Helquist. ADVOCATE 430:22, October 1, 1985.

AIDS may force re-examination of values, by R. Kerrison. HUMAN EVENTS 45:9, August 17, 1985.

AIDS may lead to a tuberculosis epidemic. DISCOVER 7:9, March 1986.

AIDS mecca of the world, by A. Jetter. MOTHER JONES 10(3):6+, April 1985.

AIDS: a medical conundrum, by R. E. Stahl, et al. JOURNAL OF CUTANEOUS PATHOLOGY 10(6):550-558, December 1983.

AIDS: a medical time bomb, by M. Stanton Evans. HUMAN EVENTS 44:7, July 14, 1984.

AIDS—meeting the challenge in the workplace. AAOHN JOURNAL 34(1):38-39+, January 1986.

—. AAOHN JOURNAL 34(6):285-290, June 1986.

AIDS meets funding drought, by W. Doherty. SCIENCE FOR PEOPLE 15(3):5, May 1983.

AIDS: minimising the occupational risks [editorial], by H. A. Waldron. BRITISH JOURNAL OF INDUSTRIAL MEDICINE 42(6):361-362, June 1985.

AIDS ministers should urge that God is not punishing. REGISTER 62:2, December 7, 1986.

AIDS: ministry issues for chaplains, by J. Bohne. PASTORAL PSYCHOLOGY 34(3): 173-192, Spring 1986.

AIDS—misplaced and better-placed hysteria, by R. Smith. MEDICAL JOURNAL OF AUSTRALIA 143(1):35, July 8, 1985.

AIDS—mobilizing to put on the pressure. BODY POLITIC 116:27, July 1985.

AIDS: Moral Majority intervenes [news], by P. David. NATURE 304(5923):201, July 21-27, 1983.

AIDS: more for research and treatment [news], by T. Beardsley. NATURE 317(6037):466, October 10-16, 1985.

AIDS: more money promised, by S. Budiansky. NATURE 303:365, June 2, 1983.

AIDS: more troubling questions, by M. Weiss. LUTHERAN FORUM 120(1):5, 1986.

AIDS: Moscow's new weapon in its secret war of smears, by I. Elliot. TIMES October 31, 1986, p. 20.

AIDS—mysteries and hidden dangers, by J. Rechy. ADVOCATE 3(83):31, December 22, 1983.

AIDS, a mysterious disease, plagues homosexual men from New York to California, by N. Faber, et al. PEOPLE WEEKLY 19:42-44, February 14, 1983.

AIDS mystery: new clues, by J. Seligmann. NEWSWEEK 101:94, May 16, 1983.

AIDS myths, by T. Barrett. CALIFORNIA NURSE 82(4):5, May 1986.

AIDS: a narrow line between complacency and alarmism, by J. Wilkinson. LISTENER February 14, 1985, p. 5-6.

AIDS, nature, and the nature of AIDS. NATIONAL REVIEW 37:18, November 1, 1985.

AIDS—the need for an integrated approach, by J. K. van Wijngaarden. NEDER-LANDS TIJDSCHRIFT VOOR GENEESKUNDE 128(22):1061-1062, June 2, 1984.

AIDS neglect, by R. Kaye. NATION 236(20):627, May 21, 1983.

AIDS: neither new nor transmissible?, by A. Berken. NEW YORK STATE JOURNAL OF MEDICINE 84(9):440-441, September 1984.

AIDS: the neurological connection, by J. Meer. PSYCHOLOGY TODAY 20:10, January 1986.

AIDS: a neurological nursing challenge, by J. A. Sunder. TOPICS IN CLINICAL NURSING 6(2):67-71, July 1984.

AIDS: new centres for clinical trials [news], by J. Palca. NATURE 322(6075):100, July 10-16, 1986.

AIDS—a new concern for blood transfusion services, by J. Leikola. KRANKEN-PFLEGE 76(10):60-61, October 1983.

AIDS: a new disease, by M. A. Conant. FRONTIERS OF RADIATION THERAPY AND ONCOLOGY 19:1-7, 1985.

—, by R. Schuppli. SCHWEIZERISCHE MONATSSCHRIFT FÜR ZAHNMEDIZIN 94(9):840-842, September 1984.

—. A nurse speaks, by F. Mignot. SOINS 469-470:31-32, January 1986.

AIDS: a new disease's deadly odyssey, by R. M. Henig. THE NEW YORK TIMES MAGAZINE February 6, 1983, p. 28-30+.

AIDS—a new immunodeficiency syndrome, by W. H. Hitzig. SCHWEIZERISCHE RUNDSCHAU FUR MEDIZIN PRAXIS 73(8):217-220, February 21, 1984.

AIDS—a new plague?, by I. Braveny. EUROPEAN JOURNAL OF CLINICAL MICRO-BIOLOGY 2(3):183-185, June 1983.

AIDS: a new problem area for nursing personnel, by J. A. Lambregts. KRANKEN-PFLEGE 39(9):335-337, September 1985.

AIDS: a new task field for nurses, by J. A. Lambregts. TIJDSCHRIFT VOOR ZIEKEN-VERPLEGING 38(6):172-182, March 12, 1985.

AIDS: new victims but maybe a treatment, by J. Arehart-Treichel. SCIENCE NEWS 124:54, July 23, 1983.

AIDS—New Zealand's position. NEW ZEALAND HOSPITAL 37(8):11, September 1985.

AIDS news update. ADVOCATE 3(75):10, September 1, 1983.

—. ADVOCATE 3(80):14, November 10, 1983.

—, by C. Heim. ADVOCATE 3(82):12, December 8, 1983.

—. ADVOCATE 3(85):12, January 10, 1984.

AIDS news update—8000 LA marchers, by S. Anderson. ADVOCATE 3(71):8, July 7, 1983.

AIDS newsletter available. CRIME CONTROL DIGEST 20(6):2, February 10, 1986.

AIDS—a nightmare in our time. ORSTERREICHISCHE KRANKENPFLEGEZEIT-SCHRIFT 38(11):271-272, November 1985.

AIDS—nightmares, by M. Perigard. GAY COMMUNITY NEWS 11(30):5, February 18, 1984.

AIDS 1976 in Cologne? [letter], by A. Konrads, et al. DEUTSCHEMEDIZINISCHE WOCHENSCHRIFT 108(35):1336, September 2, 1983.

AIDS: no need for worry in the workplace [U.S. Public Health Service report]. NEWS-WEEK 106:51, November 25, 1985.

AIDS—no relief in sight, by S. Lawrence. SCIENCE NEWS 122:202-203, September 25, 1982.

AIDS: no threat from the dead: a doctor decried special care for victims' bodies, by S. Deaton. ALBERTA REPORT 13:32+, March 31, 1986.

AIDS no threat in central service, by D. Dildine. HPN 7(10):1+, October 1983.

AIDS: no time for apathy, by W. Greaves. JOURNAL OF THE NATIONAL MEDICAL ASSOCIATION 78(2):97-98, February 1986.

AIDS: a noncommunicable cofactor [letter], by R. J. Ablin. JAMA 253(23):3398-3399, June 21, 1985.

AIDS not an opportunistic infection [letter], by A. Ellrodt, et al. LANCET 2(8351):680, September 17, 1983.

AIDS not a 'social disease' [letter]. NATURE 303(5916):371, June 2-8, 1983.

AIDS notes, by S. Hyde. GAY COMMUNITY NEWS 10(50):2, July 9, 1983.

—. GAY COMMUNITY NEWS 11(3):2, July 30, 1983.

AIDS numbers don't add up, by K. Hale. ARKANSAS TIMES 12:21-24, March 1986.

AIDS: a nurse's responsibility. Care plan for home care, by D. Dickinson. CALIFORN-IA NURSE 82(4):7, May 1986.

—. Infection precautions in the community, by G. Lusby, et al. CALIFORNIA NURSE 82(4):16, May 1986.

—. Nursing's special challenge, by C. Morrisson. CALIFORNIA NURSE 82(4):1+, May 1986.

—. Safe sex guidelines for women. CALIFORNIA NURSE 82(4):8, May 1986.

AIDS: an occupational hazard?, by R. L. Cooley, et al. JOURNAL OF THE AMERICAN DENTAL ASSOCIATION 107(1):28-31, July 1983.

AIDS: occupational implications for health care workers, by K. M. O'Laughlin, et al. OCCUPATIONAL HEALTH NURSING 32(3):134-136, March 1984.

AIDS: Ohio update and comments on diagnosis, by J. C. Neff. OHIO STATE MEDICAL JOURNAL 80(2):135-138, February 1984.

AIDS: an old disease from Africa? [letter], by C. J. Lacey, et al. BRITISH MEDICAL JOURNAL 289(6443):496, August 25, 1984.

—, by K. M. De Cock. BRITISH MEDICAL JOURNAL 289(6440):306-308, August 4, 1984.

— [letter], by K. M. De Cock. BRITISH MEDICAL JOURNAL 289(6456):1454-1455, November 24, 1984.

—, by R. Colebunders, et al. BRITISH MEDICAL JOURNAL 289(6447):765, September 22, 1984.

AIDS: an old disease under a new name? RN 47:19, March 1984.

AIDS on and off Broadway, by H. Popkin. LISTENER July 11, 1985, p. 15.

AIDS on campus: what you should know, by R. P. Keeling. AGB REPORTS 28(2):24-28, March-April 1986.

AIDS on campuses: concern goes beyond health as officials prepare to handle flood of questions, by L. Biemiller. CHRONICLE OF HIGHER EDUCATION 31(5):40-41, October 2, 1985.

AIDS on the front line. EMERGENCY MEDICINE 18(1):24-28+, January 15, 1986.

AIDS on the job: bias appears hard to defend, by F. A. Silas. AMERICAN BAR ASSOCIATION JOURNAL 76:22, January 1, 1986.

AIDS on stage, by G. Weales. COMMONWEAL 112:406-407, July 12, 1985.

AIDS on Trinidad [letter], by C. Bartholomew, et al. LANCET 1(8368):103, January 14, 1984.

AIDS: once dismissd as the "gay plague," the disease has become the No. 1 public-health menace, by M. Clark, et al. NEWSWEEK 106(7):20-24, August 12, 1985.

AIDS: one answer, many questions. SCIENCE DIGEST 93:44, January 1985.

AIDS: one man's story, by P. Morrisroe. NEW YORK 18:28-35, August 19, 1985.

AIDS: one psychosocial response, by J. P. Doherty. QRB12(8):295-297, August 1986.

AIDS: opportunism and opportunity, by M. B. Mallison. AMERICAN JOURNAL OF NURSING 86(2):115, February 1986.

AIDS or acquired immunodeficiency syndrome, by J. Leikola. REVUE DE L'INFIRMIERE 33(16):37-40, October 1983.

AIDS or not AIDS? Comments on the acquired immune deficiency syndrome, by J. E. Ollé Goig. MEDICINA CLINICA 83(6):244-248, July 14, 1984.

AIDS—organizing reporting, by C. Guilfoy. GAY COMMUNITY NEWS 11(18):3, November 19, 1983.

AIDS outcome: a first follow-up [letter], by B. E. Rivin, et al. NEW ENGLAND JOURNAL OF MEDICINE 311(13):857, September 27, 1984.

AIDS pandemic, by R. C. Gallo. DUODECIM 102(7):391-393, 1986.

AIDS panel recommends early medical discharge, by S. B. Young. AIR FORCE TIMES 47:12+, October 20, 1986.

AIDS panic, by D. Viza. NATURE 317(6035):281, September 26-October 2, 1985.

AIDS-panic: AIDS-induced psychogenic states [letter], by G. O'Brien, et al. BRITISH JOURNAL OF PSYCHIATRY 147:91, July 1985.

AIDS: panic and public policy, by J. Stryker. HEALTHSPAN 2(10):3-15, November-December 1985.

AIDS panic: are you safe?, by S. Horwitz. HARPER'S BAZAAR 116:28+, August 1983.

AIDS panic blamed in defeat of rights bill, by C. Guilfoy. GUARDIAN 38(3):5, October 16, 1985.

AIDS panic disrupts American blood banks, by I. Anderson. NEW SCIENTIST 98:927, June 30, 1983.

AIDS part 1, by R. Wells. INTERNATIONAL NURSING REVIEW 32(3/261):76-77, May-June 1985.

— part 2, by P. Nuttall. INTERNATIONAL NURSING REVIEW 32(3/261):78-79+, May-June 1985.

AIDS: Pasteur plans to pursue patent: suit on virus [news], by R. Walgate, et al. NATURE 320(6058):96, March 13-19, 1986.

AIDS: Pasteur sues over patent, by T. Beardsley. NATURE 318:595, December 19-26, 1985.

AIDS patent negotiations break down, by C. Norman. SCIENCE 232:819, May 16, 1986.

AIDS patient finds the best medicine in his struggle to survive—friends, family and faith, by S. Klein. PEOPLE WEEKLY 21:77-78+, January 30, 1984.

AIDS patient isolated in prison, by D. Van Straten. OUT 4(5):5, March 1986.

AIDS patient who died too soon, by M. Turck. HOSPITAL PRACTICE 20(1):77+, January 15, 1985.

AIDS patients allowed to serve time at home. CORRECTIONS DIGEST 17(18):10, August 27, 1986.

AIDS patients and hospitals—an update. HOSPITAL SECURITY AND SAFETY MANAGEMENT 6(7):8-10, November 1985.

AIDS patients' bills add up to trouble, by L. Punch. MODERN HEALTHCARE 14(7):49, May 15, 1984.

AIDS patients' confidentiality is medical records challenge, by C. A. Siegner. MODERN HEALTHCARE 15(24):86, November 22, 1985.

AIDS patients: dealing with legal issues surrounding diagnosis and treatment, by E. K. Murphy. AORN JOURNAL 43(6):1208-1209+, June 1986.

AIDS pill that offers hope, by J. Carey. US NEWS & WORLD REPORT 101(13): 69-70, September 29, 1986.

AIDS: a plague of fear, by D. Grady, et al. READER'S DIGEST 123:152-156, October 1983.

—. DISCOVER 4:74+, July 1983.

AIDS: a plague on all their houses? THE ECONOMIST 297:27-28, November 2, 1985.

AIDS: the plague that lays waste at noon, by J. E. Fortunato. WITNESS 68(9):6-9, September 1985.

AIDS plagued by media, by M. Adams. HERIZONS 4(1):4, January 1986.

AIDS: plan for European centre agreed [news]. NATURE 305(5937):751, October 27-November 2, 1983.

AIDS plan unveiled but funding in question by S. Hyde. GAY COMMUNITY NEWS 12(36):3, March 30, 1985.

AIDS: planning for the impact, by I. Goldstone. RNABC NEWS 17(6):20, November-December 1985.

AIDS: Poland's minister for prophylaxis, by V. Rich. NATURE 317:100, September 12, 1985.

AIDS: a police hazard?, by H. V. Walker. THE POLICE CHIEF 51(7):21, July 1984.

AIDS: the politicization of an epidemic, by D. Altman. SOCIALIST REVIEW 78:93, November 1984.

AIDS: politics of premature French claim of cure, by R. Walgate. NATURE 318:3, November 7, 1985.

AIDS: the portrait of a victim, by K. S. Edwards. OHIO STATE MEDICAL JOURNAL 81(10):706+, October 1985.

AIDS poses employer dilemma, by S. Harris. AMERICAN HEALTH CARE ASSOCIATION JOURNAL 12(2):43-44, February 1986.

AIDS poses legal questions for hospital managers, by K. B. Stickler. HOSPITAL MANAGER 13(6):1-3, November-December 1983.

AIDS poses significant legal considerations for the work place, by C. D. Stromberg. BUSINESS AND HEALTH 3(3):50-51, January-February 1986.

AIDS—a potential laboratory hazard?, by C. H. Collins. GAZETTE OF THE INSTITUTE OF MEDICAL LABORATORY SCIENCES 27(8):341-342, August 1983.

AIDS—practical guidelines, by N. I. Abdou. JOURNAL OF THE KANSAS MEDICAL SOCIETY 85(3):32-84+, March 1984.

AIDS: precautions, by B. Cox. ANNA JOURNAL 13(5):283, October 1986.

—, by C. B. Persons, et al. JOURNAL OF PRACTICAL NURSING 33(8):51-53, September-October 1983.

AIDS precautions for clinical and laboratory staff. NEBRASKA NURSE 19(1):13, February 1986.

AIDS precautions for donors. SPARE RIB 161:45, December 1985.

AIDS: precautions for health care employees, by S. Hecker. OREGON NURSE 49(1): 34-35, February-March 1984.

AIDS: precautions for health care personnel, by D. LaCamera. TOPICS IN CLINICAL NURSING 6(2):45-52, July 1984.

AIDS precautions for other high-risk groups? [letter], by R. S. Klein, et al. INFECTION CONTROL 5(10):466-467, October 1984.

AIDS: prejudice and progress, by J. Levine, et al. TIME 128(10):68, September 8, 1986.

AIDS: preschool and school issues, by J. L. Black. JOURNAL OF SCHOOL HEALTH 56(3):93-95, March 1986.

AIDS prevention and treatment, by A. Ranki. DUODECIM 102(7):429-438, 1986.

AIDS: prevention strategies, by M. A. Conant. FRONTIERS OF RADIATION THERAPY AND ONCOLOGY 19:150-154, 1985.

AIDS prevention underway in B.C., by K. Scholl. RNABC NEWS15(8):9-10, November-December 1983.

AIDS: a primary concern for the pathologist, by S. Jothy, et al. CANADIAN JOURNAL OF MEDICAL TECHNOLOGY 47(4):269-270, December 1985.

AIDS priority [letter], by L. Montagnier. NATURE 310(5977):46, August 9-15, 1984.

AIDS priority fight goes to court, by C. Norman. SCIENCE 231:11-12, January 3, 1986.

AIDS: probing the heterosexual link. NEW SCIENTIST 107:15, September 19, 1985.

AIDS: a problem for intensive care, by R. A. Banks, et al. INTENSIVE CARE MEDICINE 11(4):169-171, 1985.

AIDS problem in Africa, by R. J. Biggar. LANCET 1(8472):79-83, January 11, 1986.

AIDS: profile of an epidemic, by A. Cohen. GAY COMMUNITY NEWS 12(9):8, September 15, 1984.

AIDS prognosis is grim, by D. Walter. ADVOCATE 421:8, May 28, 1985.

AIDS: a programmer of action, by M. Adler. TIMES September 6, 1985, p. 12.

AIDS progress. Synthetic vaccine only a distant prospect [news], by T. Beardsley. NATURE 314(6013):659, April 25-May 1, 1985.

AIDS: progress at last. THE ECONOMIST 291:40, April 28, 1984.

AIDS progress report, by A. Hecht. FDA CONSUMER 20:33-35, February 1986.

AIDS project inSeattle, Washington, by S. D. Helgerson. AMERICAN JOURNAL OF PUBLIC HEALTH 74:1419, December 1984.

AIDS: the promise of alternative treatments, by C. Reuben. EAST WEST JOURNAL 16(9):52, September 1986.

AIDS: prologue. ISSUES IN SCIENCE AND TECHNOLOGY 2:39, Winter 1986.

AIDS-prompted behavior changes reported, by D. E. Riesenberg. JAMA 255:171+, January 10, 1986.

AIDS: protecting the health care worker, by A. Beaufoy, et al. RNABC NEWS 17(6):18, November-December 1985.

AIDS: protecting members' rights and health, by C. Wcislo. LABOR NOTES 91:10, September 1986.

AIDS: protecting two publics, by D. Franklin. SCIENCE 6:16-17, December 1985.

AIDS protein made, by K. Wright. NATURE 319:525, February 13, 1986.

AIDS: psychosocial needs of the health care worker, by S. Simmons-Alling. TOPICS IN CLINICAL NURSING 6(2):31-37, July 1984.

AIDS: public enemy no. 1. NEWSWEEK 101:95, June 6, 1983.

AIDS: a public health and psychological emergency, by W. F. Batchelor. AMERICAN PSYCHOLOGIST 39(11):1279-1284, November 1984.

AIDS: a public health disaster, by N. Heneson. NEW SCIENTIST 108:75-76, November 14, 1985.

AIDS, public policy and biomedical research, by S. Panem. CHEST 85(3):416-422, March 1984.

AIDS: the public reacts. PUBLIC OPINION 8:35-37, December 1985-January 1986.

—. HASTINGS CENTER REPORT 15(4):23-26, August 1985.

AIDS: public safety v. rights of victims, by N. N. Jurgens. ILLINOIS ISSUES 12:13-14, July 1986.

AIDS: putting an alternative to the test, by R. Kotsch. EAST WEST JOURNAL 16(9): 52, September 1986.

AIDS—putting the press together, by C. Patton. GAY COMMUNITY NEWS 11(23):3, December 24, 1983.

AIDS: putting the puzzle together, by J. B. Peter, et al. DIAGNOSTIC MEDICINE 7(2): 56-60+, February 1984.

AIDS quarantine measure for California ballot, by Bisticas-Cocoves. GAY COMMUNITY NEWS 13(44):1, May 31, 1986.

AIDS quarantines—government and us, by S. Hyde. GAY COMMUNITY NEWS 11(35):3, March 24, 1984.

AIDS: quest for a cure. CANADA AND THE WORLD 51:8-9, October 1985.

—, by J. Langone. DISCOVER 6:75+, January 1985.

AIDS question, by W. F. Buckley. NATIONAL REVIEW 37:63, October 18, 1985.

AIDS questions grow: lawsuits, voter initiatives, handicap laws surface, by P. Marcotte. AMERICAN BAR ASSOCIATION JOURNAL 72:28, November 1, 1986.

AIDS: a rational approach. AMERICAN FAMILY PHYSICIAN 30:298, November 1984.

AIDS reaches the Soviet Union, by B. Nahaylo. SPECTATOR October 4, 1986, p. 12-13.

AIDS: recent events, by J. G. Hellstrom, et al. PROCEEDINGS, ANNUAL MEETING OF THE MEDICAL SECTION OF THE AMERICAN COUNCIL OF LIFE INSURANCE 1985, p. 69-77.

AIDS: recent findings and their dental implications, by E. Bucci, et al. MINERVA STOMATOLOGICA 35(4):247-252, April 1986.

AIDS references for health care providers, by S. Perdew. PENNSYLVANIA NURSE 41(3):16-17, March 1986.

AIDS-related brain damage unexplained, by D. M. Barnes. SCIENCE 232:1091-1093, May 30, 1986.

AIDS related complex—conumdrum, by N. Fain. ADVOCATE 3(89):20, March 6, 1984.

AIDS-related complex in a heterosexual man seven weeks after a transfusion, by R. M. E. Fincher, et al. NEW ENGLAND JOURNAL OF MEDICINE 313:1226-1227, November 7, 1985.

AIDS-related complex with lymphoid intersitial pneumonitis [letter], by J. M. Ziza, et al. NEW ENGLAND JOURNAL OF MEDICINE 313(3):183, July 18, 1985.

AIDS-related discrimination is illegal in NewYork, by P. Freiberg. ADVOCATE 453:16, August 19, 1986.

AIDS-related lymphomas: evaluation by abdominal CT, by D. A. Nyberg, et al. RADIOLOGY 159(1):59-63, April 1986.

AIDS, related syndromes and hemophilia: the situation in France and studies in progress, by J. P. Allain. REVUE FRANCAISE DE TRANSFUSION ET IMMUNO-HEMATOLOGIE 27(4):459-461, September 1984.

AIDS related virus found. BODY POLITIC 126:23, May 1986.

AIDS: a reminder on preventing the spread of blood-borne viruses while teaching blood glucose self-monitoring, by L. C. Mullen, et al. DIABETES EDUCATOR Suppl. 12:186-187, May 1986.

AIDS—report of an epidemiological seminar, by J. M. Klopper. SOUTH AFRICAN MEDICAL JOURNAL 68(8):617-618, October 12, 1985.

AIDS—report of a site visit. ADAMHA NEWS 11(20):1+, October 1985.

AIDS reportability—confiding in gov, by C. Guilfoy. GAY COMMUNITY NEWS 11(27): 6, January 28, 1984.

AIDS reported in Eastern European countries, by P. Cummings. ADVOCATE 436: 29, December 24, 1985.

AIDS repository [letter], by R. A. Kaslow. SCIENCE 229(4708):8, July 5, 1985.

AIDS research. Big enough spending? [news], by S. Budiansky. NATURE 304(5926):478, August 11-17, 1983.

AIDS research. Is there really a virus? [news], by G. Linnebank. NATURE 305(5932): 264, September 22-28, 1983.

AIDS: a research and clinical bibliography. HEMATOLOGICAL ONCOLOGY 2(1):77-134, January-March 1984.

AIDS research and incidence on the rise. AMERICAN FAMILY PHYSICIAN 28:17, October 1983.

AIDS research and 'the window of opportunity,' by W. J. Curran. NEW ENGLAND JOURNAL OF MEDICINE 312(14):903-904, April 4, 1985.

AIDS research centers sought. ADAMHA NEWS 12(3):3, March 1986.

AIDS research: charting new directions, by E. N. Brandt, Jr. PUBLIC HEALTH RE-PORTS 99(5):433-435, September-October 1984.

AIDS: research clues for etiology, by C. Lopez. SURVEY OF IMMUNOLOGIC RE-SEARCH 3(2-3):229-232, 1984.

AIDS research funding proposals more than double. AMERICAN FAMILY PHYSICIAN 32:18, October 1985.

AIDS research funding stalled; diagnostic test advances. AMERICAN FAMILY PHYSICIAN 30:18, August 1984.

AIDS research in Britain, by D. Morris. GAY COMMUNITY NEWS 10(27):2, January 29, 1983.

AIDS research in France: different culture, same virus? by V. Elliott. SCIENCE NEWS 125:285-286, May 5, 1984.

AIDS research in new phase [news], by D. M. Barnes. SCIENCE 233(4761):282-283, July 18, 1986.

AIDS research: promising drug forces reassessment. CHEMICAL AND ENGINEER-ING NEWS 64:6-7, September 29, 1986.

AIDS research stirs bitter fight over use of experimental drugs, by M. Chase. WALL STREET JOURNAL 207:29, June 18, 1986.

AIDS research, to review or not to review: by S. Budiansky. NATURE 305:349, September 29, 1983.

AIDS research, virus both advance, J. Silberner. SCIENCE NEWS 127:7, January 5, 1985.

AIDS researcher fights eviction, by B. Nelson. GAY COMMUNITY NEWS 11(14):6, October 22, 1983.

AIDS researcher wins eviction battle, by C. Smith. GAY COMMUNITY NEWS 12(17): 3, November 10, 1984.

AIDS researchers track an elusive foe, by R. M. Baum. CHEMICAL AND ENGINEER-ING NEWS 62:15-16+, January 23, 1984.

AIDS resource list. GAY COMMUNITY NEWS 11(32):4, March 3, 1984.

AIDS: responding to the crisis. Legal implications for health care providers, by M. A. Kadzielski. HEALTH PROGRESS 67(4):48-52, May 1986.

—. Pastoral care: helping patients on an inward journey, by L. J. Tibesar. HEALTH PROGRESS 67(4):41-47, May 1986.

—. A public policy agenda, by S. W. Gamble. HEALTH PROGRESS 67(4):30-33, May 1986.

—. Will the needs be met?, by J. Cassidy. HEALTH PROGRESS 67(4):53-56, May 1986.

AIDS retrovirus antibodies in hemophiliacs treated with factor VIII or factor IX concentrates, cryorecipitate, or fresh frozen plasma: prevalence, seroconversion rate, and clinical correlations, by M. V. Ragni, et al. BLOOD 67(3):592-595, March 1986.

AIDS retrovirus (ARV-2) clone replicates in transfected human and animal fibroblasts, by J. A. Levy, et al. SCIENCE 232:998-1001, May 23, 1986.

AIDS retrovirus induced cytopathology: giant cell formation and involvement of CD4 antigen, by J. D. Lifson, et al. SCIENCE 232:1123-1127, May 30, 1986.

AIDS—a review, by J. Cohen. BRITISH JOURNAL OF HOSPITAL MEDICINE 31(4): 250-254+, April 1984.

AIDS—risk and rights—response of the trade union movement, by D. Lowe. LAMP 42(6):26-28, August 1985.

AIDS risk category broadened. FDA CONSUMER 19(9):34, November 1985.

AIDS: a risk for diabetes educators?, by C. A. Jenkins, et al. DIABETES EDUCATOR Suppl. 12:185-186, May 1986.

AIDS: the risk for women, by Farrell, et al. COMMUNIQU'ELLES 12(2):20, March 1986.

AIDS risk found low for people with working with patients. CORRECTIONS DIGEST 16(10):6-7, May 8, 1985.

—. CRIME CONTROL DIGEST 19(19):4, May 13, 1985.

AIDS risk-group profiles in whites and members of minority groups [letter], by R. Bakeman, et al. NEW ENGLAND JOURNAL OF MEDICINE 315(3):191-192, July 17, 1986.

AIDS risk groups include some women, by P. Turner. OUT 4(4):7, February 1986.

AIDS—risk groups, risk factors, measures. LAKARTIDNINGEN 82(11):958+, March 13, 1985.

AIDS: the risk to you, by W. F. Taylor. SURGICAL TECHNOLOGIST 18(4):17-20, July-August 1986.

AIDS: the risks to insurers, the threat to equity, by G. M. Oppenheimer, et al. HASTINGS CENTER REPORT 16:18-22, October 1986.

AIDS rodeo benefit, by P. Byron. GAY COMMUNITY NEWS 11(13):3, October 15, 1983.

AIDS: safeguards, not panic [editorial]. BRITISH DENTAL JOURNAL 158(6):195, March 23, 1985.

AIDS: "safer sex" is the best solution so far, by M. Jay. NEW SOCIETY December 12, 1985, p. 12-13.

AIDS—safety practices for clinical and research laboratories, by J. V. Federico, et al. INFECTION CONTROL 5(4):185-187, April 1984.

AIDS: saliva is safe. NEW SCIENTIST 105:7, February 28, 1985.

AIDS saliva link is questioned. NEW SCIENTIST 105:5, February 14, 1985.

AIDS: the saliva scare, by J. Seligmann, et al. NEWSWEEK 104(17):103, October 22, 1984.

AIDS scare prompts concern about communion, by V. F. A. Golphin. NATIONAL CATHOLIC REPORTER 22:6, November 1, 1985.

AIDS, the schools, and policy issues, by J. H. Price. JOURNAL OF SCHOOL HEALTH 56(4):137-140, April 1986.

AIDS screening: false test results raise doubts, by S. Budiansky. NATURE 312:583, December 13, 1984.

AIDS screening predicted for entire force, by P. J. Budahn. AIR FORCE TIMES 46: 1+, October 21, 1985.

AIDS screening test now available to everyone, by D. Bradford. AUSTRALIAN FAMI-LY PHYSICIAN 14(5):463, May 1985.

AIDS—selective disease or public epidemic, by R. Baumgarten, et al. ZEITSCHRIFT FUR ARZTLICHE FORTBILDUNG 79(18):761-762, 1985.

AIDS: sense not fear [editorial], by M. W. Adler, et al. BRITISH MEDICAL JOURNAL 288(6425):1177-1178, April 21, 1984.

AIDS serology testing in low- and high-risk groups, by J. R. Carlson, et al. JAMA 253(23):3405-3408, June 21, 1985.

AIDS: sharing out the spoils. NEW SCIENTIST 108:14, October 10, 1985.

AIDS—should we care, by B. Miller. SPARE RIB 141:28, April 1984.

AIDS show adapted, by S. Hachem. ADVOCATE 450:36, July 6, 1986.

AIDS: Sifting for facts about a puzzling disease, by D. H. Murphy. AMERICAN PHAR-MACY NS23(10):18-22, October 1983.

AIDS—solution: a difficult fight against prejudice, by C. Almedal. SYKEPLEIEN 73(10):24-25+, June 6, 1986.

AIDS: some unanswered questions . . . human host's response to foreign organisms, by C. Carneiro. MASSACHUSETTS NURSE 54(3):1+, March 1985.

AIDS: some unsettling questions, by R. Bier. BEST'S REVIEW 86:16+, January 1986.

AIDS—something new under the sun [editorial], by S. G. Baum. LUNG 161(4):193-194, 1983.

AIDS: special report, by J. Langone. DISCOVER 6:28-33+, December 1985.

AIDS spitting case dismissed. CRIME CONTROL DIGEST 20(33):8, August 18, 1986.

AIDS: spreading mystery disease, by R. Thompson. EDITORIAL RESEARCH REPORTS pp. 599-616, August 9, 1985.

AIDS: a spreading scourge, by C. Wallis. TIME 126:50-51, August 5, 1985.

AIDS spreads to the courts, by A. Press. NEWSWEEK 106:61, July 1, 1985.

AIDS: statistics in Puerto Rico and useful references, by J. G. Rigau-Pérez, et al. BOLETIN—ASOCIACION MEDICA DE PUERTO RICO 76(3):120-122, March 1984.

AIDS statistics released. OUT 3(4):1, February 1985.

AIDS—status 1985. Implications for sperm banks, by J. O. Nielsen. INTERNA-TIONAL JOURNAL OF ANDROLOGY 8(2):97-100, April 1985.

AIDS—still no concensus, by M. Hamilton. OCCUPATIONAL HEALTH 38(3):76, March 1986.

AIDS: the story of one family's pain, by J. McBride. US 3:38+, August 26, 1985.

AIDS stretching VA's ability to treat veterans, by J. Firshein. HOSPITALS 60(4):33-34, February 20, 1986.

AIDS-stricken inmate bites deputy; charged with attempted murder. CORRECTIONS DIGEST 17(12):3, June 4, 1986; also in CRIME CONTROL DIGEST 20(22):9-10, June 2, 1986.

AIDS strikes a star, by D. Gelman. NEWSWEEK 106:68-69, August 5, 1985.

AIDS studied among drug users. ADAMHA NEWS 11(11):1+, November 1985.

AIDS study finds virus is widespread. NEW SCIENTIST 106:3, April 25, 1985.

AIDS: a suitable place for treatment?, by N. Heneson, et al. NEW SCIENTIST 109:24, March 13, 1986.

AIDS support organizations and information services. QRB12(8):304-305, August 1986.

AIDS: a surgeon's responsibility, by M. T. Lotze. BULLETIN OF THE AMERICAN COLLEGE OF SURGEONS 70(9):6-12, September 1985.

AIDS surveillance and health education: use of previously described risk factors to identify high-risk homosexuals, by R. O. Valdiserri, et al. AMERICAN JOURNAL OF PUBLIC HEALTH 74(3):259-260, March 1984.

AIDS surveillance in haemophilia, by H. M. Daly, et al. BRITISH JOURNAL OF HAE-MATOLOGY 59(2):383-390, February 1985.

AIDS survival study, by S. Poggi. GAY COMMUNITY NEWS 13(46):2, June 14, 1986.

AIDS: a task for the churces, by E. Norman. TIMES October 13, 1986, p. 14.

AIDS-test ambiguities raise concert. BODY POLITIC 107:17, October 1984.

AIDS: test companies chosen [news], by S. Budiansky. NATURE 310(5972):6, July 5-11, 1984.

"AIDS test" guidelines issued, by N. Fain. ADVOCATE 417:26, April 2, 1985.

"AIDS" test a misnomer [letter], by A. J. Pinching. BRITISH MEDICAL JOURNAL 291(6498):821, September 21, 1985.

AIDS test: no comfort to many, by B. Bower, et al. SCIENCE NEWS 128:2, September 7, 1985.

AIDS test ordered to screen recruits, by P. Smith. AIR FORCE TIMES 46:3, September 16, 1985.

AIDS testing by insurers sparks acrimonious dabate. BEST'S REVIEW 86:100, February 1986.

AIDS testing for all troops to start September 1, by L. Famiglietti. AIR FORCE TIMES 46:1+, July 21, 1986.

AIDS testing opposed for civilians, dependents, by P. Smith. AIR FORCE TIMES 46: 4, December 9, 1985.

AIDS: testing program launched in Vancouver, by M. Rekart. RNABC NEWS 17(6): 23, November-December 1985.

AIDS testing sought. BODY POLITIC 127:23, June 1986.

AIDS tests alarm blood banks, by S. Budiansky. NATURE 313:87, January 10, 1985.

AIDS tests and cures [news]. AMERICAN FAMILY PHYSICIAN 28(6):250, December 1983.

AIDS tests could trigger world blood shortage, by O. Sattaur. NEW SCIENTIST 106: 6, May 16, 1985.

AIDS tests that could offer proof positive, by J. O. Hamilton. BUSINESS WEEK April 28, 1986, p. 27-28.

AIDS tests workplace policies. MANAGEMENT WORLD 15:4, February 1986.

AIDS that Africa could do without, by A. Veitch. GUARDIAN October 31, 1984, p. 13.

AIDS therapy by blocking CD4+ cells [letter], by A. Singer, et al. NATURE 320(6058): 113, March 13-19, 1986.

AIDS therapy: new push for clinical trials [news], by C. Norman. SCIENCE 230(4732): 1355-1358, December 20, 1985.

AIDS theapy: a step closer?, by M. Clark. NEWSWEEK 107(8):60, February 24, 1986.

AIDS: a time bomb at hospitals' door, by D. Burda, et al. HOSPITALS 60(1):54-61, January 5, 1986.

AIDS—this century's catastrophe? 1. Origin and cause, by B. A. Ostby. SYKE-PLEIEN 73(5):12-17+, March 7, 1986.

AIDS: 'This is not a little problem,' by A. W. Rogers. TEXAS HOSPITALS 41(11):10-11, April 1986.

AIDS—thorough information is never wasted, by E. Schmeltzer, et al. SYGEPLE-
JERSKEN 86(32):26-29, August 6, 1986.

AIDS: a threat to physical and psychological integrity, by L. J. Ryan. TOPICS IN CLIN-
ICAL NURSING 6(2):19-25, July 1984.

AIDS: the tip of the iceberg, by M. Helquist. ADVOCATE 427:32, June 20, 1985.

Aids to the laboratory diagnosis of AIDS [editorial], by R. Penny. PATHOLOGY 16(4):
375-377, October 1984.

AIDS to the rescue?, by M. Beauchamp. FORBES 136:72+, November 18, 1985.

AIDS to understanding [review article]. THE ECONOMIST 299:110, May 3, 1986.

AIDS toll expected to soar, by M. Helquist. ADVOCATE 453:23, August 19, 1986.

AIDS toll on hospital workers, by M. Helquist. ADVOCATE 442:25, March 18, 1986.

AIDS toll rises. US NEWS & WORLD REPORT 97:80, November 26, 1984.

AIDS: too few facts, by A. J. Fugh-Berman. OFF OUR BACKS 13(10):12+, November 11, 1983.

AIDS: too hot to study: gays protest as the U of A drops research, by T. Philip. AL-
BERTA REPORT 11:26, June 4, 1984.

AIDS: the trail of tainted blood, by M. Clark. NEWSWEEK 108(8):55, August 24,
1986.

AIDS, transfusion and hemophilia, still a mysterious relationship. Comments and hypotheses, by J. F. Bach. REVUE FRANCAISE DE TRANSFUSION ET IMMUNO-
HEMATOLOGIE 27(4):455-458, September 1984.

AIDS: transfusion patients may be at risk, by O. Sattaur. NEW SCIENTIST 97:289,
February 3, 1983.

AIDS—the transmissible immunologic deficiency disease, by U. A. Baumann, et al.
VASA 13(2):94-98, 1984.

AIDS transmission. AMERICAN FAMILY PHYSICIAN 29:388+, March 1984.

AIDS transmission [letter], by J. M. Campbell. WESTERN JOURNAL OF MEDICINE
144(1):92, January 1986.

AIDS transmission via transfusion therapy [letter], by S. C. Dereinski, et al. LANCET
1(8368):102, January 14, 1984.

AIDS transmission: what about the hepatitis B vaccine? [news], by C. Macek. JAMA
249(6):685-686, February 11, 1983.

AIDS trends: projections from limited data, by C. Norman. SCIENCE 230:1018-1021,
November 29, 1985.

AIDS triggers painful legal battles, by T. Gest. US NEWS & WORLD REPORT
100(11):73-74, March 24, 1986.

AIDS: trust not fear, by J. Imhoff. CATHOLIC WORKER 52:1+, September 1985.

AIDS: turmoil in the medical profession, by K. Weiss. NEW PHYSICIAN 32(6):13-17, June 1983.

AIDS: the twentieth century plague, by J. G. Bellows. COMPREHENSIVE THERAPY 11(11):3, November 1985.

AIDS: two British blood tests launched, by M. Clarke. NATURE 316:474, August 8, 1985.

AIDS—two years later [editorial], by J. W. Curran. NEW ENGLAND JOURNAL OF MEDICINE 309(10):609-611, September 8, 1983.

AIDS—the undeclared war, by G. Halak. OUT 2(8):5, July 1984.

AIDS: undesirable import to Japan, by D. Swinbanks. NATURE 315:8, May 2, 1985.

AIDS "unreasonable anxiety" ambiguous research. BODY POLITIC 110:18, January 1985.

AIDS update. AMERICAN FAMILY PHYSICIAN 30:322+, September 1984.

—. FDA DRUG BULLETIN 13(2):9-11, August 1983.

—. SCIENCE NEWS 128:40, July 20, 1985.

—. SCIENTIFIC AMERICAN 252:70, April 1985.

—. US NEWS & WORLD REPORT 98:48, February 18, 1985.

—, by B. Olson, et al. PRAIRIE ROSE 54(4):16, October-December 1985.

—, by L. M. Aledort. HOSPITAL PRACTICE 18(9):159-165+, September 1983.

—, by V. Gong, et al. MARYLAND MEDICAL JOURNAL 35(5):361-371, May 1986.

AIDS update: HTLV-III testing, immune globulins and employees with AIDS, by W. M. Valenti. INFECTION CONTROL 7(8):427-430, August 1986.

AIDS update: HTLV-III/LAV infection, by B. J. Cassens. PENNSYLVANIA MEDICINE 89(1):24-26, January 1986.

AIDS update: little to cheer about, by S. Hyde. GAY COMMUNITY NEWS 12(20):3, December 1, 1984.

AIDS: an update on what we know now, by D. Anderson. RN 49(3):49-54+, March 1986.

AIDS update Part 2, by W. M. Valenti. INFECTION CONTROL 6(10):421-423, October 1985.

AIDS update: search for Agent X, by P. Taulbee. SCIENCE NEWS 123:245, April 16, 1983.

AIDS ups direct-donation demand, by B. Mccormick. HOSPITALS 60(11):80, June 5, 1986.

AIDS: US administration's parsimony criticized, by S. Budiansky. NATURE 313:725, February 28, 1985.

AIDS: US and French institutes in patents struggle, by R. Walgate, et al. NATURE 317:373, October 3, 1985.

AIDS: US blood-bank test established, by T. Beardsley. NATURE 316:474, August 8, 1985.

AIDS: US company rejects UK decision, by M. Clarke. NATURE 316:759, August 29, 1985.

AIDS: US law delays drug testing, by T. Beardsley. NATURE 317:568, October 17, 1985.

AIDS: USAR testing starts in 1986, by B. Pratt. ARMY RESERVE MAGAZINE 32(2): 15, Spring 1986.

AIDS vaccine: a glimmer of hope. THE ECONOMIST 298:90, March 22, 1986.

AIDS vaccine research: promising protein, by L. Davis. SCIENCE NEWS 129:151, March 8, 1986.

AIDS versus prodromal AIDS [letter]. UGESKRIFT FOR LAEGER 146(9):673-674, February 27, 1984.

AIDS victims can obtain health cover via state pooling arrangements, by L. Kocolowski. NATIONAL UNDERWRITER 89:3, October 4, 1985.

AIDS victims can obtain health cover via state shared-risk pools, by L. Kocolowski. NATIONAL UNDERWRITER 89:4+, September 28, 1985.

AIDS victims, modern pariahs [editorial], by D. Scott. POSTGRADUATE MEDICINE 78(5):21+, October 1985.

AIDS victims pose threat to health in life, death. JET 67:37, January 28, 1985.

AIDS: victim's rights vs. the public's, by T. Philip, et al. ALBERTA REPORT 13:32-33, September 1, 1986.

AIDS victims still await vaccine, by O. Sattaur. NEW SCIENTIST 105:20, January 24, 1985.

AIDS virology: a battle on many fronts [news], by C. Norman. SCIENCE 230(4725): 518-521, November 1, 1985.

AIDS virus, by T. Kitamura. NIPPON RINSHO43(8):1783-1789, August 1985.

AIDS virus and HTLV-I differ in codon choices [letter], by P. Grantham, et al. NATURE 319(6056):727-728, February 27-March 5, 1986.

AIDS: virus clones multiply, by T. Beardsley. NATURE 311:195, September 20, 1984.

AIDS virus entry pinpointed in brain [news], by R. Lewin. SCIENCE 233(4760):160, July 11, 1986.

AIDS virus: equine similarities? by J. Silberner. SCIENCE NEWS 129:84, February 8, 1986.

AIDS virus genome sequenced, by R. Baum. CHEMICAL AND ENGINEERING NEWS 63:32-34, February 18, 1985.

AIDS virus genomes [news], by J. L. Marx. SCIENCE 227(4686):503, February 1, 1985.

AIDS virus has new name—perhaps, by J. L. Marx. SCIENCE 232:699-700, May 9, 1986.

AIDS virus: how many kinds? SCIENCE 6:8, November 1985.

AIDS virus in the brain. NEW SCIENTIST 108:29, December 5, 1985.

AIDS virus in military blood donations drops. AIR FORCE TIMES 46:18, June 23, 1986.

AIDS— a virus infection?, by J. Abb, et al. HAUTARZT 35(12):615-616, December 1984.

AIDS virus infection in Nairobi prostitutes: spread of the epidemic to East Africa, by J. K. Kreiss, et al. NEW ENGLAND JOURNAL OF MEDICINE 314:414-418, February 13, 1986.

AIDS virus infection: prognosis and transmission [letter]. JOURNAL OF THE ROYAL SOCIETY OF MEDICINE 79(2):121-123, February 1986.

AIDS virus infection: prognosis and transmission [editorial], by J. Seale. JOURNAL OF THE ROYAL SOCIETY OF MEDICINE 78(8):613-615, August 1985.

AIDS virus: infection up? SCIENCE NEWS 128:325, November 23, 1985.

AIDS: the virus is not immune, by J. Weber. NEW SCIENTIST 109:37-39, January 2, 1986.

AIDS virus is spreading and mutating, by C. Joyce. NEW SCIENTIST 104:9, October 18, 1984.

AIDS virus might cause brain disease, by O. Sattaur. NEW SCIENTIST 106:21, April 25, 1985.

AIDS virus not transmitted through tears, experts say. OHIO NURSES REVIEW 61(1):3, January 1986.

AIDS virus presents moving target, by C. Norman. SCIENCE 230:1357, December 20, 1985.

AIDS virus rarely in salive, researchers say. CORRECTIONS DIGEST 17(3):10, January 29, 1986.

AIDS virus shows a chink in its armour. THE ECONOMIST 297:105, November 16, 1985.

AIDS virus structure and disease transmission analyzed. AMERICAN FAMILY PHYSICIAN 31:275-276+, April 1985.

AIDS: waiting for cure or treatment, by J. Silberner. SCIENCE NEWS 128:229, October 12, 1985.

AIDS watch. NURSING 14:15+, July 1984.

AIDS—what is it?, by I. Goldstone. RNABC NEWS 17(6):12-15, November - December 1985.

AIDS: what is it? Who is at risk? How can it be prevented?, by W. R. Dowdle. PUBLIC WELFARE 44(3):14-19, Summer1986.

AIDS: what is now known: part 1, history and immunovirology, by P. A. Selwyn. HOSPITAL PRACTICE 21(5):67-76, May 15, 1986.

—: part 2, epidemiology, by P. A. Selwyn. HOSPITAL PRACTICE 21(6):127-129+, June 15, 1986.

—: part 3, clinical aspects, by P. A. Selwyn. HOSPITAL PRACTICE 21(9):119-131+, September 15, 1986.

—: part 4, psychosocial aspects, treatment prospects, by P. A. Selwyn. HOSPITAL PRACTICE 21(10):125-128+, October 15, 1986.

AIDS: what is our response, by H. C. McGehee, Jr. WITNESS 68(8):4, August 1985.

AIDS: what is to be done? HARPER'S 271:39-52, October 1985.

AIDS: what it does to a family, by K. Barrett. LADIES' HOME JOURNAL 100:98+, November 1983.

AIDS: what newspapers, radio and TV unfortunately grimly have to say . . . (various simple tools to fight against the spread of the virus), by L. Thiry. REVUE DE L'INFIRMIERE 36(6):30-32, March 1986.

AIDS: what precautions do you take in the hospital? by J. Bennett. AMERICAN JOURNAL OF NURSING 86(8):952-953, August 1986.

AIDS: what Sweden is doing to meet the peril of a disease that has already claimed 20,000 victims worldwide, by M. Jeffries. SWEDEN NOW 19(6):22-25, 1985.

AIDS: what women must know now!, by D. R. Zimmerman, et al. GOOD HOUSEKEEPING 201:245-246, November 1985.

AIDS: what you should know; interview by Sally Armstrong, by C. Tsoukas. CANADIAN LIVING 11:53-55, January 1986.

AIDS; the widening gyre, by J. E. Groopman, et al. NATURE 303:575-576, June 16, 1983.

AIDS will increase tenfold in the US. NEW SCIENTIST 110:26, June 19, 1986.

AIDS: winter conference update, by R. A. Kiel. CORRECTIONS TODAY 48(3):32+, May 1986.

AIDS: witchhunt aura surrounds Pentagon testing, by K. Gilberd. GUARDIAN 38(19):9, February 12, 1986.

AIDS with central nervous system toxoplasmosis [letter], by D. Moskopp. JOURNAL OF NEUROSURGERY 62(3):459-460, March 1985.

AIDS with Mycobacterium avium-intracellulare lesions resembling those of Whipple's disease [letter]. NEW ENGLAND JOURNAL OF MEDICINE 309(21):1323-1325, November 24, 1983.

AIDS—women get, more rarely give, by A. Henry. OFF OUR BACKS 15:12-13, November 1985.

AIDS work funded. OUT 3(2):4, December 1984.

AIDS worker: confentiality prime concern, by B. Egerton. OUT 2(9):5, August 1984.

AIDS: a world with no hiding place, by T. Prentice. TIMES November 19, 1986, p. 16.

Air Force plans to test 34,000 monthly for AIDS, by L. Famiglietti. AIR FORCE TIMES 46:3, May 26, 1986.

Alarm on AIDS: government bias feared, by C. Frank. AMERICAN BAR ASSOCIATION JOURNAL 71:22, December 1985.

"Alarming" AIDS policy unveiled in Cambridge, by K. Westheimer. GAY COMMUNITY NEWS 13(33):1, March 8, 1986.

Alberta's AIDS menace: doctors seek solutions as the non-homosexual public begins to panic, by S. Weatherbe. ALBERTA REPORT 12:46-51, November 25, 1985.

Alert on AIDS. FDA CONSUMER 17:2, June 1983.

Alimentary tract biopsy lesions in the acquired immune deficiency syndrome, by H. Rotterdam, et al. PATHOLOGY 17(2):181-192, April 1985.

All about AIDS. GAY COMMUNITY NEWS 10(31):11, February 26, 1983; also in USA TODAY 112:16+, October 1983.

All blood donors must be tested for AIDS, by I. Lernevall. VARDFACKET 9(11):24, June 13, 1985.

All quiet on the tabloid front, by B. Morton. THE TIMES HIGHER EDUCATION SUPPLEMENT 658:13, June 14, 1985.

All so young, by T. Fennell. ALBERTA REPORT 12:48, November 25, 1985.

All who come to its doors, by T. J. Druhot. HEALTH PROGRESS 67(4):80, May 1986.

Allogeneic leukocytes as a possible factor in induction of AIDS in homosexual men [letter], by G. M. Shearer. NEW ENGLAND JOURNAL OF MEDICINE 308(4):223-224, January 27, 1983.

Alpha-interferon administration in cytomegalovirus retinitis, by S. W. Chou, et al. ANTIMICROBIAL AGENTS AND CHEMOTHERAPY 25(1):25-28, January 1984.

Alpha interferon therapy of Kaposi's sarcoma in AIDS, by P. Volberding, et al. ANNALS OF THE NEW YORK ACADEMY OF SCIENCES 437:439-446, 1984.

Alteration of T-cell functions by infection with HTLV-I or HTLV-II, by M. Popovic, et al. SCIENCE 226:459-462, October 26, 1984.

Alterations of functional subsets of T helper and T suppressor cell populations in acquired immunodeficiency syndrome (AIDS) and chronic unexplained lymphadenopathy, by J. K. Nicholson, et al. JOURNAL OF CLINICAL IMMUNOLOGY 5(4):269-274, July 1985.

Altered distribution of T-lymphocyte subpopulations in children and adolescents with haemophilia, by N. L. Luban, et al. LANCET 1(8323):503-505, March 5, 1983.

Altered distribution of T-lymphocyte subpopulations in lymph nodes from patients with acquired immunodeficiency-like syndrome and hemophilia, by P. R. Meyer, et al. JOURNAL OF PEDIATRICS 103(3):407-410, September 1983.

Alternative care helps firms reduce costs to treat AIDS, by S. Taravella. BUSINESS INSURANCE 19(39):1+, September 30, 1985.

Alternative health approaches to AIDS: conference, by Wolhandle. GAY COMMUN-
ITY NEWS 13(34):8, March 15, 1986.

Alternative sites for screening blood for antibodies to AIDS virus [letter]. NEW ENG-
LAND JOURNAL OF MEDICINE 313(318):1157-1158, October 31, 1985.

Alternative therapies: hope for people w/AIDS?, by M. Helquist. ADVOCATE 435:43,
Decemebr 10, 1985.

AMA challenges Department of Justice ruling on employees with AIDS. CRIME
CONTROL DIGEST 20(29):4-5, July 21, 1986.

—. CORRECTIONS DIGEST 17(15):8, July 16, 1986.

Ambivalent support for AIDS vaccine, by N. Fain. ADVOCATE 419:22, April 30,
1985.

Amen corner: AIDS hysteria and the common cup: take a drink, by R. W. Horda.
WORSHIP 60:67-73, January 1986.

American AIDS team in talks with British PWAs, by A. Lumsden. NEW STATESMAN
109:5, May 24, 1985.

Americans stop talks about AIDS discovery, by S. Connor. NEW SCIENTIST 110:30,
May 15, 1986.

AMI hopes to convert Houston hospital into AIDS research and treatment center.
REVIEW OF THE FEDERATION OF AMERICAN HEALTH SYSTEMS 19(2):108-
109, March-April 1986.

Amid the debate over AIDS tests, some progress. DISCOVER 6:12, March 1985.

Amprolium for coccidiosis in AIDS [letter], by S. J. Veldhuyze van Zanten, et al. LAN-
CET 2(8398):345-346, August 1984.

ANA reaffirms position on health care for AIDS patients. PENNSYLVANIA NURSE
41(2):7, February 1986.

ANA surveys state nurses' associations on AIDS. PULSE OF THE MONTANA
STATE NURSES ASSOCIATION 23(4):1, April 1986.

ANA urges nurses to read CDC guidelines on AIDS. PENNSYLVANIA NURSE 41(2):
6+, February 1986.

ANA urges use of CDC guidelines for care of AIDS patients. FLORIDA NURSE
34(10):3, November 1985.

Anal intercourse as a possible factor in heterosexual transmission of HTLV-III to
spouses of hemophiliacs [letter],by M. Melbye, et al. NEW ENGLAND JOURNAL
OF MEDICINE 312(13):857, March 28, 1985.

Analysis of cytomegalovirus and Epstein-Barr virus antibody respOnses in treated
hemophiliacs; implications for the study of acquired immune deficiency
syndrome, by S. H. Cheeseman, et al. JAMA 252:83-85, July 6, 1984.

Analysis of the interferon system in African patients with acquired immunodeficiency
syndrome, by K. Huygen, et al. EUROPEAN JOURNAL OF CLINICAL MICROBI-
OLOGY 4(3):304-309, June 9185.

Analysis of retinal cotton-wool spots and cytomegalovirus retinitis in the acquired immunodeficiency syndrome [letter], by J. S. Pepose, et al. AMERICAN JOURNAL OF OPHTHALMOLOGY 95(1):118-120, January 1983.

Analysis of serum samples positive for HTLV-III antibodies, by J. C. Petricciani, et al. NEW ENGLAND JOURNAL OF MEDICINE 313:47-48, July 4, 1985.

Analysis of T cell subsets in different clinical subgroups of patients with the acquired immune deficiency syndrome. Comparison with the 'classic' form of Kaposi's sarcoma, by A. Mittelman, et al. AMERICAN JOURNAL OF MEDICINE 78(6, Part 1): 951-956, June 1985.

Anatomy of an epidemic, by J. Lieberson. THE NEW YORK REVIEW OF BOOKS 30: 17-22, August 18, 1983.

Anatomy of a media epidemic, by B. Odair. ALTERNATIVE MEDIA 14(3):10, Fall 1983.

Anatomy of a panic, by R. McKie, et al. OBSERVER February 24, 1985, p. 11.

Anderson closes bathhouse, cites AIDS, by Brooke, et al. ADVOCATE 424:16, July 9, 1985.

ANG joins in testing for AIDS, by P. Dalton. AIR FORCE TIMES 46:6, July 28, 1986.

ANG to begin screening members for AIDS, by P. Dalton. AIR FORCE TIMES 46:9, May 19, 1986.

Angioimmunoblastic lymphadenopathy with dysproteinemia in homosexual men with acquired immune deficiency syndrome, by W. Blumenfeld, et al. ARCHIVES OF PATHOLOGY AND LABORATORY MEDICINE 107(11):567-569, November 1983.

Angry New York doctor turns south-of-the-border smuggler to treat patients in danger of AIDS, by S. Haller. PEOPLE 23(16):139-140+, October 14, 1985.

Animal models of AIDS, by J. F. Manser. RESEARCH RESOURCES REPORTER 7(6):1-4, June 1983.

—, by N. L. Letvin, et al. SEMINARS IN ONCOLOGY 11(1):18-28, March 1984.

Another AIDS treatment , by J. Rogers. MACLEAN'S 98:61, November 11, 1985.

Another cause of diarrhea in AIDS [letter], by H. Edelstein, et al. WESTERN JOURNAL OF MEDICINE 142(2);262, February 1985.

Another cell victim of AIDS virus? SCIENCE NEWS 129:24, January 11, 1986.

Another look at the acquired immunodeficiency syndrome, by M. L. Santaella. BOLETIN—ASOCIACION MEDICA DE PUERTO RICO 76(6):249-251, June 1984.

Another scourge plagues Africa, by J. Drury. LISTENER June 5, 1986, p. 10.

Answer to AIDS/ a herpes vaccine? SCIENCE DIGEST 92:42, January 1984.

Answering the AIDS alarm, by J. Lang. RESTAURANT BUSINESS 84:108-109+, December 10, 1985.

Anti-AIDS agents show varying early results in vitro and in vivo, by D. E. Riesenberg, et al. JAMA 254:2521+, November 8, 1985.

Anti-genes attack AIDS virus, by J. Green. NEW SCIENTIST 111:23, August 28, 1986.

Anti-HTLV-III antibody incidence [letter], by J. Goldbaum. MEDICAL JOURNAL OF AUSTRALIA 143(6):261-262, September 16, 1985.

Anti-lymphocyte antibodies in patients with the acquired immune deficiency syndrome, by B. Dorsett, et al. AMERICAN JOURNAL OF MEDICINE 78(4):621-626, April 1985.

Antibodies against human T-cell leukemia virus (HTLV) in male homosexuals with acquired immunodeficiency syndrome, by R. Kurth, et al. MUENCHENER MEDIZINISCHE WOCHENSCHRIFT 125(48):1118-1123, December 2, 1983.

Antibodies against human T-cell leukemia virus type III in acquired immunodeficiency syndrome and persistent lymphadenopathy, by D. Wernicke, et al. DEUTSCHE MEDIZINISCHE WOCHENSCHRIFT 109(45):1709-1711, November 9, 1984.

Antibodies reactive with human T-lymphotropic retroviruses (HTLV-III) in the serum of patients with AIDS, by M. G. Sarngadharan,e t al. SCIENCE 224(4648):506-508, May 4, 1984.

Antibodies to adult T-cell leukemia virus (ATLV/HTLV-I) in AIDS patients and people at risk of AIDS in Germany, by G. Hunsmann, et al. MEDICAL MICROBIOLOGY AND IMMUNOLOGY 173(5):241-250, 1985.

Antibodies to AIDS-associated retrovirus distinguish between pediatric primary and acquired immunodeficiency diseases, by A. J. Ammann, et al. JAMA 253(21): 3116-3118, June 7, 1985.

Antibodies to the AIDS virus: methods of detection and clinical significance, by B. Hirschel. THERAPEUTISCHE UMSCHAU 43(2):128-132, February 1986.

Antibodies to cell membrane antigens associated with human T-cell leukemia virus in patients with AIDS, by M. Essex, et al. SCIENCE 220(4599):859-862, May 20, 1983.

Antibodies to the core protein of lymphadenopathy-associated virus (LAV) in patients with AIDS, by V. S. Kalyanaraman, et al. SCIENCE 225(4659):321-323, July 20, 1984.

Antibodies to HTLV I and III in sera from two Japanese patients, one with possible pre-AIDS [letter], by T. Aoki, et al. LANCET 2(8408):936-937, October 20, 1984.

Antibodies to HTLV-III and the lymphadenopathy syndrome in multitransfused beta-thalassemia patients, by M. DeMartino, et al. VOX SANGUINIS 49(3):230-233, 1985.

Antibodies to HTLV-III associated antigens in populations exposed to AIDS virus in France [letter], by D. Mathez, et al. LANCET a2(8400):460, August 25, 1984.

Antibodies to HTLV-III in patients with acquired immunodeficiency or lymphadenopathy syndrome in West Germany [letter], by R. Hehlmann, et al. LANCET 2(8411):1094, November 10, 1984.

Antibodies to HTLV-III in Swiss patients with AIDS and pre-AIDS and in groups at risk for AIDS, by J. Schüpbach, et al. NEW ENGLAND JOURNAL OF MEDICINE 312(5):265-270, January 31, 1985.

Antibodies to human T-cell leukemia virus membrane antigens (HTLV-MA) in hemophiliacs, by M. Essex, et al. SCIENCE 221:1061-1064, September 9, 1983.

Antibodies to human T-lymphotropic virus type III and development of the acquired immunodeficiency syndrome in homosexual men presenting with immune thrombocytopenia, by D. I. Abrams, et al. ANNALS OF INTERNAL MEDICINE 104(1): 47-50, January 1986.

Antibodies to human T lymphotropic virus type III demonstrated by a dot immunobinding assay, by G. Biberfeld, et al. SCANDINAVIAN JOURNAL OF IMMUNOLOGY 21(3):289-292, March 1985.

Antibodies to human T-lymphotropic virus type III (HTLV-III) in saliva of acquired immunodeficiency syndrome (AIDS) patients and in persons at risk for AIDS, by D. W. Archibald, et al. BLOOD 67(3):831-834, March 1986.

Antibodies to a retrovirus etiologically associated with acquired immnodeficiency syndrome (AIDS) in populations with increased incidences of the syndrome. JAMA 252:608-609, August 3, 1984; also in MMWR 33(27):377-379, July 13, 1984.

Antibodies to simian T-lymphotropic retovirus type III in African green monkeys and recognition of STLV-III viral proteins by AIDS and related sera, by P. J. Kanki, et al. LANCET 1(8441):1330-1332, June 8, 1985.

Antibody finding may hasten AIDS vaccine. CHEMICAL ENGINEERING NEWS 64:5-6, May 26, 1986.

Antibody seronegative human T-lymphotropic virus type III (HTLV-III)-infected patients with acquired immunodeficiency syndrome or related disorders, by J. E. Groopman, et al. BLOOD 66(3):742-744, September 1985.

Antibody Test Amendment passes, by M. Martinek. OUT 3(9):3, July 1985.

Antibody-test debate ranges in Atlanta, by D. Walter. ADVOCATE 420:9, May 14, 1985.

Antibody to HTLV-III in blood donors in central Africa [letter], by P. Van de Perre, et al. LANCET 1(8424):336-337, February 9, 1985.

Antibody to human T-cell leukemia virus membrane antigens, beta 2-microglobulin levels, and thymosin alpha I levels in hemophiliacs and their spouses, by J. K. Kreiss, et al. ANNALS OF INTERNAL MEDICINE 100(2):178-182, February 1984.

Antibody to human T-lymphotropic virus type III in wives of hemophiliacs. Evidence for heterosexual transmission, by J. K. Kreiss, et al. ANNALS OF INTERNAL MEDICINE 102(5):623-626, May 1985.

Antibody to lymphadenopathy-associated virus in AIDS [letter], by D. D. Ho, et al. NEW ENGLAND JOURNAL OF MEDICINE 312(10):649-650, March 7, 1985.

Antibody to lymphadenopathy-associated virus in haemophiliacs with and without AIDS [letter],by R. B. Ramsey, et al. LANCET 2(8399):397-398, August 18, 1984.

Antigay Congressman introduces AIDS bills, by D. Walter. ADVOCATE 435:20, December 10, 1985.

Antigens on HTLV-infected cells recognized by leukemia and AIDS sera are related to HTLV viral glycoprotein, by J. Schüpbach, et al. SCIENCE 224(4649):607-610, May 11, 1984.

Antilymphocyte antibodies and seropositivity for retroviruses in groups at high risk for AIDS [letter], by D. D. Kiprov, et al. NEW ENGLAND JOURNAL OF MEDICINE 312(23):1517, June 6, 1985.

Antimoniotungstate (GPA 23) treatment of three patients with AIDS and one with prodrome [letter], by W. Rozenbaum, et al. LANCET 1(8426):450-451, February 23, 1985.

Antiserum to a synthetic peptide recognizes the HTLV-III envelope glycoprotein, by R. C. Kennedy, et al. SCIENCE 231:1556-1559, March 28, 1986.

Antiviral agents join fight against AIDS. CHEMICAL AND ENGINEERING NEWS 64:6, August 11, 1986.

Antiviral chemotherapy against HTLV-III/LAV infections, by B. Oberg. JOURNAL OF ANTIMICROBIAL CHEMOTHERAPY 17(5):549-552, May 1986.

Antiviral drugs for AIDS. Current status and future prospects, by E. Sandström. DRUGS 31(6):463-466, June 1986.

Apes and AIDS, by C. Holden. SCIENCE 222:596+, November 11, 1983.

Apothecary, by J. Stamps. RFD 36:20, Fall 1983.

Apothecary—cancer, by Stamps, et al. RFD 34:24, Spring 1983.

Apparent transmission of human T-cell leukemia virus type III to a heterosexual woman with the acquired immunodeficiency syndrome, by J. E. Groopman, et al. ANNALS OF INTERNAL MEDICINE 102(1):63-66, January 1985.

Apparent transmission of human T-lymphotrophic virus type III/lymphadenopathy-associated virus from a child to a mother providing health care. MMWR 35(5):76-79, February 7, 1986; also in JAMA 255:1005+, February 28, 1986.

Approaches to AIDS therapy, by D. Klatzmann, et al. NATURE 319:10-11, January 2, 1986.

Apropos the series: threatening advice on AIDS?, by C. Allmedal, et al. SYKEPLEIEN 73(11):36-37, June 20, 1986.

Apuzzo assesses task force & community, by S. Hyde. GAY COMMUNITY NEWS 12(33):3, March 9, 1985.

Apuzzo blasts NYC/lack of money for AIDS service, by P. Freiberg. ADVOCATE 413: 9, February 5, 1985.

ARC (the AIDS-related complex [letter], by G. J. Ruiz-Argüelles, et al. REVISTA DE INVESTIGACION CLINICA 36(3):307-308, July-September 1984.

ARCW seeks input. OUT 4(4):5, February 2, 1986.

Are AIDS caregivers homophobic?, by M. Helquist. ADVOCATE 425:30, July 23, 1985.

Are victims of AIDS 'handicapped' under federal law?, by T. J. Flygare. PHI DELTA KAPPAN 67:466-467, February 1986.

Are we abandoning the AIDS patient?, by W. J. Nelson, et al. RN 47(7):18-19, July 1984.

Are you ready to die for sexual lib, by C. Shively. FAG RAG 40:1, 1983.

Army: spread of AIDS threatens readiness, by P. Smith. AIR FORCE TIMES 46:3+, August 26, 1985.

As AIDS scare hits nation's blood supply, by J. Mann. U.S. NEWS & WORLD RE-PORT 95:71-72, July 25, 1983.

As AIDS spooks the schoolroom. US NEWS & WORLD REPORT 99(13):7, September 23, 1985.

As fear of AIDS spreads, people change ways they live and work. WALL STREET JOURNAL 206:35, October 10, 1985.

As a nurse, I want to find out what the facts are on AIDS, by J. L. Phillips. CRITICAL CARE UPDATE10(9):37-38, September 1983.

Aseptic techniques for AIDS [letter], by B. E. Evans. JOURNAL OF THE AMERICAN DENTAL ASSOCIATION 107(5):706+, November 1983.

Aspects of the acquired immunodeficiency syndrome (AIDS), by V. Persaud. WEST INDIAN MEDICAL JOURNAL 32(3):119-121, September 1983.

Aspects of anal sexual practices, by J. Agnew. JOURNAL OF HOMOSEXUALITY 12(1):75, Fall 1985.

Assault on AIDS and smoking, by D. McKie. LANCET 2(8468):1371, December 14, 1985.

Assessing ophthalmic signs in patients with AIDS, by P. Stoer, et al. JOURNAL OF OPHTHALMIC NURSING AND TECHNOLOGY 4(6):6-10, November-December 1985.

Assessment of therapy for pneumocystis carinii pneumonia. PCP Therapy Project Group, by H. W. Haverkos. AMERICAN JOURNAL OF MEDICINE 76(3):501-508, March 1984.

Associated focal and segmental glomerulosclerosis in the acquired immunodeficiency syndrome, by T. K. Rao, et al. NEW ENGLAND JOURNAL OF MEDICINE 310(11):6569-673, March 15, 1984.

Association between HTLV-III/LAV infection and tuberculosis in Zaire [letter],by J. Mann, et al. JAMA 256(3):346, July 18, 1986.

Association of HTLV-III antibodies and cellular immune status of hemophiliacs, by C. Tsoukas, et al. NEW ENGLAND JOURNAL OF MEDICINE 311:1514-1515, December 6, 1984.

Association of the pX gene product of human T-cell leukemia virus type I with nucleus, by T. Kiyokawa, et al. VIROLOGY 147:462-465, December 1985.

Asymptomatic acquired immunological deficiencies. Nosologic and therapeutic problems, by J. P. Revillard. PRESSE MEDICALE 13(32):1933-1935, September 22, 1984.

Asymptomatic blood donor with a false positive HTLV-III western blot, by M. S. Saag, et al. NEW ENGLAND JOURNAL OF MEDICINE 314:118, January 9, 1986.

Asymptomatic carriage of crptosporidium in the stool of a patient with acquired immunodeficiency syndrome [letter], by F. Zar, et al. JOURNAL OF INFECTIOUS DIS-
EASES 151(1):195, January 1985.

Asymptomatic lymphadenopathy and other early presentations of AIDS, by D. I.
Abrams. FRONTIERS OF RADIATION THERAPY AND ONCOLOGY 19:59-65,
1985.

At last, hope for AIDS victims: while no cure, a new drug may prolong life,by M. Clark,
et al. NEWSWEEK 108(13):57-58, September 29, 1986.

At risk, by P. Wilsher, et al. SUNDAY TIMES November 2, 1986, p. 25.

At risk: while the Reagan administration dozes and scientists vie for glory, the deadly
AIDS [acquired immune deficiency syndrome] epidemic has put the entire nation
at risk, by D. Talbot, et al. MOTHER JONES 10:28-37, April 1985.

Atlanta AIDS conference begins, by N. Fain. ADVOCATE 420:24, May 14, 1985.

Atlanta battles gay bathhouse, by G. Cabrera. GAY COMMUNITY NEWS 12(38);1,
April 13, 1985.

ATLV in Japanese patient with AIDS [letter],by I. Miyoshi, et al. LANCET 2(8344):
275, July 30, 1983.

Attempted treatment of acquired immunodeficiency syndrome (AIDS) with thymic
humoral factor, by Y. Berner, et al. ISRAEL JOURNAL OF MEDICAL SCIENCES
20(12):1195-1196, December 1984.

Attempts at the development of vaccines against adult T-cell leukemia, by M. Hayami.
KANGO GIJUTSU 31(16):2214-2215, December 1985.

Attention, prison dentists: CDC issues warning on AIDS. CORRECTIONS DIGEST
14(19):9-10, September 7, 1983.

Attitudes toward AIDS, herpes II, and toxic shock syndrome, by L. Simkins, et al.
PSYCHOLOGICAL REPORTS 55(3):7790786, December 1984.

Attrition, not conquest, of disease [news]. NATURE 309(5963):1-2, May 3-9, 1984.

Atypical AIDS cases draw world to town, by P. Thomas. MEDICAL WORLD NEWS
27(16):7+, August 25, 1986.

Atypical Hodgkin's disease and the acquired immunodeficiency syndrome [letter],
by R. G. Scheib, et al. ANNALS OF INTERNAL MEDICINE 102(4):5544, April
1985.

Atypical infections and Kaposi's sarcoma in AIDS—radiographic findings, by M. P.
Federle. FRONTIERS OF RADIATION THERAPY AND ONCOLOGY 19:117-122,
1985.

Atypical mycobacteria and Kaposi's sarcoma in the same biopsy speciments [letter],
by T. S. Croxson, et al. NEW ENGLAND JOURNAL OF MEDICINE 308(24):1476,
June 16, 1983.

Atypical myobacterial and cytomegalovirus infection of the duodenum in a patient with
acquired immunodeficiency syndrome: endoscopic and histopathologic appearance, by J. G. Caya, et al. WISCONSIN MEDICAL JOURNAL 83(11):33-36, November 1984.

Atypical neurologic symptoms in the course of acquired immunodeficiency syndrome (AIDS), by J. Kesselring, et al. DEUTSCHE MEDIZINISCHE WOCHENSCHRIFT 111(27):1058-1060, July 4, 1986.

Atypical presentation of childhood acquired immune deficiency syndrome mimicking Crohn's disease: nutritional considerations and management, by K. J. Benkov, et al. AMERICAN JOURNAL OF GASTROENTEROLOGY 80(4):260-265, April 1985.

Atypical subcutaneous infection associated with acquired immune deficiency syndrome, by M. H. Stoler, et al. AMERICAN JOURNAL OF CLINICAL PATHOLOGY 80(5):714-718, November 1983.

Autoantibodies to T cells in adult and pediatric AIDS, by A. Rubinstein, et al. ANNALS OF THE NEW YORK ACADEMY OF SCIENCES 437:508-512, 1984.

Autoimmunity and AIDS, by M. Helquist. ADVOCATE 438:22, January 21, 1986.

Autologous blood transfusion [letter], by R. Yomtovian. JAMA 253(17):2491, May 3, 1985.

Autologous mixed lymphocyte reaction in man. XIV. Deficiency of the autologous mixed lymphocyte reaction in acquired immune deficiency syndrome (AIDS) and AIDS related complex (ARC). In vitro effect of purified interleukin-1 and interleukin-2, by S. Gupta, et al. CLINICAL AND EXPERIMENTAL IMMUNOLOGY 58(2): 395-401, November 1984.

Autopsy findings in the acquired immune deficiency syndrome, by K. Mobley, et al. PATHOLOGY ANNUAL 20(Part 1):45-65, 1985.

—, by H L. Schmidts, et al. PATOLOGE 7(1):8-21, January 1986.

—, by K. Welch, et al. JAMA 252(9):1152-1159, September 7, 1984.

Autopsy pathology in the acquired immune deficiency syndrome, by C. M. Reichert, et al. AMERICAN JOURNAL OF PATHOLOGY 112(3):357-382, September 1983.

Avalanche of new cash, by C. Norman. SCIENCE 230:1358, December 20, 1985.

Avoiding AIDS with autologous transfusions [letter], by S. E. James. BRITISH MEDICAL JOURNAL 290(6471):854, March 16, 1985.

Axelrod warns of pressure to shut bathhouses, by P. Freiberg. ADVOCATE 418:10, April 16, 1985.

B-cell abnormalities in AIDS [letter]. NEW ENGLAND JOURNAL OF MEDICINE 310(4):258-259, January 26, 1984.

B-cell immunodeficiency in acquired immune deficiency syndrome, by A. J. Ammann, et al. JAMA 251(11):1447-1449, March 16, 1984.

Babies born with AIDS, by J. Seligmann, et al. NEWSWEEK 108(12):70-71, September 22, 1986.

Backlash builds against AIDS. U.S. NEWS & WORLD REPORT 99:9, November 4, 1985.

Bacteremia and fungemia in patients with acquired immune deficiency syndrome, by R. H. Eng, et al. AMERICAN JOURNAL OF CLINICAL PATHOLOGY 86(1):105-107, July 1986.

Bacteremia and fungemia in patients with the acquired immunodeficiency syndrome, by E. Whimbey, et al. ANNALS OF INTERNAL MEDICINE 104(4):511-514, April 1986.

Bacteremia due to Mycobacterium avium-intracellulare in the acquired immunodeficiency syndrome, by A. M. Macher, et al. ANNALS OF INTERNAL MEDICINE 99(6):782-785, December 1983.

Bacterial bronchopneumopathies in patients with the acquired immunodeficiency syndrome [letter], by C. Mayaud, et al. PRESSE MEDICALE 15(16):760-761, April 19, 1986.

Bacterial expression of the acquired immunodeficiency syndrome retrovirus p24 gag protein and its use as a diagnostic reagent, by D. J. Dowbenko, et al. PROCEEDINGS OF THE NATIONAL ACADEMY OF SCIENCES 82(22):7748-7752, November 1985.

Bacterial infection in the acquired immunodeficiency syndrome of children, by L. J. Bernstein, et al. PEDIATRIC INFECTIOUS DISEASE 4(5):472-475, September-October 1985.

Bacterial pneumonia in patients with the acquired immunodeficiency syndrome, by B. Polsky, et al. ANNALS OF INTERNAL MEDICINE 104(1):38-41, January 1986.

Bad blood: "gift of life" may be also an agent of death in some AIDS [acquired immuno deficiency syndrome] cases, by M. Chase. WALL STREET JOURNAL 203:1+, March 12, 1984.

Bad blood? [screening tests for AIDS virus inconclusive]. SCIENTIFIC AMERICAN 253:78, December 1985.

Ban on gay bias proposed by Insurance Council, by Bisticas-Cocoves. GAY COMMUNITY NEWS 13(47):1, June 21, 1986.

Ban sought on gay counselors, by J. Zeh. GAY COMMUNITY NEWS 12(37):1, April 6, 1985.

Band-aids. THE ECONOMIST 288:22+, August 13-19, 1983.

Bandaids for AIDS. CULTURAL SURVIVAL QUARTERLY 3:19, Fall 1984.

Banning the baths: AIDS and gay rights, by R. O'Loughlin. GUARDIAN 37(4):5, October 24, 1984.

Basal cell carcinoma in a man with acquired immunodeficiency syndrome [letter], by L. Slazinski, et al. JOURNAL OF THE AMERICAN ACADEMY OF DERMATOLOGY 11(1):140-141, July 1984.

Basement membrane and connective tissue proteins in early lesions of Kaposi's sarcoma associated with AIDS, by R. H. Kramer, et al. JOURNAL OF INVESTIGATIVE DERMATOLOGY 84(6):516-520, June 1985.

Bathhouses reopen, but must clean up act. BODY POLITIC 110:19, January 1985.

Bathhouses—scapegoats for AIDS fear, by R. Oloughlin. ADVOCATE 3(90):16, March 20, 1984.

Battling AIDS: more misery, less mystery, by C. Wallis, et al. TIME 125(17):68, April 29, 1985.

Battling a deadly new epidemic, by C. Wallis. TIME 121:53-55, March 28,1 983.

Bay area bathowners balk at restrictions, by C. Guilfoy. GAY COMMUNITY NEWS 12(22):1, December 15, 1984.

Beating the Mardi Gras media bash, by D. Grenville. BODY POLITIC 114:19, May 1985.

Bedside bronchoalveolar lavage for the diagnosis of Pneumocystis carinii pneumonia in patients with the acquired immunodeficiency syndrome, by G. R. Flick, et al. AIDS RESEARCH 2(1):31-41, February 1986.

Behavioral and psychosocial factors in AIDS. Methodological and substantive issues, by J. L. Martin, et al. AMERICAN PSYCHOLOGIST 39(11):1303-1308, November 1984.

Behind the AIDS hysteria [editorial]. GUARDIAN 35(39):26, July 13, 1983.

Behind the mental symptoms of AIDS, by M. Norman. PSYCHOLOGY TODAY 18:12, December 1984.

Behind spreading fear of two modern "plagues" . . . acquired immune deficiency syndrome and Alzheimer's disease, by A. Trafford, et al. US NEWS & WORLD REPORT 99(7):46-47, August 12, 1985.

Being gay is a health hazard, by B. Vinocur. THE SATURDAY EVENING POST 254: 26+, October 1982.

Belated, growing response; AIDS and the churches, by B. J. Stiles. CHRISTIANITY AND CRISIS 45:534-536, Jnuary 13, 1986.

Benefits awarded to man caring for dying love,by R. Gillis. GAY COMMUNITY NEWS 13(17):1, November 9, 1985.

Bensons bomb, by S. Kulieke. ADVOCATE 3(73):18, August 4, 1983.

Beta2m: there in the beginning, by D. R. Zimmerman. MOSAIC 15(2):10-15, 1984.

Beta 2-microglobulin and the acquired immunodeficiency syndrome in a low-incidence area [letter]. JAMA 253(1):43-44, January 4, 1985.

Beta 2-microglobulin as a prognostic marker for development of AIDS [letter], by R. B. Bhalla, et al. CLINICAL CHEMISTRY 31(8):1411-1412, August 1985.

Beta-2-microglobulin in acquired immune deficiency syndrome, by P. Francioli, et al. ANTIBIOTICS AND CHEMOTHERAPY 32:147-152, 1983.

Beta-2 microglobulin: a sensitive non-specific marker for acquired immune deficiency syndrome, by P. Francioloi, et al. EUROPEAN JOURNAL OF CLINICAL MICROBIOLOGY 3(1):68-69, February 1984.

Bidirectionality of AIDS questioned. SCIENCE NEWS 129:11, January 4, 1986.

Bilateral fungal corneal ulcers in a patient with AIDS-related complex, by C. Santos, et al. AMERICAN JOURNAL OF OPHTHALMOLOGY 102(1):118-119, July 15, 1986.

Biliary tract obstruction in the acquired imunodeficiency syndrome,by S. J. Margulis, et al. ANNALS OF INTERNAL MEDICINE 105(2):207-210, August 1986.

Bill for AIDS. NEW SCIENTIST 109:21, January 16, 1986.

Billions needed for AIDS research. BODY POLITIC 118:29, September 1985.

Binding of HTLV-III/LAV to T4+ cells by a complex of the 110K viral protein and the T4 molecule, by J. S. McDougal, et al. SCIENCE 231:382-385, January 24, 1986.

Biologic health hazards: AIDS and hepatitis B, by B. Burgel. CALIFORNIA NURSE 81(6):4, July-August 1985.

Biological and biochemical characterization of a cloned Leu-3-cell surviving infection with the acquired immune deficiency syndrome retrovirus, by T. M. Folks, et al. JOURNAL OF EXPERIMENTAL MEDICINE 164(1):280-290, July 1, 1986.

Biological nature of AIDS virus, by D. Bardell. AMERICAN BIOLOGY TEACHER 48:75-77, February 1986.

Biology and therapy of Kaposi's sarcoma, by R. T. Mitsuyasu, et al. SEMINARS IN ON-COLOGY 11(10;53-59, March 1984.

Black community organizes to fight AIDS, by S. Poggi. GAY COMMUNITY NEWS 14(11):3, September 28, 1986.

Black gay man battles United for job, by C. Smith. GAY COMMUNITY NEWS 12(23):3, December 22, 1984.

Black gays—clinic—DC AIDS Forum, by U. Vaid. GAY COMMUNITY NEWS 11(12):3, October 7, 1983.

Black market forces legalisation of AIDS drug, by I. Anderson. NEW SCIENTIST 106: 6, May 16, 1985.

Blood bank now accepts lesbian, by B. Brown. WOMEN'S PRESS 13(4):2, November 1983.

Blood bank policy in Israel in relation to AIDS, by D. Michaeli. ANNALS OF THE NEW YORK ACADEMY OF SCIENCES 437:485-486, 1984.

Blood bankers send out AIDS alert, by A. Weller. PATHOLOGIST 37(6):431-432, June 1983.

Blood bankers set the AIDS record straight. COLORADO MEDICINE 80(11):318, November 1983.

Blood banking—public or private, isologous or autologous?, by R. Beal. MEDICAL JOURNAL OF AUSTRALIA 1444(8):393-394, April 14, 1986.

Blood banks and AIDS [editorial], by A. Krosnick. JOURNAL OF THE MEDICAL SOCIETY OF NEW JERSEY 81(2):105, February 1984.

Blood banks give HTLV-III test positive appraisal at five months, by C. Marwick. JAMA 254:1681-1683, October 4, 1985.

Blood banks still cope with AIDS fears and myths, by J. Riffer. HOSPITALS 60(1):74, January 5, 1986.

Blood brotherhood: a risk factor for AIDS? [letter], by L. Morfeldt-Manson, et al. LAN-CET 2(8415):1346, December 8, 1984.

Blood donation by persons at high risk of AIDS [letter], by J. J. Goedert. NEW ENG-LAND JOURNAL OF MEDICINE 312(18):1190, May 2, 1985.

Blood donor services and liability issues relating to acquired immune deficiency syn-drome, by K. S. Lipton. JOURNAL OF LEGAL MEDICINE 7(2):131-186, June 1986.

Blood donors at high risk of transmitting the acquired immune deficiency syndrome, by M. Contreras, et al. BRITISH MEDICAL JOURNAL 290(6470):749-750, March 9, 1985.

Blood drive unsettling Providence, by C. Guilfoy. GAY COMMUNITY NEWS 11(21):3, December 10, 1983.

Blood groups act to cut AIDS transmission risk. HOSPITALS 57(9):61-62, May 1, 1983.

Blood groups 'look back' for AIDS, by B. McCormick. HOSPITALS 60(16):72, August 20, 1986.

Blood product immunosuppression and the acquired immunodeficiency syndrome [letter], by R. J. Ablin, et al. ANNALS OF INTERNAL MEDICINE 104(1):130, Jan-uary 1986.

Blood shortage fails to materialize, by J. E. Fox. US MEDICINE 19(17):3+, September 1, 1983.

Blood story. Part II. AIDS—current concepts and implications for blood transfusion services and nursing staff, by C. J. Burrell, et al. AUSTRALIAN NURSES JOUR-NAL 14(7):45-47, February 1985.

Blood supply safety: NIH panel sees reduced AIDS risk. CHEMICAL AND ENGINEERING NEWS 64:4, July 14, 1986.

Blood transfusion and acquired immunodeficiency syndrome (AIDS), by B. Habibi, et al. REVUE FRANCAISE DE TRANSFUSION ET IMMUNO-HEMATOLOGIE 26(5): 447-465, Novemebr 1983.

Blood transfusion and susceptibility to AIDS [letter], by G. M. Shearer, et al. NEW ENGLAND JOURNAL OF MEDICINE 310(24):1601, June 14, 1984.

Blood transfusion, blood donation, and AIDS [editorial], by A. J. Grindon,e t al. JOUR-NAL OF THE MEDICAL ASSOCIATION OF GEORGIA 72(9):641-642, Septem-ber 193.

Blood transfusion, haemophilia, and AIDS [editorial]. LANCET 2(8417-8418):1433-1435, December 22, 1984.

Blood transfusions and the acquired immunodeficiency syndrome [letter], by J. Herman. ANNALS OF INTERNAL MEDICINE 100(3):461, March 1984.

Blood transfusions and AIDS: the facts, by P. Gadsby GOOD HOUSEKEEPING 200: 222, June 1985.

Blood treatment may not kill AIDS virus, by S. Connor. NEW SCIENTIST 109:13-14, February 20, 1986.

Blood, virus: new links to AIDS, by D. Franklin. SCIENCE NEWS 125:21, January 14, 1984.

Blood will tell—but only with difficulty, by A. Veitch. GUARDIAN May 9, 1985, p. 19.

Blood-borne agent in immune deficiency and rare infection implicated. SCIENCE NEWS 123:8, January 1, 1983.

Blood-handling precautions and the human T-leukemia virus [letter], by T. R. Franson, et al. ANNALS OF INTERNAL MEDICINE 100():765, May 1984.

Blow to research, by W. Michaud. GAY COMMUNITY NEWS 13(34):5, March 15, 1986.

Bobbi Campbell's brave fight against AIDS ends, by S. Kulieke. ADVOCATE 403:16, September 18, 1984.

Body composition studies in patients with the acquired immunodeficiency syndrome, by D. P. Kotler, et al. AMERICAN JOURNAL OF CLINICAL NUTRITION 42(6): 1255-1265, December 1985.

Body heat, by B. Thomson. EAST WEST JOURNAL 16(1):42, January 1986.

Bone marrow abnormalities in the acquired immunodeficiency syndrome [letter], by C. M. Franco, et al. ANNALS OF INTERNAL MEDICINE 101(2):275-276, August 1984.

Bone marrow biopsies in patients with the acquired immunodeficiency syndrome, by B. M. Osborne, et al. HUMAN PATHOLOGY 15(11):1048-1053, November 1984.

Bone marrow examination and culture in the diagnosis of acquird immunodeficiency syndrome (AIDS) [letter], by J. Pasternak, et al. ARCHIVES OF INTERNAL MEDICINE 143(7):1495, July 1983.

Bone marrow in the acquired immunodeficiency syndrome [letter], by R. A. Hromas, et al. ANNALS OF INTERNAL MEDICINE 101(6):877, December 1984.

Bone marrow in AIDS. A histologic, hematologic, and microbiologic study, by A. Castella, et al. AMERICAN JOURNAL OF CLINICAL PATHOLOGY 84(4):425-432, October 1985.

Bone marrow transplantation in AIDS [letter, by J. M. Hassett, et al. NEW ENGLAND JOURNAL OF MEDICINE 309(11):665, September 15, 1983.

Boston AIDS Committee receives $150,000, by s. Hyde. GAY COMMUNITY NEWS 12(32):3, March 2, 1985.

Boston AIDS Conference discusses quarantine issue, by C. Guilfoy. GAY COMMUNITY NEWS 12(41):1, May 4, 1985.

Boston City Hospital ousts man with AIDS, by C. Guilfoy. GAY COMMUNITY NEWS 12(20):1, December 1, 1984.

Boston forum calls for radical confrontation, by N. Wechsler. GAY COMMUNITY NEWS 13(24):2, Decemebr 28, 1985.

Boston hires city AIDS coordinator, by C. Guilfoy. GAY COMMUNITY NEWS 11(32):1, March 3, 1984.

Boston hospital changes AIDS policy. GAY COMMUNITY NEWS 11(14):6, October 22, 1983.

Boston official roasted—AIDS joke, by L. Goldsmith. GAY COMMUNITY NEWS 11(35):1, March 24, 1984.

Boston PWAs included in anti-viral drug study, by K. Westheimer. GAY COMMUNITY NEWS 13(50):3, July 6, 1986.

Boston quarantine proposal withdrawn, by K. Westheimer. GAY COMMUNITY NEWS 13(2):1, December 28, 1985.

Boston shows pride, by L. Goldsmith. GAY COMMUNITY NEWS 10(49):1, July 2, 1983.

Boston "walk for life" raises over $300,000, by K. Westheimer. GAY COMMUNITY NEWS 13(46):3, June 14, 1986.

Boston women meet, discuss AIDS, by S. Hyde. GAY COMMUNITY NEWS 11(11):1, October 1, 1983.

Bovine leukemia virus-related antigens in lmphocyte cultures infected with AIDS-associated viruses, by L. Thiry, et al. SCIENCE 227(4693):1482-1484, March 22, 1985.

Boys and girls come out to play? . . . shadow of AIDS has spread to the school play-ground, by C. Clementson. NURSING TIMES 82(7):19-20, February 12-18, 1986.

Boys with AIDS barred from classrooms, by L. Sherman. GAY COMMUNITY NEWS 13(7):2, August 24, 1985.

Brain biopsies in patients with acquired immune deficiency syndrome, by L. B. Moskowitz, et al. ARCHIVES OF PATHOLOGY AND LABORATORY MEDICINE 108(5):368-371, May 1984.

Brain endothelial cells infected by AIDS virus , by D. M. Barnes. SCIENCE 233(4762):418-419, July 25, 1986.

Brain function decline in children with AIDS, by D. M. Barnes. SCIENCE 232:1196, June 6, 1986.

Breakdown of P.G.E. 1 synthesis is responsible for the acquired immunodeficiency syndrome, by S. G. Marcus. MEDICAL HYPOTHESES 15(1):39-46, September 1984.

Breakthrough against a modern plague (AIDS), by P. Ohlendorf. MACLEAN'S 98:47-48, February 4, 1985.

Breakthrough of cytomegalovirus infection despite 9-(1,3-dihydroxy-2-propoxy-methyl)guanine therapy [letter],by M. C. Bach. ANNALS OF INTERNAL MEDICINE 104(4):587, April 1986.

British AIDS [news], by H. Barnes. NATURE 312(5995):583, December 13-19, 1984.

British AIDS Action Committee formed, by L. Taylor. ADVOCATE 3(81):15, November 24, 1983.

British AIDS; new cases cause alarm, by M. Clarke. NATURE 314(6006):5, March 7, 1985.

British AIDS; paper prophylaxis backfires, by H. Barnes. NATURE 312:583, December 13, 1984.

British AIDS; whose blood can now be safe? by T. Beardsley. NATURE 303:102, May 12, 1983.

British blood is almost clean. NEW SCIENTIST 109:15, February 13, 1986.

British drug set to better AZT. NEW SCIENTIST 111:17, September 25, 1986.

British hospital attempts AIDS quarantine, by P. Cummings. ADVOCATE 432:22, October 29, 1985.

British relief for AIDS victims is threatened, by S. Yanchinski. NEW SCIENTIST 98:361, May 12, 1983.

Broadway benefit raises half a million for AIDS, by S. Greco. ADVOCATE 423:49, June 25, 1985.

Bronchoalveolar lavage and transbronchial biopsy for the diagnosis of pulmonary infections in the acquired immunodeficiency syndrome, by c. Broaddus, et al. ANNALS OF INTERNAL MEDICINE 102(5)Ú747-752, June 1985.

Bronchoalveolar lavage as the exclusive diagnosic modality for Pneumocystis carinii pneumonia. A prospective study among patients with acquired immuno-deficiency syndrome, by J. A. Golden, et al. CHEST 90(1):18-22, July 1986.

Bronchoalveolar lavage cells and proteins in patients with the acquired immunodeficiency syndrome. An immunologic analysis, by K. R. Young, Jr., et al. ANNALS OF INTERNAL MEDICINE 103(4):522-533, October 1985.

Bronchoalveolar lavage in acquired immunodeficiency syndrome [letter],by A. Venet, et al. LANCET 2(8340):53, July 2, 1983.

Bronchoalveolar lavage in patients with the acquired immune deficiency syndrome (AIDS), by R. P. Baughman, et al. AIDS RESEARCH 1(2):91-97, 1983-1984.

Burkitt cell acute lymphoblastic leukemia with partial expression of T-cell markers and subclonal chromosome abnormalities in a man with acquired immunodeficiency syndrome, by M. Berman, et al. CANCER GENETICS AND CYTOGENETICS 16(4):341-347, April 15, 1985.

Burkitt lymphoma in acquired immune deficiency syndrome, by D. R. Radin, et al. JOURNAL OF COMPUTER ASSISTED TOMOGRAPHY 8(1)173-174, February 1984.

Burkitt's lymphoma in AIDS: cytogenetic study, by J. Whang-Peng, et al. BLOOD 63(4):818-822, April 1984.

California acts to protect blood, gays, by M. Lassell. ADVOCATE 419:14, April 30, 1985.

California Governor vetoes AIDS anti-discrimination. Bill, by M. Vandervelden. ADVOCATE 454:22, September 2, 1986.

California questions LaRouche signatures, by Bisticas-Cocoves. GAY COMMUNITY NEWS 13(46):1, June 14, 1986.

California Senate fails to override AIDS funding veto, by M. Helquist. ADVOCATE 427:12, August 20, 1985.

California to vote on AIDS quarantine, by J. Kiely. GAY COMMUNITY NEWS 13(50):3, July 6, 1986.

California VNAs train AIDS treatment corps. AMERICAN JOURNAL OF NURSING 84:1535, December 1984.

California wants AIDS test on organs. NEW SCIENTIST 107:19, August 1, 1985.

Californians give AIDS to monkeys, by I. Anderson. NEW SCIENTIST 101:7, March 8, 1984.

Call for quarantine, by C. Bowland. ADVOCATE 443:42, April 1, 1986.

Call to battle: a national panel urges a campaign to alert an AIDS "catastrophe", by G. J. Church, et al. TIME 128(19):18-20, November 10, 1986.

Cambridge, Boston schools revise AIDS policy, by K. Westheimer. GAY COMMUNITY NEWS 13(49):3, June 29, 1986.

Campus sex: new fears. AIDS is the latest STD to hit the nation's colleges, by M. Bruno, et al. NEWSWEEK 106(18):81-82, October 28, 1985.

Campylobacter fetus ssp fetus cholecystitis and relapsing bacteremia in a patient with acquired immunodeficiency syndrome, by E. E. Coster, et al. SOUTHERN MEDICAL JOURNAL 77(7):927-928, July 1984.

Can AIDS transmission by prevented by use of a condom? by D. T. Purtilo. JAMA 252:826, August 10, 1984.

Can contact tracing help fight AIDS? OUT 4(8);1, June 1986.

Can essential fatty acid deficiency predispose to AIDS? [letter], by U. N. Das. CANADIAN MEDICAL ASSOCIATION JOURNAL 132(8):900+, April 15, 1985.

Can hepatitis B virus and AIDS-associated retrovirus (LAV/HTLV-III) be transmitted by insects?, by T. G. Jaenson. LAKARTIDNINGEN 82(47):4133-4136, November 20, 1985.

Can sex survive AIDS?, by Arthur Kretchmer. PLAYBOY 33:48+, February 1986.

Can we help AIDS?, by A. Brown. SPECTATOR January 19, 1985, p. 16.

Can we talk?, by J. Bodis. BODY POLITIC 111:47, February 1985.

Canadian gay health groups, by T. Stroll. ADVOCATE 3(77):9, September 29, 1983.

Cancer and AIDS. 19th annual San Francisco Cancer Symposium. San Francisco, Calif., March 2-4, 1984. FRONTIERS OF RADIATION THERAPY AND ONCOLOGY 19:1-184, 1985.

Cancer trends in a population at risk of acquired immunodeficiency syndrome, by R. J. Biggar, et al. JNCI 74(4):793-797, April 1985.

Capitol report, by L. Bush. ADVOCATE 3(72):18, July 21, 1983.

—. ADVOCATE 3(73):14, August 4, 1983.

—. ADVOCATE 3(80):20, November 10, 1983.

—. ADVOCATE 3(83):24, December 22, 1983.

—. ADVOCATE 3(85):14, January 10, 1984.

Capsule-deficiency Cryptococcus neoformans in AIDS patients [letter], by D. W. Mac-kenzie, et al. LANCET 1(8429):642, March 16, 1985.

Capsule-deficient cryptococci in AIDS [letter], by E. J. Bottone, et al. LANCET 2(8454):553, September 7, 1985.

Capsule-deficient Cryptococcus neoformans in AIDS patients [letter]. LANCET 1(8435):988-997, April 27, 1985.

—, by E. J. Bottone, et al. LANCET 1(8425):400, February 16, 1985.

Cardiac abnormalities in acquired immune deficiency syndrome, by L. Fink, et al. AMERICAN JOURNAL OF CARDIOLOGY 54(8):1161-1163, November 1, 1984.

Cardiac aspergillosis in acquired immune deficiency syndrome, by S. Henochowicz, et al. AMERICAN JOURNAL OF CARDIOLOGY 55(9):1239-1240, April 15, 1985.

Cardiac involvement by Kaposi's sarcoma in acquired immune deficiency syndrome (AIDS), by M. A. Silver, et al. AMERICAN JOURNAL OF CARDIOLOGY 53(7): 983-985, March 15, 1984.

Cardiac lesions in acquired immune deficiency syndrome (AIDS), by C. Cammaro-sano, et al. JOURNAL OF THE AMERICAN COLLEGE OF CARDIOLOGY 55(3): 703-706, March 1985.

Care of pentamadine ulcers in AIDS patients, by J. R. Gottlieb, et al. PLASTIC AND RECONSTRUCTIVE SURGERY 76(4):630-632, October 1985.

Care study—HTLV-III: spread of infection via blood, by C. Emery. NURSING 3(4): 147-148, April 1986.

Care to AIDS patients: the cost impact on Medicare, by E. W. Smith. CARING 5(6):56-57, June 1986.

Caring for acquired immune deficiency syndrome patients . . . experiences of one AIDS nursing unit, by C. S. Viele, et al. ONCOLOGY NURSING FORUM 11(3):56-60, May-June 1984; also in NEW ZEALAND NURSING FORUM 13(1):7-11, February-March 1985.

Caring for the AIDS patient—fearlessly. NURSING (HORSHAM) 13(9):50-55, September 1983.

Caring for AIDS patients. NEW ZEALAND NURSING JOURNAL 77(4):5-6, April 1984.

Caring for AIDS patients in a compassionate way, by S. Butler. NURSING STANDARD 446:3, May 8, 1986.

Caring for AIDS patients: the physician's risk and responsibility [editorial], by G. N. Burrow. CANADIAN MEDICAL ASSOCIATION JOURNAL 129(11):1181, December 1, 1983.

Caring for home patients . . . AIDS, by I. Goldstone. RNABC NEWS 17(6):21-22, November-December 1985.

Caring for the infectious patient: risk factors during pregnancy, by I. Gurevich, et al. INFECTION CONTROL 5(10):482-488, October 1984.

Carl Wittman: an activist's life, by M. Bronski. GAY COMMUNITY NEWS 13(31):7, February 15, 1986.

Case for diagnosis. AIDS, by A. M. Macher, et al. MILITARY MEDICINE 151(6):M33-M40, June 1986.

—, by Y. M. Chung. MILITARY MEDICINE 149(9):518+, September 1984.

Case for heat-treated blood products [letter], by G. F. Pierce. LANCET 1(8426):451, February 23, 1985.

Case 46—1984: AIDS associated with transfusion of blood products [letter], by G. F. Leparc. NEW ENGLAND JOURNAL OF MEDICINE 312(10):648, March 7, 1985.

Case 46-1984 [a 63-year-old man with respiratory failure after an unmaintained remission of acute myelogenous leukemia], by R. E. Scully, et al. NEW ENGLAND JOURNAL OF MEDICINE 311:1303-1310, November 15, 1984.

Case history—triumph over AIDS, by F. Cantaloupe. EAST WEST JOURNAL 14(2): 46, February 1984.

Case of acquired immune deficiency syndrome (AIDS) with Pneumocystis carinii pneumonia, by A. B. Adams, et al. RESPIRATORY CARE 29(1):50-53, January 1984.

Case of AIDS in a hemophilia B patient in France , by C. Gazengel, et al. REVUE FRANCAISE DE TRANSFUSION ET IMMUNOHEMATOLOGIE 27(4):479-486, September 1984.

Case of AIDS in New Orleans, by S. R. Olive. JOURNAL OF THE LOUISIANA STATE MEDICAL SOCIETY 135(9):4-5+, September 1983.

Case of immune deficiency in a Zaire infant: AIDS?, by B. Massart, et al. REVUE MEDICALE DE LIEGE 40(10);433-438, May 15, 1985.

Case of nerves. SCIENTIFIC AMERICAN 254:65, March 1986.

Case records of the Massachusetts General Hospital. Case 2-1986 [a 58-year-old woman with fever and nodular pulmonary infiltrates], by R. E. Scully, et al. NEW ENGLAND JOURNAL OF MEDICINE 314:167-174, January 16, 1986.

Case study: a child with chronic pulmonary infiltrates. Part one, by B. Zeffren, et al. ANNALS OF ALLERGY 54(2):97-98+, February 1985.

Case study: "If I have AIDS, then let me die now," by S. Vinogradov, et al. HASTINGS CENTER REPORT 14:24-26, February 1984.

Case study in pastoral counseling, by M. E. Johson. HEALTH PROGRESS 67(4):38-40, May 1986.

Case 32-1983. Acquired immunodeficiency syndrome and cranial-nerve abnormalities. NEW ENGLAND JOURNAL OF MEDICINE 309(6):359-369, August 11, 1983.

Cases up, funding down. BODY POLITIC 125:23, April 1986.

Casual contact theories incite AIDS, by B. Nelson. GAY COMMUNITY NEWS 10(47): 3, June 18, 1983.

Catalyst for change, by R. Berkowitz. GAY COMMUNITY NEWS 11(15):5, October 29, 1983.

Catholics who fear AIDS don't have to drink from communion chalice. JET 69:28-29, December 9, 1985.

Causation of AIDs revealed, by J. E. Groopman. NATURE 308:769, April 26, 1984.

Cause of acquired immune deficiency syndrome [letter]. JAMA 251(3):341-342, January 20, 1984.

Cause of acquired immunodeficiency syndrome—is it known?, by D. P. Francis, et al. PROGRESS IN CLINICAL AND BIOLOGICAL RESEARCH 182:277-283, 1985.

Cause of AIDS? [editorial]. LANCET 1(8385):1053-1054, May 12, 1984.

Caution. AIDS virus present: handle with care! . . . ophthalmic examination equipment, by N. Garber. JOURNAL OF OPHTHALMIC NURSING AND TECHNOLOGY 4(6):22-25, November-December 1985.

Caution on AIDS viruses [letter],by J. A. Sonnabend. NATURE 310(5973):103, July 12-18, 1984.

CD4 (T4) antigen is an essential component of the receptor for the AIDS retrovirus, by A. G. Dalgleish, et al. NATURE 312(5996):763-767, December 20, 1984-January 2, 1985.

CDC advises HTLV-3 test for all "at risk", by Bisticas-Cocoves. GAY COMMUNITY NEWS 13(37):1, April 1, 1986.

CDC bans "explicit sex" from AIDS education, by K. Westheimer. GAY COMMUNITY NEWS 13(26):1, January 18, 1986.

CDC charged with sabotaging AIDS research, by Bisticas-Cocoves. GAY COMMUNITY NEWS 14(11):1, September 28, 1986.

CDC: despite RN seroconversion, AIDS precautions adequate. HOSPITAL EMPLOYEE HEALTH 4(2):17-19, February 1985.

CDC guidelines for the prevention and control of nosocomial infections. Guideline for infection control in hospital personnel, by W. W. Williams. AMERICAN JOURNAL OF INFECTION CONTROL 12(1):34-63, February 1984.

CDC guidelines: recommendations for preventing transmission of AIDS. AORN JOURNAL 43(2):528+, February 1986.

CDC: "Hands off safe sex," by J. Irving. GAY COMMUNITY NEWS 13(31):2, February 15, 1986.

CDC issues AIDS guidelines for health workers, by V. L. Bauknecht. AMERICAN NURSE 18(1):2+, January 1986.

CDC issues HTLV-III screening guidelines, by C. Guilfoy. GAY COMMUNITY NEWS 12(27):1, January 26, 1985.

CDC publishes AIDS precautions for health-care and allied professionals. EMERGENCY DEPARTMENT NEWS 5(11):17, November 1983.

CDC recommendations for preventing transmission of AIDS during invasive procedures. TEXAS NURSE 60(7):14, August 1986; also in OREGON NURSE 51(3):
10, June 1986.

CDC reports AIDS cases in U.S. top 15,000, by Bisticas-Cocoves. GAY COMMUNITY
NEWS 13(22):3, December 14, 1985.

CDC reports caution obstetric personnel, patients about AIDS virus, by A. Ropp.
NAACOG NEWSLETTER 13(6):1+, June 1986.

CDC reports first AIDS transmission from child to parent. AMERICAN FAMILY
PHYSICIAN 33:17-18, March 1986.

CDC reports 10,000 diagnosed with AIDS, by M. Cocoves. GAY COMMUNITY NEWS
12(45):1, June 1, 1985.

CDC revises AIDS risk hierarchy, by Bisticas-Cocoves. GAY COMMUNITY NEWS
14(7):3, August 24, 1986.

CDC sees no need to test health workers for AIDS; two SNA's launch campaigns "to
reduce anxiety." AMERICAN JOURNAL OF NURSING 86:200-202, February
1986.

CDC to host AIDS risk reduction conferences, by N. Fain. ADVOCATE 415:24,
March 5, 1985.

CDC updates trends in AIDS epidemic. AMERICAN FAMILY PHYSICIAN 26:290+,
November 1982.

Cela s'appelle la mort (LAV), by J. P. Richard. RELATIONS 45:244, October 1985.

Celebrating life honoring courage, by W. K. Hale. GAY COMMUNITY NEWS 11(16):
15, November 5, 1983.

Cell-mediated immune responses in AIDS [letter],by E. Buimovici-Klein,e t al. NEW
ENGLAND JOURNAL OF MEDICINE 311(5):328-329, August 2, 1984.

Cell-mediated immunity to cytomegalovirus (CMV) and herpes simplex virus (HSV)
antigens in the acquired immune deficiency syndrome: interleukin-1 and inter-
leukin-2 modify in vitro responses, by J. F. Sheridan, et al. JOURNAL OF CLIN-
ICAL IMMUNOLOGY 4(4):304-311, July 1984.

Cell replication in an immunologically stimulated cell population in human bone marrow, by M. L. Greenberg, et al. ANNALS OF THE NEW YORK ACADEMY OF SCI-
ENCES 459:67-72, 1985.

Cellular and T-lymphocyte subpopulation profiles in bronchoalveolar lavage fluid from
patients with acquired immunodeficiency syndrome and pneumonitis, by J. M.
Wallace, et al. AMERICAN REVIEW OF RESPIRATORY DISEASE 130(5):786-
790, November 1984.

Cellular immune deficiency and polylymphadenopathy in the male sexual partners of a
woman who died of acquired immunodeficiency (AIDS), by U. A. Baumann, et al.
SCHWEIZERISCHE MEDIZINISCHE WOCHENSCHRIFT 114(12):415-418,
March 24, 1984.

Cellular immunity and the acquired immune deficiency syndrome: failure to secrete
lymphokines and gamma interferon, by C. C. Hart, et al. SURVEY AND SYN-
THETICS OF PATHOLOGY RESEARH 3(5):397-408, 1984.

Cellular targets of antilymphocyte antibodies in AIDS and LAS, by R. H. Tomar, et al. CLINICAL IMMUNOLOGY AND IMMUNOPATHOLOGY 37(1):37-47, October 1985.

Central nervous system disease in acquired immunodeficiency syndrome: prospective correlation using CT, MR imaging, and pathologic studies, by M. J. Post, et al. RADIOLOGY 158(1):141-148, January 1986.

Central nervous system infections in the immunocompromised host, by D. Armstrong. INFECTION 12(Suppl. 1):S58-S64, 1984.

Central nervous system infections in patients with the acquired immune deficiency syndrome (AIDS), by A. A. Harris, et al. CLINICAL NEUROPHARMACOLOGY 8(3):201-210, 1985.

Central nervous system involvement in patients with acquired immune deficiency syndrome (AIDS), by B. S. Koppel, et al. ACTA NEUROLOGICA SCANDINAVICA 71(5):337-353, May 1985.

Central nervous system mass lesions in the acquired immunodeficiency syndrome (AIDS), by R. M. Levy, et al. JOURNAL OF NEUROSURGERY 61(1):9-16, July 1984.

Central nervous system tuberculosis with the acquired immunodeficiency syndrome and its related complex, by E. Bishburg, et al. ANNALS OF INTERNAL MEDICINE 105(2):210-213, August 1986.

Central-nervous-system toxoplasmosis in homosexual men and parenteral drug abusers, by B. Wong, et al. ANNALS OF INTERNAL MEDICINE 100(1):36-42, January 1984.

Century's catastrophe? (2) How contagious—no infection with AIDS virus?, by O. Nilsen. SYKEPLEIEN 73(6):6-11+, March 21, 1986.

Cerebral immunoblastic lymphoma and the acquired immunodeficiency syndrome, by P. F. Bidet, et al. ANNALES FRANCAISES D'ANESTHESIE ET DE REANIMATION 3(6):443-445, 1984.

Cerebral lymphoma, a complication of the acquired immunodeficiency syndrome [letter],by A. P. Blanc, et al. PRESSE MEDICALE 13(14):884, March 31, 1984.

Cerebral toxoplasmosis [letter], by J. H. Sher. LANCET 1(8335):1225, May 28, 1983.

Cerebral toxoplasmosis in acquired immune deficiency syndrome, by R. Alonso, et al. ARCHIVES OF NEUROLOGY 41(3):321-323, March 1984.

Cerebral toxoplasmosis in acquired immuno deficiency syndeome. A comparative assisted tomographic and neuropathological study of a case, by a. Gaston, et al. NEURORADIOLOGY 27(1):83-86, 1985.

Cerebral toxoplasmosis in AIDS,by F. Christ, et al. ROFO: FORTSCHRITTE AUF DEM GEBIETE DER RONTGENSTRAHLEN UND DER NUKLEARMEDIZIN 144(2): 230-231, February 1986.

Cerebral toxoplasmosis in AIDS: a simple laboratory technique for diagnosis, by A. Datry, et al. TRANSACTIONS OF THE ROYAL SOCIETY OF TROPICAL MEDICINE AND HYGIENE 78(5):679-680, 1984.

Cerebral toxoplasmosis in a patient with acquired imunodeficiency syndrome, by A. Danziger, et al. SURGICAL NEUROLOGY 20(4):332-334, October 1983.

Cerebral toxoplasmosis in two adults without known immunodeficiency [letter], by P. Hericord, et al. PRESSE MEDICALE 12(16):1017-1018, April 9, 1983.

Cervical adenopathies in relation to AIDS. Course of histological aspects. Diagnostic and prognostic value, by C. Marche, et al. ANNALES D'OTOLARYNGOLOGIE ET DE CHIRURGIE CERVICO-FACIALE 102(5):299-303, 1985.

Cetus technique detects AIDS virus. CHEMICAL AND ENGINEERING NEWS 64:8, April 21, 1986.

Challenge of the acquired immunodeficiency syndrome, by M. M. Heckler. ANNALS OF INTERNAL MEDICINE 103(5):655-656, November 1985.

Challenge of AIDS, by D. Coleman. OHIO NURSES REVIEW 61(6):11-12, June 1986.

Challenge of AIDS in a free society, by M. Arias-Klein. LAW ENFORCEMENT NEWS 12(1):8+, January 6, 1986.

Challenges and opportunities in biotechnology, by L. R. Overby. PROGRESS IN CLINICAL AND BIOLOGICAL RESEARCH 182:425-443, 1985.

Challenges in caring for the person with AIDS at home, by J. P. Martin. CARING 5(6): 12-14+, June 1986.

Chance of a lifetime, by N. Deutsch. GAY COMMUNITY NEWS 13(41):11, May 3, 1986.

Change in gay life-style, by V. Coppola. NEWSWEEK 101:80, April 18, 193.

Changes in B-lymphocytes in AIDS [letter],by G. J. Ruiz-Argüelles. SANGRE 29(2): 223-224, 1984.

Changes in sexual behaviour and fear of AIDS [letter], by M. T. Schechter, et al. LANCET 1(8389):1293, June 9, 1984.

Changing biclonal gammopathy due to different lymphocyte clones in acquired immunodeficiency syndrome with Kaposi's sarcoma, by H. Piechowiak, et al. KLINISCHE WOCHENSCHRIFT 63(20):1083-1086, October 15, 1985.

Changing patterns of acquired immunodeficiency syndrome in hemophilia patients—United States. MMWR 34(17):241-243, May 3, 1985.

—. JAMA 253:2954-2955, May 24-31, 1985.

Changing patterns of disease, by B. Lorber. TRANSACTIONS AND STUDIES OF THE COLLEGE OF PHYSICIANS OF PHILADELPHIA 7(2):117-130, June 1985.

Channeled reading of AIDS, by J. Harvey. RFD 47:23, Summer 1986.

Characteristics of the acquired immunodeficiency syndrome (AIDS) in Haiti, by J. W. Pape, et al. NEW ENGLAND JOURNAL OF MEDICINE 309(16):945-950, October 20, 1983.

Characterization of the acquired immune deficiency syndrome at the cellular and molecular level, by D. J. Barrett. MOLECULAR AND CELLULAR BIOCHEMISTRY 63(1):3-11, August 1984.

Characterization of adenovirus isolates from AIDS patients, by M. S. Horwitz, et al. ANNALS OF THE NEW YORK ACADEMY OF SCIENCES 437:161-174, 1984.

Characterization of the AIDS-associated retrovirus reverse transcriptase and optimal conditions for its detection in virions, by A. D. Hoffman, et al. VIROLOGY 147:326-235, December 1985.

Characterization of a continuous T-cell line susceptible to the cytopathic effects of the acquired immunodeficiency syndrome (AIDS)-associated retrovirus, by T. Folks, et al. PROCEEDINGS OF THE NATIONAL ACADEMY OF SCIENCES OF THE UNITED STATES OF AMERICA 82(13):4539-4543, July 1985.

Characterization of envelope and core structural gene products of HTLV-III with sera from AIDS patients, by W. G. Robey, et al. SCIENCE 228(4699):593-595, May 3, 1985.

Characterization of exogenous type D retrovirus from a fibroma of a macaque with simian AIDS and fibromatosis, by K. Stromber, et al. SCIENCE 224(4646):289-292, April 20, 1984.

Characterization of gp41 as the transmembrane protein coded by the HTLV-III/LAV envelope gene, by F. diM. Veronese, et al. SCIENCE 229:1402-1405, September 27, 1985.

Characterization of highly immunogenic p66/p51 as the reverse transcriptase of HTLV-III/LAV, by F. DiMarzo Veronese, et al. SCIENCE 231:1289-1291, March 14, 1986.

Characterization of long terminal repeat sequences of HTLV-III, by B. Starcich, et al. SCIENCE 227:538-540, February 1, 1985.

Chasing an AIDS cure, by R. Wood. GAY COMMUNITY NEWS 13(41):8, May 3, 1986.

Chemiluminescence measurement in AIDS, lymphadenopathy and hemophilia patients, by L. Stöhr, et al. ZEITSCHRIFT FÜR HAUTKRANKHEITEN 60(15):1214-1223, August 1, 1985.

Chemotherapeutic approaches to the treatment of the acquired immune deficiency syndrome (AIDS), by E. De Clercq. JOURNAL OF MEDICINAL CHEMISTRY 29(9):1561-1569, September 1986.

Childhood acquired immune deficiency syndrome manifesting as acrodermatitis enteropathica, by T. K. Tong, et al. JOURNAL OF PEDIATRICS 108(3):426-428, March 1986.

Children and AIDS: implications for child welfare, by G. R. Anderson. CHILD WELFARE 63(1):62-73, January-February 1984.

Children with AIDS: part 2, by R. M. Klug. AMERICAN JOURNAL OF NURSING 86(10):1126-1132, October 1986.

Children with AIDS: a special dilemma, by M. W. Moon. MASSACHUSETTS NURSE 55(12):1+, December 1985.

Chimps infected with AIDS-linked virus, by D. Franklin. SCIENCE NEWS 126:261, October 27, 1984.

Choosing a home volunteer for AIDS patients. An appropriate match requires sensitivity in judgement and knowledge, by G. A. Best, et al. AMERICAN JOURNAL OF HOSPICE CARE 3(2):41-43, March-April 1986.

Christian view of AIDS, by S. S. Macauley. JOURNAL OF CHRISTIAN NURSING 3(2): 32, Spring 1986.

Chromatin pattern and DNA content in acquired immune deficiency syndrome (AIDS): indicators of viral infection revealed by DNA image cytometry [letter], by W. Auffermann, et al. ANALYTICAL AND QUANTITATIVE CYTOLOGY 6(4):293-294, December 1984.

Chromosome aberrations in peripheral lymphocytes of male homosexuals, by G. Manolov, et al. CANCER GENETICS AND CYTOGENETICS 18(4):337-350, December 1985.

Chronic adenopathies in persons exposed to the risk of acquired immunodeficiency syndrome [letter], by J. P. Clauvel, et al. PRESSE MEDICALE 13(23):1456, June 2, 1984.

Chronic lymphocytic leukemia: an AIDS like disease? [letter], by N. E. Kay, et al. BRITISH JOURNAL OF HAEMATOLOGY 63(2):389-391, June 1986.

Chronicle: AIDS and the family paper, by Lisa Leff, et al. COLUMBIA JOURNALISM REVIEW 24:11+, March-April 1986.

Church as sanctuary: 1985's top story. CHRISTIAN CENTURY 102:1163-1165, December 18-25, 1985.

Church in the midst of the AIDS epidemic, by L. Ranck. ESA14(2):2-46, February 1986.

Churches and AIDS: responsibilities in mission, by L. Howell. CHRISTIANITY AND CRISIS 45:483-484, December 9, 1985.

Church's response to AIDS: is compassion waning in light of a so-called gay disease. CHRISTIANITY TODAY 29(17):50-51, November 22, 1985.

CIA/CDC/AIDS political alliance, by C. Shively. GAY COMMUNITY NEWS 10(50):5, July 9, 1983.

Cincinnati Board okays measure protecting gays,by M. Tuhus. GUARDIAN 38(41):4, August 6, 1986.

Cincinnati prepares for treatment of AIDS, by J. Zeh. GAY COMMUNITY NEWS 10(26):3, January 22, 1983.

Cincinnati rebuts threat to gay AIDS counselors, by J. Zeh. GAY COMMUNITY NEWS 12(38):1, April 13, 1985.

Cincinnatians nervous about confidentiality, by J. Zeh. GAY COMMUNITY NEWS 12(21):1, December 8, 1984.

Circulating IgA immune complexes in AIDS, by M. M. Lightfoote, et al. IMMUNOLOGICAL INVESTIGATIONS 14(4):341-345, August 1985.

Circulating immune complexes in AIDS [letter],by S. Gupta, et al. NEW ENGLAND JOURNAL OF MEDICINE 310(23):1530-1531, June 7, 1984.

City officials withdraw Cambridge AIDS policy, by K. Westheimer. GAY COMMUNITY NEWS 13(38):1, April 12, 1986.

City window. KANSAS CITY MAGAZINE 11:12-13, January 1986.

Civilian blood banks to help monitor AIDS, by P. Smith. AIR FORCE TIMES 46:24, August 26, 1985.

Civilians exempted from AIDS testing, by P. Smith. AIR FORCE TIMES 46:28, February 10, 1986.

Classification of HTLV-III infection based on 75 cases seen in a suburban community, by M. H. Kaplan, et al. CANCER RESEARCH 45(Suppl. 9):4655s-4658s, September 1985.

Classification of HTLV-III/LAV-related diseases [letter],by H. W. Haverkos, et al. JOURNAL OF INFECTIOUS DISEASES 152(5):1095, November 1985.

Classification system for human T-lymphotropic virus type III/lymphadenopathy-associated virus infections, by Centers for Disease Control, U.S. Department of Health and Human Services. ANNALS OF INTERNAL MEDICINE 105(2):234-237, August 1986.

Clinical. A new approach to combat viruses, by S. Hopkins. NURSING MIRROR 160(18):28-29, May 1, 1985.

Clinical and epidemiological survey of acquired immune deficiency syndrome in Europe, by M. P. Glauser, et al. EUROPEAN JOURNAL OF CLINICAL MICROBIOLOGY 3(1):55-58, February 1984.

Clinical and histologic findings in opportunistic ocular infections. Part of a new syndrome of acquired immunodeficiency, by N. M. Newman, et al. ARCHIVES OF OPHTHALMOLOGY 101(3):396-401, March 1983.

Clinical and immunological findings in HTLV-III infection, by K. J. Krohn, et al. CANCER RESEARCH 45(Suppl. 9):4612s-4615s, September 1985.

Clinical and laboratory findings in ten Milwaukee patients with the acquired immunodeficiency syndrome or prodromal syndromes, by P. A. Turner, et al. WISCONSIN MEDICAL JOURNAL 84(4):19-22, April 1985.

Clinical and pathologic features of an acquired immune deficiency syndrome (AIDS) in macaque monkeys, by N. L. Letvin, et al. ADVANCES IN VETERINARY SCIENCE AND COMPARATIVE MEDICINE 28:237-265, 1984.

Clinical and pathologic findings of the liver in the acquired immune deficiency syndrome (AIDS), by B. J. Glasgow, et al. AMERICAN JOURNAL OF CLINICAL PATHOLOGY 83(5):582-588, May 1985.

Clinical aspects of the acquired immune deficiency syndrome in the United Kingdom, by J. N. Weber, et al. BRITISH JOURNAL OF VENEREAL DISEASES 60(4);253-257, August 1984.

Clinical aspects of confirmed AIDS, by J. P. Coulaud, et al. BULLETIN DE L'ACADEMIE NATIONALE DE MEDECINE 168(1-2):267-270, January-February 1984.

Clinical care and research in AIDS, by P. Volberding, et al. HASTINGS CENTER REPORT 15(4):16-18, August 1985.

Clinical features of AIDS in Europe. EUROPEAN JOURNAL OF CANCER AND CLINICAL ONCOLOGY 20(2):165-167, February 1984.

Clinical features of Kaposi's sarcoma/acquired immune deficiency syndrome and its management, by B. Safai. ANTIBIOTIC CHEMOTHERAPY 32:54-70, 1983.

Clinical features of Pneumocystis pneumonia in the acquired immune deficiency syndrome, by L. A. Engelberg, et al. AMERICAN REVIEW OF RESPIRATORY DISEASE 180(4):689-694, October 1984.

Clinical features of simian acquired immunodeficiency syndrome (SAIDS) in rhesus monkeys, by R. V. Henrckson, et al. LABORATORY ANIMAL SCIENCE 34(2): 140-145, April 1984.

Clinical findings and serological evidence of HTLV-III infection in homosexual contacts of patients with AIDS and persistent generalised lymphadenopathy in London, by B. G. Gazzard, et al. LANCET 2(8401):480-483, September 1, 1984.

Clinical management of AIDS patients, by W. Melson. CALIFORNIA NURSE 82(4):10-12, May 1986.

Clinical manifestations and therapy of Isospora belli infection in patients with the acquired immunodeficiency syndrome, by J. A. DeHovitz, et al. NEW ENGLAND JOURNAL OF MEDICINE 315(2):87-90, July 10, 1986.

Clinical microbiology of acquired immune deficiency syndrome (AIDS), by C. B. Inderlied, et al. JOURNAL OF MEDICAL TECHNOLOGY 2(3):167-173+, March 1985.

Clinical pharmacokinetics of suramin in patients with HTLV-III/LAV infection, by J. M. Collins, et al. JOURNAL OF CLINICAL PHARMACOLOGY 26(1):22-26, January 1986.

Clinical picture and etiopathogenesis of AIDS, by W. Mazurkiewicz. PRZEGLAD DERMATOLOGICZNY 72(2):185-191, March-April 1985.

Clinical spectrum of the acquired immunodeficiency syndrome: implications for comprehensive patient care, by P. A. Volberding. ANNALS OF INTERNAL MEDICINE 103(5):729-733, November 1985.

Clinical spectrum of HTLV-III in humans, by J. E. Groopman. CANCER RESEARCH 45(Suppl. 9):4649s-4651s, September 1985.

Clinical spectrum of human retroviral-induced diseases, by W. J. Urba, et al. CANCER RESEARCH 45(Suppl. 9):4637s-4643s, September 1985.

Clinical spectrum of infections in patients with HTLV-III-associated diseases, by J. W. Gold. CANCER RESEARCH 45(Suppl. 9):4652s-4654s, September 1985.

Clinical symptomatology of the acquired immunodeficiency syndrome (AIDS) and related disorders, by J. E. Groopman. PROGRESS IN ALLERGY 37:182-193, 1986.

Clinical trials of interleukin-2 in the acquired immune deficiency syndrome: warning to autopsy prosectors and other health care professionals [letter], by W. M. Mitchell. HUMAN PATHOLOGY 16(1):97-98, January 1985.

Clinical work-load of HTLV-III infection [letter], by B. A. Evans, et al. LANCET 1(8442): 1388, June 15, 1985.

Clonal analysis of T lymphocytes in the acquired immunodeficiency syndrome. Evidence for an abnormality affecting individual helper and suppressor T cells, by J. B. Margolick, et al. JOURNAL OF CLINICAL INVESTIGATION 76(2):709-715, August 1985.

Clonal selection of T lymphocytes infected by cell-free human T-cell leukemia/ lymphoma virus type I: parameters of virus integration and expression, by A. DeRossi, et al. VIROLOGY 143:640-645, June 1985.

Cloning of AIDS genes brings vaccine near, by I. Anderson. NEW SCIENTIST 103:8, September 13, 1984.

Close to FDA's finish line: five AIDS-linked tests, by R. Rhein, et al. CHEMICAL WEEK 136:25-26, March 6, 1985.

Closer to an AIDS vaccine?, by C. Wallis, et al. TIME 127(14):44, April 7, 1986.

Closing the baths: where will it end?, by S. Brookie. GAY COMMUNITY NEWS 12(22): 3, December 15, 1984.

Clues to the early diagnois of Mycobacterium avium-intracellulare infection in patients with acquired immunodeficiency syndrome, by M. A. Polis, et al. ARCHIVES OF PATHOLOGY AND LABORATORY MEDICINE 109(5):465-466, May 1985.

Cluster of cases of the acquired immune deficiency syndrome. Patients linked by sexual contact, by D. M. Auerbach, et al. AMERICAN JOURNAL OF MEDICINE 76(3):487-492, March 1984.

Cluster of HTLV-III/LAV infection in an African family [letter], by T. Jonckheer, et al. LANCET 1(8425):400-401, February 16, 1985.

CMV connection, by M. Helquist. ADVOCATE 436:25, December 24, 1985.

CNS toxoplasmosis in acquired immunodeficiency syndrome, by S. L. Horowitz, et al. ARCHIVES OF NEUROLOGY 40(10):649-652, October 1983.

Coalition forms for test-site funding. OUT 4(5):6, April 1986.

Coast hospital laundry manager calls yellow alert on AIDS linen. LAUNDRY NEWS 9(8):1+, August 1983.

Coccidioidomycosis in acquired immune deficiency syndrome. Depressed humoral as well as cellular immunity, by C. J. Roberts. AMERICAN JOURNAL OF MEDICINE 76(4):734-736, April 1984.

Code forbids AIDS bids, by N. Irwin. BODY POLITIC 124:17, March 1986.

Cofactor in AIDS? SCIENCE NEWS 128:77, August 3, 1985.

Coffin as closet [editorial]. ADVOCATE 450:5, July 8, 1986.

Coincidental appearance of LAV/HTLV-III antibodies in hemophiliacs and the onset of the AIDS epidemic, by B. L. Evatt, et al. NEW ENGLAND JOURNAL OF MEDICINE 312(8):483-486, February 21, 1985.

College fears for new AIDS measures. NURSING STANDARD 390:1, March 28, 1985.

College health group sees no reason to isolate AIDS victims. THE CHRONICLE OF HIGHER EDUCATION 31:33+, October 16, 1985.

Colleges fear dual threat from AIDS, by W. Norris. THE TIMES HIGHER EDUCATION SUPPLEMENT 683:9, December 6, 1985.

Colonic biopsies have a high diagnostic yield in AIDS, by H. Rotterdam, et al. AMERICAN FAMILY PHYSICIAN 27:191, May 1983.

Colorado to keep list of HTLV-3 positives, by M. Cocoves. GAY COMMUNITY NEWS 13(11):1, September 28, 1985.

Combating AIDS. THE ECONOMIST 298:13-14, February 1, 1986.

Coming of AIDS: it didn't start with homosexuals, and it won't end with them, by J. F. Grutsch, et al. AMERICAN SPECTATOR 19(3):12-15, March 1986.

Coming of AIDS: a viral update, by J. F. Grutsch, et al. AMERICAN SPECTATOR 19:18-20, September 1986.

Coming to terms with AIDS, by J. Laurance. NEW SOCIETY November 14, 1986, p. 9-11.

Comment—need for bridge building, by Horowitz, et al. NACLA'S REPORT ON THE AMERICAS 18(2):2, March 1984.

Commentary on 'Recommendations on the prevention and control of AIDS by the Public Health Service' [letter], by N. Schmacke, et al. OFFENTLICHE GESUND-HEITSWESEN 46(8):395-396, August 1984.

Comments on the CDC Guideline for Employees Health, by W. M. Valenti. INFEC-TION CONTROL 5(4):192-194, April 1984.

Common bond of suffering, by W. A. Henry, III. TIME 125:85, May 13, 1985.

Common cup supported. CHRISTIAN CENTURY 103(6):169, February 19, 1986.

Common disinfectants kill AIDS virus. RN 49:81, January 1986.

Communicable disease report. April to June 1983. COMMUNITY MEDICINE 5(4): 330-332, November 1983.

—. October to December 1984. COMMUNITY MEDICINE 7(2):136-144, May 1985.

Community. Home AIDS, by S. Robins. NURSING MIRROR 160(8):21-22, February 1985.

Community-acquired opportunistic infections and defective cellular immunity in heter-osexual drug abusers and homosexual men, by C. B. Small, et al. AMERICAN JOURNAL OF MEDICINE 74(3):433-441, March 1983.

Community approach to AIDS through hospice. Louisiana program promotes high quality of life, by H. S. Kutzen. AMERICAN JOURNAL OF HOSPICE CARE 3(2): 17-23, March-April 1986.

Companions for men with AIDS, by A. Cohen. GAY COMMUNITY NEWS 12(19):8, November 24, 1984.

Comparative pathology of cardiac neoplasms in humans and in laboratory rodents: a review, by C. Hoch-Ligeti, et al. JOURNAL OF THE NATIONAL CANCER INSTI-TUTE 76(1):127-142, January 1986.

Comparative ultrastructural study of virions in human pre-AIDS and simian AIDS, by T. F. Warner, et al. ULTRASTRUCTURAL PATHOLOGY 7(4):251-258, 1984.

Comparison of ADCC and NK activities of peripheral blood mononuclear cells from pa-tients at risk for acquired immune deficiency syndrome (AIDS), by J. Wisecarver, et al. AIDS RESEARCH 1(5):347-352, 1983-1984.

Comparison of biopsy-proven Pneumocystis carinii pneumonia in acquired immune deficiency syndrome patients and renal allograft recipients, by R. P. Sterling, et al. ANNALS OF THORACIC SURGERY 38(5):494-499, November 1984.

Compassion for AIDS victims, by N. Mallovy. HOMEMAKERS' MAGAZINE 21:38+, March 1986.

Compassion marks church service for AIDS victims. NATIONAL CATHOLIC REPORTER 21:6, January 18, 1985.

Complacency threatens AIDS group. BODY POLITIC 403:16, September 18, 1984.

Complaint filed for AIDS/bias, by P. Byron. GAY COMMUNITY NEWS 11(7):1, September 3, 1983.

Complete nucleotide sequence of the AIDS virus, HTLV-III, by L. Ratner, et al. NATURE 313(6000):277-284, January 24-30, 1985.

Complexing AIDS, by J. Silberner. SCIENCE NEWS 128:267, October 26, 1985.

Complications of co-trimoxazole in treatment of AIDS-associated Pneumocystis carinii pneumonia in homosexual men, by H. S. Jaffe, et al. LANCET 2(8359):1109-1111, November 12, 1983.

Computerized access to clinical nursing literature on AIDS, by S. M. Sparks. TOPICS IN CLINICAL NURSING 6(2):79-82, July 1984.

Computers AIDS and literature, by R. Hall. ADVOCATE 3(76):34, September 15, 1983.

Concentric effects of the acquired immune deficiency syndrome [editorial], by E. N. Brandt, Jr. PUBLIC HEALTH REPORTS 99(1):1-2, January-February 1984.

Concerning the genesis of AIDS, by J. Morgan. MEDICAL HYPOTHESES 13(1):29-30, January 1984 and 13(4):357-358, April 1984.

Concurrent herpes simplex and cytomegalovirus retinitis and encephalitis in the acquired immune deficiency syndrome (AIDS), by J. S. Pepose, et al. OPHTHALMOLOGY 91(12):1669-1677, December 1984.

Condom mania! Sex sensation sweeping the nation, by C. Wittke. GAY COMMUNITY NEWS 13(37):6, April 1, 1986.

Condoms, by K. Orr. BODY POLITIC 109:31, December 1984.

Condoms for prisoners: would fighting AIDS promote homosexual acts?, by L. Cohen, et al. ALBERTA REPORT 12:12-13, October 7, 1985.

Condoms help stop AIDS. BODY POLITIC 123:23, February 1986.

Condoms prevent transmission of AIDS-associated retrovirus [letter], by M. Conant, et al. JAMA 255(13):1706, April 4, 1986.

Conference takes stock of diversity and unity, by Larson, et al. GAY COMMUNITY NEWS 13(20):3, November 30, 1985.

Conference vigil lobbying in Washington, by D. France. GUARDIAN 36(3):4, October 19, 1983.

Confidential matters, by S. Budiansky. NATURE 304:478, August 11, 1983.

Confidentiality in the military, by D. Walter. ADVOCATE 434:12, November 26, 1985.

Confidentiality, informed consent and untoward social consequences in research on a "new killer disease" (AIDS), by R. Purtilo, et al. CLINICAL RESEARCH 31(4):464-472, October 1983.

Congenital rubella syndrome and diabetes: a review of epidemiologic, generic, and immunologic factors, by K. A. Shaver, et al. AMERICAN ANNALS OF THE DEAF 130:526-532, December 1985.

Congregation confronts AIDS, by M. Rankin. SHMATE 13:3, Fall 1985.

Congress and AIDS legislation, by D. Walter ADVOCATE 447:14, May 27, 1986.

Congress close to doubling AIDS SPD, by L. Bush. ADVOCATE 3(71):8, July 7, 1983.

Congress eyes proposals to curb AIDS. HUMAN EVENTS 45:5, December 7, 1985.

Congress likely to halt shrinkage in AIDS funds, by C. Norman. SCIENCE 231(4744): 1364-1365, March 21, 1986.

Congress, NIH open coffers for AIDS, by G. Kolata. SCIENCE 221(4609):436+, July 29, 1983.

Congress readies AIDS funding transfusion, by C. Norman. SCIENCE 230(4724): 418-419, October 25, 1985.

Congressional Committee/AIDS funding, by D. Walter. ADVOCATE 417:12, April 2, 1985.

Congressman AIDS, by T. Johnson. LOS ANGELES 124, January 1986.

Consensus conference. The impact of routine HTLV-III antibody testing of blood and plasma donors on public health. JAMA 256(13):1778-1783, October 3, 1986.

Consent form for AIDS research urged by Brandt, by S. Kulieke. ADVOCATE 405:8, October 16, 1984.

Considerations in searching for the cause of AIDS, by J. Teas. ANNALS OF THE NEW YORK ACADEMY OF SCIENCES 437:270-272, 1984.

Considering the psychosocial aspects of AIDS, by L. J. Redouty, et al. MICHIGAN HOSPITALS 22(8):17-21, August 1986.

Conspectus. Acquired immune deficiency syndrome, by D. R. Howard. COMPRE-HENSIVE THERAPY 9(8):3-5, August 1983.

Constitutional rights of AIDS carriers. HARVARD LAW JOURNAL 99(6):1274-1292, April 1986.

Consultation and collaborative studies on AIDS offered by New Center and Registry at the Armed Forces Institute of Pathology. PUBLIC HEALTH REPORTS 101: 108, January-February 1986.

Consultation 7—here everything turns around the AIDS virus, by I. Lernevall. VARD-FACKET 9(22):10-12, December 12, 1985.

Contact tracing in the acquired immune deficiency syndrome (AIDS). Evidence for transmission of virus and disease by an asymptomatic carrier, by D. A. Cooper, et al. MEDICAL JOURNAL OF AUSTRALIA 141(9):579-582, October 27, 1984.

Containing AIDS. THE ECONOMIST 296:13-14, August 10, 1985.

Containing the AIDS epidemic [letter]. JAMA 254(15):2059-2060.

Continued risk of transfusion-transmitted AIDS, by J. Kolins. PATHOLOGIST 40(6):9-10, June 1986.

Continuing fight for all our lives, by L. Kessler. GAY COMMUNITY NEWS 11(20):5, December 3, 1983.

Continuous high-grade mycobacterium avium-intracellulare bacteremia in patients with the acquired immune deficiency syndrome, by B. Wong, et alf. AMERICAN JOURNAL OF MEDICINE 78(1):35-40, January 1985.

Contracting AIDS as a means of committing suicide [letter], by R. J. Frances, et al. AMERICAN JOURNAL OF PSYCHIATRY 142(5):656, May 1985.

Contribution of immunology to the positive and differential diagnosis of the acquired immunodeficiency syndrome. Immunologic mechanisms of the syndrome, by J. C. Gluckman, et al. BULLETIN DE L'ACADEMIE NATIONALE DE MEDECINE 168(1-2):282-287, January-February 1984.

Controlling the baths and backroom bars, by M. Callen. VILLAGE VOICE 30:36, March 12, 1985.

Controversial issues dominate Army Management Conferences—AIDS, over-40 screening. NATIONAL GUARD 40:29-30, February 1986.

Coolfont Report: a PHS plan for prevention and control of AIDS and the AIDS virus, by D. I. Macdonald. PUBLIC HEALTH REPORTS 101(4):341-348, July-August 1986.

Coombs' test and the acquired immunodeficiency syndrome [letter], by S. Gupta, et al. ANNALS OF INTERNAL MEDICINE 100(3):462, March 984.

Coordination and managment of information on AIDS, by L. S. Garden. SYGEPLE-JERSKEN 86(24):32-33+, June 1986.

Coping with AIDS, by A. Moreton. NURSING MIRROR 161(1):49-51, July 3, 1985.

Coping with AIDS: crucial considerations, by W. V. Soughton. DIMENSIONS IN HEALTH SERVICE 61(9):19-20, September 1984.

Coping with the threat of AIDS. An approach to psychosocial assessment, by J. G. Joseph, et al. AMERICAN PSYCHOLOGIST 39(11):1297-1302, November 1984.

Coping with the tragedy of AIDS, by M. Helquist. MS. 12:22, February 1984.

Corporate U.S. looks at workers with AIDS, by C. Harris. GAY COMMUNITY NEWS 13(32):3, March 1, 1986.

Correctional officials may be closing their eyes to AIDS threat. LAW ENFORCEMENT NEWS 12(1):1+, January 6, 1986.

Corrections. CRIMINAL JUSTICE NEWSLETTER 15(20):7, October 15, 1984.

Correlation between exposure to human T-cell leukemia-lymphoma virus-III and the development of AIDS, by P. D. Markham, et al. ANNALS OF THE NEW YORK ACADEMY OF SCIENCES 437:106-109, 1984.

Correlation between gallium lung scans and fiberoptic bronchoscopy in patients with suspected Pneumocystis carinii pneumonia and the acquired immune deficiency syndrome, by D. L. Coleman, et al. AMERICAN REVIEW OF RESPIRATORY DISEASE 130(6):1166-1169, December 1984.

Correlation between immunologic function and clinical subpopulations of patients with the acquired immune deficiency syndrome, by H. C. Lane, et al. AMERICAN JOURNAL OF MEDICINE 78(3):417-422, March 1985.

Correlation between serial pulmonary function tests and fiberoptic bronchoscopy in patients with Pneumocystis carinii pneumonia and the acquired immune deficiency syndrome, by D. L. Coleman, et al. AMERICAN REVIEW OF RESPIRATORY DISEASE 129(3):491-493, March 1984.

Correspondence about handling evidence in cases of acquired immune deficiency syndrome (AIDS) [letter], by J. A. Kaye. AMERICAN JOURNAL OF FORENSIC MEDICINE AND PATHOLOGY 7(1):87-88, March 1986.

Cost of AIDS, by R. Wingerter. IN THESE TIMES 10(26):22, May 28, 1986.

Cost of ignorance, by R. Davenport-Hines. TIMES LITERARY SUPPLEMENT July 18, 1986, p. 780.

Cost of transfusion in AIDS. Experience at the Claude-Bernard Hospital apropos of 28 cases, by M. Simonneau, et al. REVUE FRANCAISE DE TRANSFUSION ET IMMUNO-HEMATOLOGIE 27(4):557-560, September 1984.

Costly disease: the public bill for AIDS could be $5 billion by 1990, by G. Weiss. BARRON'S 65:32, April 22, 1985.

Could AIDS agent be a new variant of African swine fever virus? [letter], by J. Teas. LANCET 1(8330):923, April 23, 1983.

Counseling. Advice and sympathy for AIDS sufferers, by J. Sherman. HEALTH AND SOCIAL SERVICE JOURNAL 95(4976):1506-1507, November 28, 1985.

Countering AIDS . THE ECONOMIST 294:84-85, January 19, 1985.

Countertransference issues in working with persons with AIDS, by J. Dunkel, et al. SOCIAL WORK 31(2):114-117, March-April 1986.

Cranial CT in acquired immunodeficiency syndrome: spectrum of diseases and optimal contrast enhancement technique, by M. J. Post, et al. AJR 145(5):929-940, November 1985.

Crash development of AIDS test nears goal, by B. J. Culliton. SCIENCE 225(4667):1128+, September 14, 1984.

Cream City boosts AIDS support efforts, by S. Burke. OUT 3(2):6, December 1984.

Cries of plague for mysterious AIDS, by L. Wainwright. LIFE MAGAZINE 6:7, July 1983.

Crisis in public health [San Francisco], by K. Leishman. THE ATLANTIC 256:18+, October 1985.

Crisis of mounting AIDS hysteria, by D. Kline. MACLEAN'S 96:6-8, August 1, 1983.

Critical analysis of T cell subset and function evaluation in patients with persistent generalized lymphadenopathy in groups at risk for AIDS,by M. Cavaille-Coll, et al.

CLINICAL AND EXPERIMENTAL IMMUNOLOGY 57(3):511-519, September 1984.

Cry of the normal heart, by D. Smith. NEW YORK 18:42-46, June 3, 1985.

Cryptococcal arthritis in a patient with acquired immune deficiency syndrome. Case report and review of the literature, by D. D. Ricciardi, et al. JOURNAL OF RHEU-MATOLOGY 13(2):455-458, April 1986.

Cryptococcal infections in patients with acquired immune deficiency syndrome, by R. H. Eng, et al. AMERICAN JOURNAL OF MEDICINE 81(1):19-21, July 1986.

Cryptococcal meningitis, herpes genitalis and oral candidiasis in a homosexual man with acquired immunodeficiency syndrome [letter], by J. Bras,et al. NEDER-LANDS TIJDSCHRIFT VOOR GENEESKUNDE 127(34):1553-1554, August 20, 1983.

Cryptococcal meningitis, herpes genitalis and oral immunodeficiency, by L. Zegerius, et al. NEDERLANDS TIJDSCHRIFT VOOR GENEESKUNDE 127(19):817-820, May 7, 1983.

Cryptococcal myocarditis in acquired immune deficiency syndrome, by W. Lewis, et al. AMERICAN JOURNAL OF CARDIOLOGY 55(9):1240, April 15, 1985.

Cryptococcosis and torulopsidosis of the skin and lung and epidermodysplasia ver-ruciformis in AIDS (acquired immune deficiency syndrome), by I. Grimm. HAUT-ARZT 35(12):653-655, December 1984.

Cryptococcosis in the acquired immunodeficiency syndrome, by J. A. Kovacs, et al. ANNALS OF INTERNAL MEDICINE 103(4):533-538, October 1985.

Cryptosporidial enteritis in a homosexual male with an acquired immunodeficiency syndrome, by R. E. Petras, et al. CLEVELAND CLINIC QUARTERLY 50(1):41-45, Spring 1983.

Cryptosporidiosis and AIDS, by D. L. Volker. ONCOLOGY NURSING FORUM 11(3): 86, May-June 1984.

Cryptosporidiosis: assessment of chemotherapy of males with acquired immune defi-ciency syndrome (AIDS). MMWR 31(44):589-592, November 12, 1982.

Cryptosporidiosis in the acquired immune deficiency syndrome, by D. A. Cooper, et al. PATHOLOGY 16(4):455-457, October 1984.

Cryptosporidiosis in homosexual men, by R. Soave, et al. ANNALS OF INTERNAL MEDICINE 100(4):504-511, April 1984.

Cryptosporidiosis of the stomach and small intestine in patients with AIDS, by R. N. Berk, et al. AJR 143(3):549-554, September 1984.

Cryptosporidium and the enteropathy of immune deficiency, by P. Ma. JOURNAL OF PEDIATRIC GASTROENTEROLOGY AND NUTRITION 3(4):488-490, September 1984.

Cryptosporidium causing severe enteritis in a Belgian immunocompetent patient, by J. Vandepitte, et al. ACTA CLINICA BELGICA 40(1):43-47, 1985.

Cryptosporidium enterocolitis in homosexual men with AIDS, by J. Gerstoft, et al. SCANDINAVIAN JOURNAL OF INFECTIOUS DISEASES 16(4):385-388, 1984.

Cryptosporidium in acquired immunodeficiency syndrome, by J. D. Cohen, et al. DIGESTIVE DISEASES AND SCIENCES 29(8):773-777, August 1984.

Cryptosporidium in patient with acquired immunodeficiency syndrome [letter], by C. Jonas, et al. LANCET 2(8356):964, October 22, 1983.

CT biopsy of cerebral toxoplasmosis in AIDS, by B. A. Rodan, et al. JOURNAL OF THE FLORIDA MEDICAL ASSOCIATION 71(3):158-160, March 1984.

CT of acquired immunodeficiency syndrome , by E. M. Bursztyn, et al. AJNR 5(6):7110714, November-December 1984.

Culture-proven cytomegalovirus retinitis in a homosexual man with the acquired immunodeficiency syndrome, by D. M. Bachman, et al. OPHTHALMOLOGY 89(7): 797-804, July 1982.

Curious way to fight AIDS: your tax dollars at work. HUMAN EVENTS 45:6, September 21, 1985.

Current AIDS epidemiology and potential for nosocomial transmission, by D. K. Henderson. TOPICS IN CLINICAL NURSING 6(2):1-22, July 1984.

Cutaneous and lymphadenopathic Kaposi's sarcoma in Africa and the USA with observations on persistent lymphadenopathy in homosexual men at risk for the acquired immunodeficiency syndrome, by R. F. Dorfman. FRONTIERS OF RADIATION THERAPY AND ONCOLOGY 19:105-116, 1985.

Cutaneous cryptococcosis resembling molluscum contagiosum in a patient with AIDS, by M. J. Rico, et al. ARCHIVES OF DERMATOLOGY 121(7):901-902, July 1985.

Cutaneous manifestations of AIDS, by G. E. Pierard, et al. REVUE MEDICALE DE LIEGE 41(6):189-198, March 15, 1986.

Cutaneous reaction to trimethoprim-sulfamethoxazole in patients with AIDS and Kaposi's sarcoma, by R. Mituyasu, et al. NEW ENGLAND JOURNAL OF MEDICINE 308(25):1535-1537, June 2, 1983.

Cutaneous reactions to trimethoprim-sulfamethoxazole in Haitians [letter], by J. A. DeHovitz, et al. ANNALS OF INTERNAL MEDICINE 103(3):479-480, September 1985.

Cuts in AIDS funding?, by D. Walter. ADVOCATE 440:10, February 18, 1986.

Cycle for life. GAY COMMUNITY NEWS 13(42):7, May 17, 1986.

Cycle for life to visit Madison. OUT 4(8):5, June 1986.

Cyclosporin immunosuppression as the possible cause of AIDS [letter],by K. W. Sell,et al. NEW ENGLAND JOURNAL OF MEDICINE 309(17):1065, October 27, 1983.

Cyclosporine-like substances not detected in patients with AIDS [letter],by H. F. Schran, et al. NEW ENGLAND JOURNAL OF MEDICINE 310(20):1324, May 17, 1984.

Cytofluorographic analysis of lymph nodes from patients with the persistent generalized lymphadenopathy (PGL) syndrome, by N. Levy, et al. DIAGNOSTIC IMMUNOLOGY 3(1):15-23, 1985.

Cytologic diagnosis of Pneumocystis carinii infection by bronchoalveolar lavage in acquired immune deficiency syndrome, by M. Orenstein, et al. ACTA CYTOLOGICA 29(5):727-731, September-October 1985.

Cytologic findings in homosexual males with acquired immunodeficiency, by S. W. Lobenthal, et al. ACTA CYTOLOGICA 27(6):597-604, November-December 1983.

Cytomegalovirus and carcinogenesis, by F. Rapp. JOURNAL OF THE NATIONAL CANCER INSTITUTE 72(4):783-787, April 1984.

Cytomegalovirus- and Cryptosporidium-associated acalculous gangrenous cholecystitis, by R. S. Blumberg, et al. AMERICAN JOURNAL OF MEDICINE 76(6):1118-1123, June 1984.

Cytomegalovirus and herpes simplex virus ascending myelitis in a patient with acquired immune deficiency syndrome, by T. Tucker, et al. ANNALS OF NEUROLOGY 18(1):74-79, July 1985.

Cytomegalovirus colitis. Report of the clinical, endoscopic, and pathologic findings in two patients with the acquired immune deficiency syndrome, by M. S. Meiselman, et al. GASTROENTEROLOGY 88(1, Part 1):171-175, January 1985.

Cytomegalovirus colitis in acquired immunodeficiency syndrome—a chronic disease with varying manifestations, by W. Levinson, et al. AMERICAN JOURNAL OF GASTROENTEROLOGY 80(6):445-447, June 1985.

Cytomegalovirus colitis in AIDS: radiographic findings in 11 patients, by E. J. Balthazar, et al. RADIOLOGY 155(3):585-589, June 1985.

Cytomegalovirus encephalitis in acquired immunodeficiency syndrome, by D. A. Hawley, et al. AMERICAN JOURNAL OF CLINICAL PATHOLOGY 80(6):874-877, December 1983.

Cytomegalovirus encephalitis in a patient with acquired immunodeficiency syndrome [letter], by C. Vital, et al. ARCHIVES OF PATHOLOGY AND LABORATORY MEDICINE 109(2):105-106, February 1985.

Cytomegalovirus esophagitis and gastritis in AIDS, by E. J. Balthazar, et al. AJR 144(6):1201-1204, June 1985.

Cytomegalovirus esophagogastritis in a patient with acquired immunodeficiency syndrome,by P. G. Freedman, et al. AMERICAN JOURNAL OF GASTROENTEROLOGY 80(6):434-437, June 1985.

Cytomegalovirus-induced demyelination associated with acquired immune deficiency syndrome, by L. B. Moskowitz, et al. ARCHIVES OF PATHOLOGY AND LABORATORY MEDICINE 108(11):873-877, November 1984.

Cytomegalovirus-induced immunosuppression, by M. S. Hirsch, et al. ANNALS OF THE NEW YORK ACADEMY OF SCIENCES 478:8-15, 1984.

Cytomegalovirus infection, ascending myelitis, and pulmonary embolus [letter], by P. H. Bagley, et al. ANNALS OF INTERNAL MEDICINE 104(4):587, April 1986.

Cytomegalovirus infection in homosexual men—relationship to AIDS, by W. L. Drew. FRONTIERS OF RADIATION THERAPY AND ONCOLOGY 19:38-42, 1985.

Cytomegalovirus infections in AIDS [letter], by H. L. Schmidts, et al. DEUTSCHE MEDIZINISCHE WOCHENSCHRIFT 110(20):818, May 17, 1985.

Cytomegalovirus meningoencephalitis in a homosexual man with Kaposi's sarcoma: isolatin of CMV from CSF cells, by R. H. Edwards, et al. NEUROLOGY 35(4):560-562, April 1985.

Cytomegalovirus pyloric obstruction in a child with acquired immunodeficiency syndrome, by M. S. Victoria, et al. PEDIATRIC INFECTIOUS DISEASE 4(5):550-552, September-October 1985.

Cytomegalovirus retinitis in the acquired immunodeficiency syndrome (AIDS). Light-microscopical, ultrastructural and immunohistochemical examination of a case, by O. A. Jensen, et al. ACTA OPHTHALMOLOGICA 62(1):1-9, February 1984.

Cytomegalovirus retinitis in a young homosexual male with acquired immunodeficiency, by J. Neuwirth, et al. OPHTHALMOLOGY 89(7):805-808, July 1982.

Cytomegalovirus retinitis: a manifestation of the acquired immune deficiency syndrome (AIDS), by A. H. Friedman, et al. BRITISH JOURNAL OF OPHTHALMOLOGY 67(6):372-380, June 1983.

Cytotoxic effector mechanisms in AIDS, by S. Cunningham-Rundles, et al. ADVANCES IN EXPERIMENTAL MEDICINE AND BIOLOGY 187:97-110, 1985.

Damage control. TIME 126:25, November 4, 1985.

Dapsone for AIDS-associated Kaposi's sarcoma [letter], by G. J. Hruza, et al. LANCET 1(8429):642, March 16, 1985.

Dateline: San Francisco: a crisis of mounting AIDS hysteria, by D. Kline. MACLEAN'S 96:6-8, August 1, 1983.

David's story. READERS DIGEST (CANADA) 127:50-55, August 1985.

DC Council enacts tough insurance law, by D. Walter. ADVOCATE 449:12, June 24, 1986.

D.C. Insurance Law enacted, by D. Walter. ADVOCATE 454:22, September 2, 1986.

D.C. Insurance Law surviving, by J. McKnight. GAY COMMUNITY NEWS 14(7):1, August 24, 1986.

DC insurers barred from testing for AIDS, by J. Firshein. HOSPITALS 60(13):50+, July 5, 1986.

Deadline moved up for overseas AIDS tests, by L. Famiglietti. AIR FORCE TIMES 47: 1+, September 22, 1986.

Deadly spread of AIDS, by C. Wallis. TIME 120:55, September 6, 1982.

Dealing with AIDS, by C. Hays. NATIONAL CATHOLIC REGISTER 63:1+, March 16, 1986.

Death and the erotic imagination, by M. Bronski. GAY COMMUNITY NEWS 14(8):8, September 7, 1986.

Death in the AIDS patient: role of cytomegalovirus [letter], by A. M. Macher, et al. NEW ENGLAND JOURNAL OF MEDICINE 309(23):1454, December 8, 1983.

Death in the family, by L. Van Gelder. ROLLING STONE February 3, 1983, p. 18-20+.

Deathly ill at centre stage, by A. Nelson. MACLEAN'S 98:58, June 24, 1985.

Debate continues over treatment of workers with AIDS. SAVINGS INSTITUTIONS 107:76-77, January 1986.

Decision backs phone employee, by K. Westheimer. GAY COMMUNITY NEWS 13(41):1, May 3, 1986.

Deconstructing a syndrome. GAY COMMUNITY NEWS 13:30, Fall 1983.

Decreased expression of human class II antigens on monocytes from patients with acquired immune deficiency syndrome. Increased expression with interferon-gamma, by W. Heagy, et al. JOURNAL OF CLINICAL INVESTIGATION 74(6):2089-2096, December 1984.

Decreased 5' nucleotidase activity in lymphocytes from asymptomatic sexually active homosexual men and patients with the acquired immune deficiency syndrome, by J. L. Murray, et al. BLOOD 64(5):1016-1021, November 1984.

Decreased helper T lymphocytes in homosexual men. I. Sexual contact in high-incidence areas for the acquired immunodeficiency syndrome, by J. J. Goedert, et al. AMERICAN JOURNAL OF EPIDEMIOLOGY 121(5):629-636, May 1985.

—. II. Sexual practices, by J. J. Goedert, et al. AMERICAN JOURNAL OF EPIDEMIOLOGY 121(5):637-644, May 1985.

Decreased incidence of syphilis among homosexual men as a consequence of AIDS?, by L. Hellström, et al. LAKARTIDNINGEN 82(28-29):2529-2530, July 10, 1985.

Decreased population of Leu-7+ natural killer cells in lymph nodes of homosexual men with AIDS-related persistent lymphadenopathy, by S. Jothy, et al. CANADIAN MEDICAL ASSOCIATION JOURNAL 132(2):141-144, January 15, 1985.

Dedicated soldier: in war against AIDS, Samuel Broder serves as general and private, by M. Chase. WALL STREET JOURNAL 208:1+, October 17, 1986.

Defective B-lymphocyte function in homosexual men in relation to the acquired immunodeficiency syndrome, by S. G. Pahwa, et al. ANNALS OF INTERNAL MEDICINE 101(6):757-763, December 1984.

Defective humoral immunity in pediatric acquired immune deficiency syndrome, by L. J. Bernstein, et al. JOURNAL OF PEDIATRICS 107(3):352-357, September 1985.

Defective in vitro T cell colony formation in the acquired immunodeficiency syndrome, by A. Winkelstein, et al. JOURNAL OF IMMUNOLOGY 134(1):151-156, January 1985.

Defective monocyte function in acquired immune deficiency syndrome (AIDS): evidence from a monocyte-dependent T-cell proliferative system, by H. E. Prince, et al. JOURNAL OF CLINICAL IMMUNOLOGY 5(1):21-25, January 1985.

Defective polymorphonuclear leukocyte migration in AIDS [letter], by G. J. Ras, et al. SOUTH AFRICAN MEDICAL JOURNAL 68(5):292-293, August 31, 1985.

Defective regulation of Epstein-Barr virus infection in patients with acquired immunodeficiency syndrome (AIDS) or AIDS-related disorders,by D. L. Birx, et al. NEW ENGLAND JOURNAL OF MEDICINE 314(14):874-879, April 3, 1986.

116

Defective reticuloendothelial system Fc-receptor function in patients with acquired immunodeficiency syndrome, by B. S. Bender, et al. JOURNAL OF INFECTIOUS DISEASES 152(2):409-412, August 1985.

Defective T-cell response to PHA and mitogenic monoclonal antibodies in male homosexuals with acquired immunodeficiency syndrome and its in vitro correction by interleukin 2, by N. Ciobanu, et al. JOURNAL OF CLINICAL IMMUNOLOGY 3(4):332-340, October 1983.

Deficiency in dietary gamma-linolenic and/or eicosapentaenoic acids may determine individual susceptibility to AIDS, by M. E. Bégin, et al. MEDICAL HYPOTHESES 20(1):1-8, May 1986.

Deficiency of interferon-alpha generating capacity is associated with susceptibility to opportunistic infections in patients with AIDS, by C. Lopez, et al. ANNALS OF THE NEW YORK ACADEMY OF SCIENCES 437:39-48, 1984.

Deficient, HLA-restricted, cytomegalovirus-specific cytotoxic T cells and natural killer cells in patients with the acquired immunodeficiency syndrome, by A. H. Rook, et al. JOURNAL OF INFECTIOUS DISEASES 152(3):627-630, September 1985.

Deficient LAV I neutralising capacity of sera from patients with AIDS or related syndromes [letter], by F. Clavel, et al. LANCET 1(8433):879-880, April 13, 1985.

Deficient OKT4 epitope on helper T cells in a patient with SLE: confusion with AIDS, by W. Stohl. NEW ENGLAND JOURNAL OF MEDICINE 310:1531, June 7, 1984.

Defuse AIDS panic!, by H. Cole. RFD 45:34, Winter 1985.

Delta AIDS regulation takes quick nosedive, by D. Walter. ADVOCATE 416:14, March 19, 1985.

Delta backs down on AIDS policy, by C. Guilfoy. GAY COMMUNITY NEWS 12(31):1, February 23, 1985.

Delta bumps PWA from flight, later apologizes, by P. Freiberg. ADVOCATE 455:14, September 16, 1985.

Dementia and AIDS. AMERICAN FAMILY PHYSICIAN 32:239+, August 1985.

Demonstration of Isospora belli by acid-fast stain in a patient with acquired immune deficiency syndrome, by E. Ng, et al. JOURNAL OF CLINICAL MICROBIOLOGY 20(3):384-386, September 1984.

Demonstration of serum antibodies to cryptosporidium sp. in normal and immunodeficiency humans with confirmed infections, by P. N. Campbell,e t al. JOURNAL OF CLINICAL MICROBIOLOGY 18(1):165-169, July 1983.

Dendritic reticulum cells in AIDS-related lymphadenopathy, by M. Alavaikko, et al. EXPERIENTIA 41(9):1173-1175, September 15, 1985.

Dental care for the AIDS patient: the dentist's perspective, by L. Brooks. TEXAS HOSPITALS 40(6):9, November 1984.

Dental care for the AIDS patient: the infection control practitioner's perspective, by C. Hardy. TEXAS HOSPITALS 40(5):9-10, October 1984.

Depressed interleukin 2 receptor expression in acquired immune deficiency and lymphadenopathy syndromes, by H. E. Prince, et al. JOURNAL OF IMMUNOLOGY 133(3):1313-1317, Septemeber 1984.

Deregulation of interleukin-2 receptor gene expression in HTLV-I-induced adult T-cell leukemia, by M. Krönke, et al. SCIENCE 228:1215-1217, June 7, 1985.

Description of an emerging epidemic: the acquired immunodeficiency syndrome (AIDS), by F. M. Muggia. GAN TO KAGAKU RYOHO 10(12):2429-2441, December 1983.

Desire and Mr. Hayhoe, by A. Lumsden. NEW STATESMAN 110:14-15, November 29, 1985.

Desperate American AIDS victims journey to Paris, hoping that a new drug can stave off death, by J. Jarvis, et al. PEOPLE 24(7):42-43, August 12, 1985.

Desperate living—analysis—gay health. RFD 36:21, Fall 1983.

Despite increase in cases, AIDS not a public risk. WORLD HEALTH March 1984, p. 30-31.

Detaining patients with AIDS. BRITISH MEDICAL JOURNAL 291(6502):1102, October 19, 1985.

Detection, isolation, and continuous production of cytopathic retroviruses (HTLV-III) from patients with AIDS and pre-AIDS, by M. Popovic, et al. SCIENCE 224:497-500, May 4, 1984.

Detection of AIDS virus in macrophages in brain tissue from AIDS patients with encephalopathy, by S. Koenig, et al. SCIENCE 233:1089-1093, September 5, 1986.

Detection of anti-HTLV-III antibodies in gammaglobulin preparations for intramuscular injection [letter], by N. Scheiermann, et al. DEUTSCHE MEDIZINISCHE WOCHENSCHRIFT 110(49):1912-1913, December 6, 1985.

Detection of anti-HTLV-III/LAV antibody by enzyme-linked immunosorbent assay in high-risk individuals in Switzerland 1974-1985, by J. Stroun, et al. EUROPEAN JOURNAL OF CLINICAL MICROBIOLOGY 4(6):583-586, December 1985.

Detection of coronavirus-like particles in homosexual men with acquired immunodeficiency and related lymphadenopathy syndrome, by P. Kern, et al. KLINISCHE WOCHENSCHRIFT 63(2):68-72, January 15, 1985.

Detection of IgG antibodies to lymphadenopathy-associated virus in patients with AIDS or lymphadenopathy syndrome,by F. Brun-Vezinet, et al. LANCET 1(8389):1253-1256, June 9, 1984.

Detection of infectious HTLV-III/LAV virus in cell-free plasma from AIDS patients [letter], by D. Zagury, et al. LANCET 2(8453):505-506, August 31, 1985.

Detection of terminal deoxynucleotidyl transferase [letter],by R. D. Barr, et al. BLOOD 66(4):1006-1007, October 1985.

Detection of two human T cell leukemia/lymphotropic viruses in cultured lymphocytes of a hemophiliac with acquired immunodeficiency syndrome, by E. L. Palmer, et al. JOURNAL OF INFECTIOUS DISEASES 151(3):559-563, March 1985.

Determination of a splice acceptor site of pX gene in HTLV-I infected cells, by T. Okamoto, et al. VIROLOGY 143:636-639, June 1985.

Development and early natural history of HTLV-III antibodies in persons with hemophilia, by M. E. Eyster, et al. JAMA 253:2219-2223, April 19, 1985.

Developmental abnormalities in infants and children with acquired immune deficiency syndrome (AIDS) and AIDS-related complex, by M. H. Ultmann, et al. DEVELOPMENTAL MEDICINE AND CHILD NEUROLOGY 27(5):563-571, October 1985.

Diagnosis and management of acquired immune deficiency syndrome in intravenous drug users, by D. Shine. ADVANCES IN ALCOHOL AND SUBSTANCE ABUSE 5(1-2):25-34, 1985-1986.

Diagnosis and management of mycobacterial infection and disease in persons with human T-lymphotropic virus type III/lymphadenopathy-associated virus infection. MMWR 35(28):448-452, July 18, 1986.

Diagnosis for interstitial lung disease in patients with acquired immunodeficiency syndrome (AIDS): a prospective comparison of bronchial washing, alveolar lavage, transbronchial lung biopsy, and open-lung biopsy, by R. J. McKenna, Jr., et al. ANNALS OF THORACIC SURGERY 41(3):318-321, March 1986.

Diagnosis of HTLV-III infection by ultrastructural examination of germinal centers in lymph node—a case report, by T. F. Warner, et al. AIDS RESEARCH 2(1):43-50, February 1986.

Diagnosis of intracranial lesions in AIDS [letter], by I. C. Denton, Jr., et al. JAMA 253(23):3398, June 21, 1985.

Diagnosis of Pneumocystis carinii pneumonia in patients with the acquired immunodeficiency syndrome using subsegmental bronchoalveolar lavage, by F. P. Ognibene, et al. AMERICAN REVIEW OF RESPIRATORY DISEASE 129(6):929-932, June 1984.

Diagnosis of pulmonary complications of the acquired immune deficiency syndrome, by M. J. Rosen, et al. THORAX 40(8):571-575, August 1985.

Diagnosis of pulmonary disease in acquired immune deficiency syndrome (AIDS) [letter], by R. Kern, et al. AMERICAN REVIEW OF RESPIRATORY DISEASE 131(5): 802-803, May 1985.

Diagnosis of pulmonary disease in acquired immune deficiency syndrome (AIDS). Role of bronchoscopy and bronchoalveolar lavage, by D. E. Stover, et al. AMERICAN REVIEW OF RESPIRATORY DISEASE 130(4):659-662, October 1984.

Diagnosis of Toxoplasma encephalitis in absence of neurological signs by early computerised tomographic scanning in patients with AIDS [letter], by R. Roué, et al. LANCET 2(8417-8418):1472, December 22, 1984.

Diagnostic pathology in the acquired immunodeficiency syndrome. Surgical pathology and cytology experience with 67 patients, by J. B. Amberson, et al. ARCHIVES OF PATHOLOGY AND LABORATORY MEDICINE 109(4):345-351, April 1985.

Diagnostic potential for human malignancies of bacterially produced HTLV-I envelope protein, by K. P. Samuel, et al. SCIENCE 226:1074-1097, November 30, 1984.

Diagnostic utility of fiberoptic bronchoscopy in patients with Pneumocystis carinii pneumonia and the acquired immune deficiency syndrome, by D. L. Coleman, et al. AMERICAN REVIEW OF RESPIRATORY DISEASE 128(5):795-799, November 1983.

Diagnostic value of the determination of an interferon-induced enzyme activity: decreased 2',5'-oligoadenylate dependent binding protein activity in AIDS patient lymphocytes, by J. M. Wu, et al. AIDS RESEARCH 2(2):127-131, Spring 1986.

Diarrhea and the acquired immunodeficiency syndrome, by C. Bories, et al. GASTROENTEROLOGIE CLINIQUE ET BIOLOGIQUE 9(4):354-360, April 1985.

Diarrhea and malabsorption associated with the acquired immunodeficiency syndrome (AIDS). NUTRITION REVIEWS 43:235-237, August 1985.

Diarrhea and malabsorption in acquired immune deficiency syndrome: a study of four cases with special emphasis on opportunistic protozoan infestations, by R. Modigliani, et al. GUT 26(2):179-187, February 1985.

Diarrhea caused by 'nonpathogenic amoebae' in patients with AIDS [letter], by K. V. Rolston, et al. NEW ENGLAND JOURNAL OF MEDICINE 315(3):192, July 17, 1986.

Difference in the behavior of T-lymphocyte populations in heroin and methadone addicts, by M. A. Brugo, et al. BOLLETTINO DELL ISTITUTO SIEROTERAPICO MILANESE 62(6):517-523, 1983.

Different kind of AIDS fight: scientists engage in a heated transatlantic duel, by C. Wallis, et al. TIME 127(19):86, May 12, 1986.

Different view of AIDS,by C. R. Tennison, Jr. NORTH CAROLINA MEDICAL JOURNAL 44(7):457-458, July 1983.

Differential antibody responses of individuals infected with AIDS-associated retroviruses surveyed using the viral core antigen p25 ga expressed in bacteria, by K. S. Steimer, et al. VIROLOGY 150(1):283-290, April 15, 1986.

Differential diagnosis at the bedside. Mycoplasma pneumonia or AIDS?, by O. Karg, et al. MUENCHENER MEDIZINISCHE WOCHENSCHRIFT 125(35):72-73, September 2, 1983.

Differential effects of interferon-alpha 2 and interleukin-2 on natural killer cell activity in patients with acquired immune deficiency syndrome, by M. M. Reddy, et al. JOURNAL OF BIOLOGICAL RESPONSE MODIFIERS 3(4):379-386, August 1984.

Differential susceptibility to the acquired immunodeficiency syndrome retrovirus in cloned cells of human leukemic T-cell line Molt-4, by R. Kikukawa, et al. JOURNAL OF VIROLOGY 57(3):159-1162, March 1986.

Difficulties in the diagnosis of acquired immune deficiency syndrome [letter], by E. G. Wilkins, et al. JOURNAL OF CLINICAL PATHOLOGY 37(11):1316-1317, November 1984.

Diffuse alveolar damage and interstitial fibrosis in acquired immunodeficiency syndrome patients without concurrent pulmonary infection, by G. Ramaswamy , et al. ARCHIVES OF PATHOLOGY AND LABORATORY MEDICINE 109(5):408-412, May 1985.

Diffuse immunoblastic sarcoma from benign lymphoid proliferation [letter], by J. L. Wade, 3d, et al. ANNALS OF INTERNAL MEDICINE 10094):765, May 1984.

Diffuse pulmonary gallium accumulation with a normal chest radiogram in a homosexual man with Pneumocystis carinii pneumonia. A case report, by S. C. Moses, et al. CLINICAL NUCLEAR MEDICINE 8(12):608-609, December 1983.

Diffuse toxoplasmic retinchoroiditis in a patient with AIDS, by D. W. Parke, 2d, et al. ARCHIVES OF OPHTHALMOLOGY 104(4):571-575, April 1986.

Digestive manifestations of the acquired immunodeficiency syndrome (AIDS): study in 26 patients, by E. René , et al. GASTROENTEROLOGIE CLINIQUE ET BIOLO-GIQUE 9(4):327-335, April 1985.

Dioceses' ministries gear up for AIDS epidemic, by Bill Kenkelen. NATIONAL CATH-OLIC REPORTER 23:1+, December 12, 1986.

Direct polyclonal activation of human B lymphocytes by the acquired immune deficiency syndrome virus, by S. M. Schnittman, et al. SCIENCE 233:1084-1086, September 5, 1986.

Directed blood program to prevent AIDS contamination? AMERICAN FAMILY PHY-SICIAN 33:253, February 1986.

Disabling fear of AIDS responsive to imipramine, by M. A. Jenike, et al. PSYCHO-SOMATICS 27(2):143-144, February 1986.

Disease in many guises, by C. Norman. SCIENCE 230:1019, November 29, 1985.

Disease-specific and tissue-specific production of unintegrated feline leukaemia virus variant DNA in feline AIDS, by J. I. Mullins, et al. NATURE 319:333-336, January 23, 1986.

Disinfection in LAV/HTLV-III infections. KRANKENPFLEGE. SOINS INFIRMIERS 79(5):40-42+, May 1986.

Disproportionate expansion of a minor T cell subset in patients with lymphadenopathy syndrome and acquired immunodeficiency syndrome, by D. e. Lewis, et al. JOURNAL OF INFECTIOUS DISEASES 151(3):555-559, March 1985.

Dispute over AIDS patient priority, by T. Beardsley. NATURE 310:174, July 19, 1984.

Disseminated bilateral chorioretinitis due to Histoplasma capsulatum in a patient with the acquired immunodeficiency syndrome, by A. Macher, et al. OPHTHALMOL-OGY 92(8):1159-1164, August 1985.

Disseminated CMV infection [letter], by D. P. Kotler, et al. JAMA 253(21):3093-3094, June 7, 1985.

Disseminated coccidioidomycosis in AIDS [letter], by D. I. Abrams, et al. NEW ENG-LAND JOURNAL OF MEDICINE 310(15):986-987, April 12, 1984.

Disseminated coccidioidomycosis in a patient with acquired immune deficiency syn-drome, by A. Kovacs, et al. WESTERN JOURNAL OF MEDICINE 140(3):447-449, March 1984.

Disseminated cryptococcal infection, AIDS, Kaposi's sarcoma, chronic diarrhea, hepa-titis B carrier, and cytomegalovirus, by M. Vongxaiburana. WEST VIRGINIA MEDI-CAL JOURNAL 81(11):248-251, November 1985.

Disseminated cryptococcosis in two AIDS patients. A contribution to cryptococcosis diagnosis in AIDS, by F. Staib, et al. DEUTSCHE MEDIZINISCHE WOCHEN-SCHRIFT 111(27):1061-1065, July 4, 1986.

Disseminated cryptococcosis presenting as herpetiform lesions in a homosexual man with acquired immunodeficiency syndrome, by L. K. Borton, et al. JOURNAL OF

THE AMERICAN ACADEMY OF DERMATOLOGY 10(2 Pt 2):387-390, February 1984.

Disseminated histoplasmosis associated with the acquired imune deficiency syndrome,by M. N. Taylor, et al. AMERICAN JOURNAL OF MEDICINE 77(3):579-580, September 1984.

Disseminated histoplasmosis in the acquired immune deficiency syndrome, by L. J. Wheat, et al. ARCHIVES OF INTERNAL MEDICINE144(11):2147-2149, November 1984.

Disseminated histoplasmosis in patients with the acquired immune deficiency syndrome, by J. R. Bonner, et al. ARCHIVES OF INTERNAL MEDICINE 144(11): 2178-2181, Novembr 1984.

Disseminated histoplasmosis, invasive pulmonary aspergillosis, and other opportunistic infections in a homosexual patient with acquired immune deficiency syndrome, by P. G. Jones, et al. SEXUALLY TRANSMITTED DISEASES 10(4):202-204, October-December 1983.

Disseminated infection due to mycobacterium avium-intreacellulare complex [letter], by B. C. West, et al. CHEST 85(5):710-711, May 1984.

Disseminated Kaposi's sarcoma associated with cytomegalic infection and systemic candidiasis in a male homosexual patient (acquired immunodeficiency syndrome), by E. Simó-Camps. MEDICINA CLINICA 83(19):807-811, December 8, 1984.

Disseminated Kaposi's sarcoma in pregnancy: a manifestation of acquired immune deficiency syndrome, by K. F. Rawlinson, et al. OBSTETRICS AND GYNECOLOGY 63(Suppl. 3):2S-6S, March 1984.

Disseminated Kaposi-sarcoma within the framework of acquired immunodeficiency syndrome, by H. Mensing, et al. IMMUNITAT UND INFEKTION 12(5):253-255, October 1984.

Disseminated Mycobacterium avium-intracellulare infection in acquired immunodeficiency syndrome mimicking Whipple's disease,by J. S. Gillin, et al. GASTROENTEROLOGY 85(5):1187-1191, November 1983.

Disseminated Mycobacterium avium-intracellulare infection in homosexual men dying of acquired immunodeficiency, by P. Zakowski, et al. JAMA 248(22):2980-2982, December 10, 1982.

Disseminated Mycobacterium avium-intracellulare infection in homosexual men with acquired cell-mediated immunodeficiency: a histologic and immunologic study of two cases, by C. C. Sohn, et al. AMERICAN JOURNAL OF CLINICAL PATHOLOGY 79(2):247-252, February 1983.

Disseminated Mycobacterium bovis infection from BCG vaccination of a patient with acquired immunodeficiency syndrome. MMWR 34(16):227-228, April 26, 1985.

Disseminated talc granulomatosis. An unusual finding in a patient with acquired immunodeficiency syndrome and fatal cytomegalovirus infection, by J. H. Lewis, et al. ARCHIVES OF PATHOLOGY AND LABORATORY MEDICINE 109(2);147-150, February 1985.

Disseminated tuberculosis and the acquired immunodeficiency syndrome [letter] by A. E. Pitchenik, et al. ANNALS OF INTERNAL MEDICINE 98(1):112, January 1983.

Disseminated tubuloreticular inclusions in acquired immunodeficiency syndrome (AIDS), by M. Kostianovsky, et al. ULTRASTRUCTURAL PATHOLOGY 4(4):331-336, June 1983.

Dissenter in the AIDS capital of the world [Belle Glade, Fla.; views of Mark Whiteside]. DISCOVER 6:48, December 1985.

Distinct IgG recognition patterns during progression of subclinical and clinical infection with lymphadenopathy associated virus/human T lymphotropic virus, by J. M. Lange, et al. BRITISH MEDICAL JOURNAL 292(6515):228-230, January 25, 1986.

Distinctive follicular hyperplasia in the acquired immune deficiency syndrome (AIDS) and the AIDS related complex. A pre-lymphomatous state for B cell lymphomas, by P. R. Meyer, et al. HEMATOLOGICAL ONCOLOGY 2(4):319-347, October-December 1984.

Distribution of the level of antibody to AIDS-assocated virus (LAV) in sera from AIDS or AIDS-related complex and Japanese hemophiliacs infected with AIDS-associated virus, by H. Tsuchie, et al. MICROBIOLOGYAND IMMUNOLOGY 29(11):1083-1087, 1985.

Distribution of type D retrovirus sequences in tissues of macaques with simian acquired immune deficiency and retroperitoneal fibromatosis, by M. L. Bryant, et al. VIROLOGY 150(1):149-160, April 15, 1986.

Diversity of clinical spectrum of HTLV-III infection, by S. L. Valle, et al. LANCET 1(8424):301-304, February 9, 1985.

DNCB data released, by M. Helquist. ADVOCATE 443:21, April 1, 1986.

Do human retroviruses cause multiple sclerosis? NEW SCIENTIST 108:30, December 5, 1985.

Do not go gently, by W. Blumenfeld. GAY COMMUNITY NEWS 11(16):8, November 5, 1983.

Do these primates have AIDS?, by C. Macek. JAMA 249(13):1696-1697, April 1, 1983.

Doctor urges LA County to triple AIDS funding, by J. Cort. ADVOCATE 406:23, October 30, 1984.

Doctors' efforts to control AIDS spark battles over civil liberties, by M. Chase. WALL STREET JOURNAL 205:23+, February 8, 1985.

Doctors explode myths about AIDS. JET 68:24-27, August 19, 1985.

DOD: 40 with AIDS virus denied enlistment, by P. Smith. AIR FORCE TIMES 46:19, December 16, 1985.

DOD says two die from AIDS, over dozen afflicted, by P. Smith. AIR FORCE TIMES 44:10, February 6, 1984.

DOD seeks suggestions on monitoring AIDS, by P. Smith. AIR FORCE TIMES 46:1+, August 12, 1985.

DOD won't punish donors who have AIDS, by P. Smith. AIR FORCE TIMES 45:4, May 20, 1985.

Does antibody screening of donors increase the risk of transfusion-associated AIDS? [letter], by J. T. Perkins, et al. NEW ENGLAND JOURNAL OF MEDICINE 313(2): 115-116, July 11, 1985.

Does prostaglandin aid the AIDS virus?, by B. Johnstone. NEW SCIENTIST 110:28, April 10, 1986.

Does quinine facilitate AIDS?, by V. Ruocco,e t al. ANTIBIOTIC CHEMOTHERAPY 32:159-160, 1983.

Doing research in an epidemic: confidentiality, by K. Mayer. GAY COMMUNITY NEWS 12(36):5, March 30, 1985.

DOJ opinion fuels AIDS firing debate, by D. Burda. HOSPITALS 60(15):30, August 5, 1986.

Domestic AIDS cases clear 4000 mark, by C. Guilfoy. GAY COMMUNITY NEWS 12(1): 1, July 14, 1984.

Don't shy away from a friend, by W. Handy. OUT 4(2):7, December 1985.

Double agent. SCIENTIFIC AMERICAN 251:66+, July 1984.

Double life of an AIDS victim, by G. Clarke. TIME 126:106, October 14, 1985.

Doubts over AIDs precautions spur RN resignation. AMERICAN JOURNAL OF NURSING 83:1258+, September 1983.

Dr. Alfred Katz says fear, not AIDS, is causing a Red Cross blood loss, by M. Ryan. PEOPLE 20:32-33, July 11, 1983.

Dr. Cornwall was obsessed with AIDS . . . the most difficult person I've worked with, by L. Moran. NURSINGLIFE 5(1):30-31, January-February 1985.

Dr. Robert Gallo, the medical sleuth who tracked the cause of AIDS, now tries to find the cure, by M. Brower. PEOPLE 22:49-50+, September 24, 1984.

Draconian law or human decencies, by L. Gostin. NEW STATESMAN June 20, 1986, p. 17-18.

Drug abuse and AIDS: troubling connections, by G. De Stafano. ADVOCATE 449: 47, June 24, 1986.

Drug abusers 'most likely' to spread AIDS virus by needles, by N. Casey. NURSING STANDARD 433:8, February 6, 1986.

Drug hike protestors claim they were sold out, by S. Poggi. GAY COMMUNITY NEWS 13(44):2, May 31, 1986.

Drug-linked AIDS cases up. CORRECTIONS DIGEST 17(10):10, May 7, 1986; also in NARCOTICS CONTROL DIGEST 16(9):2, April 30, 1986.

Drug test advances, civil rights abuses. BODY POLITIC 128:22, July 1986.

Drug therapy for the opportunistic diseases associated with AIDS, by D. Glickman, et al. AMERICAN PHARMACY NS23(10):23-28, October 1983.

Drug trials: four stages of testing, by M. Helquist. ADVOCATE 450:23, July 8, 1986.

Dual diagnosis: AIDS and addiction, by L. Caputo. SOCIAL WORK 30:360-364, July-August 1985.

Dubious test approved; funding cuts loom. BODY POLITIC 113:21, April 1985.

Dukakis announces $1.8 million AIDS grant, by S. Hyde. GAY COMMUNITY NEWS 13(7):3, August 24, 1985.

Dukakis presence at AIDS event draws fire, by S. Poggi. GAY COMMUNITY NEWS 13(2):3, October 5, 1985.

Dumped AIDS patient dies in SF, by D. France. GAY COMMUNITY NEWS 11(16):3, November 5, 1983.

Duties, fears and physicians, by E. H. Loewy. SOCIAL SCIENCE & MEDICINE 22(12):1363-1366, 1986.

Dying to live/reflection on the Black Death, by G. Hannon. BODY POLITIC 117:27, August 1985.

Early data about AIDS infections, by M. Helquist. ADVOCATE 424:26, July 9, 1985.

Early experience and difficulties with bronchoalveolar lavage and transbronchial biopsy in the diagnosis of AIDS associated pneumonia in Britain, by c. R. Swinburn, et al. THORAX 40(3):166-170, March 1985.

Early frost: the story behind NBC's AIDS dram, by A. Block. ADVOCATE 434:43, November 26, 1985.

Early results show drug helps patients to fight AIDS. NEW SCIENTIST 109:23, March 20, 1986.

Early tests find fewer than 240 with AIDS, by P. Smith. AIR FORCE TIMES 46:3, May 26, 1986.

Eastern AIDS, by V. Rich. NATURE 308(5955):105, March 8, 1984.

Economic impact of the first 10,000 cases of acquired immunodeficiency syndrome in the United States, by A. M. Hardy, et al. JAMA 255:209-211, January 10, 1986.

Economic implications: acquired immunodeficiency syndrome [editorial[, by C. H. Ramírez-Ronda. BOLETIN—ASOCIACION MEDICA DE PUERTO RICO 77(4): 132-133, April 1985.

Educating about AIDS, by J. Kosterlitz. NATIONAL JOURNAL 18:2044-2049, August 30, 1986.

Educating staff about AIDS eases hysteria. HOSPITALS 58(3):40+, February 1, 1984.

Education and foster care of children infected with human T-lymphotropic virus type III/lymphadenopathy-associated virus. JAMA 254:1430+, September 20, 1985; also in MMWR 34(34):517-521, August 30, 1985.

Education blitz necessary to reduce fear of AIDS, says infection control nurse, by J. Banning. CANADIAN NURSE 81(10):10, November 1985.

Education For All Handicapped Children Act: coverage of children with acquired immune deficiency syndrome (AIDS), by N. L. Jones. JOURNAL OF LAW AND EDUCATION 15(2):195-206, Spring 1986.

Education: a forum for attacking fear, by R. Wilkinson, et al. HOSPITALS 60(1):60, January 1986.

Education still essential in fighting fear of AIDS. MEDICAL PRODUCTS SALES 16(11):77-78+, November 1985.

Effect of the acquired immune deficiency syndrome (AIDS) on blood transfusion and donation patterns in the state of Minnesota, by E. P. Scott, et al. MINNESOTA MEDICINE 68(9):665-669, September 1985.

Effect of Cohn fractionation conditions on infectivity of the AIDS virus, by A. M. Prince, et al. NEW ENGLAND JOURNAL OF MEDICINE 314:386, February 6, 1986.

Effect of death fear on decadence of the 1970s, by M. Bronski. ADVOCATE 437:8, January 7, 1986.

Effective rehabilitation of immune deficiency, by R. Miles. RFD 45:36, Winter 1985.

Effects of the acquired immune deficiency syndrome on gay lifestyle and the gay individual, by D. A. Hirsch, et al. ANNALS OF THE NEW YORK ACADEMY OF SCIENCES 437:273-282, 1984.

Effects of AIDS on various aspects of blood banking, by M. Kuriyan, et al. JOURNAL OF THE MEDICAL SOCIETY OF NEW JERSEY 81(10):875--877, October 1984.

Effects of alcohol on immune system, by T. Prugh. ADAMHA NEWS 12(1):3, January 1986.

Effects of exposure to factor concentrates containing donations from identified AIDS patients. A matched cohort study, by J. Jason, et al. JAMA 256(13):1758-1762, October 3, 1986.

Effects of intravenous recombinant gamma-interferon on the respiratory burst of blood monocytes from patients with AIDS, by J. e. Pennington, et al. JOURNAL OF INFECTIOUS DISEASES 153(3):609-612, March 1986.

Effects of a novel compound (AL 721) on HTLV-III infectivity in vitro, by P. S. Sarin, et al. NEW ENGLAND JOURNAL OF MEDICINE 313:1289-1290, November 14, 1985.

Effects of suramin on HTLV-III/LAV infection presenting as Kaposi's sarcoma or AIDS-related complex: clinical pharmacology and suppression of virus replication in vivo, by S. Broder, et al. LANCET 2(8456):627-630, September 21, 1985.

Electron microscopic diagnosis of cerebral toxoplasmosis. Case report, by L. Cerezo, et al. JOURNAL OF NEUROSURGERY 63(3):470-472, September 1985.

Electron microscopic evidence of non-A, non-B hepatitis markers and virus-like particles in immunocompromised humans, by S. Watanabe, et al. HEPATOLOGY 4(4):628-632, July-August 1984.

Electron microscopy of the intestine and rectum in acquired immunodeficiency syndrome, by W. O. Dobbins, 3d, et al. GASTROENTEROLOGY 88(3):738-749, March 1985.

Elevated adenosine deaminase and purine nucleoside phosphorylase activity in peripheral blood null lymphocytes from patients with acquired immune deficiency syndrome, by J. L. Murray, et al. BLOOD 65(6):1318-1324, June 1985.

Elevated beta 2-microglobulin and lysozyme levels in patients with acquired immune deficiency syndrome,by M. H. Grieco, et al. CLINICAL IMMUNOLOGY AND IMMU-NOPATHOLOGY 32(2):174-184, August 1984.

Elevated erythrocyte adenosine deaminase activity in patients with acquired immuno-deficiency syndrome, by M. J. Cowan, et al. PROCEEDINGS OF THE NATIONAL ACADEMY OF SCIENCES USA 83(4):1089-1091, February 1986.

Elevated levels of interferon-induced 2'-5' oligoadenylate synthetase in generalized persistent lymphadenopathy and the acquired immunodeficiency syndrome, by S. E. Read, et al. JOURNAL OF INFECTIOUS DISEASES 152(3):66-472, Sep-tember 1985.

Elevated urinary neopterin levels in patients with the acquired immunodeficiency syndrome (AIDS). A priliminary report, by H. Wachter, et al. HOPPE-SEYLER'S ZEITSCHRIFT FUER PHYSIOLOGISCHE CHEMIE 364(9):1345-1346, Septem-ber 1983.

Emergence of acquired immune deficiency syndrome, by K. R. McBride. QUEEN'S QUARTERLY 92(3):530-534, 1985.

Emerging importance of infections due to the Mycobacterium avium-intracellulare complex [editorial], by D. Y. Rosenzweig. NEW YORK STATE JOURNAL OF MEDICINE 84(6):290, June 1984.

Emotional hearings on AIDS held in S.F., by M. Helquist. ADVOCATE 426:15, Aug-ust 6, 1985.

Employer seeks insurance money/man fired /AIDS, by S. Ager. ADVOCATE 417:17, April 2, 1985.

Employers can fire AIDS victims to keep the disease from spreading, DOJ rules. JUVENILE JUSTICE DIGEST 14(12):7-8, June 30, 1986; also in CRIME CONTROL DIGEST 20(26):8, June 30, 1986.

Encephalopathy in patients with LAV-HTLV-III infections, by J. Goudsmit, et al. NED-ERLANDS TIJDSCHRIFT VOOR GENEESKUNDE 130(22):998-999, May 31, 1986.

Endemic acquired immunodeficiency syndrome [letter], by W. M. Valenti, et al. AN-NALS OF INTERNAL MEDICINE 101(3):399-400, September 1984.

Endemic Kaposi's sarcoma vs. Kaposi's sarcoma in AIDS: a brief communication, by J. A. Malliwah, et al. HIROSHIMA JOURNAL OF MEDICIAL SCIENCES 34(3):201-296, September 1985.

Ensuring quality hospice care for the person with AIDS, by J. P. Martin. QRB 12(10): 353-358, October 1986.

Enteric coccidiosis among patients with the acquired immunodeficiency syndrome, by M. E. Whiteside, et al. AMERICAN JOURNAL OF TROPICAL MEDICINE AND HYGIENE 33(6):1065-1072, November 1984.

Enteropathy associated with the acquired immunodeficiency syndrome,by D. P. Kot-ler, et al. ANNALS OF INTERNAL MEDICINE 101(4):421-428, October 1984.

Entirely new hygienic guidelines for care of AIDS patients, by M. Meyer. SYGEPLE-JERSKEN 85(45):20-22, November 6, 1985.

Envelope gene-derived recombinant peptide in the serodiagnosis of human immunodeficiency virus infection [letter], by T. F. Schulz, et al. LANCET 2(8498):111-112, July 12, 1986.

Eosinophilic pustular folliculitis in patients with acquired immunodeficiency syndrome. Report of three cases, by F. F. Soeprono, et al. JOURNAL OF THE AMERICAN ACADEMY OF DERMATOLOGY 14(6):1020-1022, June 1986.

Epidemic acquired immune deficiency syndrome: epidemiologic evidence for a transmissible agent, by D. P. Francis, et al. JOURNAL OF THE NATIONAL CANCER INSTITUTE 71(1):1-4, July 1983.

Epidemic Kaposi's sarcoma and opportunistic infections, by D. A. Cooper. MEDICAL JOURNAL OF AUSTRALIA 1(12):564-566, June 11, 1983.

Epidemic Kaposi's sarcoma: a manifestation of the acquired immune deficiency syndrome, by A. E. Friedman-Kien. JOURNAL OF DERMATOLOGIC SURGERY AND ONCOLOGY 9(8):637-640, August 1983.

Epidemic of acquired immune deficiency syndrome (AIDS) and Kaposi's sarcoma. First workshop of the European Study Group on AIDS/KS, Naples, June 25, 1983. ANTIBIOTICS AND CHEMOTHERAPY 32:1-164, 1983.

Epidemic of acquired immunodeficiency in rhesus monkeys, by R. V. Henrickson, et al. LANCET 1(8321):388-390, February 19, 1983.

Epidemic of acquired immunodeficiency syndrome (AIDS) and suggestions for its control in drug abusers, by M. Marmor, et al. JOURNAL OF SUBSTANCE ABUSE AND TREATMENT 1(4):237-247, 1984.

Epidemic of the acquired immunodeficiency syndrome: a need for economic and social planning, by J. E. Groopman, et al. ANNALS OF INTERNAL MEDICINE 99(2):259-261, August 1983.

Epidemic of acquired immunodeficiency syndrome triggering psychotic-psychogenic reactions, by M. Assel, et al. HAREFUAH 108(9):431-433, May 1, 1985.

Epidemic of AIDS related virus (HTLV-III/LAV) infection among intravenous drug abusers, by J. r. Robertson, et al. BRITISH MEDICAL JOURNAL 292(6519):527-529, Feburary 22, 1986.

Epidemic of AIDS related virus infection among intravenous drug abusers [letter],by R. P. Brettle. BRITISH MEDICAL JOURNAL 292(6336):1671, June 21, 1986.

Epidemic of the 80s: AIDS, by D. M. Price, et al. CANCER NURSING 7(4):283-290, August 1984.

Epidemic of fear (AIDS), by J. Barber. MACLEAN'S 98:61+, September 23, 1985.

Epidemic proportions, by J. Fishman. GAY COMMUNITY NEWS 11(7):5, September 3, 1983.

Epidemic spreads, by C. Doyle. OBSERVER May 1, 1983, p. 27.

Epidemiologic and clinical aspects of the acquired immune deficiency syndrome, by T. C. Quinn. DELAWARE MEDICAL JOURNAL 56(12):721-730, December 1984.

Epidemics and the Government, by G. Wilson. THE GAO REVIEW 19(2):26-27+, Spring 1984.

Epidemic's unsung heroes, by C. Norman. SCIENCE 230:1020, November 29, 1985.

Epidemiologic and pathogenic aspects of AIDS, by G. Melino, et al. CLINICA TERA-PEUTICA 112(6):537-546, March 31, 1985.

Epidemiologic aspects of acquired immunodeficiency syndrome (AIDS) in the United States: cases associated with transfusions, by J. W. Curran, et al. PROGRESS IN CLINICAL AND BIOLOGICAL RESEARCH 182:259-269, 1985.

Epidemiologic aspects of an outbreak of acquired immunodeficiency in rhesus monkeys (Macaca mulatta), by N. W. Lerche, et al. LABORATORY ANIMAL SCIENCE 34(2):146-150, April 1984.

Epidemiologic designs for the study of acquired immunodeficiency disease: options and obstacles, by A. S. Monto. REVIEWS OF INFECTIOUS DISEASES 6(5):720-725, September-October 1984.

Epidemiologic lessons from viral hepatitis B, by W. T. London. ANNALS OF THE NEW YORK ACADEMY OF SCIENCES 437:100-105, 1984.

Epidemiological and clinical aspects of acquired immunodeficiency syndrome, by N. Clumeck. REVUE MEDICALE DE BRUXELLES 7(4):271-274, April 1986.

Epidemiological aspects of acquired immune deficiency syndrome in France, by J. B. Brunet, et al. ANNALS OF THE NEW YORK ACADEMY OF SCIENCES 437:334-339, 1984.

Epidemiological investigation of AIDS, by K. H. Mayer. HASTINGS CENTER RE-PORT 15(Suppl. 12-15), August 1985.

Epidemiological trends of AIDS in the United States,by J. W. Curran, et al. CANCER RESEARCH 45(Suppl. 9):4602s-4604s, September 1985.

Epidemiology and prevention of the acquired immunodeficiency syndrome, by J. W. Curran. ANNALS OF INTERNAL MEDICINE 103(5):657-662, November 1985.

Epidemiology of acquired immune deficiency syndrome, by H. W. Haverkos. ANTI-BIOTIC CHEMOTHERAPY 32:18-26, 1983.

—, by H. W. Haverkos, et al. DIAGNOSTIC IMMUNOLOGY 2(2):67-72, 1984.

—. FRONTIERS OF RADIATION THERAPY AND ONCOLOGY 19:8-13, 1985.

—, by T. J. Spira, et al. PROGRESS IN ALLERGY 37:65-80, 1986.

Epidemiology of the acquired immune deficiency syndrome (A.I.D.S.), by M. McEvoy. JOURNAL OF THE ROYAL SOCIETY OF HEALTH 105(3):88-90, June 1985.

—, by T. A. Peterman, et al. EPIDEMIOLOGIC REVIEWS 7:1-21, 1985.

Epidemiology of the Acquired Immunodeficiency Syndrome in intravenous drug abusers, by J. P. Koplan, et al. ADVANCES IN ALCOHOL AND SUBSTANCE ABUSE 5(1 & 2):13-23, Fall 1985-Winter 1986.

Epidemiology of the acquired immunodeficiency syndrome (AIDS) in the United States, by J. R. Allen. SEMINARS IN ONCOLOGY 11(1):4-11, March 1984.

Epidemiology of AIDS [letter], by G. Hunsmann, et al. KLINISCHE WOCHEN-SCHRIFT 63(13):616-617, July 1, 1985.

—, by J. L'age-Stehr. OFFENTLICHE GESUNDHEITSWESEN 47(8):343-348, August 1985.

—, by J. Seale. ZEITSCHRIFT FUR HAUTKRANKHEITEN 59(8):525-528, April 15, 1984.

—, by L. Pamnany. MEDICAL JOURNAL OF AUSTRALIA 140(8):506, April 14, 1984.

—, by W. R. Dowdle. PUBLIC HEALTH REPORTS 98(4):308-312, July-August 1983.

Epidemiology of AIDS: current status and future prospects, by J. W. Curran, et al. SCIENCE 229(4720):1352-1357, September 27, 1985.

Epidemiology of AIDS in Europe. EUROPEAN JOURNAL OF CANCER AND CLINI-CAL ONCOLOGY 20(2):157-164, February 1984.

Epidemiology of human lymphotrophic retroviruses: an overview, by W. A. Blattner, et al. CANCER RESEARCH 45(Suppl. 9):4598s-4601s, September 1985.

Epidemiology of human T-lymphotropic virus type III and the risk of the acquired im-munodeficiency syndrome, by W. A. Blattner, et al. ANNALS OF INTERNAL MEDICINE 103(5):665-670, November 1985.

Epidemiology of pediatric acquired immunodeficiency syndrome, by A. Rubinstein, et al. CLINICAL IMMUNOLOGY AND IMMUNOPATHOLOGY 40(1):115-121, July 1986.

Epstein-Barr virus and chronic lymphadenomegaly in male homosexuals with ac-quired immunodeficiency syndrome (AIDS), by H. Lipscomb, et al. AIDS RE-SEARCH 1(1):59-82, 1983-1984.

Epstein-Barr virus infection in a child with acquired immunodeficiency syndrome, by J. C. Jackler, et al. AMERICAN JOURNAL OF DISEASES OF CHILDREN 139(10): 1000-1004, October 1985.

Equine infectious anemia virus *gag* and *pol* genes: relatedness to visna and AIDS virus, by R. M. Stephens, et al. SCIENCE 231:589-594, February 7,1986.

Equipment handling risks from common and exotic pathogens, by J. Jeffries. JOURNAL OF STERILE SERVICE MANAGEMENT 3(6):4-8, April 1986.

ERD rules AIDS ban discriminatory. OUT 4(8):3, June 1986.

Eroticizing safe sex, "south-of-Market" style, by B. Beuse. ADVOCATE 452:30, Aug-ust 5, 1986.

Erythroblastopenia in acquired immunodeficiency syndrome (AIDS) [letter], by Y. N. Berner, et al. ACTA HAEMATOLOGICA 70(4):273, 1983.

Estimating AIDS (UK) [letter], by M. McEvoy. LANCET 2(8466):1248, November 30, 1985.

Estimation of risk of outcomes of HTLV-III infection [letter], by D. J. Hunter, et al. LAN-CET 1(8482):677-678, March 22, 1986.

Ethical dilemmas in caring for patients with the acquired immunodeficiency syndrome, by R. Steinbrook, et al. ANNALS OF INTERNAL MEDICINE 103(5):787-790, November 1985.

Ethical issues in AIDS research, by M. A. Grodin, et al. QRB12(10):347-352, October 1986.

Ethical issues in the care of patients with AIDS, by M. Cooke. QRB 12(10):343-346, October 1986.

Ethics and AIDS, by A. Jonsen. BULLETIN OF THE AMERICAN COLLEGE OF SURGEONS 70(6):16-18, June 1985.

Ethics of AIDS, by G. Allen. MACLEAN'S 98:44-48, November 18, 1985.

Ethics of AIDS research, by C. Patto. GAY COMMUNITY NEWS 12(33):8, March 9, 1985.

Ethics of a new disease, by G. Copello. ST LUKE'S JOURNAL OF THEOLOGY 29(2): 91-95, March 1986.

Etiology of acquired immunodeficiency syndrome, by Kh. Odiseev. VUTRESHNI BOLESTI 24(2):7-9, 1985.

Etiology of AIDS [letter],by A. J. Ammann. JAMA 252(10):1281-1282, September 14, 1984.

Etiology of AIDS, by J. A. Sonnabend. AIDS RESEARCH 1(1):1-12, 1983-1984.

Etiology of AIDS: biological and biochemical characteristics of HTLV-III, by P. D. Markham, et al. ADVANCES IN EXPERIMENTAL MEDICINE AND BIOLOGY 187:13-34, 1985.

Etiquette for an epidemic: when someone has AIDS, by R. Boucheron. ADVOCATE 434:9, November 26, 1985.

Etoposide in AIDS therapy. AMERICAN FAMILY PHYSICIAN 31:276, March 1985.

Europe convenes 1st AIDS Conference, by N. Fain. ADVOCATE 3(89):20, March 6, 1984.

European AIDS cases double annually, by P. Cumings. ADVOCATE 429:18, September 17, 1985.

Europeans confer—increase slows. BODY POLITIC 1(1):17, March 1984.

Evaluation of abdominal pain in the AIDS patient, by D. A. Potter, et al. ANNALS OF SURGERY 199(3):332-339, March 1984.

Evaluation of the acquired immunodeficiency syndrome (AIDS) reported in health-care personnel—United States. MMWR 32(27):358-360, July 15, 1983.

Evaluation of body weight and nutritional status among AIDS patients, by P. O'Sullivan, et al. AMERICAN DIETETIC ASSOCIATION JOURNAL 85:1483-1484, November 1985.

Evaluation of cerebral mass lesions in acquired immunodeficiency syndrome [letter], by A. E. Pitchenik, et al. NEW ENGLAND JOURNAL OF MEDICINE 308(18): 1099, May 5, 1983.

Evaluation of commercial AIDS screening test kits [letter], by J. R. Carlson, et al. LANCET 1(8442):1388, June 15, 1985.

Evaluation of natural killer cell activity in patients with persistent generalized lymphadenopathy and acquired immunodeficiency syndrome, by P. C. Creemers, et al.
CLINICAL IMMUNOLOGY AND IMMUNOPATHOLOGY 36(2):141-150, August
1985.

Evaluation of patients with the acquired immunodeficiency syndrome (AIDS) by fiberoptic bronchoscopy, by C. Harcup, et al. ENDOSCOPY 17(6):217-220, November 1985.

Evaluation of serologic tests for Pneumocystis carinii antibody and antigenemia in patients with acquired immunodeficiency syndrome, by S. E. Maddison, et al. DIAG-
NOSTIC MICROBIOLOGY AND INFECTIOUS DISEASE 2(1):69-73, January
1984.

Everybody out of the pool. THE PROGRESSIVE 47:11-12, September 1983.

Everything you need to know about AIDS, by C. L. Carney. PARENTS 61(4):105-
108+, April 1986.

Evidence against transmission of human T-lymphotropic virus/lymphadenopathy-
associated virus (HTLV-III/LAV) in families of children with the acquired immunodeficiency syndrome, by J. E. Kaplan, et al. PEDIATRIC INFECTIOUS DISEASE
4(5):468-471, September-October 1985.

Evidence for exposure to HTLV-III in Uganda before 1973, by W. C. Saxinger, et al.
SCIENCE 227:1036-1038, March 1, 1985.

Evidence for HTLV-III in T-cells from semen of AIDS patients: expression in primary
cell culture, long-term mitogen-stimulated cell cultures, and cocultures with a permissive T-cell line, by D. Zagury, et al. CANCER RESEARCH 45(Suppl. 9):
4595s-4597s, September 1985.

Evidence for a 1980 HTLV-III infection in a currently asymptomatic B hemophiliac in
Italy, by O. E. Vernier, et al. JAMA 254:1449-1450, September 20, 1985.

Evidence of a virus in multiple sclerosis. NEW SCIENTIST 108:30, November 21,
1985.

Evidence that immune deficiency after marrow transplantation is not caused by AIDS-
associated retrovirus [letter], by K. Atkinson, et al. NEW ENGLAND JOURNAL
OF MEDICINE 313(3):182-183, July 18, 1985.

Ex-Carter official hired by gay group, by L. Bush. ADVOCATE 3(75):8, September 1,
1983.

Excessive concern about AIDS in two bisexual men, by G. P. Lippert. CANADIAN
JOURNAL OF PSYCHIATRY 31(1):63-65, February 1986.

Exchange on AIDS, by J. Lieberson. THE NEW YORK REVIEW OF BOOKS 30:43-
45, October 13, 1983.

Excommunicated. CHRISTIAN CENTURY 103(5):112, February 5-12, 1986.

Exogenous interleukin-2 and mitogen responses in AIDS patients [letter], by M.
Cavaille-Coll, et al. LANCET a1(8388):1245, June 2, 1984.

Experiences in the Cologne AIDS consultation, by L. Häusermann, et al. ZEIT-
SCHRIFT FUR HAUTKRANKHEITEN 59(6):353-354, March 15, 1984.

Experimental infection of chimpanzees with lymphadenopathy-associated virus. JAMA 252:995, August 24, 1984.

Experimental transmission of macaque AIDS by means of inoculation of macaque lymphoma tissue, by N. L. Letvin, et al. LANCET 2(8350):599-602, September 10, 1983.

Experimental transmission of simian acquired immunodeficiency syndrome (SAIDS) and Kaposi-like skin lesions, by W. T. London,e t al. LANCET 2(8355):869-873, October 15, 1983.

Explaining AIDS/Health Workers Forum, by L. Goldsmith. GAY COMMUNITY NEWS 10(27):3, January 29, 1983.

Exploited for headlines. BODY POLITIC 126:22, May 1986.

Expression in Escherichia coli of open reading frame gene segments of HTLV-III, by N. T. Chang, et al. SCIENCE 228:93-96, April 5, 1985.

Expression of beta 2 microglobulin on the surface of mononuclear cells in patients with acquired immune deficiency syndrome (AIDS, and AIDS-related complex (ARC), by S. Gupta. ADVANCES IN EXPERIMENTAL MEDICINE AND BIOLOGY 187:111-115, 1985.

Expression of endothelial cell surface antigens by AIDS-associated Kaposi's sarcoma. Evidence for a vascular endothelial cell origin, by J. L. Rutgers, et al. AMERICAN JOURNAL OF PATHOLOGY 122(3):493-499, March 1986.

Expression of human immunodeficiency virus antigen (HIV-Ag) in serum and cerebrospinal fluid during acute and chronic infection, by J. Goudsmit, et al. LANCET 2(8500):177--180, July 26, 1986.

Expression of the *pX* gene of HTLV-I: general splicing mechanism in the HTLV family, by M. Seiki, et al. SCIENCE 228:1532-1534, June 28, 1985.

Expression of the 3' terminal region of human T-cell leukemia viruses, by W. Wachsman, et al. SCIENCE 226:177-179, October 12, 1984.

Expressions of HTLV-III infection in a pediatric population, by S. Pahwa, et al. ADVANCES IN EXPERIENTAL MEDICINE AND BIOLOGY 187:45-51, 1985.

Extracorporeal perfusion of plasma over immobilized protein A in a patient with Kaposi's sarcoma and acquired immunodeficiency, by D. D. Kiprov, et al. JOURNAL OF BIOLOGICAL RESPONSE MODIFIERS 3(3):341-346, 1984.

Eye disorders in 4 patients with acquired immunodeficiency syndrome, by M. F. Hoogesteger, et al. NEDERLANDS TIJDSCHRIFT VOOR GENEESKUNDE 129(1):24-25, January 5, 1985.

Facing a common enemy, by E. Jackson. BODY POLITIC 116:13, July 1985.

Facing a fatal disease, by B. Levin. MACLEAN'S 99:48-49, January 6, 1986.

Facing it: a novel of AIDS, by J. Andriote. ADVOCATE 423:43, June 25, 1985.

Factor VIII products and disordered immune regulation [letter], by R. S. Gordon, Jr. LANCET 1(8331):991, April 30, 1983.

Facts about acquired immune deficiency syndrome (AIDS). WISCONSIN MEDICAL JOURNAL 82(11):15-18, November 1983.

Facts about acquired immune deficiency syndrome, by the AIDS Task Force. HEALTHRIGHT 4:27-29, May 1985.

Facts about AIDS. NEW ZEALAND NURSING JOURNAL 77(4):1-4, April 1984.

—. PLASTIC SURGICAL NURSING 3(3):73-75, Fall 1983.

—, by J. Nelson. ESSENCE 16:56+, August 1985.

Facts about AIDS: a detention training program, by L. D. Carlin. TRAINING AIDS DIGEST 10(11):1+, November 1985.

Facts that stay concealed, by D. Anderson. TIMES August 19, 1986, p. 10.

Failure (and danger) of mitozantrone in AIDS-related Kaposi's sarcoma [letter], by L. Kaplan, et al. LANCET 2(8451):396, August 17, 1985.

Failure to thrive due to fear of AIDS [letter], by W. L. Henley. LANCET 2(8498):112-113, July 12, 1986.

Faith, hope and bigotry, by O. Sattaur. NEW SCIENTIST 106:45, May 16, 1985.

False-positive results in the detection of anti-LAV/HTLV-III antibodies by enzyme immunoassay, by H. Näher, et al. HAUTARZT 37(6):338-340 June 1986.

Falwell launches (another) anti-gay campaign, by M. Godwin. GAY COMMUNITY NEWS 13(3):2, July 27, 1985.

Falwell on antigay AIDS crusade, by M. Henson. GUARDIAN 35(40):5, July 27, 1983.

Falwell speaks—Cincinnati responds, by S. Hyde. GAY COMMUNITY NEWS 11(2):3, July 23, 1983.

Falwell's claim of God's judgement, by J. Real. ADVOCATE 3(73):10, August 4, 1983.

Family gives refuge to a son who has AIDS, by J. Seligman,e t al. NEWSWEEK 106:24, August 12, 1985.

Family of human T-lymphotropic leukemia viruses: HTLV-I as the cause of adult T cell leukemia and HTLV-III as the cause of acquired immunodeficincy syndrome, by F. Wong-Staal, et al. BLOOD 65(2):253-263, February 1985.

Farewell, sexual revolution. Hello, new Victorianism, by E. Cornish. THE FUTURIST 20:2+, January-February 1986.

'Fast-buck' artists are making a killing on AIDS, by S. Ticer. BUSINESS WEEK December 2, 1985, p. 85-86.

Fatal AIDS in a haemophiliac in the UK [letter], by H. M. Daly, et al. LANCET 2(8360):1190, November 19, 1983.

Fatal AIDS in a UK haemophiliac [letter],by H. M. Daly, et al. LANCET 1(8367):44, January 1984.

Fatal cryptosporidiosis complicating Kaposi's sarcoma in an immunocompromised man, by M. Wittner, et al. AMERICAN JOURNAL OF THE MEDICAL SCIENCES 287(2):47-48, March-April 1984.

Fatal pulmonary pneumocystosis 2 years after multiple transfusions [letter], by G. Offenstadt, et al. PRESSE MEDICALE 13(39):2388-2389, November 3, 1984.

Fatal toxoplasmosis of the central nervous system in a heroin user with acquired immunodeficiency disease, by S. K. Murthy, et al. NEW YORK STATE JOURNAL OF MEDICINE 84(9):464-466, September 1984.

FDA advises blood centers on phase-in of AIDS test. MLO17(4):21-23, April 1985.

FDA approves blood screen for AIDS, by C. Foty. OFF OUR BACKS 15(4):2, April 1985.

FDA approves Pasteur's AIDS test kit, by C. Norman. SCIENCE 231:1063, March 7, 1986.

FDA issues guidelines to protect transfusion recipients from AIDS. HOSPITALS 57(12):59-60, June 16, 1983.

FDA postpones licensing of HTLV-III test, by c. Guilfoy. GAY COMMUNITY NEWS 12(32):1, March 2, 1985.

FDA responses to the challenges of AIDS, by H. M. Meyer, Jr. PUBLIC HEALTH REPORTS 98(4):320-323, July-August 1983.

Fear about confidentiality jeopardizes study, by J. Cort. ADVOCATE 4(8):10, November 27, 1984.

Fear and healing in the AIDS crisis, by L. Hancock. CHRISTIANITY AND CRISIS 45: 255-258, June 24, 1985.

Fear and loathing in the workplace: what managers can do about AIDS, by I. Pave. BUSINESS WEEK November 25, 1985, p. 126.

Fear and loathing . . . lack of compassion in dealing with AIDS victims, by J. Neuberer. NURSING TIMES 82(6):22, February 5-11, 1986.

Fear in San Francisco, by Nora Gallagher. CALIFORNIA MAGAZINE 11:93+, March 1 1986.

Fear—loving in NYC—life after AIDS, by J. Fouralt. BODY POLITIC 1:37, January 1984.

Fear of AIDS, by M. P. Rowe, et al. HARVARD BUSINESS REVIEW 64(4):28-30+, July-August 1986.

Fear of AIDS and gonorrhea rates in homosexual men [letter],by F. N. Judson. LANCET 2(8342):159-160, July 16, 1983.

Fear of AIDS causes crisis in blood banks across nation. JET 69:28-29, December 16, 1985.

Fear of AIDS: illness as a metaphor, by E. M. Gjersten SYKEPLEIEN 72(18):16-17+, October 21, 1985.

Fear of AIDS infects the nation. U.S. NEWS & WORLD REPORT 94:13, June 27, 1983.

Fear of dying. THE ECONOMIST 296:29-30, September 14, 1985.

Fear rules as officials slap classroom ban on AIDS boy [United States], by B. Norris. THE TIMES EDUCATIONAL SUPPLEMENT 3606:11, August 9, 1985.

Fears/frustrations stymie patients, by P. Byron. GAY COMMUNITY NEWS 11(10):3, September 24, 1983.

Federal Government intensifies its efforts in the mental health aspects of AIDS, by B. Runck. HOSPITAL AND COMMUNITY PSYCHIATRY 37(3):219-221, March 1986.

Federal officials back use of consent forms, by C. Guilfoy. GAY COMMUNITY NEWS 12(10):1, September 22, 1984.

Federal response to the AIDS epidemic, by P. R. Lee, et al. HEALTH POLICY 6(3):259-267, 1986.

Feds AIDS action lacking, by L. Bush. ADVOCATE 3(76):8, September 15, 1983.

Feds open hotline on AIDS. CORRECTIONS DIGEST 14(15):8, July 13, 1983.

—. CRIME CONTROL DIGEST 17(28):6, July 18, 1983.

Feds to rush AIDS drugs, by K. Popert. BODY POLITIC 129:15, August 1986.

FeLV-induced feline acquired immune deficiency syndrome. A model for human AIDS, by W. D. Hardy, Jr., et al. PROGRESS IN ALLERGY 37:353-376, 1986.

Female prostitutes: a risk group for infection with human T-cell lymphotropic virus type III, by P. Van de Perre, et al. LANCET 2(8454):524-527, September 7, 1985.

Female-to-male AIDS link found, by J. Silberner. SCIENCE NEWS 129:164-165, March 15, 1986.

Female-to-male transmission of AIDS [letter], by B. F. Polk. JAMA 254(22):3177-3178, December 13, 1985.

—, by H. W. Haverkos, et al. JAMA 254(8):1035-1036, August 23-30, 1985.

Female-to-male transmission of AIDS: a reexamination of the African sex ratio of cases [letter], by N. Padian, et al. JAMA 256(5):590, August 1, 1986.

Female-to-male transmission of HTLV-III [letter]. JAMA 255(13):1703-1706, April 4, 1986.

Fetal transmission of AIDS through the mother's womb, by A. Rubinstein. COMPRE-HENSIVE THERAPY 11(5):6-11, May 1985.

Fever all through the night: is disease shaping a new sexual ethic? by N. Gallagher. MOTHER JONES 7:36-43, November 1982.

Fever, cough, anal ulcer in a heterosexual man, by P. J. de Caprariis, et al. HOSPITAL PRACTICE 19(4):122+, April 1984.

Few companies have special policies for AIDS. COMPENSATION AND BENEFITS REVIEW 18:6-7, March-April 1986.

Fight against AIDS. First-level information and education. KRANKENPFLEGE. SOINS INFIRMIERS 78(10):49, October 1985.

Fighting AIDS: the search for a cure, by J. Wilkinson. LISTENER October 17, 1985, p. 7-8.

Fighting AIDS with the facts and sound aseptic practice. OR MANAGER 1(9):1+, December 1985.

Fighting back against AIDS, by P. J. Collins. PATIENT CARE 19(19):131+, November 15, 1985.

Fighting the backlash/AIDS network, by P. Albert. GUILD NOTES 9(3):12, Summer 1985.

Fighting for life [motion picture and television artists' views], by S. Haller. PEOPLE 24:28-33, September 23, 1985.

Fighting for our lives, by C. Sorrel. OFF OUR BACKS 13:10, November 1983.

Fighting for their lives, by B. Egerton. OUT 3(1):1, November 1984.

Fighting off AIDS. NEW SCIENTIST 108:13, October 31, 1985.

Fighting off a killer called Slim, by T. Prentice. TIMES October 27, 1986, p 14.

Fighting a scourge: gains against AIDS have come rapidly, but a cure is distant; need for effective therapies is urgent as cases rise, by M. Case. WALL STREET JOURNAL 206:1+, August 5, 1985.

Figure it out, by A. Lumsden. NEW STATESMAN November 7, 1986, p. 8-9.

Figures don't lie, they tell half-truths, by E. Jackson. BODY POLITIC 116:14, July 1985.

Filmmaker Arthur Bressa on AIDS, by M. Bronski. GAY COMMUNITY NEWS 13(17): 10, November 9, 1985.

Financial implications of AIDS, by S. D. Sedaka, et al. CARING 5(6):38-39+, June 1986.

Financing extinction in the tropics, by D. Coules. NOT MAN APART 15(4):14, May 1985.

Findings in psychiatric consultations with patients with acquired immune deficiency syndrome, by J. W. Dilley, et al. AMERICAN JOURNAL OF PSYCHIATRY 142(1): 82-86, January 1985.

Fires, by M. Totke. BODY POLITIC 128:31, July 1986.

Firing employees who have AIDS brings on new round of legal action, by C. R. Goerth. OCCUPATIONAL HEALTH AND SAFETY 54(10):28, October 1985.

Firing of AIDS victims in Florida touches off national policy debate. CRIME CONTROL DIGEST 19(5):10, February 4, 1985.

First AIDS, by J. McQuaid. THE NEW REPUBLIC 189:16, August 1, 1983.

—, by J. Melville. GUARDIAN September 24, 1986, p. 11.

First AIDS death in military gets cautious response, by K. Popert. BODY POLITIC 124:15, March 1986.

First AIDS death reported in Maryland prison system. CORRECTIONS DIGEST 15(20):4-5, September 26, 1984.

First AIDS hospital set to open in July. MEDICAL WORLD NEWS 27(11):133-134, June 9, 1986.

First case in Italy of fatal AIDS in a hemophiliac, by R. Kal Bo Zanon, et al. ACTA HAEMATOLOGICA 75(1):34-37, 1986.

First case of AIDS in a homosexual in Israel. Results of different therapeutic regimens, by R. Marilus, et al. ISRAEL JOURNAL OF MEDICAL SCIENCES 20(3): 249-251, March 1984.

First case of AIDS in Hong Kong [letter], by a. Y. Chan, et al. JAMA 254(6):751, August 9, 1985.

First case of AIDS in Salzburg. Important diagnostic hint by determination of neopterin, by K. Wessely, et al. WIENER KLINISCHE WOCHENSCHRIFT 97(2):88-90, January 18, 1985.

First case of AIDS in the Tyrol, by I. Auhuber, et al. WIENER KLINISCHE WOCHEN-SCHRIFT 96(11):426-427, May 25, 1984.

First chimp infected with AIDS virus. SCIENCE NEWS 126:121, August 25, 1984.

First International Conference on the Acquired Immunodeficiency Syndrome, by I. H. Frazer, et al. MEDICAL JOURNAL OF AUSTRALIA 143(1):31-3, July 8, 1985.

First Nat'l Canadian Conference on AIDS, by S. Poggi. GAY COMMUNITY NEWS 12(50):2, July 6, 1985.

First two fatal cases of AIDS in Sweden—diagnostic and therapeutic experiences, by E. Asbrink, et al. LAKARTIDNINGEN 81(15):1513-1516, April 11, 1984.

Fitz-Hugh and Curtis syndrome in a homosexual man with impaired cell mediated immunity, by W. P. Winkler, et al. GASTROINTESTINAL ENDOSCOPY 31(1):28-30, February 1985.

Flight attendants with AIDS fight friendly skies, by S. Kulieke. ADVOCATE 411:9, January 8, 1985.

Florida AIDS victim deported, by D. France. GUARDIAN 36(6):4, November 9, 1983.

Florida county fired AIDS victims illegally. CIVIL LIBERTIES 356:3, Winter 1986.

Florida fires workers who have AIDS, by C. Guilfoy GAY COMUNITY NEWS 12(29):1, February 9, 1985.

Florida man wins AIDS discrimination appeal, by D. Walter. ADVOCATE 438:17, January 21, 1986.

Florida test case challenge of Justice Dept. ruling, by D. Walter. ADVOCATE 454:16, September 2, 1986.

Follicular dendritic cells and virus-like particles in AIDS-related lymphadenopathy, by J. A. Armstrong, et al. LANCET 2(8399):370-372, August 18, 1984.

Follow-up at 41/2 years on homosexual men with generalized lymphadenopathy [letter], by U. Mathur-Wagh, et al. NEW ENGLAND JOURNAL OF MEDICINE 313(24):1542-1543, December 12, 1985.

Footing the bill, by B. Maschinot. IN THESE TIMES 9(37):4, October 2, 1985.

Forum advocates AIDS ministry, by K. Smith. NATIONAL CATHOLIC REPORTER 21:19, March 8, 1985.

Forum: the costs of treatment, by J. Gildea. HEALTH COST MANAGEMENT 3(1):16-18, January-February 1986.

Forum looks at fear among health workers, by K. Westheimer. GAY COMMUNITY NEWS 13(19):2, November 23, 1985.

Foster mom may sue to get AIDS kid in school. JET 68:23, April 15, 1985.

Four more AIDS cases in Britain. NEW SCIENTIST 98:609, June 2, 1983.

Four theories about a mystery disease. ROLLING STONE p.20, February 3, 1983.

14q+ abnormality with probable t(8;14)(q24;q32) in a young Haitian immigrant with acquired immunodeficiency syndrome and concomitant Burkitt's-like lymphoma, by M. Gyger, et al. CANCER GENETICS AND CYTOGENETICS 17(4):283-288, August 1985.

14th century black death type scenario, by P. Forbes. NEW STATESMAN November 7, 1986, p. 6-8.

Fourth case of AIDS in haemophiliac children in Seville [letter], by P. Noguerol, et al. LANCET 2(8409):986, October 27, 1984.

France packs AIDs kit. NEW SCIENTIST 104:5, December 6, 1984.

Free AIDS information materials available. PUBLIC HEALTH REPORTS 99:390, July-August 1984.

Free needles for drug users weighed as anti-AIDS tactic. CRIMINAL JUSTICE NEWS-LETTER 16(24):4-5, December 16, 1985.

"Free" needles for intravenous drug users at risk for AIDS: current developments in New York City, by D. C. Des Larlais, et al. NEW ENGLAND JOURNAL OF MEDI-CINE 313:1476, December 5, 1985.

French believe AIDS discovery is theirs, by A. Lloyd. NEW SCIENTIST 102:6, April 26, 1984.

French claim on AIDS testing, by R. Rhein, et al. CHEMICAL WEEK 137:11, October 16, 1985.

French doctors ban American blood imports. NEW SCIENTIST 98:529, May 26, 1983.

French, US viral isolates compared in search for cause of AIDS [news], by C. Marwick, et al. JAMA 251(22):2901-2903+, June 8, 1984.

Frequency and anatomic distribution of lymphadenopathic Kaposi's sarcoma in the acquired immunodeficiency syndrome: an autopsy series, by L. B. Moskowitz, et al. HUMAN PATHOLOGY 16(5):447-456, May 1985.

Frequent detection and isolation of cytopathic retroviruses (HTLV-III) from patients with AIDS and at risk for AIDS, by R. C. Gallo, et al. SCIENCE 224(4648):500-503, May 4, 1984.

Frequent transmission of HTLV-III among spouses of patients with AIDS-related complex and AIDS, by R. R. Redfield, et al. JAMA 253(11):1571-1573, March 15, 1985.

Fresh lead. THE ECONOMIST 287:94-95, May 28-June 3, 1983.

Fresno police deputies adopt masks to guard against AIDS. CORRECTIONS DIGEST 16(22):6-7, October 23, 1985; also in CRIME CONTROL DIGEST 19(43):7, September 28, 1985.

Friends gone with the wind, by A. Kantrowitz. ADVOCATE 454:43, September 2, 1986.

Frighten and be fired. THE ECONOMIST 299:29-30, June 28, 1986.

Frightened,suffering and resented, by D. France. GUARDIAN 36(21):6, February 29, 1984.

From the editor's desk. ADVOCATE 449:5, June 24, 1986.

From New York, by S. Jacoby. PRESENT TENSE 13:45-47, Winter 1986.

From The National Institutes of Health. Summary of the National Institutes of Health Research Workshop on the Epidemiology of the Acquired Immunodeficiency Syndrome (AIDS), by R. Edelman. JOURNAL OF INFECTIOUS DISEASES 150(2):295-303, August 1984.

Frontlines: schools flunk on AIDS instruction, by Laura Fraser. MOTHER JONES 11:8, June 1986.

Functional integrity of T, B, and natural killer cells in homosexual subjects with prodromata and in patients with AIDS, by J. G. Bekesi, et al. ANNALS OF THE NEW YORK ACADEMY OF SCIENCES 437:28-38, 1984.

Functional properties of antigen-specific T cells infected by human T-cell leukemia-lymphoma virus (HTLV-I), by H. Mitsuya, et al. SCIENCE 225:1484-1486, September 28, 1984.

Functional relation between HTLV-III x and adenovirus EIA proteins in transcriptional activation, by I.S. Y. Chen, et al. SCIENCE 230:570-573, November 1, 1985.

Functional T lymphocyte immune deficiency in a population of homosexual men who do not exhibit symptoms of acuqired immune deficiency syndrome, by G. M. Shearer, et al. JOURNAL OF CLINICAL INVESTIGATION 74(2):496-506, August 1984.

Funding improves for AIDS groups, by K. Popert. BODY POLITIC 1(6):11, September 1984.

Fungal agent: microbiologist sites plant mould as possible cause of AIDS, by A. Lukits. EQUINOX 3:18, March-April 1984.

Fungal infections in patients with AIDS and AIDS-related complex, by K. Holmberg, et al. SCANDINAVIAN JOURNAL OF INFECTIOUS DISEASES. 18(3):179-192, 1986.

Fungal stains in the acquired immunodeficiency syndrome [letter], by R. E. Stahl, et al. ANNALS OF INTERNAL MEDICINE 102(3):413, March 1985.

Furor over an AIDS announcement, by c. Wallis, et al. TIME 126(19):77, November 11, 1985.

Further anxieties about AIDS, by J. Maddox. NATURE 319:9, January 2, 1986.

Future shock [New York City], by L. Glynn. MACLEAN'S 98:52, November 18, 1985.

Ga-67 studies in a patient with acquired immunodeficiency syndrome and disseminated mycobacterial infection, by C. M. Malhotra, et al. CLINICAL NUCLEAR MEDICINE 10(2):96-98, February 1985.

Gala night for singing [opera stage benefit in East Hampton, N.Y.]. OPERA NEWS 50:32, November 1985.

Gala with a grim side [Hollywood fundraiser], by W. R. Doerner. TIME 126:30+, September 30, 1985.

Gallium-67 scintigraphy in acquired immune deficiency syndrome complicated by Pneumocystis carinii pneumonia, by F. R. Graybeal, Jr., et al. CLINICAL NUCLEAR MEDICINE 10(9):669-670, September 1985.

Gallo cautious about vaccine, by C. Guilfoy. GAY COMMUNITY NEWS 13(17):3, November 9, 1985.

Gallo testing new drug. BODY POLITIC 121:25, December 1985.

Gamma interferon and AIDS [letter], by J. L. Moore, et al. NEW ENGLAND JOURNAL OF MEDICINE 312(7):442-443, February 14, 1985.

Gastrointestinal cryptosporidiosis and sytomegalovirus enterocolitis, by d. F. Altman. FRONTIERS OF RADIATION THERAPY AND ONCOLOGY 19:88-90, 1985.

Gastrointestinal histoplasmosis in suspected acquired immunodeficiency syndrome, by C. M. Haggerty, et al. WESTERN JOURNAL OF MEDICINE 143(2):244-246, August 1985.

Gastrointestinal infections during AIDS [letter], by E. René, et al. LANCET 1(8382): 915, April 2, 1984.

Gastrointestinal involvement in acquired immunologic deficiency syndrome (AIDS), by R. Münch, et al. ZEITSCHRIFT FUR GASTROENTEROLOGIE 24(5):235-244, May 1986.

Gastrointestinal Kaposi's sarcoma in AIDS: radiographic manifestations, by S. D. Wall, et al. JOURNAL OF CLINICAL GASTROENTEROLOGY 6(2):165-171, April 1984.

Gastrointestinal Kaposi's sarcoma in patients with acquired immunodeficiency syndrome. Endoscopic and autopsy findings, by S. L. Friedman, et al. GASTROENTEROLOGY 89(1):102-108, July 1985.

Gastrointestinal manifestations of the acquired immunodeficiency syndrome: a review of 22 cases, by B. Dworkin, et al. AMERICAN JOURNAL OF GASTROENTEROLOGY 80(10):774-778, October 1985.

Gastrointestinal manifestations of AIDS, by E. René, et al. ANNALES DE GASTROENTEROLOGIE ET D'HEPATOLOGIE 21(6):389-391, December 1985.

Gastrointestinal sytomegalovirus infection in a homosexual man with severe acquired immunodeficiency syndrome, by S. L. Gertler, et al. GASTROENTEROLOGY 85(6):1403-1406, December 1983.

Gay America in transition, by T. Morganthau. NEWSWEEK 102:30-36+, August 8, 1983.

Gay Anti-Defamation League forms in NY, by P. Freiberg. ADVOCATE 436:14, December 24, 1985.

Gay body politics, by R. Kaye. IN THESE TIMES 7(39):12, October 29, 1983.

Gay business: the impact of AIDS, by P. Freiberg. ADVOCATE 437:10, January 7, 1986.

Gay cancer isn't gay anymore, by M. Horosko. DANCE MAGAZINE 57:72, February 1983.

Gay Catholic activist makes life, AIDS death educational opportunity for Baltimore church, by F. A. Vincent. NATIONAL CHURCH REPORTER 21:6-7, September 27, 1985.

Gay compromise syndrome, by J. McGlynn. NURSING MIRROR 156(12):20-22, March 23, 1983.

Gay crisis, crisis for all [editorial]. GUARDIAN 38(39):22, July 9, 1986.

Gay dramatists pen new works/ "Age of AIDS", by M. Kearns. ADVOCATE 412:24, January 22, 1985.

Gay erotic fantasies: don't let AIDS destroy, by E. Ingle. ADVOCATE 449:9, June 24, 1986.

Gay father ordered to take HTLV-3 test, by P. Freiberg. ADVOCATE 448:D15, June 10, 1986.

Gay group sets 1984 for global actn, by D. France. GAY COMMUNITY NEWS 11(5):3, August 13, 1983.

Gay health organizations, by S. Kleinberg. ADVOCATE 3(98):24, July 10, 1984.

Gay leaders ask Congress for more AIDS funding, by D. Walter. ADVOCATE 422:16, June 11, 1985.

Gay man with AIDS wins discharge BT, by J. Ryan. GAY COMMUNITY NEWS 11(33): 1, March 10, 1984.

Gay men challenge dentists on AIDS, Hep B, by C. Guilfoy. GAY COMMUNITY NEWS 13(4):3, August 3, 1985.

Gay men urged not to take AIDS-virus test,by D. Walter. ADVOCATE 414:12, February 19, 1985.

Gay papers bicker over AIDS coverage, by R. Oloughlin. MEDIAFILE 3(12):1, June 1983.

Gay perspective on AIDS, by R. Evans. NORTHWEST PASSAGE 23(11):10, June 1983.

Gay plague, by M. VerMeulen. NEW YORK 15:52-54+, May 31, 1982.

Gay plague is invading Alberta, by J. Westaway. ALBERTA REPORT 10:33, February 21, 1983.

Gay plague takes a life in Alberta, by F. Orr. ALBERTA REPORT 10:36, June 27, 1983.

Gay recruits needed for AIDS research, by K. Popert. BODY POLITIC 109:9, December 1984.

Gay representatives lobby for AIDS policy, by J. Ryan. GAY COMMUNITY NEWS 12(24):1, December 29, 1984.

Gay rights groups divided over HHS investigation, by D. Walter. ADVOCATE 449:17, June 24, 1986.

Gay rights victories . . . and setbacks. OFF OUR BACKS 17(8):10, August 1986.

Gay times and diseases, by Patrick J. Buchanan, et al. AMERICAN SPECTATOR 17:15+, August 1984.

Gay writers on disease & health, by Mitzel. GAY COMMUNITY NEWS 45:8, June 7, 1986.

Gay/lesbian community statement on HTLV-III test. GAY COMMUNITY NEWS 12(33): 9, March 9, 1985.

Gays and the stigma of bad blood, by R. Bayer. HASTINGS CENTER REPORT 13(2): 5-7, April 1983.

Gays must not take the rap for straight fears, by S. Anderson. ADVOCATE 444:9, April 15, 1986.

Gene-cloners may have treatment for AIDS, by N. Heneson. NEW SCIENTIST 98: 843, June 23, 1983.

General strategy for the use of allogeneic lymphocyte infusions in the treatment of disorders characterized by impaired helper or suppressor T cell function: autoimmune diseases and the acquired immunodeficiency syndrome (AIDS), by M. F. McCarty. MEDICAL HYPOTHESES 16(3):189-206, March 1985.

Generalized lymphadenopathy in homosexual men: an update of the New York experience, by C. E. Metroka, et al. ANNALS OF THE NEW YORK ACADEMY OF SCIENCES 437:400-411, 1984.

Generalized lymphadenopathy syndrome related to AIDS. Histopatholgic aspects of the lymph nodes, by C. Marche, et al. BULLETIN DE L'ACADEMIE NATIONALE DE MEDECINE 168(1-2):271-277, January-February 1984.

Generalized tuberculosis in a patient with acquired immunodeficiency syndrome, by A. de la Loma, et al. JOURNAL OF INFECTION 10(1):57-59, January 1985.

Genes of AIDS-linked virus cloned, by D. Franklin. SCIENCE NEWS 126:164, September 15, 1984.

Genes of likely AIDS virus cloned. CHEMICAL AND ENGINEERING NEWS 62:7, September 17, 1984.

Genetic variability of the AIDS virus: nucleotide sequence analysis of two isolates from African patients, by M. Alizon, et al. CELL 46(1):63-74, July 4, 1986.

Genetic variation in HTLV-III/LAV over time in patients with AIDS or at risk for AIDS, by B. H. Hahn, et al. SCIENCE 232:1548-1553, June 20, 1986.

Genomic diversity of the acquired immune deficiency syndrome virus HTLV-III: different viruses exhibit greatest divergence in their envelope genes, by B. H. Hahn, et al. PROCEEDINGS OF THE NATIONAL ACADEMY OF SCIENCES USA 82(14):4813-4817, July 1985.

Genomic diversity of human T-lymphotropic virus type III (HTLV-III), by F. Wong-Staal, et al. SCIENCE 229:759-762, August 23, 1985.

Genomic heterogeneity of AIDS retroviral isolates from North America and Zaire, by S. Benn, et al. SCIENCE 230:949-951, November 22, 1985.

Germ of doubt, by A. Veitch. GUARDIAN December 20, 1985, p. 15.

Ginsberg meditates on death and eternity, by E. Shively. GAY COMMUNITY NEWS 13(34):7, March 15, 1986.

Giving researchers a hand, by M. Helquist. ADVOCATE 434:20, November 26, 1985.

GLC promises cash help to AIDS voluntary effort, by J. Meldrum. NEW STATESMAN 108:8, December 21, 1984.

GLCS and the HTLV-III, by Varnum, et al. GAY COMMUNITY NEWS 13(16):5, November 2, 1985.

Glimmer of hope; AIDS vaccine. THE ECONOMIST 298:90, March 22, 1986.

Glomerular lesions in the acquired immunodeficiency syndrome, by V. Pardo,e t al. ANNALS OF INTERNAL MEDICINE 101(4):429-434, October 1984.

Gloom in the Palais des Congres: an AIDS conference offers little hope for a cure, by J. Murphy, et al. TIME 128():51, July 7, 1986.

God and the AIDS victim: Anglicans offer sympathy and debate morality, by W. Harbeck, et al. ALBERTA REPORT 13:40-41, March 24, 1986.

God as judge, God as savior, by H. S. Shoemaker. CHRISTIAN MINISTRY 17(1):24-26, January 1986.

Gonorrhoea in homosexual men and media coverage of the acquired immune deficiency syndrome in London 1982-3, by I. V. Weller, et al. BRITISH MEDICAL JOURNAL 289(6451):1041, October 20, 1984.

"Good" and "bad" of California's 40 AIDS bills, by Bisticas-Cocoves. GAY COMMUNITY NEWS 13(44):3, May 31, 1986.

Good friends: raising funds for AIDS. ADVOCATE 3(74):25, August 18, 1983.

Good news, bad news: 21 views on AIDS. UTNE READER 17:70, August 1986.

Goodbye to promiscuity, by W. J. Weatherby. GUARDIAN August 30, 1985, p. 13.

GOP Senators hold briefing on AIDS, by D. Walter. ADVOCATE 428:18, September 3, 1985.

Government awards $100 million to study AIDS drug, by D. Walter. ADVOCATE 453:14, August 19, 1986.

Government irresponsible on AIDS, says Fettner. OUT 3(12):3, October 1985.

Government's response to fears about acquired immunodeficiency syndrome, by R. Deitch. LANCET 1(8427):530-531, March 2, 1985.

Governor compromises on vetoed AIDS funds, by M. Helquist. ADVOCATE 431:23, October 15, 1985.

Governor flipflops on AIDS funding, by B. Nelson. GAY COMMUNITY NEWS 10(50): 3, July 9, 1983. 10(50):2, July 9, 1983.

Grants to study ADM aspects of AIDS. ADAMHA NEWS 12(1):1+, January 1986.

Granulomatous involvement of the liver in patients with AIDS, by M. S. Orenstein, et al. GUT 26(11):1220-1225, November 1985.

Grassroots action/Gov. vagueness, by E. Jackson. BODY POLITIC 96:15, September 1983.

Grassroots petition demands AIDS response, by M. Cocoves. GAY COMMUNITY NEWS 12(47):3, June 15, 1985.

Great AIDS race: testing the test, by J. Silberner. SCIENCE NEWS 127:36, January 19, 1985.

Great Calgary AIDS debate: wrath of God or mystery disease: Christians divide, by M. McKinley. ALBERTA REPORT 10:30, September 5, 1983.

Green door to peace of mind, by M. Dynes, et al. TIMES November 17, 1986, p. 14.

Greetings—with a brief look back [editorial], by T. F. Zuck. TRANSFUSION 23(6):459, November-December 1983.

Grim ABC's of AIDS: a government report says children must be told about the disease, by B. Kantrowitz, et al. NEWSWEEK 108(18):66-67, November 3, 1986.

Grim projections for AIDS epidemic, by D. M. Barnes. SCIENCE 232:1589-1590, June 27, 1986.

Group-fantasy origins of AIDS, by C. G. Schmidt. JOURNAL OF PSYCHOHISTORY 12(1):37-78, 1984.

Group health insurers do not exclude AIDS cover. BUSINESS INSURANCE 19:61, September 30, 1985.

Groups at high risk for AIDS [letter], by J. E. Ollé-Goig, et al. NEW ENGLAND JOURNAL OF MEDICINE 311(2):124, July 12, 1984.

Growing Canadian AIDS alarm, by S. McKay. MACLEAN'S 96:34-35, July 11, 1983.

Guardian angel, by P. Morrisroe. NEW YORK 18:46-49+, December 9, 1985.

Guidance on AIDS in bid to quell fears, by S. Ellis. NURSING STANDARD 311:3, September 1, 1983.

Guide to the investigation and treatment of patients with AIDS and AIDS-related disorders, by F. A. Shepherd, et al. CANADIAN MEDICAL ASSOCIATION JOURNAL 134(9):999-1008, May 1, 1986.

Guidelines for the care of patients with AIDS [letter], by J. P. Paul. NEW ENGLAND JOURNAL OF MEDICINE 310(18):1194, May 3, 1984.

Guidelines for caring for the AIDS patient in the home setting, by E. C. Garvey. NITA 8(6):481-483, November-December 1985.

Guidelines for enrolling children with AIDS set up in two states. PHI DELTA KAPPAN 66:448-449, February 1985.

Guidelines for people responsible for education and day care of children with HTLV-III/LAV infection, by G. F. Smith. CANADIAN MEDICAL ASSOCIATION JOURNAL 135(2):134-136, July 15, 1986.

Guidelines for working with blood in Stockholm County. JORDEMODERN 99(6):216-217, June 1986.

Guidelines to protect nurses from AIDS. NURSING STANDARD 379:1, January 10, 1985.

Guild lawyers oppose San Francisco's sex police, by M. Burtle. GUILD NOTES 9(1):2, Winter 1985.

Haemophilia and AIDS [letter], by A. G. Bird, et al. LANCET 1(8421):162-163, January 19, 1985.

—, by A. L. Bloom. LANCET 1(8424):336, February 9, 1985.

Haemophilia, blood products and AIDS [letter], by D. G. Woodfield. NEW ZEALAND MEDICAL JOURNAL 97(748):51-52, January 25, 1984.

—, by E. W. Berry, et al. NEW ZEALAND MEDICAL JOURNAL 96(744):986, November 23, 1983.

Haemophilia, blood transfusion, and the AIDS virus [editorial], by J. S. Lilleyman. ARCHIVES OF DISEASE IN CHILDHOOD 61(2):105-107, February 1986.

Haemophiliac sues over AIDS. NEW SCIENTIST 102:5, May 17, 1984.

Haiti—AIDS stigma, by M. Cooley. NACLA'S REPORT ON THE AMERICAS 17(5):47, September 1983.

Haiti and the acquired immunodeficiency syndrome [letter]. ANNALS OF INTERNAL MEDICINE 99(4):565, October 1983.

Haiti and the acquired immunodeficiency syndrome, by J. R. Leonidas, et al. ANNALS OF INTERNAL MEDICINE 98(6):1020-1021, June 1983.

Haiti and the AIDS connection, By M. Barry, et al. JOURNAL OF CHRONIC DISEASES 37(7):593-595, 1984.

Haiti and the stigma of AIDS [letter],by R. S. Greco. LANCET 2(8348):515-516, August 27, 1983.

Haitian Ambassador deplores AIDS connection [letter], by S. Sherman. NEW ENGLAND JOURNAL OF MEDICINE 309(11):668-669, September 15, 1983.

Haitian connection. THE ECONOMIST 286:77, January 29-February 4, 1983.

Haitian liason for AIDS group, by C. Guilfoy. GAY COMMUNITY NEWS 12(34):1, March 16, 1985.

Haitians and AIDS. AMERICAN FAMILY PHYSICIAN 31:241, June 1985.

Haitians wrongly labeled but hyster. GUARDIAN 35(41):9, August 10, 1983.b

Halifax: getting together to battle AIDS, by D. Henderson. BODY POLITIC 109:14, December 1984.

Hart disappointing on gay issues, by J. Ryan. GAY COMMUNITY NEWS 11(36):3, March 31, 1984.

Hastings Center initiates AIDS study, by M. F. Goldsmith. JAMA 254:2527, November 8, 1985.

Hate, fear and Rock Hudson, by J. Brady. ADVERTISING AGE 56:39, August 15, 1985.

Haven for AIDS outcasts. LIFE 7:78-82, January 1984.

Hawaii report. A lesson in AIDS hysteria, by C. Ikegami. JOSANPU ZASSHI 37(10): 860-863, October 1983.

HB vaccine study. AMERICAN FAMILY PHYSICIAN 31:274, March 1985.

Head and neck presentations of acquired immunodeficiency syndrome,by R. A. Rosenberg, et al. LARYNGOSCOPE 94(5, Part 1):642-646, May 1984.

Head lice linked with AIDS, by H. Wilce. THE TIMES EDUCATIONAL SUPPLEMENT 3636:7, March 7, 1986.

Health, by N. Fain. ADVOCATE 3(72):20, July 21, 1983; also in subsequent issues.

Health: AIDS: epidemic of the '80s, by M. Horosko. DANCE MAGAZINE 60:76-78+, January 1986.

Health-AIDS—the gold rush, by N. Fain. ADVOCATE 3(74):22, August 18, 1983.

Health care advocacy for AIDS patients, by R. L. Cecchi. QRB12(8):297-303, August 1986.

Health care and the politics of AIDS, by N. Freudenberg. HEALTH PAC BULLETIN 16(3):29, May 1985.

Health care employees with AIDS—set policies before problems arise, by A. Dong. DIMENSIONS IN HEALTH SERVICE 63(6):43, September 1986.

Health care personnel and AIDS [letter], by L. Siegel. ARCHIVES OF INTERNAL MEDICINE 144(12):2431, December 1984.

Health care system under AIDS siege, by W. Curry. PHYSICIAN EXECUTIVE 12(2):4-6, March-April 1986.

Health care workers with AIDS [letter], by M. S. Cord. CANADIAN MEDICAL ASSOCIATION JOURNAL 134(6):573, March 15, 1986.

Health concerns and the common cup; Bishops liturgy committee. ORIGINS 15:475-477, January 2, 1986.

Health Conference aims for diversity, by C. Irvine. GAY COMMUNITY NEWS 12(1):3, July 14, 1984.

Health—creative responses from all, by N. Fain. ADVOCATE 3(81):22, November 24, 1983.

Health crisis: AIDS is now becoming a legal epidemic, too, by J. Hyatt. INC. 7:19-20, December 1985.

Health Director closes Bay Area sex businesses, by C. Guilfoy. GAY COMMUNITY NEWS 12(14):1, October 20, 1984.

Health Director resigns, by J. Ryan. GAY COMMUNITY NEWS 12(15):1, October 27, 1984.

Health education: the advertising myth, by M. Pownall. NURSING TIMES 82(34):19-20, August 20-26, 1986.

Health education and the politics of AIDS, by N. Freundenberg. HEALTH PAC BUL-LETIN 16(3):29-30, May-June 1985.

Health experts call for improved HIV testing , by D. Walter. ADVOCATE 453:22, August 19, 1986.

Health office set up/Koch pressured, by B. Nelson. GAY COMMUNITY NEWS 10(36): 1, April 2, 1983.

Health officials close baths and sex clubs. BODY POLITIC 1(8):17, November 1984.

Health officials recommend contact tracing/HTLV3, by D. Walter. ADVOCATE 449: 15, June 24, 1986.

Health officials seek ways to halt AIDS, by J. L. Marx. SCIENCE 219:271-272, January 21, 1983.

Health personnel may have gotten AIDS from patients. RN 48:6, December 1985.

Health—two kinds of answers to AIDS, by N. Fain. ADVOCATE 3(76):16, September 15, 1983.

Health worker's AIDS prompts investigation, by C. Guilfoy. GAY COMMUNITY NEWS 12(24):2, December 29, 1984.

Hearing held in PWA case, by J. Kiely. GAY COMMUNITY NEWS 14(2):1, July 20, 1986.

Heated sera and laboratory tests [letter], by S. I. Vas, et al. ANNALS OF INTERNAL MEDICINE 103(2)308, August 1985.

Heckler finally meets with gay leaders, by D. Walter. ADVOCATE 411:11, January 8, 1985.

Heckler stand on AIDS hit. GAY COMMUNITY NEWS 12(43):3, May 18, 1985.

Help for AIDS victims. CHRISTIAN CENTURY 103(7):201-202, February 26, 1986.

Helper suppressor T cells—AIDS, by N. Fain. ADVOCATE 3(78):22, October 13, 1983.

Helping AIDS patients through unconditional love, by K. Mrgudic. AMERICAN JOURNAL OF HOSPICE CARE 3(2):5, March-April 1986.

Helping AIDS victims. CHRISTIANITY TODAY 30(2):59, February 7, 1986.

Helping battle AIDS, by J. Fierman. FORTUNE 111:57-58, April 15, 1985.

Helping gay AIDS patients in crisis, by D. J. Lopez, et al. SOCIAL CASEWORK 65(7): 387-394, 1984.

Helping out the hot line, by N. Fain. ADVOCATE 3(77):23, September 29, 1983.

Helquist report, by M. Helquist. ADVOCATE 445:21, April 29, 1986; also in 447:21, 448:21, 452:21, 455:21.

Helquist report—is oral sex safe?, by M. Helquist. ADVOCATE 444:23, April 15, 1986.

Helquist report—round two for cyclosporin, by M. Helquist. ADVOCATE 449:21, June 24, 1986.

Hematogenous hexamitiasis in a macaque monkey with an immunodeficiency syndrome [letter], by N. L. Letvin, et al. JOURNAL OF INFECTIOUS DISEASES 149(5):828, May 1984.

Hematologic abnormalities in the acquired immune deficiency syndrome by J. L. Spivak, et al. AMERICAN JOURNAL OF MEDICINE 77(2):224-228, August 1984.

Hematologic care of the surgical patient, by S. A. Berkman. HOSPITAL PRACTICE 21(2):124DD+, Feburary 15, 1986.

Hematologic manifestations in homosexual men with Kaposi's sarcoma,by D. I. Abrams, et al. AMERICAN JOURNAL OF CLINICAL PATHOLOGY 81(1):13-18, January 1984.

Hemolytic-uremic syndrome with the acquired immunodeficiency syndrome [letter], by R. V. Boccia, et al. ANNALS OF INTERNAL MEDICINE 101(5):716-717, November 1984.

Hemophilia, AIDS and hepatitis. AMERICAN FAMILY PHYSICIAN 29:313-314, May 1984.

Hemophilia and acquired immune deficiency syndrome, by P. H. Levine, et al. PROGRESS IN CLINICAL AND BIOLOGICAL RESEARCH 182:287-296, 1985.

Hemophilia and the acquired immune deficiency syndrome (AIDS), by E. J. Sjamsoedin-Visser, et al. NEDERLANDS TIJDSCHRIFT VOOR GENEESKUNDE 127(23): 1008-1009, June 4, 1983.

Hemophilia and the acquired immunodeficiency syndrome [letter], by O. D. Ratnoff, et al. ANNALS OF INTERNAL MEDICINE 102(3):412, March 1985.

Hemophilia and AIDS. AMERICAN FAMILY PHYSICIAN 31:318, January 1985.

Hemophilia and thrombocytopenia in a patient with impaired cellular immunity. A case report, by U. Zeithuber, et al. BLUT 48(6):392-395, June 1984.

Hemophilia, hepatitis, and the acquired immunodeficiency syndrome, by G. C. White, 2d, et al. ANNALS OF INTERNAL MEDICINE 98(3):403-404, March 1983.

Hemophilus influenzae bactermia in a patient with immunodeficiency caused by HTLV-III [letter], by D. L. Garbowit, et al. NEW ENGLAND JOURNAL OF MEDICINE 314(1):56, January 2, 1986.

149

Hepatic involvement in the acquired immunodeficiency syndrome. Study of 20 cases, by J. F. Devars du Mayne, et al. PRESSE MEDICALE 14(21):1177-1180, May 25, 1985.

Hepatic lesions in AIDS, by C. Marche, et al. ARCHIVES D'ANATOMIE ET DE CYTOLOGIE PATHOLOGIQUES 32(2):120-121, 1984.

Hepatic vascular lesions in AIDS [letter], by J. F. Devars du Mayne. JAMA 254(1):53-54, July 5, 1985.

Hepatitis B and AIDS in Africa [letter], by J. F. Cook. MEDICAL JOURNAL OF AUSTRALIA 142(12):661, June 10, 1985.

Hepatitis B immune globulin as treatment of CMV infections in patients with AIDS, by W. C. Jordan. JOURNAL OF THE NATIONAL MEDICAL ASSOCIATION 78(1): 61-62, January 1986.

Hepatitis B immunization and AIDS, by R. Thomssen, et al. DEUTSCHE MEDIZINISCHE WOCHENSCHRIFT 108(36):1373-1374, September 9, 1983.

Hepatitis B surface antigen could harbour the infective agent of AIDS, by M. I. McDonald, et al. LANCET 2(8355):882-884, October 15, 1983.

Hepatitis B vaccination and AIDS [letter], by S. Kato, et al. JAMA 254(1):53, July 5, 1985.

Hepatitis B vaccination: the danger of AIDS transmission, by R. Scheier. ZEITSCHRIFT FUR HAUTKRANKHEITEN 59(8):502-506, April 15, 1984.

Hepatitis "B" vaccine. MEDICAL BULLETIN OF THE U.S. ARMY, EUROPE 41(2):14, February 1984.

—. Pasteur Institute in AIDS fracas ,by R. Walgate. NATURE 304(5922):104, July 14-20, 1983.

Hepatitis B vaccine and AIDS. AMERICAN FAMILY PHYSICIAN 33:312, March 1986.

— [letter], by J. B. Epstein. CANADIAN DENTAL ASSOCIATION JOURNAL 5(2):115, February 1986.

Hepatitis B vaccine does not transmit AIDS. AMERICAN JOURNAL OF NURSING 83:1196, August 1983.

Hepatitis B vaccine: evidence confirming lack of AIDS transmission, by B. Poiesz, et al. JAMA 253:21-22, January 4, 1985; also in MMWR 33(49):685-687, December 1, 1984.

Hepatitis B virus and the prevention of primary cancer of the liver, by B. S. Blumberg, et al. JOURNAL OF THE NATIONAL CANCER INSTITUTE 74(2):267-273, February 1985.

Hepatitis B virus DNA sequences in lymphoid cells from patients with AIDS and AIDS-related complex, by F. Laure, et al. SCIENCE 229(4713):561-563, August 9, 1985.

Hepatitis B virus (HBV) DNA in leucocytes in acquired immune deficiency syndrome (AIDS), by L. E. Lie-Injo, et al. CYTOBIOS 44(176):119-128, 1985.

Hepatitis B virus in AIDS [letter],by L. E. Lie-Injo. LANCET 1(8367):54, January 7, 1984.

150

Hepatitis B virus infection in the acquired immunodeficiency syndrome, by V. K. Rustgi, et al. ANNALS OF INTERNAL MEDICINE 101(6):795-797, December 1984.

Hepatitis in children with acquired immune deficiency syndrome. Histopathologic and immunocytologic features, by L. F. Duffy, et al. GASTROENTEROLOGY 90(1): 173-181, January 1986.

Hepatitis vaccine and the acquired immunodeficiency syndrome [letter], by A. M. Schwartz, et al. ANNALS OF INTERNAL MEDICINE 99(4):567-568, October 1983.

Herpes may be a factor in getting AIDS: study. JET 66:35, July 30, 1984.

Herpes virus infections in the acquired immune deficiency syndrome, by G. V. Quinnan, Jr., et al. JAMA 252(1):72-77, July 6, 1984.

Herpes virus may have role in AIDS. AMERICAN FAMILY PHYSICIAN 27:268-269, April 1983.

Herpes without vesicles: limited, recurrent genital lesions in an immunodebilitated host, by H. Schneiderman, et al. SOUTHERN MEDICAL JOURNAL 79(3):368-370, March 1986.

Herpes zoster and the acquired immunodeficienty syndrome [letter],by L. A. Cone, et al. ANNALS OF INTERNAL MEDICINE 100(3):462, March 1984.

Herpes zoster ophthalmicus and acquired immune deficiency syndrome, by E. L. Cole, et al. ARCHIVES OF OPHTHALMOLOGY 102(7):1027-1029, July 1984.

Herpes zoster ophthalmicus in patients at risk for AIDS [letter], by W. Sandor, et al. NEW ENGLAND JOURNAL OF MEDICINE 310(17):1118-1119, April 26, 1984.

Herpes zoster: a possible early clinical sign for development of acquired immunodeficiency syndrome in high-risk individuals, by A. E. Friedman-Kien, et al. JOURNAL OF THE AMERICAN ACADEMY OF DERMATOLOGY 14(6):1023-1028, June 1986.

Heterogeneity of epidemic Kaposi's sarcoma. Implications for therapy, by R. T. Mitsu-yasu, et al. CANCER 57(Suppl. 8):1657-1661, April 15, 1986.

Heterosexual AIDS panic: a quear paradigm, by C. Patto. GAY COMMUNITY NEWS 12(29):3, February 9, 1985.

Heterosexual and homosexual patients with the acquired immunodeficiency syndrome. A comparison of surveillance, interview, and laboratory data, by M. E. Guinan, et al. ANNALS OF INTERNAL MEDICINE 100(2):213-218, February 1984.

Heterosexual partners: a large risk group for AIDS [letter], by D. C. Des Jarlais, et al. LANCET 2(8416):1346-1347, December 8, 1984.

Heterosexual promiscuity among African patients with AIDS [letter], by N. Clumck, et al. NEW ENGLAND JOURNAL OF MEDICINE 313(3):182, July 18, 1985.

Heterosexual transmission of the acquired immunodeficiency syndrome (AIDS), by M. Vogt, et al. DEUTSCHE MEDIZINISCHE WOCHENSCHRIFT 110(39):1483-1487, September 27, 1985.

Heterosexual transmission of AIDS [letter],by R. B. Pearce. JAMA 256(5):90-591, August 1, 1986.

Heterosexual transmission of human T-lymphotropic virus type III/lymphadenopathy-associated virus. JAMA 254:2051-2052, October 18, 1985; also in MMWR 34(37): 561-563, September 20, 1985.

Heterosexually acquired HTLV-III/LAV disease (AIDS-related complex and AIDS). Epidemiologic evidence for female-to-male transmission, by R. R. Redfield, et al. JAMA 254(15):2094-2096, October 18, 1985.

HHS announces new contract award, research initiatives in fight against AIDS. PUBLIC HEALTH REPORTS 98(6):622-623, November-December 1983.

HHS investigations centered on AIDS, by E. N. Brandt, Jr. US MEDICINE 20(2):67-69, January 15, 1984.

HHS official resigns over AIDS policy, by C. Linebarger. ADVOCATE 443:14, April 1, 1986.

HHS rejects proposed ban on HTLV-3 test, by Bisticas-Cocoves. GAY COMMUNITY NEWS 12(44):1, May 25, 1985.

HHS to screen new immigrants for HTLV-III, by Bisticas-Cocoves. GAY COMMUNITY NEWS 13(31):1, February 22, 1986.

High-grade non-Hodgkin's lymphoma in patients with AIDS, by J. L. Ziegler, et al. ANNALS OF THE NEW YORK ACADEMY OF SCIENCES 437:412-419, 1984.

High school students' perceptions and misperceptions of aAIDS, by J. H. Price, et al. JOURNAL OF SCHOOL HEALTH 55(3):107-109, March 1985.

High-stakes race is on to develop blood test to detect AIDS virus, by A. Cooper. NATIONAL JOURNAL 16:1470-1472, August 4, 1984.

Higher AIDS budget proposed, by Bisticas-Cocoves. GAY COMMUNITY NEWS 13(5):1, August 10, 1985.

Highly abnormal B-cell function found in AIDS. HOSPITAL PRACTICE 18(10): 32+, October 1983.

Hill bars 'adverse action' against AIDS carriers, by P. J. Budahn. AIR FORCE TIMES 47:10, November 3, 1986.

Histological study of retinal necrosis due to cytomeglovirus in AIDS , by P. Dhermy, et al. BULLETIN DES SOCIETES D'OPHTHALMOLOGIE DE FRANCE 84(4):381-384, April 1984.

Histopathologic changes in macaques with an acquired immunodeficiency syndrome (AIDS), by W. King, et al. AMERICAN JOURNAL OF PATHOLOGY 113(3):382-388, December 1983.

Histopathological aspects of lymph nodes in the prodromal phase of the acquired immunodeficiency syndrome and related conditions, by J. Diebold, et al. ARCHIVES D'ANATOMIE ET DE CYTOLOGIE PATHOLOGIQUES 32(4):253-254, 1984.

Histopathological changes in the thymus gland in the acquired immune deficiency syndrome, by A. E. Davis, Jr. ANNALS OF THE NEW YORK ACADEMY OF SCIENCES 437:493-502, 1984.

Histopathological studies of lymphadenopathy in AIDS: tentative classification. Preliminary report, by C. Marche, et al. ANTIBIOTIC CHEMOTHERAPY 32:76-86, 1983.

Histopathological study of lymph nodes in patients with lymphadenopathy or acquired immune deficiency syndrome, by c. Marche, et al. EUROPEAN JOURNAL OF CLINICAL MICROBIOLOGY 3(1):75-76, February 1984.

Histopathology of the acquired immune deficiency syndrome, by C. Urmacher, et al. PATHOLOGY ANNUAL 20(Part 1):197-220, 1985.

Histoplasmosis diagnosed on peripheral blood smear from a patient with AIDS, by S. Henochowicz, et al. JAMA 253(21):3148, June 7, 1985.

Histoplasmosis in the acquired immune deficiency syndrome, by L. J. Wheat, et al. AMERICAN JOURNAL OF MEDICINE 78(2):203-210, February 1985.

Histoplasmosis in acquired immunodeficiency syndrome (AIDS): diagnosis by bone marrow examination [letter], by J. Pasternak, et al. ARCHIVES OF INTERNAL MEDICINE 143(10):2024, October 1983.

Histoplasmosis presenting with unusual skin lesions in acquired immunodeficiency syndrome (AIDS), by J. A. Hazelhurst, et al. BRITISH JOURNAL OF DERMATOLOGY 113·3):345-348, September 1985.

History of an epidemic, by R. Bazell. THE NEW REPUBLIC 189:14-15+, August 1, 1983.

HIV infection with seroconversion after a superficial needlestick injury to the finger, by E. Oksenhendler, et al. NEW ENGLAND JOURNAL OF MEDICINE 315(9):582, August 28, 1986.

HLA studies in acquired immune deficiency syndrome patients with Kaposi's sarcoma, by H. E. Prince, et al. JOURNAL OF CLINICAL IMMUNOLOGY 4(3):242-245, May 1984.

HLA-A,B,C and DR antigen frequencies in acquired immunodeficiency syndrome (AIDS) patients with opportunistic infections, by M. S. Pollack, et al. HUMAN IMMUNOLOGY 11(2):99-103, October 1984.

Hodgkin's disease and the acquired immunodeficiency syndrome [letter], by H. L. Ioachim, et al. ANNALS OF INTERNAL MEDICINE 101(6):876-877, December 1984.

—,by N. J. Robert, et al. ANNALS OF INTERNAL MEDICINE 101(1):142-143, July 1984.

Hodgkin's disease in AIDS complex patients. Report of four cases and tissue immunologic marker studies, by P. D. Unger, et al. CANCER 58(4):821-825, August 15, 1986.

Holistic aid for AIDS, by C. McPartland. NEW AGE 9(4):17, November 1983.

Holistic antidote to the epidemic of fear, by C. Hall. RFD 45:46, Winter 1985.

Holistic care of the AIDS victim, by A. Gillis. HEALTH CARE 26(3):34-35, April 1984.

Holistic health: one approach to AIDS. OUT 4(6):3, May 1986.

Holistic hyperbole, by R. Trow. BODY POLITIC 93:38, May 1983.

Hollywood bash to combat AIDS, by B. Barol. NEWSWEEK 106:80-81, September 30, 1985.

Hollywood Bowl AIDS benefit, by S. Anderson. ADVOCATE 3(78):13, October 13, 1983.

Hollywood faces AIDS, by S. Rosenthal. US 3:27+, October 7, 1985.

Hollywood love scenes: the scares, laughs, romance, by M. Murphy, et al. TV GUIDE 34:4+, February 8, 1986.

Home AIDS . . . district nurse's role in caring for the patient with acquired immune deficiency syndrome in his own home, by S. Robins. NURSING MIRROR 160(8):21-22, February 20, 1985.

Home care dealers help combat AIDS fears, by E. Beck. MEDICAL PRODUCTS SALES 16(12):21+, December 1985.

Home care for the AIDS patient: safety first, by K. Dhundale, et al. NURSING 16(9):34-36, September 1986.

Home care/hospice for the AIDS patient, by P. M. Gibbons. MASSACHUSETTS NURSE 54(7):5-6, July 1985.

Home care hospice program . . . AIDS, by J. Lieberman. CALIFORNIA NURSE 82(4):6-7, May 1986.

Home care of the client with AIDS, by J. K. Bryant. JOURNAL OF COMMUNITY HEALTH NURSING 3(2):69-74, 1986.

Home care plan for AIDS, by H. Schietinger. AMERICAN JOURNAL OF NURSING 86(9):1021-1028, September 1986.

Homology of genome of AIDS-associated virus with genomes of human T-cell leukemia viruses, by S. K. Arya, et al. SCIENCE 225:927-930, August 31, 1984.

Homophobia among physicians and nurses: an empirical study, by C. J. Douglas, et al. HOSPITAL AND COMMUNITY PSYCHIATRY 36(12):1309-1311, December 1985.

Homosexual plague strikes new victims, by E. Keerdoja. NEWSWEEK 100:10, August 23, 1982.

Homosexual promiscuity and the fear of AIDS [letter],by R. Golubjatnikov, et al. LANCET 2(8351):681, September 17, 1983.

Homosexuality and sexually transmitted diseases, including the acquired immunologic deficiency syndrome, by C. H. Coester, et al. INTERNIST 24():334-345, June 1983.

Homosexuality: kick and kickback [editorial], by J. L. Fletcher. SOUTHERN MEDICAL JOURNAL 77(2):149-150, Febraury 1984.

Hope for therapies in 1986, by M. Helquist. ADVOCATE 437:21, January 7, 1986.

Hopes for an AIDS vaccine are fading fast, by S. Connor. NEW SCIENTIST 111:28-29, July 3, 1986.

Hospice, AIDS and the community . . . workshop on AIDS for the community, by C. J. Sheehan. CARING 5(6):34-37, June 1986.

Hospice care endorsed for AIDS patients. Michigan Hospice Organization. MICHI-GAN HOSPITALS 22(8):25, August 1986.

Hospital guidelines on AIDS developed at UCSF. INFECTION CONTROL DIGEST 4(8):3-4, August 1983.

Hospital hygiene. AIDS: preventing contamination in the hospital, by G. Ducel. KRANKENPFLEGE. SOINS INFIRMIERS 79(5):67-70, May 1986.

—. Notice of the Expert Federal Commission for AIDS on procedures to adopt in regard to patients with AIDS and to persons carrying anti-LAV/HTLV-III antibodies. KRANKENPFLEGE. SOINS INFIRMIERS 79(5):74-75, May 1986.

Hospital report admits failings in AID case,by C. Guilfoy. GAY COMMUNITY NEWS 12(32):3, March 2, 1985.

Hospital waste: states confront task of disposal, by L. Lehrer. PROFESSIONAL SAN-ITATION MANAGEMENT 17(3):39, October0November 1985.

Hospital workers with AIDS not in high-risk group. CORRECTIONS DIGEST 14(16):6-7, July 27, 1983.

Hospitals face legal issues involving AIDS patients, employees, by J. D. Epstein, et al. TEXAS HOSPITALS 41(11):12-15, April 1986.

Hospitals may be AIDS victims too. MEDICAL WORLD NEWS 26(23):92-93, December 9, 1985.

Hospitals stepping up effort to protect staff from AIDS. AMERICAN JOURNAL OF NURSING 83:1468+, October 1983.

Hospitalwide approach to AIDS. Recommendations of the Advisory Committee on Infections within Hospitals, by the American Hospital Association. INFECTION CONTROL 5(5):242-248, May 1984.

Hot on the trail of the cause and cure of AIDS, by O. Timbs, et al. TIMES April 6, 1984, p. 11.

House Committee doubles '86 AIDS research money, by M. Cocoves. GAY COM-MUNITY NEWS 13(11):3, September 28, 1985.

House OKs record AIDS funding, by Bush, et al. ADVOCATE 3(79):8, October 27, 1983.

House panel holds hearing on AIDS and IV drug abuse. NARCOTICS CONTROL DI-GEST 15(25-26):5-6, December 11, 1985.

Houston gay rights squashed in referendum, by S. Hyde. GAY COMMUNITY NEWS 12(28):1, February 2, 1985.

How adult T-cell leukaemia spread in Japan, by J. Bell. NEW SCIENTIST 105:22, March 7, 1985.

How the AIDS ruling affects us. DISABILITY 7(5):26, September 1986.

How AIDS threatens all of us, by T. Stuttaford. SPECTATOR November 15, 1986, p. 9-11.

How America nurtured AIDS. NEW SCIENTIST 110:25, May 29, 1986.

How blood traders could have launched AIDS. NEW SCIENTIST 105:7, March 28, 1985.

How common is HTLV-III infection in the United States? by S. L. Sivak, et al. NEW ENGLAND JOURNAL OF MEDICINE 313:1352, November 21, 1985.

How dangerous is AIDS?, by G. Jörgensen. KRANKENPFLEGE JOURNAL 24(6):12-14+, June 1, 1986.

How do you get AIDS, by N. Fain. ADVOCATE 3(79):20, October 27, 1983.

How does the medical profession protect itself? by W. Williams. JOURNAL OF THE LOUISIANA STATE MEDICAL SOCIETY 137(9):53-55, September 1985.

How fast we forget, by F. S. Welch. PHOENIX 21:192, January 1986.

How Gallo got credit for AIDS discovery, by O. Sattaur. NEW SCIENTIST 105:3-4, February 7, 1985.

How HTLV causes leukaemia, by O. Sattaur. NEW SCIENTIST 103:35, August 2, 1984.

How should Catholic hospitals respond to the AIDS problem? HOSPITAL PRO-GRESS 65:49-50, May 1984.

How should we handle the ethical questions regarding information to donors and pa-tients and the practical implications regarding deferral of donors and handling of donated blood in the event of introducing a screening test for HTLV-III as in order to prevent transmission of AIDS by blood transfusion?, by J. R. Bove, et al. VOX SANGUINIS 49(3):234-239, 1985.

How to avoid catching AIDS, by A. Veitch, et al. GUARDIAN November 21, 1986, p. 21.

How to care for an AIDS patient,by D. A. Coleman. RN 49(7):16-21, July 1986.

How to explain the fears, by C. Phillips. CHATELAINE 59:40, November 1986.

How to prevent spreading AIDS via blood transfusions. RN 46:11-12, April 1983.

How to reduce the AIDS hysteria in central service, by S. Romey. HOSPITAL TOPICS 61(6):34, November-December 1983.

How to safeguard against AIDS, by C. Joyce. NEW SCIENTIST 102:8, May 31, 1984.

How to turn a disease into VD, by J. Seale. NEW SCIENTIST 106:38-41, June 20, 1985.

How a virus that is very hard to catch crossed the world; AIDS and public health, by J. Meldrum. NEW STATESMAN 110:14-15, September 27, 1985.

How will the law respond to AIDS?, by A. Affriol, et al.. JOURNAL OF PRACTICAL NURSING 35(4):31, December 1985.

HTLV and AIDS. AMERICAN FAMILY PHYSICIAN 28:255, July 1983.

— [editorial]. LANCET 1(8335):1200, May 28, 1983.

HTLV and AIDS in France [letter], by D. Mathez, et al. LANCET 1(8380):799, April 7, 1984.

HTLV and AIDS in West Germany [letter],by M. Born, et al. LANCET 1(8370):222, January 28, 1984.

HTLV exposure and AIDS. AMERICAN FAMILY PHYSICIAN 33:358, March 1986.

HTLV-I antibodies in childhood leukemia, by D. L. Williams, et al. JAMA 253:2496, May 3, 1985.

HTLV-I antibody status in hemophilia patients treated with factor concentrates prepared from U.S. plasma sources and in hemophilia patients with AIDS, by T. L. Chorba, et al. THROMBOSIS AND HAEMOSTASIS 53(2):180-182, April 22, 1985.

HTLV-I-specific antibody in AIDS patients and others at risk, by M. Robert-Guroff, et al. LANCET 2(8395):128-131, July 21, 1984.

HTLV-positive T-cell lymphoma/leukaemia in an AIDS patient [letter], by M. Kobayashi, et al. LANCET 1(8390):1361-1362, June 16, 1984.

HTLV/III, AIDS, and the brain [editorial], by P. H. Black. NEW ENGLAND JOURNAL OF MEDICINE 313(2):1538-1540, December 12, 1985.

HTLV-III AIDS link, by J. A. Bennett. AMERICAN JOURNAL OF NURSING 85(10): 1086-1089, October 1985.

HTLV-III and blood donors [editorial]. LANCET 1(8433):856, April 13, 1985.

HTLV/III and the etiology of AIDS, by R. C. Gallo, et al. PROGRESS IN ALLERGY 37: 1-45, 1986.

HTLV-III and LAV: similar, or identical? by C. Norman. SCIENCE 230:643, November 8, 1985.

HTLV-III and psychiatric disturbance [letter], by c. S. Thomas, et al. LANCET 2(8451): 395-396, August 17, 1985.

HTLV-III antibodies and immunological alterations in hemophilia patients, by E. Seifried, et al. KLINISCHE WOCHENSCHRIFT 64(3):115-124, February 3, 1986.

HTLV-III antibodies in haematology staff [letter], by P. Jones, et al. LANCET 1(8422): 217, January 26, 1985.

HTLV-III antibodies in US Army blood donors in West Germany, by J. J. James. JAMA 254:1449, September 20, 1985.

HTLV-III antibody in East Africa [letter]. NEW ENGLAND JOURNAL OF MEDICINE 315(4):259-260, July 24, 1986.

HTLV-III antibody in Sydney homosexual men [letter], by P. W. Robertson, et al. MEDICAL JOURNAL OF AUSTRALIA 143(6):261, September 16, 1985.

HTLV-III antibody status and immunological abnormalities in haemophilic patients [letter], by E. H. Moffat, et al. LANCET 1(8434):935, April 20, 1985.

HTLV-III antibody test is licensed, by Freiberg, et al. ADVOCATE 417:11, April 2, 1985.

HTLV-III antibody test: what it can and cannot do. CHART 83(5):5, May-June 1986.

HTLV-III antibody testing in Spain [letter], by R. Nájera, et al. LANCET 2(8458):783, October 5, 1985.

HTLV-III env gene products synthesized in E. coli are recognized by antibodies present in the sera of AIDS patients, by R. Crowl, et al. CELL 41(3):979-986, July 1985.

HTLV-III exposure among drug users, by H. M. Ginzburg, et al. CANCER RESEARCH 45(Suppl. 9):4605s-4608s, September 1985.

HTLV-III exposure during cardiopulmonary resuscitation [letter], by S. M. Saviteer, et al. NEW ENGLAND JOURNAL OF MEDICINE 313(25):1606-1607, December 19, 1985.

HTLV-III gag protein is processed in yeast cells by the virus pol-protease, by R. A. Kramer, et al. SCIENCE 231:1580-1584, March 28, 1986.

HTLV-III in cells cultured from semen of two patients with AIDS, by D. Zagury, et al. SCIENCE 226(4673):449-451, October 26, 1984.

HTLV-III in persons with intravenous drug abuse. Correlation of antibodies against HTLV-III with neopterin and TH/TS, by P. Hengster, et al. DEUTSCHE MEDIZIN-ISCHE WOCHENSCHRIFT 111(12):453-457, March 21, 1986.

HTLV-III in saliva of people with AIDS-related complex and healthy homosexual men at risk for AIDS, by J. E. Groopman, et al. SCIENCE 226(4673):447-449, October 26, 1984.

HTLV/III in the semen and blood of a healthy homosexual man, by D. D. Ho, et al. SCIENCE 226(4673):451-453, October 26, 1984.

HTLV-III in symptom-free seronegative persons, by S. Z. Salaguddin, et al. LANCET 2(8417-8418):1418-1420, December 22, 1984.

HTLV-III infection among health care workers. Association with needle-stick injuries, by S. H. Weiss, et al. JAMA 254(15):2089-2093, October 18, 1985.

HTLV-III infection and AIDS in a Zambian nurse resident in Britain [letter], by A. E. Raine, et al. LANCET 2(8409):985, October 27, 1984.

HTLV-III infection and epitope recognition by OKT4 monoclonal antibody [letter], by T. Hattori, et al. NEW ENGLAND JOURNAL OF MEDICINE 313(24):1543-1544, December 12, 1985.

HTLV-III infection in brains of children and adults with AIDS encephalopathy, by G. M. Shaw, et al. SCIENCE 227:177-181, January 11, 1985.

HTLV-III infection in kidney transplant recipients [letter], by J. L'age-Stehr, et al. LANCET 2(8468):1361-1362, December 14, 1985.

HTLV-III infections and AIDS—current epidemiology and serology, by G. Biberfeld, et al. LAKARTIDNINGEN 82(20):1867-1870, May 15, 1985.

HTLV-III/LAV antibody and immune status of household contacts and sexual partners of persons with hemophilia, by J. M. Jason, et al. JAMA 255:212-215, January 10, 1986.

HTLV-III/LAV-antibody-positive soldiers in Berlin [letter], by J. J. James, et al. NEW ENGLAND JOURNAL OF MEDICINE 314(1):55-56, January 2, 1986.

HTLV-III, LAV, ARV are variants of same AIDS virus [letter], by L. Ratner, et al. NATURE 313(6004):636-637, February 21-27, 1985.

HTLV-III/LAV-like retrovirus particles in the brains of patients with AIDS encephalopathy, by L. G. Epstein, et al. AIDS RESEARCH 1(6):447-454, 1984-1985.

HTLV-III/LAV-seronegative, virus-negative sexual partners and household contacts of hemophiliacs [letter], by T. McFadden, et al. JAMA 255(13):1702, April 4, 1986.

HTLV3 list proposal sparks debate, by C. Guilfoy. GAY COMMUNITY NEWS 12(8):3, September 8, 1984.

HTLV-III-neutralizing antibodies in patients with AIDS and AIDS-related complex, by M. Robert-Guroff, et al. NATURE 316(6023):72-74, July 4-10, 1985.

HTLV-III peptide produced by recombinant DNA is immunoreactive with sera from patients with AIDS, by N. T. Chang, et al. NATURE 315(6015):151-154, May 9-15, 1985.

HTLV3 screening—a cautious perspective, by B. Andrews. GAY COMMUNITY NEWS 12(4):5, August 4, 1984.

HTLV-3 screening: problematic but available, by C. Guilfoy. GAY COMMUNITY NEWS 12(2):3, July 21, 1984.

HTLV-III seroconversion associated with heat-treated factor VIII concentrate [letter], by G. C. White, 2d, et al. LANCET 1(8481):611-612, March 15, 1986.

HTLV-III seropositivity in AIDS [letter],by W. M. Behan, et al. LANCET 1(8389):1292, June 9, 1984.

HTLV-III: should testing ever be routine?,by D. Miller, et al. BRITISH MEDICAL JOURNAL 292(6525):941-943, April 5, 1986.

HTLV-3 test availability elicits mixed response, by C. Guilfoy. GAY COMMUNITY NEWS 12(40):3, April 27, 1985.

HTLV-III test sought as basis for insurance, by M. Cocoves. GAY COMMUNITY NEWS 13(10):1, September 21, 1985.

HTLV-III testing of donor blood imminent; complex issues remain, by M. F. Goldsmith. JAMA 253:173-175+, January 11, 1985.

HTLV-III transmission [editorial], by L. D. Grouse. JAMA 254(15):2130-2131, October 18, 1985.

HTLV-III viremia in homosexual men with generalized lymphadenopathy, by J. E. Kaplan, et al. NEW ENGLAND JOURNAL OF MEDICINE 312:1572-1573, June 13, 1985.

Hudson and AIDS—in retrospect, by M. Bronski. GAY COMMUNITY NEWS 13(13):3, October 12, 1985.

Hug an AIDS victim—he is safe. NEW SCIENTIST 109:15, February 13, 1986.

Human alpha- and beta-interferon but not gamma- suppress the in vitro replication of LAV, HTLV-III, and ARV-2, by J. K. Yamamoto, et al. JOURNAL OF INTERFERON RESEARCH 6(2):143-152, April 1986.

Human cryptosporidiosis in the acquired immune deficiency syndrome, by L. A. Guarda, et al. ARCHIVES OF PATHOLOGY AND LABORATORY MEDICINE 107(11):562-566, November 1983.

Human cryptosporidiosis: spectrum of disease. Report of six cases and review of the literature, by S. D. Pitlik, et al. ARCHIVES OF INTERNAL MEDICINE 143(12): 2269-2275, December 1983.

Human immunodeficiency virus and the adrenal medulla [letter]by C. D. Weiss. AN-NALS OF INTERNAL MEDICINE 105(2):300, August 1986.

Human immunodeficiency virus infection in transplant recipients [letter], by C. Hiesse, et al. ANNALS OF INTERNAL MEDICINE 105(2):301, August 1986.

Human immunodeficiency viruses, by J. Coffin, et al. SCIENCE 232:697, May 9, 1986.

Human interferon-alpha production in homosexual men with the acquired immune deficiency syndrome [letter], by J. Abb, et al. JOURNAL OF INFECTIOUS DISEAS-ES 150(1):158-189, July 1984.

Human lymphoblastoid interferon treatment of Kaposi's sarcoma in the acquired immune deficiency syndrome. Clinical response and prognostic parameters, by E. P. Gelmann, et al. AMERICAN JOURNAL OF MEDICINE 78(5):737-741, May 1985.

Human lymphocyte subpopulations in lymphadenopathies in homosexual men, by P. Rácz, et al. ADVANCES IN EXPERIMENTAL MEDICINE AND BIOLOGY 186:1069-1076, 1985.

Human lymphocytopathic retroviruses (HLRV)? by J. W. Shields. NATURE 317:480, October 10, 1985.

Human recombinant interleukin-2 partly reconstitutes deficiency in-vitro immune responses of lyphocytes from patients with AIDS, by J. D. Lifson,e t al. LANCET 1(8379):698-702, March 1984.

Human T-cell leukemia/lymphoma syndrome [serology positive for HTLV-I antibodies], by E. S. Christian, et al. AMERICAN FAMILY PHYSICIAN 32:155-1260, July 1985.

Human T-cell leukemia/lymphoma viruses: clinical and epidemiologic features, by W. A. Blattner, et al. CURRENT TOPICS IN MICROBIOLOGY AND IMMUNOLOGY 115:67-88, 1985.

Human T-cell leukemia (lymphotropic) retroviruses and their causative role in T-cell malignancies and acquired immune deficiency syndrome, by R. C. Gallo. CAN-CER 55(10):2317-2323, May 15, 1985.

Human T-cell leukemia/lymphotropic retroviruses (HTLV) family: past, present, and future, by R. C. Gallo. CANCER RESEARCH 45(Suppl. 9):4524s-4533s, Septem-ber 1985.

Human T-cell leukemia/lymphotropic virus type III in the conjunctival epithelium of a patient with AIDS, by L. S. Fujikawa, et al. AMERICAN JOURNAL OF OPHTHAL-MOLOGY 100(4):507-509, October 15, 1985.

Human T-cell leukemia virus and AIDS [letter],by P. H. Black, et al. NEW ENGLAND JOURNAL OF MEDICINE 309(14):856, October 6, 1983.

Human T-cell leukemia virus family, adult T cell leukemia, and AIDS, by R. C. Gallo, et al. HAMATOLOGIE UND BLUTTRANSFUSION 29:317-325, 1985.

Human T-cell leukemia virus (HTLV-I) antibodies in Africa, by W. Saxinger, et al. SCIENCE 225:1473-1476, September 28, 1984.

Human T-cell leukemia virus in acquired immune deficiency syndrome: preliminary observation. JAMA 249(21)L2878-2879, June 3, 1983.

Human T-cell leukemia virus in lymphocytes of two hemophiliacs with the acquired immunodeficiency syndrome, by E. L. Palmer, et al. ANNALS OF INTERNAL MEDICINE 101(3):293-297, September 1984.

Human T-cell leukemia virus infection in patients with acquired immune deficiency syndrome: preliminary observations. MMWR 32(18):233-234, May 13, 1983.

Human T-cell leukemia virus linked to AIDS, by J. L. Marx. SCIENCE 220(4599):806-809, May 20, 1983.

Human T-cell leukemia virus type I is a member of the African subtype of simian viruses (STLV), by T. Watanabe, et al. VIROLOGY 148:385-388, January 30, 1986.

Human T-cell leukemia virus type II: primary structure analysis of the major internal protein, p24 and the nucleic acid binding protein, p15, by S. G. Devare, et al. VIROLOGY 142:206-210, April 15, 1985.

Human T cell leukemia virus type III antibody, lymphadenopathy, and acquired immune deficiency syndrome in hemophiliac subjects. Results of a prospective study, by J. K. Kreiss, et al. AMERICAN JOURNAL OF MEDICINE 80(3):345-350, March 1986.

Human T-cell leukemia viruses (HTLV): a unique family of pathogenic retroviruses, by S. Broder, et al. ANNUAL REVIEW OF IMMUNOLOGY 3:321-336, 1985.

Human T-cell lymphotropic virus antibody screening: data survey on 33,603 German blood donors correlated to confirmatory tests,by P. Kühnl, et al. VOX SANGUINIS 49(5):327-330, 1985.

Human T-cell lymphotropic virus type-I antibodies in Falashas and other ethnic groups in Israel, by Z. Ben-Ishai, et al. NATURE 315:665-666, June 20, 1985.

Human T-cell lymphotropic virus type III associated disorders. The spectrum in the heterosexual population, by P. S. Gill, et al. ARCHIVES OF INTERNAL MEDICINE 146(8):1501-1504, Augus 1986.

Human 'T' leukemia virus still suspected in AIDS [interview by John Maurice], by R. C. Gallo. JAMA 250(8):1015+, August 26, 1983.

Human T-lymphotropic retrovirus and AIDS. HTLV-III is probably the cause of acquired immunodeficiency syndrome, by J. H. Dobloug. TIDSSKRIFT FOR DEN NORSKE LAEGEFORENING 105(1):50-52, January 10, 1985.

Human T-lymphotropic retrovirus (HTLV-III) as the cause of the acquired immunodeficiency syndrome, by R. C. Gallo, et al. ANNALS OF INTERNAL MEDICINE 103(5):679-689, November 1985.

Human T-lymphotropic retrovirus type III/lymphadenopathy-associated virus antibody: association with hemopiliacs' immune status and blood component usage, by J. Jason, et al. JAMA 253:3409-3415, June 21, 1985.

161

Human T-lymphotropic retroviruses, by F. Wong-Staal, et al. NATURE 317:395-403, October 3, 1985.

Human T-lymphotropic retroviruses in adult T-cell leukemia-lymphoma and acquired immune deficiency syndrome, by P. S. Sarin, et al. JOURNAL OF CLINICAL IMMUNOLOGY 4(6):415-423, November 1984.

Human T-lymphotropic virus type III (HTLV-III) infection in seronegative haemophiliacs after transfusion of factor VIII, by C. A. Ludlam, et al. LANCET 2(8449):233-236, August 3, 1985.

Human T lymphotropic virus type III infection of human alveolar macrophages, by S. Z. Salahuddin, et al. BLOOD 68(1):281-284, July 1986.

Humoral and cellular immunity in uremia, by C. Irkec, et al. MIKROBIYOLOJI BULTENI 16(3):191-195, July 1982.

Humoral immune responses in healthy heterosexual, homosexual and vasectomized men and in homosexual men with the acquired immune deficiency syndrome, by S. S. Witkin, et al. AIDS RESEARCH 1(1):31-44, 1983-1984.

Humoral response to disseminated infection by Mycobacterium avium-Mycobacterium intracellulare in acquired immunodeficiency syndrome and hairy cell leukemia, by S. M. Winter, et al. JOURNAL OF INFECTIOUS DISEASES 151(3):523-527, March 1985.

Humoral responses to Pneumocystis carinii in patients with acquired immunodeficiency syndrome and in immunocompromised homosexual men, by B. Hofmann, et al. JOURNAL OF INFECTIOUS DISEASES 152(4):838-840, October 1985.

Hunting down AIDS, by B. Henker, et al. ALBERTA REPORT 12:39-40, March 18, 1985.

Hunting for the hidden killers, by W. Isaacson. TIME 122:50-55, July 4, 1983.

Hygeia's comments, by D. Sage. I KNOW YOU KNOW 1(5):9, April 1985.

Hyperalgesic pseudothrombophlebitis. New syndrome in male homosexual, by S. B. Abramson, et al. AMERICAN JOURNAL OF MEDICINE 78(2):317-320, February 1985.

Hypercalcemia and disseminated cytomegalovirus infection in the acquired immunodeficiency syndrome, by G. P. Zaloga, et al. ANNALS OF INTERNAL MEDICINE 102(3);331-333, March 1985.

Hypervascular follicular hyperplasia and Kaposi's sarcoma in patients at risk for AIDS [letter], by N. L. Harris. NEW ENGLAND JOURNAL OF MEDICINE 10(7):462-463, February 16, 1984.

Hypoalbuminemia, diarrhea, and the acquired immunodeficiency syndrome [letter], by R. R. Brinson. ANNALS OF INTERNAL MEDICINE 102(3):413, March 1985.

Hypoglycemic coma from pentamadine in an AIDS patient [letter], by M. P. Spadafora, et al. AMERICAN JOURNAL OF EMERGENCY MEDICINE 4(4):384, July 1986.

Hypothesis: AIDS: AAIDS (acquired autoimmune immunodeficiency syndrome)?, by P. A. Paciucci, et al. AIDS RESEARCH 1(2):149-155, 1983-1984.

Hypothesis: fungal toxins are involved in aspergillosis and AIDS, by R. D. Eichner, et al. AUSTRALIAN JOURNAL OF EXPERIMENTAL BIOLOGY AND MEDICAL SCIENCE 62(Part 4):479-484, August 1984.

Hypothesis: the pathogenesis of AIDS. Activation of the T- and B-cell cascades, by A. S. Evans. YALE JOURNAL OF BIOLOGY AND MEDICINE 57(3):317-327, May-June 1984.

IASP (or IBA), not AIDS [letter],by J. F. Soothill. LANCET 1(8323):526, March 5, 1983.

Iatrogenic AIDS? 2 possible cases in Barcelona [letter]. MEDICINA CLINICA 82(8): 380-381, March 3, 1984.

Icelandic research. Slow virus infections and AIDS, by G. Pétursson, et al. NORDISK MEDICIN 101(5):160-161+, 1986.

Identification and antigenicity of the major envelope glycoprotein of lymphadeno-pathy-associated virus, by L. Montagnier, et al. VIROLOGY 144:283-239, July 15, 1985.

Identification of C or D virus-type particles in the germinal centers of lymph nodes sampled at the lymphadenopathy stage of the acquired immunodeficiency syndrome [letter], by a. Le Tourneau, et al. PRESSE MEDICALE 15(3):121, January 25, 1986.

Identification of Cryptosporidium in patients with the acquired immunologic syndrome [letter],by P. Payne, et al. NEW ENGLAND JOURNAL OF MEDICINE 309(10): 613-614, September 8, 1983.

Identification of the gene responsible for human T-cell leukaemia virus transcriptional regulation, by A. J. Cann, et al. NATURE 318:571-574, December 12, 1985.

Identification of HTLV-III/LAV or gene product and detection of antibodies in human sera, by N. C. Kan, et al. SCIENCE 231:1553-1555, March 28, 1986.

Identification of multiple cytomegalovirus strains in homosexual men with acquired immunodeficiency syndrome, by S. A. Spector, et al. JOURNAL OF INFECTIOUS DISEASES 150(6):953-956, December 1984.

Identification of the putative transforming protein of the human T-cell leukemia viruses HTLV-I and HTLV-II, by D. J. Slamon, et al. SCIENCE 226:61-65, October 5, 1984.

Idiopathic thrombocytopenic purpura in homosexual men, by S. Karpatkin. ANNALS OF THE NEW YORK ACADEMY OF SCIENCES 237:58-64, 1984.

Idiotypes and AIDS [letter], by J. Gheuens. LANCET 2(8393):41, July 7, 1984.

"If I have AIDS, then let me die now!" [case study], by S. Vinogradov, et al. HASTINGS CENTER REPORT 14:24-26, February 1984.

—. Commentary, by A. J. Levinson. HASTINGS CENTER REPORT 14(1):26, February 1984.

If your partner contracts AIDS. RN 47:15, February 1984.

IgA deficiency and AIDS [letter], by M. Hepner, et al. JAMA 254(7):912, August 16,1985.

163

IgG-antibodies to HTLV-III in patients with AIDS, LAS, and persons at risk of AIDS in West Germany, by R. Hehlmann, et al. BLUT 50(1):13-18, January 1985.

IgG subglass deficiencies in children with suspected AIDS [letter],by J. A. Church, et al. LANCET 1(8371):279, February 4, 1984.

IgM and IgG antibodies to HTLV-III in the lymphadenopathy syndrome and subjects at risk for AIDS [letter], by P. Pouletty, et al. BRITISH MEDICAL JOURNAL 291(6497):741, September 14, 1985.

IgM and IgG antibodies to human T cell lymphotropic retrovirus (HTLV-III) in lymphadenopathy syndrome and subjects at risk for AIDS in Italy, by F. Aiuti, et al. BRITISH MEDICAL JOURNAL 291(6489):165-166, July 20, 1985.

IL-2 production and response in vitro by the leukocytes of patients with acquired immune deficiency syndrome, by J. M. Reuben, et al. LYMPHOKINE RESEARCH 4(2):103-116, Spring 1985.

Immature sinus histiocytes in the lymphadenopathic stage of AIDS: relationship to polyclonal B-cell activation? [letter], by J. J. Van den Oord, et al. JOURNAL OF PATHOLOGY 145(1):63-64, January 1985.

Immediate causes of death in acquired immunodeficiency syndrome, by L. Moskowitz, et al. ARCHIVES OF PATHOLOGY AND LABORATORY MEDICINE 109(8): 735-738, August 1985.

Immune-cell augmentation (with altered T-subset ratio) is common in healthy homosexual men [letter], by J. L. Fahey, et al. NEW ENGLAND JOURNAL OF MEDICINE 308(14):842-843, April 7, 1983.

Immune complexes in the acquired immunodeficiency syndrome (AIDS): relationship to disease manifestation, risk group, and immunologic defect, by J. S. McDougal, et al. JOURNAL OF CLINICAL IMMUNOLOGY 5(2):130-138, March 1985.

Immune defects in simian acquired immunodeficiency syndrome, by D. H. Maul, et al. VETERINARY IMMUNOLOGY AND IMMUNOPATHOLOGY 8(3):201-214, February 1985.

Immune deficiency presenting as disseminated sporotrichosis,by S. E. Matter, et al. JOURNAL OF THE OKLAHOMA STATE MEDICAL ASSOCIATION 77(4):114-117, April 1984.

Immune deficiency syndrome in children [letter], by F. Rosner, et al. JAMA 250(22): 3046, December 9, 1983.

—, by J. Oleske, et al. JAMA 249(17):2345-2349, May 6, 1983.

Immune derangements in asymptomatic male homosexuals in Israel: a pre-AIDS condition?, by Z. T. Handzel, et al. ANNALS OF THE NEW YORK ACADEMY OF SCIENCES 437:549-553, 1984.

Immune function and dysfunction in AIDS,by F. P. Siegal. SEMINARS IN ONCOLOGY 11(1):29-39, March 1984.

Immune status of AIDS patients in France: relationship with lymphadenopathy associated virus tropism, by D. Klatzmann, et al. ANNALS OF THE NEW YORK ACADEMY OF SCIENCES 437:228-237, 1984.

Immune system in AIDS, by J. Laurence. SCIENTIFIC AMERICAN 253(6):84-92, December 1985.

Immune thrombocytopenia in homosexual men [letter]. ANNALS OF INTERNAL MEDICINE 104(4):583-584, April 1986.

Immunity syndrome: new test, new ideas, by J. A. Miller. SCIENCE NEWS 123:197, March 26, 1983.

Immunocompromise syndrome in homosexual men. Prevalence of possible risk factors and screening for the prodrome using an accurate white cell count, by D. Goldmeier, et al. BRITISH JOURNAL OF VENEREAL DISEASES 59(2):127-130, April 1983.

Immunodeficiency among female sexual partners of males with acquired immune deficiency syndrome (AIDS)—New York. MMWR 31(52):697-698, January 7, 1983.

Immunodeficiency in female sexual partners of men with the acquired immunodeficiency syndrome, by C. Harris, et al. NEW ENGLAND JOURNAL OF MEDICINE 308(20):1181-1184, May 19, 1983.

Immunodeficiency syndrome, by W. A. Blattner, et al. ANNALS OF INTERNAL MEDICINE 103(5):665-670, November 1985.

Immunodeficiency syndrome, acquired post-transfusionally in a non-hemophilac (letter), by M. F. Legrand, et al. PRESSE MEDICALE 14(30):1609-1610, September 14, 1985.

Immunodeficient and 'backward' child, by G. Kliman, et al. HOSPITAL PRACTICE 19(5):108-110, 112, 114, May 1984.

Immunogen for herpes, AIDS? by C. Wenz. NATURE 311(5985):404, October 4, 1984.

Immunoglobulin subclasses of antibodies to human T-cell leukemia/lymphoma virus I-associated antigens in acquired immune deficiency syndrome and lymphadeno-pathy syndrome, by J. Goudsmit, et al. JOURNAL OF VIROLOGY 53(1):287-291, January 1985.

Immunoglobulins in the acquired immunodeficiency syndrome [letter], by M. Fiorilli, et al. ANNALS OF INTERNAL MEDICINE 102(6):862-863, June 1985.

Immunohistochemical reactivity of anti-LAV p18 monoclonal antibody in lymph nodes from PGL and AIDS patients, by C. L. Parravicini, et al. BOLLETTINO DELL ISTI-TUTO SIEROTERAPICO MILANESE 64(5):422-424, 1985.

Immunohistological approach to persistent lymphadenopathy and its relevance to AIDS, by G. Janossy, et al. CLINICAL AND EXPERIMENTAL IMMUNOLOGY 59(2):257-266, February 1985.

Immunohistology of non-T cells in the acquired immunodeficiency syndrome, by G. S. Wood, et al. AMERICAN JOURNAL OF PATHOLOGY 120(3):371-379, September 1985.

Immunohistopathology of lymph nodes in HTLV-III infected homosexuals with persistent adenopathy or AIDS, by P. Biberfeld, et al. CANCER RESEARCH 45(Suppl. 9):4665s-4670s, September 1985.

Immunologic abnormalities among male homosexuals in New York City: changes over time, by M. Marmor, et al. ANNALS OF THE NEW YORK ACADEMY OF SCIENCES 437:312-319, 1984.

Immunologic abnormalities in the acquired immunodeficiency syndrome, by D. L. Bowen, et al. PROGRESS IN ALLERGY 37:207-223, 1986.

—, by H. C. Lane, et al. ANNUAL REVIEW OF IMMUNOLOGY 3:477-500, 1985.

Immunologic alterations in acquired immune deficiency syndrome, by M. S. Gottlieb, et al. ANTIOBIOTIC CHEMOTHERAPY 32:99-104, 1983.

Immunologic alterations in brochoalveolar lavage fluid in the acquired immunodeficiency syndrome (AIDS), by J. A. Rankin, et al. AMERICAN REVIEW OF RESPIRATORY DISEASE 128(1):189-194, July 1983.

Immunologic alterations in monkeys with simian acquired immunodeficiency syndrome (SAIDS), by D. B. Budzko, et al. PROCEEDINGS OF THE SOCIETY FOR EXPERIMENTAL BIOLOGY AND MEDICINE 179(2):227-231, June 1985.

Immunologic aspects of AIDS, by M. S. Gottlieb. FRONTIERS OF RADIATION THERAPY AND ONCOLOGY 19:33-37, 1985.

—, by L. Hammarström, et al. LAKARTIDNINGEN 80(7):530+, February 16, 1983.

Immunologic characteristics of acquired immunodeficiency syndrome,by M. Velasco. REVISTA MEDICA DE CHILE 111(12):1299-1300, December 1983.

Immunologic dysfunction in infants infected through transfusion with HTLV-III, by R. F. Wykoff, et al. NEW ENGLAND JOURNAL OF MEDICINE 312(5):294-296, January 31, 1985.

Immunologic dysfunction in patients with classic hemophilia receiving lyophilized factor VIII concentrates and cryoprecipitate, by C. Tsoukas, et al. CANADIAN MEDICAL ASSOCIATION JOURNAL 129(7):713-717, October 1, 1983.

Immunologic evaluation of hemophilia patients and their wives. Relationships to the acquired immunodeficiency syndrome, by R. D. deShazo, et al. ANNALS OF INTERNAL MEDICINE 99(2):159-164, August 1983.

Immunologic findings in healthy Haitians in Montreal, by A. Adrien, et al. CANADIAN MEDICAL ASSOCIATION JOURNAL 133(5):401-406, September 1, 1985.

Immunologic findings in homosexual males with generalized lymphadenopathy. Prodromal state of acquired immunodeficiency syndrome?,by J. R. Kalden,e t al. KLINISCHE WOCHENSCHRIFT 61(21):1067-1073, November 2, 1983.

Immunologic findings in Texas homosexual men: relationship to the acquired immune deficiency syndrome, by J. T. Newman, et al. TEXAS MEDICINE 79(11):44-47, November 1983.

Immunologic laboratory tests in acquired immunodeficiency syndrome (AIDS) and suspected AIDS, by H. I. Joller-Jemelka, et al. SCHWEIZERISCHE MEDIZINISCHE WOCHENSCHRIFT 115(4):125-132, January 26, 1985.

Immunologic profiles of adults with congenital bleeding disorders, by J. C. Goldsmith, et al. AIDS RESEARCH 1(3):163-179, 1983-1984.

Immunologic reconstitution in the acquired immunodeficiency syndrome, by H. C. Lane, et al. ANNALS OF INTERNAL MEDICINE 103(5):714-718, November 1985.

Immunologic studies in asymptomatic hemophilia patients. Relationship to acquired immune deficiency syndrome (AIDS), by A. Landay, et al. JOURNAL OF CLINICAL INVESTIGATION 71(5):1500-1504, May 1983.

Immunologic studies of the acquired immune deficiency syndrome: relationship of immunodeficiency to extent of disease, by E. M. Hersh, et al. ANNALS OF THE NEW YORK ACADEMY OF SCIENCES 437:364-372, 1984.

Immunologic studies on the definition of impaired resistance in AIDS, by P. Kern, et al. OFFENTLICHE GESUNDHEITSWESEN 46(9):445-448, September 1984.

Immunologic study of spouses and siblings of asymptomatic hemophiliacs, by M. V. Ragni, et al. SCANDINAVIAN JOURNAL OF HAEMATOLOGY. SUPPLEMENTUM 40:373, 1984.

Immunological abnormalities in patients with the acquired immune deficiency syndrome (AIDS)—a review, by J. M. Dwyer, et al. CLINICAL IMMUNOLOGY REVIEWS 3(1):25-129, 1984.

Immunological abnormalities in South African homosexual men, by R. Anderson, et al. SOUTH AFRICAN MEDICAL JOURNAL 64(4):119-122, July 23, 1983.

Immunological abnormalities in South African homosexuals—a non-infectious cofactor? [letter], by R. J. Ablin, et al. SOUTH AFRICAN MEDICAL JOURNAL 67(2): 40-41, January 12, 1985.

Immunological and virological investigation in patients with lymphoadenopathy syndrome and in a population at risk for acquired immunodeficiency syndrome (AIDS), with particular focus on the detection of antibodies to human T-lymphotropic retroviruses (HTLV III), by M. C. Sirianni, et al. JOURNAL OF CLINICAL IMMUNOLOGY 5(4):261-268, July 1985.

Immunological and virological studies in a risk population for AIDS in Rome, by F. Aiuti, et al. ANNALS OF THE NEW YORK ACADEMY OF SCIENCES 437:554-558, 1984.

Immunological changes in HTLV-III infections and AIDS, by K. Krohn, et al. DUODECIM 102(7):413-422, 1986.

Immunological characterizations of patients with acquired immune deficiency syndrome, acquired immune deficiency syndrome-related symptom complex, and a related life-style, by E. M. Hersh, et al. CANCER RESEARCH 44(12, Part 1): 5894-5901, December 1984.

Immunological control of Epstein-Barr virus infection: possible lessons for AIDS, by M. A. Epstein. ANNALS OF THE NEW YORK ACADEMY OF SCIENCES 437:1-7, 1984.

Immunological evaluation of acquired immune deficiency syndrome patients in France: preliminary results, by M. Cavaille-Coll, et al. ANTIOBIOTIC CHEMOTHERAPY 32:105-111, 1983.

Immunological findings associated with HTLV-III antibody positivity, by J. Antonen. ANNALS OF CLINICAL RESEARCH 17(2):81-85, 1985.

Immunological properties of the Gag protein p24 of the acquired immunodeficiency syndrome retrovirus (human T-cell leukemia virus type III, by M. G. Sarngadharan, et al. PROCEEDINGS OF THE NATIONAL ACADEMY OF SCIENCES USA 82(10):3481-3484, May 1985.

Immunological properties of HTLV-III antigens recognized by sera of patients with AIDS and AIDS-related complex and of asymptomatic carriers of HTLV-III infection, by M. G. Sarngadharan, et al. CANCER RESEARCH 45(Suppl. 9):4574s-4577s, September 1985.

Immunological studies in acquired immunodeficiency syndrome. Functional studies of lymphocyte subpopulations, by B. Hofmann, et al. SCANDINAVIAN JOURNAL OF IMMUNOLOGY 21(3):235-243, March 1985.

Immunological studies in patients with acquired immune deficiency syndrome, by H. S. Panitch, et al. ANNALS OF THE NEW YORK ACADEMY OF SCIENCES 437: 513-517, 1984.

Immunological studies of homosexual men with immunodeficiency and Kaposi's sarcoma, by R. W. Schroff, et al. CLINICAL IMMUNOLOGY AND IMMUNO-PATHOLOGY 27(3):300-314, June 1983.

Immunological studies of male homosexuals with the prodrome of the acquired immunodeficiency syndrome (AIDS),by E. M. Hershe t al. ADVANCES IN EXPERI-MENTAL MEDICINE AND BIOLOGY 166:285-293, 1983.

Immunological variablies as predictors of prognosis in patients with Kaposi's sarcoma and the acquired immunodeficiency syndrome, by S. Vadhan-Raj, et al. CANCER RESEARCH 46(1):417-425, January 1986.

Immunologically oriented concept of the genesis of acquired immunodeficiency syndrome, by A. S. Mark, et al. MEDICAL HYPOTHESES 17(2):167-173, June 1985.

Immunology of the acquired immunodeficiency syndrome, by P. W. McLaughlin, et al. HENRY FORD HOSPITAL MEDICAL JOURNAL 32(3):107-115, 1984.

Immunology of groups at risk for acquired immune deficiency syndrome, by W. Lang. FRONTIERS OF RADIATION THERAPY AND ONCOLOGY 19:43-51, 1985.

Immunopathogenesis of the acquired immunodeficiency syndrome, by D. L. Bowen, et al. ANNALS OF INTERNAL MEDICINE 103(5):704-709, November 1985.

Immunopathogenesis of AIDS, by A. J. Lewandowski. JOURNAL OF MEDICAL TECHNOLOGY 3(3):145-148+, March 1986.

Immunopathologic evaluation of lymph nodes from monkey and man with acquired immune deficiency syndrome and related conditions, by P. R. Meyer, et al. HEMATOLOGICAL ONCOLOGY 3(3):199-210, July-September 1985.

Immunoperoxidase evaluation of lymph nodes from acquired immune deficiency patients, by M. Mangkornkanok-Mark, et al. CLINICAL AND EXPERIMENTAL IMMU-NOLOGY 55(3):581-586, March 1984.

Immunopotentiation of impaired lymphocyte functions in vitro by isoprinosine in prodromal subjects and AIDS patients, by P. Tsang, et al. INTERNATIONAL JOURNAL OF IMMUNOPHARMACOLOGY 7(4):511-514, 1985.

Immunopurinogenic enzymatic activity in the acquired immunodeficiency syndrome, by E. Mejias, et al. ADVANCES IN EXPERIMENTAL MEDICINE AND BIOLOGY 295(Part A):275-280, 1986.

Immunoregulatory circuits in the acquired immune deficiency syndrome and related complex. Production of and response to interleukins 1 and 2, NK function and its enhancement by interleukin-2 and kinetics of the autologous mixed lymphocyte reaction, by J. Alcocer-Varela, et al. CLINICAL AND EXPERIMENTAL IMMUNOL-OGY 60(1):31-38, April 1985.

Immunoregulatory lymphokines of T hybridomas from AIDS patients: constitutive and inducible suppressor factors, by J. Laurence, et al. SCIENCE 225(4657):66-69, July 6, 1984.

Immunoregulatory T cells in men with a new acquired immunodeficiency syndrome, by E. Benveniste, et al. JOURNAL OF CLINICAL IMMUNOLOGY 3(4):359-367, October 1983.

Immunosuppressants in patients with AIDS [letter], by A. Hausen, et al. NATURE 320(6058):114, March 13-19, 1986.

Immunotherapy and therapy of complications of AIDS, by H. Masur. TOPICS IN CLIN-ICAL NURSING 6(2):53-60, July 1984.

Immunotoxins to combat AIDS [letter],by A. Surolia, et al. NATURE 322(6075):119-120, July 10-16, 1986.

Impact of the acquired immunodeficiency syndrome on medical residency training, by R. M. Wachter. NEW ENGLAND JOURNAL OF MEDICINE 314:177-180, January 16, 1986.

Impact of the AIDS epidemic on corneal transplantation [editorial], by J. S. Pepose, et al. AMERICAN JOURNAL OF OPHTHALMOLOGY 100(4):610-613, October 15, 1985.

Impact of AIDS on blood services in the United States, by S. G. Sandler, et al. VOX SANGUINIS 46(1):1-7, 1984.

Impact of AIDS on health care personnel, by K. H. Mayer. JOURNAL OF MEDICAL TECHNOLOGY 3(3):156-158+, March 1986.

Impact of A.I.D.S. on laboratory medicine, by R. P. Rennie. CANADIAN JOURNAL OF MEDICAL TECHNOLOGY 47(4):266, December 1985.

Impact of AIDS on the voluntary blood donor system: a preliminary analysis, by A. J. Katz, et al. ANNALS OF THE NEW YORK ACADEMY OF SCIENCES 437:487-492, 1984.

Impact of AIDS-related cases on an inpatient therapeutic milieu, by H. J. Polan, et al. HOSPITAL AND COMMUNITY PSYCHIATRY 36(2):173-176, February 1985.

Impact of the first gay AIDS patient on hopice staff, by S. Geis, et al. HOSPICE JOUR-NAL 1(3):17-36, Fall 1985.

Impaired immune regulation in children and adolescents with hemophilia and thalas-semia in Israel, by T. Umiel, et al. AMERICAN JOURNAL OF PEDIATRIC HEMA-TOLOGY/ONCOLOGY 6(4):371-378, Winter 1984.

Impaired in vitro interferon, blastogenic, and natural killer cell responses to viral stimu-lation in acquired immune deficiency syndrome, by E. M. Hersh, et al. CANCER RESEARCH 45(1):406-410, January 1985.

Impaired mononuclear-cell proliferation in patients with the acquired immune defi-ciency syndrome results from abnormalities of both T lymphocytes and adherent mononuclear cells, by K. Shannon, et al. JOURNAL OF CLINICAL IMMUNOL-OGY 5(4):239-245, July 1985.

169

Impaired production of lymphokines and immune (gamma) interferon in the acquired immunodeficiency syndrome, by H. W. Murray, et al. NEW ENGLAND JOURNAL OF MEDICINE 310(14):883-889, April 5, 1984.

Implications of the acquired immunodeficiency syndrome for health policy, by E. N. Brandt, Jr. ANNALS OF INTERNAL MEDICINE 103(5):771-773, November 1985.

Implications of the discovery of HTLV-III for the treatment of AIDS, by R. Yarchoan, et al. CANCER RESARCH 45(Suppl. 9):4685s-4688s, September 1985.

In fear of AIDS, by T. Allis. D MAGAZINE 12:136+, October 1985.

In-hospital needlesticks and other significant blood exposures to blood from patients with acquired immunodeficiency syndrome and lymphadenopathy syndrome, by F. S. Rhame. AMERICAN JOURNAL OF INFECTION CONTROL 12(20:69-75, April 1984.

In memoriam, by P. Wynne. ISSUES IN RADICAL THERAPY 11(3):8, 1984.

In memoriam: Bobbi Campbell 1952-1984. GAY COMMUNITY NEWS 12(8):11, September 8, 1984.

In New Jersey a pediatrician tends the littlest victims, by G. Breu. PEOPLE 23:46-47, June 17, 1985.

In the news: AIDS, by J. Richters. HEALTHRIGHT 2:4-7, August 1983.

In prison with AIDS, by J. Jones. GUARDIAN 38(10):1, December 4, 1985.

In pursuit of AIDS. NEW SCIENTIST 105:2, February 7, 1985.

In search of the best drugs against AIDS, by D. M. Barnes. SCIENCE 233(4762):419, July 25, 1986.

In situ quantitation of lymph node helper, suppressor, and cytotoxic T cell subsets in AIDS, by G. S. Wood, et al. BLOOD 67(3):596-603, March 1986.

In vitro and in vivo studies with interleukin 2 (IL-2) and various immunostimulants in a patient with AIDS, by P. Vaith, et al. IMMUNITÄT UND INFEKTION 13(2):51-63, April 1985.

In vitro augmentation of interleukin-2 production and lymphocytes with the TAC antigen marker in patients with AIDS [letter],by K. Y. Tsang, et al. NEW ENGLAND JOURNAL OF MEDICINE 310(15):987, April 12, 1984.

In-vivo immunomodulation by isoprinosine in patients with the acquired immunodeficiency syndrome and related complexes, by M. H. Grieco,e t al. ANNALS OF INTERNAL MEDICINE 101(2):206-207, August 1984.

INA Board acts on AIDS recommendations. CHART 83(5):3, May-June 1986.

Inactivation by wet and dry heat of AIDS-associated retroviruses during factor VIII purification from plasma [letter], by J. A. Levy, et al. LANCET 1(8443):1456-1457, June 22, 1985.

Inactivation of the AIDS-causing retrovirus and other human viruses in antihemophilic plasma protein preparations by pasteurization, by J. Hilfenhaus, et al. VOX SANGUINIS 50(4):208-211, 1986.

Inactivation of AIDS virus in clothing, by I. H. Linden, et al. JAMA 253:2580, May 3, 1985.

Inactivation of human T-cell lymphotropic retrovirus (HTLV-III) by LDtm, by P. S. Sarin, et al. NEW ENGLAND JOURNAL OF MEDICINE 313:1416, November 28, 1985.

Inadequate reaction to AIDS, by B. Tivey. BODY POLITIC 124:17, March 1986.

Incidence and risk of transmission of HTLV III infections to staff at a London hospital, 1982-85, by D. C. Shanson, et al. JOURNAL OF HOSPITAL INFECTION 6(Suppl. C):15-22, December 1985.

Incidence of the acquired immunodeficiency syndrome in San Francisco, 1980-1983, by A. R. Moss, et al. JOURNAL OF INFECTIOUS DISEASES 152(1):152-161, July 1985.

—. FRONTIERS OF RADIATION THERAPY AND ONCOLOGY 19:14-20, 1985.

Incidence of AIDS [letter], by P. R. Gustafson. JAMA 254(6):751-752, August 9, 1985.

Incidence of AIDS cases in the Federal Republic of Germany and in Munich, by F. D. Goebel. KRANKENPFLEGE JOURNAL 24(7):32-33, July 1, 1986.

Incidence of Kaposi's sarcoma and mycosis fungoides in the United States including Puerto Rico, 1973-81, by R. J. Biggar, et al. JOURNAL OF THE NATIONAL CANCER INSTITUTE 73(1):89-94, July 1984.

Incidence rate of acquired immunodeficiency syndrome in selected populations, by A. M. Hardy, et al. JAMA 253(2):215-220, January 11, 1985.

Incidents dramatize level of fear. LAW ENFORCEMENT NEWS 12(1):1+, January 6, 1986.

Incognito in Colorado, by B. Maschinot. IN THESE TIMES 9(38):4, October 9, 1985.

Increase in AIDS cases—anomaly or trend?, by Bill Kenkelen. NATIONAL CATHOLIC REPORTER 22:32, May 16, 1986.

Increase in high-grade lymphomas in young men, by C. C. Boring, et al. LANCET 1(8433):857-859, April 13, 1985.

Increased frequency of HLA-DR5 in lymphadenopathy stage of AIDS [letter],by R. W. Enlow, et al. LANCET 2(8340):51-52, July 2, 1983.

India against AIDS, by K. S. Jayaraman. NATURE 318(6043):201, November 21, 1985.

Indications for and diagnostic efficacy of open-lung biopsy in the patient with acquired immunodeficiency syndrome (AIDS),by H. I. Pass, et al. ANNALS OF THORACIC SURGERY 41(3):307-312, March 1986.

Indications of a new virus in MS patients, by J. L. Marx. SCIENCE 230:1028, November 29, 1985.

Indiscriminate killer, by J. Barber. MACLEAN'S 98:38, August 12, 1985.

Induction of AIDS-like disease in macaque monkeys with T-cell tropic retrovirus STLV-III, by N. L. Letvin, et al. SCIENCE 230(4721):71-73, October 4, 1985.

Induction of antibody to asialo GM1 by spermatozoa and its occurrence in the sera of homosexual men with the acquired immune deficiency syndrome (AIDS), by S. S. Witkin, et al. CLINICAL AND EXPERIMENTAL IMMUNOLOGY 54(2):346-350, November 1983.

Induction of cytolytic activity by anti-T3 monoclonal antibody. Activation of alloimmune memory cells and natural killer cells from normal and immunodeficiency individuals, by M. Suthanthiran, et al. JOURNAL OF CLINICAL INVESTIGATION 74(6):2263-2271, December 1984.

Induction of HTLV-III/LAV from a nonvirus-producing T-cell lime: implications for latency, by T. Folks, et al. SCIENCE231:600-602, February 7, 1986.

Induction of immunodeficiency in mice by injection with syngeneic splenocytes immune to semi-allogeneic hybrid cells, by B. S. Kim. CELLULAR IMMUNOLOGY 88(1):222-227, October 1, 1984.

Industry trade groups give money for AIDS education and research. THE NATIONAL UNDERWRITER (LIFE & HEALTH INSURANCE EDITION) 90:2, March 22, 1986.

Industry worry: is AIDS in the red bag?, by T. Naber. WASTE AGE 16(10):48-49, October 1985.

Inevitable love, by M. Bronski. GAY COMMUNITY NEWS 13(41):11, May 3, 1986.

Infected by the AIDS panic, by N. von Hoffman. SPECTATOR September 28, 1985, p. 9-10.

Infection and T lymphocyte subpopulations: changes associated with bacteremia and the acquired immunodeficiency syndrome, by J. A. Fishman, et al. DIAGNOSTIC IMMUNOLOGY 1(3):261-265, 1983.

Infection by the LAV virus and the acquired immunodeficiency syndrome, by J. C. Gluckman, et al. PRESSE MEDICALE 14(27):1451-1453, July 6, 1985.

Infection by the retrovirus associated with the acquired immunodeficiency syndrome. Clinical, biological, and molecular features, by J. A. Levy, et al. ANNALS OF INTERNAL MEDICINE 103(5):694-699, November 1985.

Infection control. EMS reacts—and overreacts—to the AIDS panic, by B. Smith. JOURNAL OF EMERGENCY MEDICAL SERVICE 8(8):24-29, August 1983.

Infection control and employee health: update on AIDS, by W. M. Valenti. INFECTION CONTROL 6(2):85-86, February 1985.

Infection control and the hospitalized AIDS patient, by A. Adams, et al. INFECTION CONTROL 6(5):200-201, May 1985.

Infection control and the pregnant health care worker, by W. M. Valenti. AMERICAN JOURNAL OF INFECTION CONTROL 14(1):20-27, February 1986.

Infection control at home, by G. Lusby, et al. AMERICAN JOURNAL OF HOSPITAL CARE 3(2):24-27, March-April 1986.

Infection control: gays and medicine age of AIDS, by E. Collins. BORDERLINES 4:4, Winter 1985.

Infection-control guidelines for patients with the acquired immunodeficiency syndrome (AIDS), by J. E. Conte, Jr., et al. NEW ENGLAND JOURNAL OF MEDICINE 309(12):740-744, September 22, 1983.

Infection control in the patient with AIDS, by P. J. Ungvarski. JOURNAL OF HOSPITAL INFECTION 5(Suppl. A):111-113, December 1984.

Infection control—a progress report, by R. P. Wenzel, et al. INFECTION CONTROL 6(1):9-10, January 1985.

Infection control update: AIDS, by P. Jemison-Smith, et al. CRITICAL CARE UPDATE 10(3):30-31, March 1983.

Infection, immunity, and blood transfusion [editorial], by L. J. Bruce-Chwatt. BRITISH MEDICAL JOURNAL 288(6433):1782-1783, June 16, 1984.

Infection, immunity, and blood transfusion. Proceedings of the XVIth Annual Scientific Symposium of the American Red Cross. Washington, DC, May 9-11, 1984. PROGRESS IN CLINICAL AND BIOLOGICAL RESEARCH 182:1-464, 1985.

Infection in the immunocompromised host, by J. Ô. Leyden. ARCHIVES OF DERMATOLOGY 121(7):855-857, July 1985.

Infection mechanism? by J. Palca. NATURE 319:170, January 16, 1986.

Infection of chimpanzees by human T-lymphotropic retoviruses in brain and other tissues from AIDS patients [letter], by D. C. Gajdusek, et al. LANCET 1(8419):55-56, January 5, 1985.

Infection of chimpanzees with lymphadenopathy-associated virus [letter], by D. P. Francis, et al. LANCET 2(8414):1276-1277, December 1, 1984.

Infection of HTLV-III/LAV in HTLV-I-carrying cells MT-2 and MT-4 and application in plaque assay, by S. Harada, et al. SCIENCE 229:563-566, August 9, 1985.

Infection of human T-lymphotropic virus type I (HTLV-I)-bearing MT-4 cells with HTLV-III (AIDS virus): chronological studies of early events, by S. Harada, et al. VIROLOGY 146:272-281, October 30, 1985.

Infection precautions in the community . . . at home, by G. Lusby, et al. CALIFORNIA NURSE 82(4):16, May 1986.

Infection with HTLV-III/LAV and transfusion-associated acquired immunodeficiency syndrome. Serologic evidence of an association, by H. W. Jaffe, et al. JAMA 254(6):770-773, August 9, 1985.

Infection with human T-lymphotropic virus type III/lymphadenopathy-associated virus: considerations for transmission in the child day care setting, by K. L. MacDonald, et al. REVIEWS OF INFECTIOUS DISEASES 8(4):606-612, July-August 1986.

Infection with Rhodococcus equi in AIDS [letter], by D. C. Sane, et al. NEW ENGLAND JOURNAL OF MEDICINE 314(1):56-57, January 2, 1986.

Infection with two genotypes of Epstein-Barr virus in an infant with AIDS and lymphoma of the central nervous system, by B. Z. Katz, et al. JOURNAL OF INFECTIOUS DISEASES 153(3):601-604, March 1986.

Infections due to Pneumocystis carinii and Mycobacterium avium-intracellulare in patients with acquired immune deficiency syndrome, by J. H. Shelhamer, et al. ANNALS OF THE NEW YORK ACADEMY OF SCIENCES 437:394-399, 1984.

Infections in AIDS patients, by J. Dryjanski, et al. CLINICAL HAEMATOLOGY 13(3): 709-726, October 1984.

Infections in homosexual men, by S. Iwarson, et al. LAKARTIDNINGEN 80(7):548-552, February 16, 1983.

Infectious complications of the acquired immune deficiency syndrome, by J. W. Gold, et al. ANNALS OF THE NEW YORK ACADEMY OF SCIENCES 437:383-393, 1984.

Infectious complications of blood transfusions, by S. A. Berkman. SEMINARS IN ONCOLOGY 11(1):68-76, March 1984.

Infectious mutants of HTLV-III with changes in the 3' region and markedly reduced cytopathic effects, by A. G. Fisher, et al. SCIENCE 233(4764):655-659, August 8, 1986.

Inflammatory neuropathy in homosexual men with lymphadenopathy, by W. I. Lipkin, et al. NEUROLOGY 35(10):1479-1483, October 1985.

Information, consideration needed—Brandt, by C. Marwick. JAMA 253(23):376-3377, June 21, 1985.

Informed consent/choices about AIDS, by L. Fishman. GAY COMMUNITY NEWS 10(42):8, May 14, 1983.

Infrequency of isolation of HTLV-III virus from saliva in AIDS [letter], by D. D. Ho, et al. NEW ENGLAND JOURNAL OF MEDICINE 313(24):1606, December 19, 1985.

Inhalation-induced immunosuppression: sniffing out the volatile nitrite-AIDS connection [editorial], by K. H. Mayer. PHARMACOTHERARPY 4(5):235-236, September-October 1984.

Inhibition of in vitro lymphocyte proliferation by serum from acquired immune deficiency syndrome patients depends on the ratio of cells to serum in culture, by A. K. Henning, et al. CLINICAL IMMUNOLOGY AND IMMUNOPATHOLOGY 33(2):258-267, November 1984.

Inhibitors of retroviral DNA polymerase: their implication in the treatment of AIDS, by P. Chandra, et al. CANCER RESEARCH 45(Suppl. 9):4677s-4684s, September 1985.

Iniquity of the fathers upon the children [editorial], by M. E. Alberts. JOURNAL OF THE IOWA MEDICAL SOCIETY 73(6):226, June 1983.

Initial European AIDS symposium, by S. Gesenhues. ZFA 60(2):82-83, January 20, 1984.

Initial observations of the effect of radiotherapy on epidemic Kaposi's sarcoma, by J. S. Cooper, et al. JAMA 252(7):934-935, August 17, 1984.

Injunct against NY march denied, by P. Byron. GAY COMMUNITY NEWS 10(49);1, July 2, 1983.

Inmates dying from AIDS disease. CORRECTIONS DIGEST 14(13):7, June 15, 1983.

Inoculation of cryptococcosis without transmission of the acquired immunodeficiency syndrome [letter], by J. B. Glaser, et al. NEW ENGLAND JOURNAL OF MEDICINE 313(4):266, July 25, 1985.

Insect-borne transmission of AIDS?, by D. P. Drotman. JAMA 254:1085, August 23-30, 1985.

Inside a bathhouse [gay bathhouse in New York City], by P. Weiss. THE NEW RE-
PUBLIC 193:12-13, December 2, 1985.

Inside the billion-dollar business of blood, by A. Rock. MONEY 15:152-154+, March
1986.

Institute of Medicine launches assessment of AIDS programs, by C. Norman.
SCIENCE 231:1500, March 28, 1986.

Insurance against AIDS?, by R. Blaun. NEW YORK 18:62-65, June 3, 1985.

Insurance industry must combat threat of AIDS to solvency, by L. s. Howard.
NATIONAL UNDERWRITER 90:1+, March 22, 1986.

Insurers contend AIDS victims treated same as other policyholders, by M. J. Fisher.
NATIONAL UNDERWRITER 89:1+, November 9, 1985.

Insurers gear up to examine impact of AIDS, by L. Kocolowski. NATIONAL UN-
DERWRITER 89:4+, September 21, 1985.

Insurers need AIDS tests, doctor says. THE NATIONAL UNDERWRITER (LIFE &
HEALTH INSURANCE EDITION) 89:4+, October 5, 1985.

Insurers: watchful but not worried, by T. Shahoda, et al. HOSPITALS 60(1):58, January 5, 1986.

Interdisciplinary approach to dealing with the problems of AIDS patients at a tertiary
medical center, by A. A. Cote, et al. HOSPITAL TOPICS 62(5):28-30,
September-October 1984.

Interferon and interferon inactivators in patients with acquired immune deficiency syndrome and Kaposi's sarcoma. A preliminary report, by M. G. Ikossi-O'Connor, et
al. RESEARCH COMMUNICATIONS IN CHEMICAL PATHOLOGY AND PHAR-
MACOLOGY 45(2):271-277, August 1984.

Interferon helps AIDS victims. NEW SCIENTIST 98:681, June 9, 1983.

Interferon-induced 2'-5' oligoadenylate synthetase during interferon-alpha therapy in
homosexual men with Kaposi's sarcoma: marked deficiency in biochemical response to interferon in patients with acquired imunodeficiency syndrome, by O.
T. Preble, et al. JOURNAL OF INFECTIOUS DISEASES 152(3):457-465, September 1985.

Interferon may help AIDS victims. NEW SCIENTIST 100:324, November 3, 1983.

Interferon may help some AIDS patients with Kaposi's sarcoma, researchers report.
PUBLIC HEALTH REPORTS 98(3):228, May-June 1983.

Interferon production in male homosexuals with the acquired immune deficiency syndrome (AIDS) or generalized lymphadenopathy, by J. Abb, et al. INFECTION
12(4):240-242, July-August 1984.

Interferon-related leukocyte inclusions in acquired immune deficiency syndrome: localization in T cells, by P. M. Grimley, et al. AMERICAN JOURNAL OF CLINICAL
PATHOLOGY 81(2):147-155, February 1984.

Interferons and other biological response modifiers in the treatment of Kaposi's sarcoma, by S. E. Krown, et al. FRONTIERS OF RADIATION THERAPY AND ONCOL-
OGY 19:138-149, 1985.

Interim advice from the Public Health Council concerning patients with acquired immunodeficiency syndrome, by S. A. Danner. NEDERLANDS TIJDSCHRIFT VOOR GENEESKUNDE 128(42):2001-2002, October 20, 1984.

Interleukin regulation of the immune system (IRIS) in male homosexuals with acquired immune deficiency disease syndrome, by M. A. Palladino, et al. ANNALS OF THE NEW YORK ACADEMY OF SCIENCES 437:535-539, 1984.

Interleukin 2 augmentation of natural killer cell activity in homosexual men with acquired immune deficiency syndrome, by M. M. Reddy, et al. INFECTION AND IMMUNITY 44(2):339-343, May 1984.

Interleukin-2 enhances the depressed natural killer and cytomegalovirus-specific cytotoxic activities of lymphocytes from patients with the acquired immune deficiency syndrome, by A. H. Rook, et al. JOURNAL OF CLINICAL INVESTIGATION 72(1):398-403, July 1983.

Interleukin 2 enhances the natural killer cell activity of acquired immunodeficiency syndrome patients through a gamma-interferon-independent mechanism, by A. H. Rook, et al. JOURNAL OF IMMUNOLOGY 134(3):1503-1507, March 1985.

Interleukin-2 production and response to exogenous interleukin-2 in a patient with the acquired immune deficiency syndrome (AIDS), by G. J. Hauser, et al. CLINICAL AND EXPERIMENTAL IMMUNOLOGY 56(1):14-17, April 1984.

Interleukin-2 production by persons with the generalized lymphadenopathy syndrome or the acquired immune deficiency syndrome, by C. H. Kirkpatrick, et al. JOURNAL OF CLINICAL IMMUNOLOGY 5(1):31-37, January 1985.

Interleukin 2 therapy in infectious diseases: ratinale and prospects, by J. P. Siegel, et al. INFECTION 12(4):298-302, July-August 1984.

Interleukin 2 trial will try to spark flagging immunity of AIDS patients [news], by C. Marwick. JAMA 250(9):1125, September 2, 1983.

International Conference on Acquired Immunodeficiency Syndrome. 14-17 April 1985, Atlanta, Georgia. ANNALS OF INTERNAL MEDICINE 103(5):653-781, November 1985.

International issues at AAPHR Conference, by M Helquist. ADVOCATE 429:11, September 17, 1985.

International occurrence of the acquired immunodeficiency syndrome, by J. B. Brunet, et al. ANNALS OF INTERNAL MEDICINE 103(5):670-674, November 1985.

Interventions to minimize AIDS [letter], by M. W. Ross. MEDICAL JOURNAL OF AUSTRALIA 142(4):279-280, February 18, 1985.

Interview [M. Krim], by B. Lawren. OMNI 8:76-78+, November 1985.

Interview: Michael Hennessey—Sheriff of San Francisco County, Calif., and authority on AIDS behind bars, by J. Nislow. LAW ENFORCEMENT NEWS 12(1):9-11+, January 6, 1986.

Interview with Bobbi Campbell, by R. Evans. NORTHWEST PASSAGE 24(2):7, September 1983.

Interview with Dr. W. Stille, Frankfurt. Will AIDS-suspected blood donors soon be identifiable?, by W. Stille. MUENCHENER MEDIZINISCHE WOCHENSCHRIFT 125(48):Suppl. 2, December 2, 1983.

Intestinal infection with Mycobacterium avium in acquired immune deficiency syndrome (AIDS). Histological and clinical comparison with Whipple's disease, by R. I. Roth, et al. DIGESTIVE DISEASES AND SCIENCES 30(5):497-504, May 1985.

Intestinal perforation associated with cytomegalovirus infection in patients with acquired immune deficiency syndrome,by D. Frank, et al. AMERICAN JOURNAL OF GASTROENTEROLOGY 79(3):201-205, March 1984.

Intestinal protozoal infections in AIDS [letter],by R. B. Pearce. LANCET 2(8340):51, July 2, 1983.

Intra-blood-brain-barrier synthesis of HTLV-III-specific IgG in patients with neurologic symptoms associated with AIDS or AIDS-related complex, by L. Resnick, et al. NEW ENGLAND JOURNAL OF MEDICINE 313:1498-1504, December 12, 1985.

Intracerebral-mass lesions in the acquired immunodeficiency syndrome (AIDS) [letter], by R. M. Levy, et al. NEW ENGLAND JOURNAL OF MEDICINE 309(23): 1454-1455, December 8, 1983.

Intracerebral toxoplasmosis in patients with acquired immune deficiency syndrome, by M. Handler, et al. JOURNAL OF NEUROSURGERY 59(6):994-1001, December 1983.

Intracranial lesions in the acquired imunodeficiency syndrome. Radiological (computed tomographic) features, by C. M. Elkin, et al. JAMA 253(3):393-396, January 18, 1985.

Intracranial lesions in AIDS. AMERICAN FAMILY PHYSICIAN 32:206+, September 1985.

Intracranial space-occupying lesions in acquired immune deficiency syndrome patients, by R. B. Snow, et al. NEUROSURGERY 165(2):148-153, February 1985.

Intrathoracic adenopathy: differential feature of AIDS and diffuse lymphadenopathy syndrome by R. G. Ster,e t al. AJR 142(4):689-692, April 1984.

Intravenous amphetamine abuse, primary cerebral mucormycosis, and acquired immunodeficiency, by M. S. Micozzi, et al. JOURNAL OF FORENSIC SCIENCES 30(2):504-510, April 1985.

Intravenous drug abusers and the acquired immunodeficiency syndrome (AIDS). Demographic, drug use, and needle-sharing patterns, by g. H. Friedland, et al. ARCHIVES OF INTERNAL MEDICINE 145(8):1413-1417, August 1985.

Intravenous drug users and the acquired immune deficiency syndrome, by H. M. Ginzburg. PUBLIC HEALTH REPORTS 99(2):206-212, March -April 1984.

Intravenous gammaglobulin, thrombocytopenia, and the acquired immunodeficiency syndrome [letter], by J. F. Delfraissy, et al. ANNALS OF INTERNAL MEDICINE 103(3):478-479, September 1985.

Introduction of lymphotropic virus (LAV/HTLV-III) into the male homosexual community in Amsterdam, by R. A. Coutinho, et al. GENITOURINARY MEDICINE 62(1):38-43, February 1986.

Investigation begins into spread of new AIDS virus. NEW SCIENTIST 110:25, April 10, 1986.

Investigators combine work to find key to AIDS. AMERICAN FAMILY PHYSICIAN 29:17, May 1984.

Investigators study AIDs epidemiology and drug treatment. AMERICAN FAMILY PHYSICIAN 32:206, December 1985.

Investing in hope on AIDS, by D. Dorfman. NEW YORK 18:21, September 9, 1985.

Involvement of cytomegalovirus in acquired immune deficiency syndrome and Kaposi's sarcoma, by g. Giraldo, et al. PROGRESS IN ALLERGY 37:319-331, 1986.

Iron and iron binding proteins in persistent generalised lymphadenopathy and AIDS [letter],by B. S. Blumberg, et al. LANCET 1(8372):347, February 11, 1984.

Iron, ferritin, and AIDS [letter], by I. Kushner. LANCET 1(8377):633, March 17, 1984.

Is AIDS an epidemic form of African Kaposi's sarcoma? Discussion paper, by J. Weber. JOURNAL OF THE ROYAL SOCIETY OF MEDICINE 77(7):572-576, July 1984.

Is AIDS caused by a neurotropic virus? [letter], by W. Radding. JAMA 253(19):2831, May 17, 1985.

Is the AIDS virus recombinant?, by H. Toh, et al. NATURE 316(6023):21-22, July 4-10, 1985.

Is human T-cell leukemia virus the cause of acquired immunodeficiency syndrome?, by Z. M. Rupniewska. ACTA HAEMATOLOGICA POLONICA 15(1-2):69-77, January-June 1984.

Is it possible to contain the danger of AIDS to health care personnel?, by G. Melino, et al. NUOVI ANNALI D IGIENE E MICROBIOLOGIA 35(5):327-335, September-October 1984.

Is nobody safe from AIDS? ECONOMIST 298:79-81, February 1, 1986.

Is our blood supply safe?, by R. D. Fritz, et al. WISCONSIN MEDICAL JOURNAL 82(11):26-27, November 1983.

Is presence of interferon predictive for AIDS? [letter], by E. Buimovici-Klein, et al. LANCET 2(8345):344, August 6, 1983.

Is school for all? AIDS victims spark dilemma, by F. A. Silas. AMERICAN BAR ASSOCIATION JOURNAL 71:18-19, November 1985.

Is there an acquired immune deficiency syndrome in infants and children?, by A. J. Ammann. PEDIATRICS 72(3):430-432, September 1983.

Is there an "AIDS plague"? HUMAN EVENTS 45:6+, May 18, 1985.

Is there correlation of T cell proliferative functions and surface marker phenotypes in patients with acquired immune deficiency syndrome or lymphadenopathy syndrome?, by J. C. Gluckman, et al. CLINICAL AND EXPERIMENTAL IMMUNOLOGY 60(1):8-16, April 1985.

Is there death after sex?, by B. D. Colen. ROLLING STONE February 3, 1983, p. 17.

Is there gay life after AIDS?, by R. King. COSMOPOLITAN 199:198+, December 1985.

Is there life after sex?, by B. D. Colen. ROLLING STONE February 3, 1983, p. 17.

Is there a risk of AIDS for health care personnel?, by G. Melino, et al. NUOVI ANNALI D IGIENE E MICROBIOLOGIA 35(4):249-268, July-August 1984.

Is there risk to health care workers? AMERICAN JOURNAL OF NURSING 85:972, September 1985.

Is there safe sex?, by R. Bebout. BODY POLITIC 99:33, December 1983.

Is there unwarranted risk in cohorting AIDS patients? [letter], by C. B. Burrus. INFECTION CONTROL 6(10):389, October 1985.

Is this any way to run a movement? 6 leaders, by L. Giteck. ADVOCATE 448:42, June 10, 1986.

Is this brochure "vile and disgusting"? OUT 4(3):5, January 1986.

Is your facility an 'AIDS hospital,'? MODERN HEALTHCARE 15(22):5, October 25, 1985.

Is your organization ready for AIDS? TRAINING 23:87-88, March 1986.

Isobutyl nitrite and AIDS. AMERICAN FAMILY PHYSICIAN 32:272, November 1985.

Isolation and identification of a novel virus from patients with AIDS, by S. C. Lo. AMERICAN JOURNAL OF TROPICAL MEDICINE AND HYGIENE 35(4):675-676, July 1986.

Isolation of AIDS-associated retrovirus from genital secretions of women with antibodies to the virus, by C. B. Wofsy, et al. LANCET 1(8480):527-529, March 8, 1986.

Isolation of AIDS-associated retroviruses from cerebrospinal fluid and brain of patients with neurological symptoms, by J. a. Levy, et al. LANCET 2(8455):586-588, September 14, 1985.

Isolation of AIDS virus from cell-free breast milk of three healthy virus carriers [letter], by L. Thiry, et al. LANCET 2(8460):891-892, October 19, 1985.

Isolation of HTLV-III from cerebrospinal fluid and neural tissues of patients with neurologic syndromes related to the acquired immunodeficiency syndorme, by D. D. Ho, et al. NEW ENGLAND JOURNAL OF MEDICINE 313(24):1493-1497, December 12, 1985.

Isolation of HTLV-III/LAV from cervical secretions of women at risk for AIDS, by M. W. Vogt, et al. LANCET 1(8480):525-527, March 8, 1986.

Isolation of HTLV-III/LAV from samples of serum proteins given to cancer patients—Bahamas. JAMA 254:1139, September 6, 1985.

Isolation of human T-cell leukemia virus in acquired immune deficiency syndrome (AIDS), by R. C. Gallo, et al. SCIENCE 220(4599):865-867, May 20, 1983.

Isolation of human T-lyphotropic retrovirus (LAV) from Zairian married couple, one with AIDS, one with prodromes, by A. Ellrodt, et al. LANCET 1(8391):1383-1385, June 23, 1984.

Isolation of human T-lymphotropic virus type III from the tears of a patient with the acquired immunodeficiency syndrome, by L. S. Fujikawa, et al. LANCET 2(8454): 529-530, September 7, 1985.

Isolation of infectious human T-cell leukemia/lymphotropic virus type III (HTLV-III) from patients with acquired immunodeficiency syndrome (AIDS) or AIDS-related complex (ARC) and from healthy carriers: a study of risk groups and tissue sources, by S. Z. Salahuddin, et al. PROCEEDINGS OF THE NATIONAL ACADEMY OF SCIENCES USA82(16):5530-5534, August 1985.

Isolation of LAV/HTLV-III from a patient with amyotrophic lateral sclerosis [letter], by P. M. Hoffman, et al. NEW ENGLAND JOURNAL OF MEDICINE 313(5):324-325, August 1, 1985.

Isolation of a lymphadenopathy-associated virus from a patient with the acquired immune deficiency syndrome, by M. L. Bechker, et al. SOUTH AFRICAN MEDICAL JOURNAL 68(3):144-147, August 3, 1985.

Isolation of lymphadenopathy-associated virus (LAV) and detection of LAV antibodies from US patients with AIDS, by F. Barré-Sinoussi, et al. JAMA 253(12):1737-1739, March 22-29, 1985.

Isolation of lymphocytopahic retroviruses from San Francisco patients with AIDS, by J. A. Levy, et al. SCIENCE 225(4664):840-842, August 24, 1984.

Isolation of a new human retrovirus from West African patients with AIDS, by F. Clavel, et al. SCIENCE 233(4761):343-346, July 18, 1986.

Isolation of new lymphotropic retrovirus from two siblings with haemophilia B, one with AIDS, by E. Vilmer, et al. LANCET 1(8380):753-757, April 7, 1984.

Isolation of a new retrovirus in a patient at risk for acquired immunodeficiency syndrome, by J. C. Chermann, et al. ANTIBIOTIC CHEMOTHERAPY 32:48-53, 1983.

Isolation of T-cell tropic HTLV-III-like retrovirus from macaques, by M. D. Daniel, et al. SCIENCE 228(4704):1201-1204, June 7, 1985.

Isolation of a T-lymphotropic retrovirus from a patient at risk for acquired immune deficiency syndrome (AIDS), by F. Barré-Sinoussi, et al. SCIENCE 220(4599):868-871, May 20, 1983.

Isolation of T-lymphotropic retrovirus related to HTLV-III/LAV from wild-caught African Green monkeys, by P. J. Kanki, et al. SCIENCE 230:951-954, November 22, 1985.

Isoprinosine and Imuthiol, two potentially active compounds in patients with AIDS-related complex symptoms, by a. Pompidou, et al. CANCER RESEARCH 45(Suppl. 9):4671s-4673s, Setpember 1985.

Isoprinosine unproven. FDA CONSUMER 19:37-38, September 1985.

Isospora belli in a patient with acquired immunodeficiency syndrome, by R. Shein, et al. JOURNAL OF CLINICAL GASTROENTEROLOGY 6(6):525-528, December 1984.

Issues of morality dominate Houston's politics, by B. Sablatura. IN THESE TIMES 9(41):8, October 30, 1985.

Japan blames US blood for AIDS cases, by B. Johnstone. NEW SCIENTIST 106:22, July 4, 1985.

Japan buys British 'litmus test' for AIDS, by S. Connor. NEW SCIENTIST 111:16, August 28, 1986.

Japan screens donated blood, by D. Swinbanks. NATURE 319(6055):610, February 20-26, 1986.

Jogging past the AIDS clinic, by P. Yancey. CHRISTIANITY TODAY 30(4):64, March 7, 1986.

Joint statement on acquired immune deficiency syndrome (AIDS) related to transfusion. TRANSFUSION 23(2):87-88, March-April 1983.

Journal of a plague year, by D. K. Mano. NATIONAL REVIEW 35:836-837, July 8, 1983.

Judge backs New York AIDS policy, by B. Norris. THE TIMES EDUCATIONAL SUPPLEMENT 3635:13, February 28, 1986.

Judge intervenes in bathhouse controversy, by S. Brooke. GAY COMMUNITY NEWS 12(15):1, October 27, 1984.

Jumping guns? by S. Budiansky. NATURE 309:106, May 10, 1984.

Just be a friend. NURSING 16(8):71 August 1986.

Justice, compassion needed in treating AIDS patients, by J. M. Cox. HEALTH PROGRESS 67(4):34-37, May 1986.

Justice Department: PWAs may be fired, by D. Walter. ADVOCATE 451:13, Juy 22, 1986.

Justification of Rock Hudson: AIDS has a dual message for Christians, by C. Plantinga, Jr. CHRISTIANITY TODAY 15:16-17, October 18, 1985.

Kaplan memorial lecture. The family of human lymphotropic retroviruses called HTLV: HTLV-I in adult T-cell leukemia (ATL), HTLV-II in hairy cell leukemias, and HTLV-III in AIDS, by R. C. Gallo. INTERNATIONAL SYMPOSIUM OF THE PRINCESS TAKAMATSU CANCER RESEARCH FUND 15:13-38, 1984.

Kaposi sarcoma and lymphadenopathy syndrome: limitations of abnominal CT in acquired immunodeficiency syndrome, by K. L. Moon, Jr., et al. RADIOLOGY 150(2):479-483, February 1984.

Kaposi sarcoma in acquired immune deficiency syndrome (AIDS). I: Clinical findings and laboratory diagnosis], by H. Weidauer, et al. LARYNGOLOGIE, RHINOLOGIE, OTOLOGIE 64(8):418-422, August 1985.

Kaposi sarcoma in two infants with acquired immune deficiency syndrome, by B. E. Buck, et al. JOURNAL OF PEDIATRICS 103(6):911-913, December 1983.

Kaposi's sarcoma—an acquired immunodeficiency syndrome, by J. A. Price, et al. OHIO STATE MEDICAL JOURNAL 80(2):143-145, February 1984.

Kaposi's sarcoma/AIDS surveillance in the UK [letter], by B. H. O.Connor, et al. LANCET 1(8329):872, April 16, 1983.

Kaposi's sarcoma—alpha-fetoprotein in amniotic fluid, by K. Shibusawa. KANGO 37(6):98-99, May 1985.

Kaposi's sarcoma among four different AIDS risk groups [letter],by D. C. De Jarlais, et al. NEW ENGLAND JOURNAL OF MEDICINE 310(17):119, April 26, 1984.

Kaposi's sarcoma and the acquired immune deficiency syndrome. Treatment with recombinant interferon alpha and analysis of prognostic factors, by S. E. Krown, et al. CANCER 57(Suppl. 8):1662-1665, April 15, 1986.

Kaposi's sarcoma and acquired immune deficiency syndrome—the British experience, by N. P. Smith. ANTIBIOTIC CHEMOTHERAPY 32:71-75, 1983.

Kaposi's sarcoma and the acquired immunodeficiency syndrome [letter],by R. R. Bailey. NEW ZEALAND MEDICAL JOURNAL 97(748):50, January 25, 1984.

Kaposi's sarcoma and acquired immunodeficiency syndrome (AIDS), by I. Frydecka, et al. POLSKI TYGODNIK LEKARSKI 40(39):1109-1111, September 30, 1985.

Kaposi's sarcoma and AIDS. AMERICAN FAMILY PHYSICIAN 30:268, October 1984.

—, by F. M. Muggia, et al. MEDICAL CLINICS OF NORTH AMERICA 70(1):139-154, January 1986.

—, by H. Reich, et al. KLINISCHE MONATSBLATTER FUR AUGENHEILKUNDE 187(1):1-8, July 1985.

—, by W. Rozenbaum. BULLETIN DE LA SOCIETE DE PATHOLOGIE EXOTIQUE ET DE SES FILIALES 77(4, Part 2):589-591, 1984.

Kaposi's sarcoma and community-acquired immune deficiency syndrome, by E. Abemayor, et al. ARCHIVES OF OTOLARYNGOLOGY 109(8):536-542, August 1983.

Kaposi's sarcoma and the diagnosis of acquired immunodeficiency syndrome. Case report and brief review, by M. A Kielhofner, et al. MISSOURI MEDICINE 81(10): 662-666, October 1984.

Kaposi's sarcoma and fatal opportunistic infections in a homosexual man with immunodeficiency, by M. F. Prummel, et al. NEDERLANDS TIJDSCHRIFT VOOR GENEESKUNDE 127(19):820-824, May 7, 1983.

Kaposi's sarcoma and HTLV-III infection. Virus-like particles in skin lesions: experimental observations, by P. Cuneo Crovari, et al. BOLLETTINO DELL ISTITUTO SIEROTERAPICO MILANESE 64(5):353-362, 1985.

Kaposi's sarcoma and immunoblastic sarcoma in the acquired immune deficiency syndrome [letter], by R. A. Figlin, et al. JAMA 251(3):342-343, January 20, 1984.

Kaposi's sarcoma and malignant lymphoma in AIDS, by H. J. Leu, et al. VIRCHOWS ARCHIV. A. PATHOLOGICAL ANATOMY AND HISTOPATHOLOGY 903(2):205-212, 1984.

Kaposi's sarcoma and T-cell lymphoma in an immunodeficienct woman: a case report, by M. T. Sabatini, et al. AIDS RESEARCH 1(2):135-137, 1983-1984.

Kaposi's sarcoma and variably acid-fast bacteria in vivo in two homosexual men, by A. R. Cantwell, Jr. CUTIS 32(1):58-61+, July 1983.

Kaposi's sarcoma, aplastic pancytopenia, and multiple infections in a homosexual [letter], by W. Sterry, et al. LANCET 1(8330):924-925, April 23, 1983.

Kaposi's sarcoma associated with AIDS in a woman from Uganda [letter], by D. Edwards, et al. LANCET 1(8377):631-632, March 17, 1984.

Kaposi's sarcoma causing pulmonary infiltrates and respiratory failure in the acquired immunodeficiency syndrome, by F. P. Ognibene, et al. ANNALS OF INTERNAL MEDICINE 102(4):471-475, April 1985.

Kaposi's sarcoma, chronic ulcerative herpes simplex, and acquired immunodeficiency, by W. I. Dotz, et al. ARCHIVES OF DERMATOLOGY 119(1):93-94, January 1983.

Kaposi's sarcoma: a comparison of classical, endemic, and epidemic forms, by J. L. Ziegler, et al. SEMINARS IN ONCOLOGY 11(1):47-52, March 1984.

Kaposi's sarcoma: gastrointestinal manifestations, by D. F. Altman. FRONTIERS OF RADIATION THERAPY AND ONCOLOGY 19:123-125, 1985.

Kaposi's sarcoma: immunoperoxidase staining for cytomegalovirus, by J. Civantos, et al. AIDS RESEARCH 1(2):121-125, 1983-1984.

Kaposi's sarcoma in the acquired immune deficiency syndrome, by W. Leslie, et al. MEDICAL PEDIATRICS AND ONCOLOGY 12(4):336-342, 1984.

Kaposi's sarcoma in acquired immune deficiency syndrome (AIDS), by N. D. Francis, et al. JOURNAL OF CLINICAL PATHOLOGY 39(5):469-474, May 1986.

Kaposi's sarcoma in AIDS, by J. H. Dobloug, et al. TIDSSKRIFT FOR DEN NORSKE LAEGEFORENING 105(28):1964-1968, October 10, 1985.

Kaposi's sarcoma in AIDS: the role of radiation therapy, by J. W. Harris, et al. FRONTIERS OF RADIATION THERAPY AND ONCOLOGY 19:126-132, 1985.

Kaposi's sarcoma in Burundi and the Central Arican Republic in the framework of acquired immunodeficiency syndrome (AIDS), by R. Laroche, et al. MEDECINE TROPICALE 46(2):121-129, April-June 1986.

Kaposi's sarcoma in Los Angeles, California, by R. K. Ross, et al. JOURNAL OF THE NATIONAL CANCER INSTITUTE 75(6):1011-1015, December 1985.

Kaposi's sarcoma in the light of epidemiologic and immunologic studies, by B. Toruniowa, et al. WIADOMOSCI LEKARSKIE 37(19):1537-1543, October 1, 1984.

Kaposi's sarcoma in a patient with acquired immune deficiency syndrome, by G. B. Nickles, et al. JOURNAL OF ORAL AND MAXILLOFACIAL SURGERY 42(1):56-60, January 1984.

Kaposi's sarcoma in transfusion-associated AIDS [letter], by E. Vélez-García, et al. NEW ENGLAND JOURNAL OF MEDICINE 312(10):648, March 7, 1985.

Kaposi's sarcoma in young male homosexuals. Report of 2 cases, by V. Petri, et al. AMB 30(7-8):161-164, July-August 1984.

Kaposi's sarcoma: a new staging classification, by R. L. Krigel, et al. CANCER TREATMENT REPORTS 67(6):531-534, June 1983.

Kaposi's sarcoma of the head and neck in the acquired immune deficiency syndrome, by C. A. Patow, et al. OTOLARYNGOLOGY—HEAD AND NECK SURGERY 92(3):255-260, June 1984.

Kaposi's sarcoma of the skin and its relation to AIDS, by W. Meigel, et al. OFFENT-LICHE GESUNDHEITSWESEN 46(10);519-521, October 1984.

Kaposi's sarcoma: an oncologic looking glass, by J. E. Groopman, et al. NATURE 299:103-104, September 9, 1982.

Kaposi's sarcoma presenting as homogeneous pulmonary infiltrates in a patient with acquired immunodeficiency syndrome, by L. Rucker, et al. WESTERN JOURNAL OF MEDICINE 142(6):831-833, June 1985.

Kaposi's sarcoma presenting as pulmonary disease in the acquired immunodeficiency syndrome:diagnosis by lung biopsy, by G. Nash, et al. HUMAN PATHOLOGY 15(10):999-1001, October 1984.

Kaposi's sarcoma, tuberculosis and Hodgkin's lymphoma in a lymph node—possible acquired immunodeficiency syndrome. A case report, by M. M. Hayes, et al. SOUTH AFRICAN MEDICAL JOURNAL 66(6):226-229, August 11, 1984.

Keep common cup. CHRISTIAN CENTURY 103(1):9, January 1-8, 1986.

Keep insurer AIDS tests: MD. THE NATIONAL UNDERWRITER (PROPERTY & CAS-UALTY INSURANCE EDITION) 89:3+, October 4, 1985.

Keeping AIDS at bay, by R. McKie, et al. OBSERVER November 9, 1986, p. 11.

Keeping the AIDS virus out of blood supply, by D. M. Barnes. SCIENCE 233:514-515, August 1, 1986.

Keeping the blood supply safe. WISCONSIN MEDICAL JOURNAL 82(11):26, November 1983.

Keeping confidential, by P. H. Ridout, et al. POLICY OPTIONS/OPTIONS POLIT-IQUES 7:41-43, July-August 1986.

Kennedy introduces $25M AIDS package, by K. Westheimer. GAY COMMUNITY NEWS 13(41):1, May 3, 1986.

Ketoconazole therapy for AIDS patients with disseminated histoplasmosis [letter], by P. R. Gustafson, et al. ARCHIVES OF INTERNAL MEDICINE 145(12):2272, December 1985.

KGB: Pentagon is responsible for AIDS, by Ralph de Toledano. HUMAN EVENTS 46:9, March 29, 1986.

Killer spit? Dentists worry about catching AIDS, by C. Milner, et al. ALBERTA RE-PORT 12:21, September 2, 1985.

Kiss is still a kiss?, by N. Fain. VILLAGE VOICE 29:11, October 9, 1984.

Know the enemy. THE ECONOMIST 300:74-75, July 5, 1986.

Knowing the face of the enemy, by C. Wallis, et al. TIME 123(18):66-67, April 30, 1984.

Knowing Ron. P. L. Spechko. JAMA 253:985, February 15, 1985.

Koch asks Cuomo to curb insurance discrimination, by P. Freiberg. ADVOCATE 438:17, January 21, 1986.

Koch official defends city's AIDS spending,by P. Freiberg. ADVOCATE 416:12, March 19, 1985.

Koch raises NY AIDS funding, by P. Freiberg. ADVOCATE 419:16, April 30, 1985.

Koch's postulates and the search for the AIDS agent, by R. M. Krause. PUBLIC HEALTH REPORTS 99(3):291-299, May-June 1984.

—, by R. M. Krause. REVIEWS OF INFECTIOUS DISEASES 6(2):270-279, March-April 1984.

Kramer v. cruising; "The Normal Heart" [play review]. THE ECONOMIST 299:104, April 5, 1986.

LA Councilman proposes law banning AIDS bias,by Brooke, et al. ADVOCATE 425: 21, July 23, 1985.

LA ordinance seeks to stop leper syndrome, by R. Hippler. GUARDIAN 37(45):5, Septemebr 18, 1985.

LA, West Hollywood ban AIDS discrimination, by Brooke, et al. ADVOCATE 429:13, September 17, 1985.

Lab assistants at AIDS syposium, by I Lernevall. VARDFACKET 10(6):10, March 20, 1986.

Laboratory and serological studies argue against possible transmission of AIDS by hepatitis B vaccine [letter], by F. Barré-Sinoussi, et al. LANCET 2(8449):274, August 1985.

Laboratory evaluation of AIDS, by D. A. Bergeron. JOURNAL OF MEDICAL TECH-NOLOGY 3(3):152-155+, March 1986.

Laboratory investigation of pediatric acquired immunodeficiency syndrome, by A. J. Ammann, et al. CLINICAL IMMUNOLOGY AND IMMUNOPATHOLOGY 40(1):122-127, July 1986.

Lack of antibodies to adult T-cell leukaemia virus and to AIDS virus in Israeli Falashas [letter], by A. Karpas, et al. NATURE 319(6056):794, February 27-March 5, 1986.

Lack of correlation between promiscuity and seropositivity to HTLV-III from a low-incidence area for AIDS, by L. H. Calabrese, et al. NEW ENGLAND JOURNAL OF MEDICINE 312:1256-1257, May 9, 1985.

Lack of effect of hepatitis B vaccine on T-cell phenotypes, by I. M. Jacobson, et al. NEW ENGLAND JOURNAL OF MEDICINE 311:1030-1032, October 18, 1984.

Lack of evidence of HTLV-III endemicity in southern Africa, by S. F. Lyons, et al. NEW ENGLAND JOURNAL OF MEDICINE 312:1257-1258, May 9, 1985.

Lack of specific cell mediated immunity to cytomegalovirus in people at risk for AIDS, by M. C. Sirianni, et al. AIDS RESEARCH 1(2):99-105, 1983-1984.

Lack of transmission of HTLV-III/LAV infection to household contacts of patients with AIDS or AIDS-related complex with oral candidiasis, by G. H. Friedland, et al. NEW ENGLAND JOURNAL OF MEDICINE 314:344-349, February 6, 1986.

185

Langerhans cell, as a representative of the accessory cell system, in health and disease, by G. J. Thorbecke, et al. IMMUNOBIOLOGY 168(3-5):313-324, December 1984.

Large-scale AIDS testing program delayed, by L. Famiglietti. AIR FORCE TIMES 46: 10, June 16, 1986.

LaRouche advocates "spread panic, not AIDS", by D. Walter. ADVOCATE 435:21, December 10, 1985.

LaRouche AIDS initiative, by P. Freiberg. ADVOCATE 453:10, August 19, 1986.

LaRouche behind bigoted Calif. AIDS referendum. GUARDIAN 38(39):5, July 9, 1986.

LaRouche quarantine on November ballot. BODY POLITIC 129:19, August 1986.

LaRouche-supported initiative on AIDS policy in California spurs debate on handling disease, by J. R. Emshwiller. WALL STREET JOURNAL 208:38, August 11, 1986.

Last minute withdrawal, by Armstrong, et al. BODY POLITIC 121:37, December 1985.

Last weeks of an AIDS sufferer at Berkeley: a friend remembers, by L. Biemiller. THE CHRONICLE OF HIGHER EDUCATION 31:1+, December 4, 1985.

Last word on avoiding AIDS, by J. H. Tanne. NEW YORK 18:28-34, October 7, 1985.

Latency period in transfusion-related AIDS may exceed five years. AMERICAN FAMILY PHYSICIAN 32:144, July 1985.

Latest great idea from Mayor Koch is a real winner! NARCOTICS CONTROL DIGEST 15(20):7, October 2, 1985.

Laundry workers need AIDS guidelines. LAUNDRY NEWS 11(10):24, October 1985.

LAV/HTLV-III infection after a one-time sexual contact with an AIDS patient, by P. Reiss, et al. NEDERLANDS TIJDSCHRIFT VOOR GENEESKUNDE 129(40): 1933-1934, October 5, 1985.

LAV/HTLV-III—new discoveries on its properties, isolation, vaccination and therapy, by B. Asjö, et al. LAKARTIDNINGEN 82(20):1870-1875, May 15, 1985.

LAV/HTLV-III seroconversion and disease in hemophiliacs treated in France, by D. Mathez, et al. NEW ENGLAND JOURNAL OF MEDICINE 314:118-119, January 9, 1986.

LAV type II: a second retrovirus associated with AIDS in West Africa, by F. Clavel, et al. COMPTES RENDUS DE L'ACADEMIE DES SCIENCES. SERIE III, SCIENCES DE LA VIE 302(13):485-488, 1986.

Law-medicine notes—AIDS research and 'the window of opportunity' [letter]. NEW ENGLAND JOURNAL OF MEDICINE 313(8):515-517, August 22, 1985.

Law review offers articles on legal aspects of AIDS. CRIME CONTROL DIGEST 20(45):10, November 10, 1986.

Lawsuit on AIDS. NEWSWEEK 106:65, December 23, 1985.

Lawsuit over Rock's estate exposes scandal—and asserts a lover's right to know [case of M. Christian], by S. Haller. PEOPLE 24:52-54+, November 25, 1985.

Lawyers oppose most AIDS-related discrimination, by L. R. Reskin. AMERICAN BAR ASSOCIATION JOURNAL 72:34, June 1, 1986.

Laying the groundwork for neturalizing AIDS-linked virus, by J. E. Groopman. NATURE 316:12, July 4, 1985.

Leading edge. FINANCIAL WORLD 154:47, May 15-28, 1985.

Learn more about AIDS, by M. Fearns. NURSING STANDARD 436:5, February 27, 1986.

Learning from AIDS, by J. Wilson. GAY COMMUNITY NEWS 11(5):6, August 13, 1983.

Learning to care for clients with AIDS—the practicum controversy by M. N. Bremner, et al. NURSING AND HEALTH CARE 7(5):250-253, May 1986.

Learning to live with AIDS, by J. Interrante. GAY COMMUNITY NEWS 12(32):6, March 2, 1985.

—, by P. Ungvarski. NURSING MIRROR 160(2):20-22, May 22, 1985.

Learning to talk about an unspeakable disease, by R. Summerbell. BODY POLITIC 126:37, May 1986.

Legal: AIDS-related litigation looms over employers, by D. B. Thompson. INDUSTRY WEEK 227:26-28, December 9, 1985.

Legal aspects of AIDS part 1, by H. Creighton. NURSING MANAGEMENT 17(11):14+, November 1986.

Legal implications for health care providers, by M. a. Kadzielski. HEALTH PROG-RESS 67(4):48-52, May 1986.

Legal issues around the AIDS crisis, by P. Bucalo. CALIFORNIA NURSE 82(4):14-15, May 1986.

Legal issues of AIDS, by A. D Hagerty. MICHIGAN HOSPITALS 22(8):22-24, August 1986.

Legionellosis in the acquired immunodeficiency syndrome [letter], by O. Guenot, et al. PRESSE MEDICALE 13(35):2150-2151, October 6, 1984.

Legislating AIDS away [editorial], by J. M. Dwyer. MEDICAL JOURNAL OF AUSTRALIA 143(7):276-277, September 30, 1985.

Legislation affecting nursing practice. Legislation affecting occupational allied health groups. Legislation related to acquired immune deficiency syndrome, by C. La-Bar. STATE NURSING LEGISLATION QUARTERLY 4(2):1-23, Summer 1986.

Legislation/confidentiality in AID research. ADVOCATE 416:109, March 19, 1985.

Legitimacy and paternity—HLA test—self-incrimination—AIDS. THE FAMILY LAW REPORTER: COURT OPINIONS 11(40):1515, August 20, 1985.

Leishmaniasis or AIDS? [letter], by A. de la Loma, et al. TRANSACTIONS OF THE ROYAL SOCIETY OF TROPICAL MEDICINE AND HYGIENE 79(3):421-422, 1985.

Lesbian/Gay Health Conference, by J. Thomas, et al. OFF OUR BACKS 16(5):1, May 1986.

Lesbians and AIDS, by J. Sky. LESBIAN INSIDER INSIGHTER INCITER 2(1):6, February 1986.

Lesbians/gays, by J. Hall. NORTHWEST PASSAGE 25(10):10, June 1985.

Lesbians take aim against AIDS, by K. Mcalister. LONGEST REVOLUTION 7:6, August 1983.

Lesions of the digestive mucosa in AIDS, by c. Marche, et al. ARCHIVES D'ANATOMIE ET DE CYTOLOGIE PATHOLOGIQUES 32(2):122-123, 1984.

Lessening fears: contact does not spread AIDS, by C. Wallis, et al. TIME 127(7):90, February 17, 1986.

Lesser AIDS and tuberculosis [letter], by J. J. Goedert, et al. LANCET 2(8445):52, July 6, 1985.

Let's face it—we're frightened about AIDS, by M. J. Carpenter. LAW ENFORCEMENT NEWS 12(1):8, January 6, 1986.

Letter from Commissioner Young, by F. E. Young. FDA DRUG BULLETIN 3:26, October 1985.

Letter from London, by N. DeJongh. ADVOCATE 450:28, July 8, 1986.

Leu 3a/TQ 1 and leu 2a/leu 15 double marker studies of AIDS and ARC patients [letter], by M. J. Warzynski, et al. AIDS RESEARCH 1(6):vi-ix, 1984-1985.

Leukemia virus linked to AIDS. NEW SCIENTIST 98:439, May 19, 1983.

Leukemia virus variant fingered as likely AIDS cause, by D. Franklin. SCIENCE NEWS 125:260, April 28, 1984.

Leukocyte subset analysis and related immunological findings in acquired immunodeficiency disease syndrome (AIDS) and malignancies, by E. M. Hersh, et al. DIAGNOSTIC IMMUNOLOGY 1(3):168-173, 1983.

Leukopenia, trimethoprim-sulfamethoxazole, and folinic acid [letter], by H. Hollander. ANNALS OF INTERNAL MEDICINE 102(1):138, January 1985.

Levamisole, immunostimulation, and the acquired immunodeficiency syndrome [letter], by N. Surapaneni, et al. ANNALS OF INTERNAL MEDICINE 102(2):137, January 1985.

Leveraging AIDS [race to develop reliable blood test], by R. Teitelman. FORBES 135:115, April 8, 1985.

Life and love after AIDS, by R. Joyce. BODY POLITIC 126:13, May 1986.

Life firm using disputed AIDS test, by L. Kocolowski. NATIONAL UNDERWRITER 89:31, November 1, 1985.

Life industry to plan fight against AIDS. NATIONAL UNDERWRITER 90:18, January 4, 1986.

Life-sustaining care, by M. Helquist. ADVOCATE 443:21, April 1, 1986.

Life table analysis of children with acquired immunodeficiency syndrome, by R. Lampert, et al. PEDIATRIC INFECTIOUS DISEASE 5(3):374-375, May-June 1986.

Life-threatening bacterial pneumonia in male homosexuals with laboratory features of the acquired immunodeficiency syndrome, by S. White, et al. CHEST 87(4):486-488, April 1985.

Like sheep virus, AIDS virus infects brain, by D. D. Bennett. SCIENCE NEWS 127:22, January 12, 1985.

Likely explanation of the etiology of AIDS, by S. Iwarson. NORDISK MEDICIN 99(8-9): 200-201, 1984.

Limited usefulness of lymphocytopenia in screening for AIDS in hospital patients, by W. J. Boyko, et al. CANADIAN MEDICAL ASSOCIATION JOURNAL 133(4):293, August 15, 1985.

Limiting factor VIII cryoprecipitate selection to female donors [letter], by A. Shore, et al. LANCET 1(8420):98-99, January 12, 1985.

Limiting right of insurers to use AIDS data called discrimination by ACLI, HIA. THE NATIONAL UNDERWRITER (LIFE & HEALTH INSURANCE EDITION) 90:2+, February 1, 1986.

Listeria monocytogenes bacteremia in the acquired immunodeficiency syndrome [letter], by f. X. Real, et al. ANNALS OF INTERNAL MEDICINE 101(6):883, December 1984.

Listeria monocytogenes meningitis in AIDS, by K. Koziol, et al. CANADIAN MEDICAL ASSOCIATION JOURNAL 135(1):43-44, July 1, 1986.

Listeria monocytogenes sepsis and small cell carcinoma of the rectum: an unusual presentation of the acquired immunodeficiency syndrome, by E. J. read, et al. AMERICAN JOURNAL OF CLINICAL PATHOLOGY 83(3):385-389, March 1985.

Listeria sepsis in AIDS [letter],by M. Thiel, et al. DEUTSCHE MEDIZINISCHE WO-CHENSCHRIFT 111(8):316-317, Feburary 21, 1986.

Listeriosis and AIDS: an unfounded assumption [letter],by M. Boucher, et al. AMERI-CAN JOURNAL OF OBSTETRICS AND GYNECOLOGY 149(7):804-806, August 1, 1984.

Listeriosis as a cause of maternal death: an obstetric complication of the acquired im-munodeficiency syndrome (AIDS), by C. V. Wetli, et al. AMERICAN JOURNAL OF OBSTETRICS AND GYNECOLOGY 147(1):7-9, September 1, 1983.

Little knowledge, dangerous thing [editorial]. BODY POLITIC 121:8, December 1985.

Liver in the acquired immunodeficiency syndrome: a clinical and histologic study, by E. Lebovics, et al. HEPATOLOGY 5(2):293-298, March-April 1985.

Living and dying day-by-day, by M. Bronski. GAY COMMUNITY NEWS 45:9, June 7, 1986.

Living as we do, by A. O'Connor. BODY POLITIC 123:31, February 1986.

Living with AIDS, by C. Maves. ADVOCATE 421:30, May 28, 1985.

—, by M. Herron. WHOLE EARTH REVIEW 48:34-53, Fall 1985.

Living with AIDS [editorial], by L. Watson. MEDICAL JOURNAL OF AUSTRALIA 141(9):559-560, October 27, 1984.

Living with AIDS: a mother's perspective, by B. Peabody. AMERICAN JOURNAL OF NURSING 86(1):45-46, January 1986.

Living with AIDS on the job, by S. Koepp, et al. TIME 128(8):48, August 25, 1986.

Living with AIDS: when the system fails, by R. Cecchi. AMERICAN JOURNAL OF NURSING 86(1):45+, January 1986.

Localization of cytomegalovirus proteins and genome during fulminant central nervous system infection in an AIDS patient, by C. A. Wiley, et al. JOURNAL OF NEUROPATHOLOGY AND EXPERIMENTAL NEUROLOGY 45(2):127-139, March 1986.

Locally synthesized antibodies in cerebrospinal fluid of patients with AIDS, by R. Ackermann, et al. JOURNAL OF NEUROLOGY 233(3):140-141, June 1986.

Location of the *trans*-activating region on the genome of human T-cell lymphotropic virus type III, by J. Sodroski, et al. SCIENCE 229:74-77, July 5, 1985.

Lodging of patients with AIDS as your guests: case studies are presented to discuss the role of nurses, by S. P. Hotzemer. AMERICAN JOURNAL OF HOSPICE CARE 3(2):28-31, March-April 1986.

Long shots: the race to develop vaccine against AIDS mobilizes researchers, by M. Chase. WALL STREET JOURNAL 204:1+ September 4, 1984.

Long-term cultivation of T-cell subsets from patients with acquired immune deficiency syndrome, by J. A. Levy, et al. CLINICAL IMMUNOLOGY AND IMMUNOPATHOLOGY 35(3):328-336, June 1985.

Long-term cultures of HTLV-III-infected T cells: a model of cytopathology of T-cell depletion in AIDS, by D. Zagury, et al. SCIENCE 231:850-853, February 21, 1986.

Longitudinal assessment of persistent generalized lymphadenopathy (PGL) in homosexual men, by U. Mathur-Wagh, et al. ADVANCES IN EXPERIMENTAL MEDICINE AND BIOLOGY 187:93-96, 1985.

Longitudinal immunological studies on a cohort of initially symptom-free homosexual men in London with respect to HTLV-III serology, by A. J. Pinching, et al. ADVANCES IN EXPERIMENTAL MEDICINE AND BIOLOGY 187:67-72, 1985.

Longitudinal study of a patient with acquired immunodeficiency syndrome using T cell subset analysis, by R. L. Siegel, et al. ADVANCES IN EXPERIMENTAL MEDICINE AND BIOLOGY 166:295-303, 1983.

Longitudinal study of persistent generalised lymphadenopathy in homosexual men: relation to acquired immunodeficiency syndrome, by U. Mathur-Wagh,e t al. LANCET 1(8385):1033-1038, May 12, 1984.

Look at AIDS inside: coming soon to a prison, by E. Mead. NORTHWEST PASSAGE 26(4):5, December 1985.

Looking death in the face, by B. Mahoney. AMERICAN PHOTOGRAPHER 16:98-102, April 1986.

Looking for an answer: the AIDS test. NEW YORK 18:31, October 7, 1985.

'Looking' for the cause of AIDS [editorial], by D. Zucker-Franklin. NEW ENGLAND JOURNAL OF MEDICINE 308(14):837-838, April 7, 1983.

Looking for rhyme and reason, by J. Aynsley. BODY POLITIC 124:14, March 1986.

Looking for the virus overlooking other causes, by K. Kelley. GUARDIAN 37(39):7, July 10, 1985.

Los Angeles bans anti-AIDS discrimination, by M. Cocoves. GAY COMMUNITY NEWS 13(8):1, August 31, 1985.

Louise Hay—can she really help people?, by G. DeStefano. ADVOCATE 452:50, August 5, 1986.

Love, growth and friendship: being an AIDS buddy, by G. Dale. ADVOCATE 448:8, June 10, 1986.

Love in a chilling climate, by J. Sherman, et al. TIMES November 5, 1986, p. 14.

Lovers of AIDS victims: psychosocial stresses and counseling needs, by S. B. Geis, et al. DEATH STUDIES 10(1):43-53, 1986.

Low circulating thymulin-like activity in children with AIDS and AIDS-related complex, by G. S. Incefy, et al. AIDS RESEARCH 2(2):109-116, Spring 1986.

Low prevalence in the UK of HTLV-I and HTLV-II infection in subjects with AIDS, with extended lymphadenopathy, and at risk of AIDS, by R. S. Tedder, et al. LANCET 2(8395):125-128, July 21, 1984.

Low serum thymic hormone levels in patients with acquired immunodeficiency syndrome [letter], by M. Dardenne, et al. NEW ENGLAND JOURNAL OF MEDICINE 309(1):48-49, July 7, 1983.

Lung complications in AIDS, by R. Weiske, et al. RADIOLOGE 26(1):3-9, January 1986.

Lupus anticoagulant in the acquired immunodeficiency syndrome, by E. J. Bloom, et al. JAMA 256(4):491-493, July 25, 1986.

Lurking killer without a cure, by A. Veitch. GUARDIAN November 2, 1983, p. 13.

Lymph node biopsy in lymphadenopathy syndrome and AIDS [letter], by H. Müller, et al. DEUTCHE MEDIZINISCHE WOCHENSCHRIFT 110(36):1391, September 6, 1985.

Lymph node involvement in AIDS [letter]. UGESKRIFT FOR LAEGER 146(9):672-673, February 27, 1984.

Lymph node pathology of HTLV and HTLV-associated neoplasms, by E. S. Jaffe, et al. CANCER RESEARCH 45(Suppl. 9):4662s-4664s, September 1985.

Lymphadenopathic and oropharyngeal Kaposi's sarcoma in a drug addict with acquired immunodeficiency syndrome. Immunological abnormalities in peripheral blood and lymphoid tissue, by F. Facchetti, et al. APPLIED PATHOLOGY 2(2): 103-109, 1984.

Lymphadenopathies in homosexual men. Relationships with the acquired immune deficiency syndrome, by H. L. Ioachim, et al. JAMA 250(10):1316-1309, September 9, 1983.

Lymphadenopathy. AMERICAN FAMILY PHYSICIAN 29:257+, February 1984.

Lymphadenopathy and antibodies to HTLV-III in homosexual men. Clinical, laboratory and epidemiological features, by U. Bienzle, et al. KLINISCHE WOCHEN-SCHRIFT 63(13):597-602, July 1, 1985.

Lymphadenopathy and a lower T-helper/suppressor cell (Th/Ts) ration in homosexual men in West Germany. Studies of 147 patients to evaluate the individual risk of acquiring AIDS, by M. Heitmann, et al. HAUTARZT 36(2):90-95, February 1985.

Lymphadenopathy-associated viral antibody in AIDS. Immune correlations and definition of a carrier state, by J. Laurence, et al. NEW ENGLAND JOURNAL OF MEDICINE 311(20):1269-1273, November 15, 1984.

Lymphadenopathy associated virus and its etiological role in AIDS, by L. Montagnier, et al. INTERNATIONAL SYMPOSIUM OF THE PRINCESS TAKAMATSU CANCER RESEARCH FUND 15:319-331, 1984.

Lymphadenopathy-associated virus: from molecular biology to pathogenicity, by L. Montagnier. ANNALS OF INTERNAL MEDICINE 103(5):689-693, November 1985.

Lymphadenopathy associated virus in AIDS, lymphadenopathy associated syndrome, and classic Kaposi patients in Greece [letter],by G. Papaevangelou, et al. LANCET 2(8403):642, September 15, 1984.

Lymphadenopathy-associated-virus infection and acquired immunodeficiency syndrome, by J. C. Gluckman, et al. ANNUAL REVIEW OF IMMUNOLOGY 4:97-117, 1986.

Lymphadenopathy associated virus infection of a blood donor-recipient pair with acquired immunodeficiency syndrome, by P. M. Feorino, et al. SCIENCE 225:69-72, July 6, 1984.

Lymphadenopathy-associated virus isolated from bronchoalveolar lavage fluid in AIDS-related complex with lymphoid interstitial pneumonitis, by J. M. Ziza, et al. NEW ENGLAND JOURNAL OF MEDICINE 313:183, July 18, 1985.

Lymphadenopathy associated virus: its role in the pathogenesis of AIDS and related diseases, by L. Montagnier. PROGRESS IN ALLERGY 37:46-64, 1986.

Lymphadenopathy associated virus (L.A.V.): its association with AIDS or prodromes, by F. Barré-Sinoussi, et al. ADVANCES IN EXPERIMENTAL MEDICINE AND BIOLOGY 187:35-43, 1985.

Lymphadenopathy: endpoint or prodrome? Update of a 24-month prospective study, by D. I. Abrams, et al. ANNALS OF THE NEW YORK ACADEMY OF SCIENCES 437:207-215, 1984.

—? Update of a 36-month prospective study, by D. I. Abrams, et al. ADVANCES IN EXPERIMENTAL MEDICINE AND BIOLOGY 187:73-84, 1985.

Lymphadenopathy in a heterogenous population at risk for the acquired immunodeficiency syndrome (AIDS)—a morphologic study, by J. Domingo, et al. AMERICAN JOURNAL OF CLINICAL PATHOLOGY 80(4):649-654, November 1983.

Lymphadenopathy in patients at risk for acquired immunodeficiency syndrome. Histopathology and histochemistry, by M. Raphael, et al. ARCHIVES OF PATHOLOGY AND LABORATORY MEDICINE 109(2):128-132, February 1985.

Lymphadenopathy syndrome in two thalassemic patients after LAV contamination by blood transfusion, by F. Boiteux, et al. NEW ENGLAND JOURNAL OF MEDICINE 312:648-649, March 7, 1985.

Lymphocyte phenotypes in patients with highly reduced T inducer to T cytotoxic/suppressor ratio, by f. Herrman. CLINICAL AND EXPERIMENTAL IMMUNOLOGY 56(2):476-478, May 1984.

Lymphocyte phenotyping by fluorescence microscopy and flow cytometry: results in homosexual men and heterosexual controls, by J. T. Newman,e t al. AIDS RESEARCH 1(2):127-134, 1983-1984.

Lymphocyte populations in hemophilia A and B. Relatin to acquired immunodeficiency syndrome and therapeutic implications, by V. Vicente, et al. SANGRE 28(3):318-329, 1983.

Lymphocyte-reactive antibodies in acquired imune deficiency syndrome, by R. C. Williams, Jr., et al. JOURNAL OF CLINICAL IMMUNOLOGY 4(2):118-123, March 1984.

Lymphocyte subsets in patients with acquired immunodeficiency syndrome (AIDS), aids-related complex (ARC), and acute viral infections, by D. E. Lewis, et al. TRANSACTIONS OF THE ASSOCIATION OF AMERICAN PHYSICIANS 97:197-204, 1984.

Lymphocyte transfusion in case of acquired immunodeficiency syndrome [letter],by K. C. Davis, et al. LANCET 1(8324):599-600, March 12, 1983.

Lymphocytic interstitial pneumonia associated with the acquired immune deficiency syndrome, by M. H. Grieco, et al. AMERICAN REVIEW OF RESPIRATORY DISEASE 131(6)952-955, June 1985.

Lymphocytic subsets in the acquired immunodeficiency syndrome [letter], by S. Gupta, et al. ANNALS OF INTERNAL MEDICINE 99(4):566-567, October 1983.

Lymphocytotoxic antibodies against peripheral blood B and T lymphocytes in homosexuals with AIDS and ARC, by W. Pruzanski, et al. AIDS RESEARCH 1(3):211-220, 1983-1984.

Lymphocytotoxic antibodies to non-HLA antigens in the sera of patients with acquired immunodeficiency syndrome (AIDS), by M. S. Pollack, et al. PROGRESS IN CLINICAL AND BIOLOGICAL RESEARCH 133:209-213, 1983.

Lymphoid interstitial pneumonitis in acquired immunodeficiency syndrome-related complex, by P. Solal-Celigny, et al. AMERICAN REVIEW OF RESPIRATORY DISEASE 131(6):956-960, June 1985.

Lymphoid lesions associated with the acquired immunodeficiency syndrome, by H. L. Iochim, et al. AMERICAN JOURNAL OF SURGICAL PATHOLOGY 7(6):543-553, September 1983.

Lymphoma in macaques: association with virus of human T lymphotrophic family, by T. Homma, et al. SCIENCE 225:716-718, August 17, 1984.

Lymphoma presenting as a traumatic hematoma in HTLV-III antibody-positive hemophiliac, by M. V. Ragni, et al. NEW ENGLAND JOURNAL OF MEDICINE 313:640, September 5, 1985.

Lymphoma versus AIDS [letter],by J. H. Mead, et al. AMERICAN JOURNAL OF CLINICAL PATHOLOGY 80(4):546-547, October 1983.

Lymphoreticular malignancies in the setting of acquired immunodeficiency syndrome (AIDS). A potential model for evolution of hyman lymphid neoplasma, by A. Khojasteh, et al. MISSOURI MEDICINE 82(9):599-602, September 1985.

Lymphotropic retroviruses (HTLV-I, -II, -III), by P. J. Fischinger, et el. CANCER RESEARCH 45(Suppl. 9):4694s-4699s, September 1985.

Lymphotropic virus type III, by D. P. Francis, et al. ANNALS OF INTERNAL MEDICINE 103(5):719-722, November 1985.

Lyndon La Rouche initiative: AIDS quarantine, by P. Freiberg. ADVOCATE 446:12, May 13, 1986.

Lyphocytoxic antibodies in the acquired immune deficiency syndrome (AIDS), by B. E. Kloster, et al. CLINICAL IMMUNOLOGY AND IMMUNOPATHOLOGY 30(2): 330-335, February 1984.

Lytic infection by British AIDS virus and development of rapid cell test for antiviral antibodies, by A. Karpas, et al. LANCET 2(8457):695-697, September 28, 1985.

MAAFS-NEAFS combined meeting, Atlantic City, New Jersey, April 25-27, 1984. CRIME LABORATORY DIGEST 11(3):57, July 1984.

Maculopapular rash in a patient with acquired immunodeficiency syndrome. Disseminated histoplasmosis in acquired immunodeficiency syndrome (AIDS), by D. C. Kalter, et al. ARCHIVES OF DERMATOLOGY 121(11):1455-1456+, November 1985.

Major glycoprotein antigens that induce antibodies in AIDS patients are encoded by HLTV-III, by J. S. Allan, et al. SCIENCE 228:1091-1094, May 31, 1985.

Major medical problems and detoxification treatment of parenteral drug-abusing alcoholics, by D. M. Novick. ADVANCES IN ALCOHOL AND SUBSTANCE ABUSE 3(4):87-105, 1984.

Making a buck off AIDS, by J. Irving. GAY COMMUNITY NEWS 13(28):2, February 1, 1986.

Making capital out of AIDS, by R. Butt. TIMES November 20, 1986, p. 20.

Making sense of AIDS, by M. Amis. OBSERVER June 23, 1985, p. 17-18.

Making sure you don't miss AIDS, by A. S. Brodoff. PATIENT CARE 18(1):166-167+, January 15, 1984.

Malabsorption and mucosal abnormalities of the small intestine in the acquired immunodeficiency syndrome, by J. S. Gillin, et al. ANNALS OF INTERNAL MEDICINE 102(5):619-622, May 1985.

Malign neglect, by D. Altman. VILLAGE VOICE 30:181, April 2, 1985.

Malignancies in the AIDS patient: natural history, treatment strategies, and preliminary results, by D. L. Longo, et al. ANNALS OF THE NEW YORK ACADEMY OF SCIENCES 237:421-430, 1984.

Malignant catarrhal fever parallel with AIDS. THE VETERINARY RECORD 117:351-352, October 5, 1985.

Malignant lymphoma presenting as Kaposi's sarcoma in a homosexual man with the acquired immunodeficiency syndrome, by S. E. Lind, et al. ANNALS OF INTERNAL MEDICINE 102(3):338-340, March 1985.

Malignant lymphoreticular lesions in patients with immune disorders resembling acquired immunodeficiency syndrome (AIDS): review of 80 cases, by A. Khojasteh, et al. SOUTHERN MEDICAL JOURNAL 79(9):1070-1075, September 1986.

Malignant rabbit fibroma syndrome. A possible model for acquired immunodeficiency syndrome (AIDS), by D. S. Strayer, et al. AMERICAN JOURNAL OF PATHOLOGY 120(1):170-171, July 1985.

Malnutrition and concomitant herpesvirus infection as a possible cause of immunodeficiency syndrome in Haitian infants [letter], by J. Goudsmit. NEW ENGLAND JOURNAL OF MEDICINE 309(9):554-555, September 1, 1983.

Malnutrition or AIDS in Haiti? [letter], by J. W. Mellors, et al. NEW ENGLAND JOURNAL OF MEDICINE 310(17):1119-1120, April 26, 1984.

Man who found the AIDS virus [Robert Gallo], by S. Schiefelbein. SCIENCE DIGEST 92:62-65+, July 1984.

Man who may shut the tabs, by B. Averill. VILLAGE VOICE 30:36, January 22, 1985.

Man with ARC cites confidentiality breach, by C. Guilfoy. GAY COMMUNITY NEWS 13(8):3, August 31, 1985.

Management of an AIDS patient in a nursing home, by H. J. Cools, et al. NEDERLANDS TIJDSCHRIFT VOOR GENEESKUNDE 130(28):1285-1287, July 12, 1986.

Management of AIDS pneumonia, by A. L. Pozniak, et al. BRITISH JOURNAL OF DISEASES OF THE CHEST 79(2):105-114, April 1985.

Management of infectious complications in acquired immunodeficiency syndrome, by I. H. Grant, et al. AMERICAN JOURNAL OF MEDICINE 81(1A):59-72, July 28, 1986.

Management of opportunistic pneumonia in AIDS, by A. s. Teirstein, et al. ANNALS OF THE NEW YORK ACADEMY OF SCIENCES 437:461-465, 1984.

Management of suspected AIDS patients, by D. B. Stough, et al. JOURNAL OF THE ARKANSAS MEDICAL SOCIETY 80(4):169-172, September 1983.

Managing AIDS and AIDS hysteria in hospitals. HOSPITAL SECURITY AND SAFETY MANAGEMENT 4(8):5-12, Decembe 1983.

Managing AIDS in children, by M. Boland, et al. MCN 9(6):384-389, November-December 1984.

Manner of speaking—Quebec AIDS Conference, by Courte, et al. BODY POLITIC 128:19, July 1986.

Many groups offer AIDS information, support, by M. F. Goldsmith. JAMA 254:2522-2523, November 8, 1985.

Mark Halberstadt. GAY COMMUNITY NEWS 12(5):6, August 11, 1984.

MASN to expand, hires coordinators. OUT 4(6):5, May 1986.

Mason-Pfizer monkey virus and simian AIDS [letter], by D. L. Fine. LANCET 1(8372): 335, February 11, 1984.

Massachusetts AIDS caseload rises to 296, by C. Guilfoy. GAY COMMUNITY NEWS 13(3):3, July 27, 1985.

Massachusetts AIDS policy defuses school furor, by C. Guilfoy. GAY COMMUNITY NEWS 13(10):3, September 21, 1985.

Massachusetts cuts AIDS funding, by C. Guilfoy. GAY COMMUNITY NEWS 12(48):1, June 22, 1985.

Massachusetts House crushes Gay Rights Bill, 88-65, by C. Gulfoy. GAY COMMUNITY NEWS 13(12):1, October 5, 1985.

Massachusetts House passes Bill for HTLV-3 confidentiality, by S. Poggi. GAY COMMUNITY NEWS 13(44):1, May 31, 1986.

Massachusetts passes law to grant HTLV-3 confidentiality, by K. Westheimer. GAY COMMUNITY NEWS 14(2):1, July 20, 1986.

Massachusetts sets sites for HTLV-3 test, by C. Guilfoy. GAY COMMUNITY NEWS 12(39):6, April 20, 1985.

Maternal transmission of acquired immune deficiency syndrome, by M. J. Cowan, et al. PEDIATRICS 73(3):382-386, March 1984.

Maternal transmission of AIDS studied. RESEARCH RESOURCES REPORTER 9(2): 11-12, February 1985.

Matlovich may push for D.C. ban on sex in baths, by D. Walter. ADVOCATE 420:10, May 14, 1985.

Maxillofacial manifestations of acquired immunodeficiency syndrome, by P. Goudot, et al. REVUE DE STOMATOLOGIE ET DE CHIRURGIE MAXILLO-FACIALE 86(1):3-8, 1985.

May a blood bank refuse donations to prevent the spread of AIDS?, by L. G. Smith, et al. JOURNAL OF THE MEDICAL SOCIETY OF NEW JERSEY 81(2):125-129, February 1984.

MD diagnosed with bias, by A. Lesk. BODY POLITIC 125:19, April 1986.

Meanwhile at the NCI, by N. Fain. ADVOCATE 3(78):23, October 13, 1983.

Measures to decrease the risk of acquired immunodeficiency syndrome transmission by blood transfusion. Evidence of volunteer blood donor cooperation, by J. Pindyck, et al. TRANSFUSION 25(1):3-9, January-February 1985.

Measuring antibodies may predict disease, by D. M. Barnes. SCIENCE 233:419, July 25, 1986.

Mechanism and modulation of immune dysfunction in AIDS associated syndromes, by J. G. Bekesi, et al. ADVANCES IN EXPERIMENTAL MEDICINE AND BIOLOGY 187:141-150, 1985.

Mechanisms of T-cell functional deficiency in the acquired immunodeficiency syndrome, by G. V. Quinnan Jr, et al. ANNALS OF INTERNAL MEDICINE 103(5): 710-714, November 1985.

Media hypes AIDS breakthrough/NIH, by N. Fain. ADVOCATE 3(75):14, September 1, 1983.

Media indicts woman—rumored AIDS, by C. Guilfoy. GAY COMMUNITY NEWS 11(35):7, March 24, 1984.

Media seething over bad blood, by E. Jackson. BODY POLITIC 92:11, April 1983.

Medical anthropology and the AIDS epidemic: a case study in San Francisco, by N. Spencer. URBAN ANTHROPOLOGY 12:141-159, Summer 1983.

Medical caution/political judgment [editorial]. BODY POLITIC 93:8, May 1983.

Medical editor revises AIDS testing remark, by K. Westheimer. GAY COMMUNITY NEWS 13(40):1, April 26, 1986.

Medical expert views potential for abuse in AIDS screening, by R. L. Cohen. THE NATIONAL PRISON PROJECT JOURNAL 6:5-6, Winter 1985.

Medical experts challenge Justice Dept. memo, by D. Walter. ADVOCATE 454:14, September 2, 1986.

Medical pathology conference. Respiratory failure in a 54-year-old man with hemophilia A, by J. H. Garcia, et al. ALABAMA JOURNAL OF MEDICAL SCIENCES 20(2):164-170, April 1983.

Medical research: band-aids. THE ECONOMIST 288:22+, August 13, 1983.

Medical response to AIDS epidemics [letter],by B. S. Bender, et al. NEW ENGLAND JOURNAL OF MEDICINE 310(6):389, February 9, 1984.

Medicine's fearsome new public enemy (acquired immune deficiency syndrome), by D. Grady, et al. READERS DIGEST 123:145-146+, October 1983.

Meeting the AIDS challenge in Illinois. CHART 83(5):4-5, May-June 1986.

Memorandum from the Swiss Professional Commission for AIDS Problems on how to deal with AIDS patients and persons with antibodies to LAV/HTLV-III. KRANKEN-PFLEGE. SOINS INFIRMIERS 79(2):74-75, February 1986.

Men with AIDS: dying of red tape, by S. Hyde. GAY COMMUNITY NEWS 11(5):1, August 13, 1983.

Menace of AIDS, by L. Cohen. ALBERTA REPORT 11:39, September 10, 1984.

Message from Secretary Heckler, by M. M. Heckler. FDA DRUG BULLETIN 15(3):26, October 1985.

Metastatic small-cell carcinoma of the lung in a patient with AIDS [letter], by N. J. Nusbaum. NEW ENGLAND JOURNAL OF MEDICINE 312(26):1706, June 27, 1985.

Miami: cycles of fear, by M. E. Schoonover. CHRISTIANITY AND CRISIS 46(8):174-175, May 19, 1986.

Michael Gottlieb, M.D.: challenge of AIDS research, by M. Helquist. ADVOCATE 451: 32, July 22, 1986.

Microsporidiosis myositis in a patient with the acquired immunodeficiency syndrome, by D. K. Ledford, et al. ANNALS OF INTERNAL MEDICINE 102(5):628-630, May 1985.

Microvascular aspects of acquired immune deficiency syndrome retinopathy, by D. A. Newsome, et al. AMERICAN JOURNAL OF OPHTHALMOLOGY 98(5):590-61, November 1984.

Military AIDS testing offers research bonus, by C. Norman. SCIENCE 232:818-820, May 16, 1986.

Military seeking test results, by M. Cocoves. GAY COMMUNITY NEWS 12(41):1, May 4, 1985.

Military test for viril antibodies: anti-gay, by T. Ensign. GUARDIAN 38(6):3, November 6, 1985.

Military to screen recruits for HTLV-III, by S. Poggi. GAY COMMUNITY NEWS 13(9):1, September 14, 1985.

Mind set for the fight against AIDS, by P. Tatchell. GUARDIAN September 5, 1986, p. 17.

Minimal risk of transmission of AIDS-associated retrovirus infection by oral-genital contact [letter], by D. Lyman, et al. JAMA 255(13):1703, April 4, 1986.

Minimizing the risk of contracting AIDS, by J. L. Marx. SCIENCE 219:1301, March 18, 1983.

Ministerial ethics and AIDS, by G. T. Miller. CHRISTIAN MINISTRY 17(3):22-24, May 1986.

Ministers back AIDS education. NEW SCIENTIST 108:21, October 3, 1985.

Ministers delayed launch of AIDS test. NEW SCIENTIST107:16, August 8, 1985.

Ministry to AIDS victims, by Francis A. Quinn. ORIGINS 16:224-226, September 4, 1986.

Minnesota Board to seek sex partner notification, by Bisticas-Cocoves. GAY COMMUNITY NEWS 13(41):1, May 3, 1986.

Minority access: still shut out. MEDIAFILE 5(4):8, November 1984.

Minute foci of Kaposi's sarcoma in a patient with acquired immunodeficiency syndrome [letter], by S. H. Swerdlow, et al. ARCHIVES OF PATHOLOGY AND LABORATORY MEDICINE 109(2):106-107, Feburary 1985.

Miracle cure; holism or hokum?, by K. Schneider. NEW AGE September 1985, p. 14.

Mixed results found in Boston HTLV-III project, by S. Hyde. GAY COMMUNITY NEWS 12(35):6, March 23, 1985.

Mobilizing to treat AIDS . . . nursing home staff, by R. C. Marlowe. PROVIDER 12(4): 49-50, April 1986.

Modern-day plague: the AIDS virus has found a niche in our society, and it acts as if it wants to stay, by J. Kaplan. NATURAL HISTORY 95:28+, February 1986.

Modern life, by C. Ratcliff. ARTFORUM 24:8, January 1986.

Modulation in vitro of immune parameters in homosexual males with the preclinical complex of symptoms related to acquired immune deficiency syndrome by azimexon, by Y. Z. Patt, et al. JOURNAL OF BIOLOGICAL RESPONSE MODIFIERS 5(3):263-269, June 1986.

Modulation of T- and B-lymphocyte functions by isoprinosine in homosexual subjects with prodromata and in patients with acquired immune deficiency syndrome (AIDS), by P. H. Tsang, et al. JOURNAL OF CLINICAL IMMUNOLOGY 4(6):469-478, November 1984.

Modulation of virus-specific immunity in vitro by the addition of interleukin-1 and interleukin-2 in patients with the acquired immune deficiency syndrome, by J. F. Sheridan, et al. ANNALS OF THE NEW YORK ACADEMY OF SCIENCES 437:53-534, 1984.

Molecular biology of human T-lymphotropic retroviruses, by F. Wong-Staal, et al. CANCER RESEARCH 45(Suppl. 9):4539s-4544s, September 1985.

Molecular biology of human T-lymphotropic retroviruses (HTLV), by F. Dorner, et al. WIENER MEDIZINISCHE WOCHENSCHRIFT 36(708):181-188, April 30, 1986.

Molecular biology of viruses associated with AIDS and current attempts to prevent its spread, by J. Holy. CASOPIS LEKARU CESKYCH 125(16):496-498, April 18, 1986.

Molecular characterization of human T-cell leukemia (lymphotropic) virus III in the acquired immune deficiency syndrome, by G. M. Shaw, et al. SCIENCE 226:1165-1171, December 7, 1984.

Molecular clone of HTLV-III with biological activity, by A. G. Fisher, et al. NATURE 316:262-265, July 18, 1985.

Molecular cloning and characterization of the HTLV-III virus associated with AIDS, by B. H. Hahn, et al. NATURE 312(5990):166-169, November 8-14, 1984.

Molecular cloning of AIDS-associated retrovirus, by P. A. Luciw, et al. NATURE 312(5996):760-763, December 20, 1984-January 2, 1985.

Molecular cloning of lymphadenopathy-associated virus, by M. Alizon, et al. NATURE 312(5996):757-760, December 20, 1984-January 2, 1985.

Molecular comparison of retroviruses associated with human and simian AIDS, by M. L. Bryant, et al. HEMATOLOGICAL ONCOLOGY 3(3):187-197, July-September 1985.

Molecular level view gives immune system clues [news], by C. Marwick. JAMA 253(23):3371+, June 21, 1985.

Molecular studies of human T cell leukemia/lymphotropic retroviruses, by F. Wong-Staal. HAMATOLOGIE UND BLUTTRANSFUSION 29:326-330, 1985.

Molluscum contagiosum and the acquired immunodeficiency syndrome [letter], by M. Katzman, et al. ANNALS OF INTERNAL MEDICINE 102(3);413-414, March 1985.

—, by P. C. Lombardo, et al. ARCHIVES OF DEROMATOLOGY 121(7):834-835, July 1985.

Mondale—need education—gay issues, by J. Ryan. GAY COMMUNITY NEWS 11(31):1, February 25, 1984.

Money for AIDS; British spending too little, US research will need control. NATURE 304:671-672, August 25, 1983.

Monilial enteritis in acquired immunodeficiency syndrome,by D. R. Radin, et al. AJR. AMERICAN JOURNAL OF ROENTGENOLOGY 141(6):1289-1290, December 1983.

Monkey AIDS, by T. Gauntt. OMNI 6:22, April 1984.

Monkey business in AIDS research. NEW SCIENTIST 97:747, March 17, 1983.

Monkey puzzle. TIME 123:60, March 12, 1984.

Monkeys possible source of human AIDS [African green monkeys; research by Max Essex, et al.], by J. Silberner. SCIENCE NEWS 127:245, April 20, 1985.

Monkeys too: relentless immunity disease, by J. A. Miller. SCIENCE NEWS 123:151, March 5, 1983.

Monoclonal antibody-defined beta 2-microglobulin-positive mononuclear cells in acquired immune deficiency syndrome, by S. Gupta. SCANDINAVIAN JOURNAL OF IMMUNOLOGY 22(4):357-361, October 1985.

Monoclonal immunoglobulins in HTLV-III-Positive sera [letter],by P. G. Sala, et al. CLINICAL CHEMISTRY 32(3):574, March 1986.

Monocyte function in the acquired immune deficiency syndrome. Defective chemotaxis, by P. D. Smith, et al. JOURNAL OF CLINICAL INVESTIGATION 74(6):2121-2128, December 1984.

Monocyte function in intravenous drug abusers with lymphadenopathy syndrome and in patients with acquired immunodeficiency syndrome: selective impairment of chemotaxis, by G. Po.i, et al. CLINICAL AND EXPERIMENTAL IMMUNOLOGY 62(1):136-142, October 1985.

Monocytoid B lymphocytes: their relation to the patterns of the acquired immunodeficiency syndrome (AIDS) and AIDS-related lymphadenopathy, by C. C. Sohn, et al. HUMAN PATHOLOGY 16(10):979-985, October 1985.

Mononuclear and polymorphonuclear leucocyte dysfunction in male homosexuals with the acquired immunodeficiency syndrome (AIDS), by G. J. Ras, et al. SOUTH AFRICAN MEDICAL JOURNAL 66(21):806-809, November 24, 1984.

Moral, ethical, and legal aspects of infection control, by B. Parent. AMERICAN JOURNAL OF INFECTION CONTROL 13(6):278-280, December 1985.

"Morals", medicine, and the AIDS epidemic, by P. M. Kayal. JOURNAL OF RELIGION AND HEALTH 24:218-238, Fall 1985.

More about the HTLV's and how they act, by J. L. Marx. SCIENCE 229:37-38, July 5, 1985.

More AIDS appears in Alberta, by S. McCarthy, et al. ALBERTA REPORT 11:30, March 5, 1984.

More AIDS money , by S. Budiansky. NATURE 304(5928):677, August 25-31, 1983.

—, by T. Beardsley. NATURE 318(6044):306, November 28-December 4, 1985.

More AIDS, more questions. SCIENCE NEWS 127:173, March 16, 1985.

More effective and less costly AIDS health services, by D. Altman. CARING 5(6):52-55, June 1986.

More evidence for brain disease in AIDS, by O. Sattaur. NEW SCIENTIST 108:26, October 10, 1985.

More federal AIDS research grants, by N. Fain. ADVOCATE 3(71):18, July 7, 1983.

More for AIDS in '85 budget request, by J. Ryan. GAY COMMUNITY NEWS 11(30):1, February 18, 1984.

More funding needed in rising AIDS crisis, by S. Martz. IN THESE TIMES 9(36):3, September 25, 1985.

More heterosexual spread of HTLV-III virus seen , by M. F. Goldsmith. JAMA 253(23):3377-3379, June 21, 1985.

More on AIDS from blood. DISCOVER 6:13, July 1985.

More on blood transfusion and AIDS [letter], by R. S. Gordon, Jr. NEW ENGLAND JOURNAL OF MEDICINE 310(26):1742, June 28, 1984.

More on ultrastructure of AIDS lymph nodes [letter], by S. P. Hammar, et al. NEW ENGLAND JOURNAL OF MEDICINE 310(14):924, April 5, 1984.

More progress on the HTLV family, by J. L. Marx. SCIENCE 227:156-157, January 11, 1985.

More teens, women infected by AIDS virus, study shows, by P. Smith. AIR FORCE TIMES 46:6, July 28, 1986.

More US funds for AIDS , by T. Beardsley. NATURE 316(6027):384, August 1-7, 1985.

Morphologic changes in lymph nodes of macaques with an immunodeficiency syndrome, by L. V. Chalifoux, et al. LABORATORY INVESTIGATION 51(1):22-26, July 1984.

Morphological alterations in the lymphoreticular system in acquired immunodeficiency syndrome, by P. I. Liu, et al. ANNALS OF CLINICAL AND LABORATORY SCIENCE 15(3):212-218, May-June 1985.

Morphological findings in the lymphadenopathy syndrome (LAS) and acquired immunodeficiency syndrome (AIDS), by S. Falk et al. DEUTSCHE MEDIZINISCHE WOCHENSCHRIFT 111(18):714-718, May 2, 1986.

201

Morphology of the retroviruses associated with AIDS and SAIDS, by G. Lecatsas, et al. PROCEEDINGS OF THE SOCIETY FOR EXPERIMENTAL BIOLOGY AND MEDICINE 177(3):495-498, December 1984.

Mortality associated with mode of presentation in the acquired immune deficiency syndrome, by a. R. Moss, et al. JNCI 73(6):1281-1284, December 1984.

Mother cares . . . and so does Zelda!, by M. Daniels. ADVOCATE 448:50, June 10, 1986.

Mother tells how a blood donation, the gift of life, led to her young son's death from AIDS, by H. Kushnick. PEOPLE 21:62+, June 4, 1984.

Mother with AIDS prompts school policy, by M. Schwartz. GAY COMMUNITY NEWS 12(46):2, June 8, 1985.

Mothers of infants with the acquired immunodeficiency syndrome: evidence for both symptomatic and assymptomatic carriers, by G. B. Scott, et al. JAMA 253:363-366, January 18, 1985.

Mothers on the front lines, by M. Helquist. ADVOCATE 438:22, January 21, 1986.

Move to repeal DC AIDS insur. protect. rebuffed, by D. Walter. ADVOCATE 453:22, August 19, 1986.

Moving target. SCIENTIFIC AMERICAN 253:85, October 1985.

Moving to meet needs of Haitians with AIDS, by A. Cohen. GAY COMMUNITY NEWS 13(15):1, October 26, 1985.

Moynihan Bill requires PHS provide funds: AIDS, by D. Walter. ADVOCATE 427:21, August 20, 1985.

Much ado about HTLV-III saliva study, by C. Guilfoy. GAY COMMUNITY NEWS 12(14): 1, October 20, 1984.

Multicentric angiofollicular lymph node hyperplasia (Castleman's disease) followed by Kaposi's sarcoma in two homosexual males with the acquired immunodeficiency syndrome (AIDS), by N. A. Lachant, et al. AMERICAN JOURNAL OF CLINICAL PATHOLOGY 83(1):27-33, January 1985.

Multicentric Kaposi's sarcoma of the conjunctiva in a male homosexual with the acquired immunodeficiency syndrome, by A. M. Macher, et al. OPHTHALMOLOGY 90(8):879-884, August 1983.

Multifactorial model for the development of AIDS in homosexual men, by J. A. Sonnabend, et al. ANNALS OF THE NEW YORK ACADEMY OF SCIENCES 437: 177-183, 1984.

Multifocal abnormalities of the gatrointestinal tract in AIDS, by S. D. Wall, et al. AJR. AMERICAN JOURNAL OF ROENTGENOLOGY 146(1):1-5, January 1986.

Multinucleated giant cells and HTLV-III in AIDS encephalopathy, by L. R. Sharer, et al. HUMAN PATHOLOGY 16(8):760, August 1985.

Multiple infections and death in a homosexual man [clinical conference]. AMERICAN JOURNAL OF MEDICINE 75(5):855-867, November 1983.

Multiple infections by cytomegalovirus in patients with acquired immunodeficiency syndrome: documentation by Southern blot hybridizatin, by W. L. Drew, et al. JOURNAL OF INFECTIOUS DISEASES 150(6):952-953, December 1984.

Multiple myeloma in a homosexual man with chronic lymphadenopathy, by L. A. Vandermolen, et al. ARCHIVES OF INTERNAL MEDICINE 145(4):745-746, April 1985.

Multiple opportunistic infection due to AIDS in a previously healthy black woman from Zaire [letter], by G. Offenstadt, et al. NEW ENGLAND JOURNAL OF MEDICINE 308(13):775, March 31, 1983.

Multiple opportunistic infections and neoplasms in the acquired immunodeficiency syndrome [editorial], by G. P. Wormser. JAMA 253(23)3441-3442, June 21, 1985.

Multiple sclerosis and human T-cell lymphotropic retroviruses, by H. Koprowski, et al. NATURE 318:154-160, November 14, 1985.

Multiple sclerosis and viruses, by P. Newmark. NATURE 318:101, November 14, 1985.

Multivesicular rosettes, a possible marker of acquired immunodeficiency syndrome (AIDS) in the endothelial cells of the splenic sinusoids [letter], by E. Feliu, et al. MEDICINA CLINICA 83(3):129, June 16, 1984.

Mutant virus worries vaccine researchers. NEW SCIENTIST 110:26, June 26, 1986.

My first AIDS patient, by L. Hadden. RN 49(3):51, March 1986.

My husband has AIDS, by G. Blair. FAMILY CIRCLE 99:52+, February 11, 1986.

My personal experience with AIDS, by A. J. Ferrara. AMERICAN PSYCHOLOGIST 39(11):1285-1287, November 1984.

Mycobacterial culture in acquired immunodeficiency syndrome [letter], by J. A. Girón, et al. ANNALS OF INTERNAL MEDICINE 98(6):1028-1029, June 1983.

Mycobacteriosis and AIDS in hospitals, by G. E. Noel. CANADIAN MEDICAL ASSOCIATION JOURNAL 135(2):136, July 15, 1986.

Mycobacteriosis in AIDS: easy to miss the correct diagnosis, by R. Grubb, et al. LAK-ARTIDNINGEN 82(25):2349-2351, June 19, 1985.

Mycobacterium avium-complex infections and development of the acquired immuno-deficiency syndrome: casual opportunist or causal cofactor?, by F. M. Collins. INTERNATIONAL JOURNAL OF LEPROSY AND OTHER MYCOBACTERIAL DISEASES 54(3):458-474, September 1986.

Mycobacterium avium complex infections in patients with the acquired immunodeficiency syndrome, by C. C. Hawkins, et al. ANNALS OF INTERNAL MEDICINE 105(2):184-188, August 1986.

Mycobacterium avium-intracellulare: another scourge for individuals with the acquired immunodeficiency syndrome [editorial], by H. Masur. JAMA 248(22):3013, December 10, 1982.

Mycobacterium avium-intracellulare-associated colitis in a patient with the acquired immunodeficiency syndrome, by A. Wolke, et al. JOURNAL OF CLINICAL GASTROENTEROLOGY 6(3):225-229, June 1984.

Mycobacterium avium-intracellulare complex enteritis: pseudo-Whipple disease in AIDS, by M. E. Vincent, et al. AJR 144(5):921-922, May 1985.

Mycobacterium avium-intracellulare infection and possibly venereal transmission [letter], by P. J. de Caprariis, et al. ANNALS OF INTERNAL MEDICINE 101(5):721, November 1984.

Mycobacterium avium-Mycobacterium intracellulare from the intestinal tracts of patients with the acquired immunodeficiency syndrome: concepts regarding acquisition and pathogenesis, by B. Damsker, et al. JOURNAL OF INFECTIOUS DISEASES 151(1):179-181, January 1985.

Mycobacterium avium: a pathogen of patients with acquired immunodeficiency syndrome, by O. G. Berlin, et al. DIAGNOSTIC MICROBIOLOGY AND INFECTIOUS DISEASE 2(3):213-218, June 1984.

Mycobacterium gordonae in the acquired immunodeficiency syndrome [letter],by J. Chan, et al. ANNALS OF INTERNAL MEDICINE 101(3):400, September 1984.

Mycobacterium tuberculosis bacteremia in the acquired immunodeficiency syndrome, by B. R. Saltzman,e t al. JAMA 256(3):390-391, July 18, 1986.

Mycobacterium xenopi and the acquired immunodeficiency syndrome [letter], by F. T. Tecson-Tumang, et al. ANNALS OF INTERNAL MEDICINE 100(3):461-462, March 1984.

Mycobacterium xenopi infection in a patient with acquired imunodeficiency syndrome, by R. H. Eng, et al. CHEST 86(1):145-147, July 1984.

Myelodysplasia in the acquired immune deficiency syndrome, by D. R. Schneider, et al. AMERICAN JOURNAL OF CLINICAL PATHOLOGY 84(2):144-152, August 1985.

Mystery immune disorder; the Haitian connection. ECONOMIST 286:77, January 29, 1983.

Mystery of AIDS. AFRICA 165:71, May 1985.

—, by N. Castleman. MEDICAL SELF CARE 20:32, Spring 1983.

Mystery of AIDS could be solved [T-cell leukaemia virus type III (HTLV III)]. NEW SCIENTIST 102:3, April 19, 1984.

Mystery of AIDS [most asked questions and answers], by B. Rensberger. SCIENCE DIGEST 94:40-41+, January 1986.

Myth and ideology of AIDS, by B. Kochis. NORTHWEST PASSAGE 26(4):3, December 1985.

Name for AIDS virus [letter], by F. Wong-Staal. NATURE 314(6012):574, April 18-24, 1985.

Nasty new epidemic, by J. Seligmann. NEWSWEEK 105:72-73, February 4, 1985.

National AIDS candlelight vigil. ADVOCATE 3(78):17, October 13, 1983.

National AIDS Research Foundation formed, by M. Daniels. ADVOCATE 432:11, October 29, 1985.

National AIDS vigil: at a low time, by J. Irvine. GAY COMMUNITY NEWS 11(12):1, October 7, 1983.

National AIDS vigil set for Oct. 8. GAY COMMUNITY NEWS 11(9):1, September 17, 1983.

National case-control study of Kaposi's sarcoma and Pneumocystis carinii pneumonia in homosexual men: Part I. Epidemiologic results, by H. W. Jaffe, et al. ANNALS OF INTERNAL MEDICINE 99(2):145151, August 1983.

—: Part 2. Laboratory results, by M. F. Rogers, et al. ANNALS OF INTERNAL MEDICINE 99(2):151-158, August 1983.

National Institutes of Health and Research into the acquired immune deficiency syndrome, by F. P. Witti, et al. PUBLIC HEALTH REPORTS 98(4):312-319, July-August 1983.

National Social Welfare Board's directions and general recommendations concerning AIDS. JORDEMODERN 98(7-8):246-251, July-August 1985.

Nationwide AIDS report/checking up, by E. Jackson. BODY POLITIC 95:12, July 1983.

Native Americans, PWA's protest health costs , by Bisticas-Cocoves. GAY COMMUNITY NEWS 13(13):1, October 12, 1985.

Natural history of the AIDS related complex in hemophilia—relationships to Epstein Barr virus, by F. Gervais, et al. AIDS RESEARCH 1(3):197-209, 1983-1984.

Natural history of HTLV-III infection is studied, by S. H. Weiss. AMERICAN FAMILY PHYSICIAN 32:176, August 1985.

Natural history of human T lymphotropic virus-III infection: the cause of AIDS, by M. Melbye. BRITISH MEDICAL JOURNAL 292(6512):5-12, January 4, 1986.

Natural history of infection with the lymphadenopathy-associated virus/human T-lymphotropic virus type III, by D. P. Francis, et al. ANNALS OF INTERNAL MEDICINE 103(5):719-722, November 1985.

Natural history of Kaposi's sarcoma in the acquired immunodeficiency syndrome, by B. Safai, et al. ANNALS OF INTERNAL MEDICINE 103(5):744-750, November 1985.

Natural history of primary infection with LAV in multitranfused patients, by the AIDS-Hemophilia French Study Group. BLOOD 68(1):89-94, July 1986.

Natural killer cell function and modulation by alpha IFN and IL2 in AIDS patients and prodromal subjects, by F. Lew, et al. JOURNAL OF CLINICAL AND LABORATORY IMMUNOLOGY 14(3):115-121, July 1984.

Natural killer cells in intravenous drug abusers with lymphadenopathy syndrome, by G. Poli, et al. CLINICAL AND EXPERIMENTAL IMMUNOLOGY 62(1):128-135, October 1985.

Natural resistance to parental T-lymphocyte-induced immunosuppression in F1 hybrid mice: implications for acquired immune deficiency syndrome (AIDS),by G. M. Shearer. IMMUNOLOGICAL REVIEWS 73:115-126, 1983.

Naturally occurring antibodies reactive with sperm proteins: apparent deficiency in AIDS sera, by T. C. Rodman, et al. SCIENCE 228(4704):1211-1215, June 7, 1985.

Nature's deadly experiment, by S. DeGarmo. SCIENCE DIGEST 91:6, December 1983.

NBC movie helped AIDS cause, gay leaders say, by B. Kenkelen. NATIONAL CATHOLIC REPORTER 22:6, November 22, 1985.

NEA sets guidelines to handle AIDS in schools. JET 69:37, October 28, 1985.

Necropsy findings in acquired immunodeficiency syndrome: a comparison of premortem diagnoses with postmortem findings, by A. N. Hui, et al. HUMAN PATHOLOGY 15(7):670-676, July 1984.

Necroscopic findings of variably acid-fast bacteria in a fatal case of acquired immunodeficiency syndrome and Kaposi's sarcoma,by A. R. Cantwell, Jr. GROWTH 47(2):129-134, Summer 1983.

Need for psychosocial research on AIDS and counseling laterrentions for AIDS victims, by R. T. Kinnier. JOURNAL OF COUNSELING AND DEVELOPMENT 64(7):472-473, March 1986.

Needle-prick injury and AIDS. NEW ZEALAND NURSING FORUM 14(2):3, August 1986.

Needle-stick injuries during the care of patients with AIDS [letter], by G. P. Wormser, et al. NEW ENGLAND JOURNAL OF MEDICINE 310(22):1461-1462, May 31, 1984.

Needlestick transmission of AIDS and Africa [letter], by J. Desmyter. LANCET 1(8422):217, January 26, 1985.

Needlestick transmission of HTLV-III from a patient infected in Africa [editorial]. LANCET 2(8416):1376-1377, December 15, 1984.

Neither sensationalism nor balanced discussion has resulted in a good strategy on AIDS, by D. Borley. NURSING STANDARD 387:5, March 7, 1985.

Neurologic complications in acquired immunodeficiency syndrome (AIDS), by C. B. Britton, et al. NEUROLOGICAL CLINIC 2(2):315-339, May 1984.

Neurologic complications in acquired immunodeficiency syndrome (AIDS). A clinical, computer tomographic and neuropathologic case presentation with a review of the literature, by S. M. Pulst. NERVENARZT 55(8):407-412, August 1984.

Neurologic manifestations in acquired immunodeficiency syndrome (AIDS), by J. Kesselring. DEUTSCHE MEDIZINISCHE WOCHENSCHRIFT 111(27):1068-1073, July 4, 1986.

Neurologic manifestations of the acquired immunodeficiency syndrome, by G. Fenelon, et al. REVUE NEUROLOGIQUE 142(2):97-106, 1986.

Neurological complications appear often in AIDS, by C. Marwick. JAMA 253:3379+, June 21, 1985.

Neurological complications in infants and children with acquired immune deficiency syndrome, by A. L. Belman, et al. ANNALS OF NEUROLOGY 18(5):560-566, November 1985.

Neurological complications now characterizing many AIDS victims [news], by P. Gapen. JAMA 248(22):2941-2942, December 10, 1982.

Neurological complications of acquired immune deficiency syndrome: analysis of 50 patients, by W. D. Snider, et al. ANNALS OF NEUROLOGY 14(4);403-418, October 1983.

Neurological disorders and AIDS. ADVOCATE 454:23, Septemebr 2, 1986.

Neurological manifestations of acquired immunodeficiency syndrome,by J. H. McArthur, et al. JOURNAL OF NEUROSCIENCE NURSING 18(5):242-249, October 1986.

Neurological manifestations of the acquired immunodeficiency syndrome (AIDS): experience at UCSF and review of the literature, by R. M. Levy, et al. JOURNAL OF NEUROSURGERY 62(4):475-495, April 1985.

Neurological syndromes complicating AIDS, by B. D. Jordan, et al. FRONTIERS OF RADIATION THERAPY AND ONCOLOGY 19:82-87, 1985.

Neuropathologic findings in the acquired immunodeficiency syndrome (AIDS), by K. Anders, et al. CLINICAL NEUROPATHOLOGY 5(1):1-20, January-February 1986.

Neuropathologic observations in acquired immunodeficiency syndrome (AIDS), by L. R. Sharer, et al. ACTA NEUROPATHOLOGICA 66(3):188-198, 1985.

Neuropathology of acquired immune deficiency syndrome, by L. B. Moskowitz, et al. ARCHIVES OF PATHOLOGY AND LABORATORY MEDICINE 108(11):867-872, November 1984.

Neuropathology of AIDS, by A. Hirano, et al. NO TO SHINKEI 36(11):1136-1137, November 1984.

Neuropsychiatric aspects of acquired immune deficiency syndrome, by R. J. Loewenstein, et al. INTERNATIONAL JOURNAL OF PSYCHIATRY IN MEDICINE 13(4):255-260, 1983-1984.

Neuropsychiatric complications of AIDS, by R. S. Hoffman. PSYCHOSOMATICS 25(5):393-395+, May 1984.

Neuropsychiatric complications of AIDS: a literature review, by W. M. Detmer, et al. INTERNATIONAL JOURNAL OF PSYCHIATRY IN MEDICINE 16(1):21-29, 1986-1987.

Neutralization of the AIDS retrovirus by antibodies to a recombinant envelope glycoprotein, by L. A. Lasky, et al. SCIENCE 233(4760):209-212, July 11, 1986.

Neutralization of HTLV-III/LAV replication by antiserum to thymosin a_1, by P. S. Sarin, et al. SCIENCE 232:1135-1137, May 30, 1986.

Neutralization of human T-lymphotropic virus type III by sera of AIDS and AIDS-risk patients, by R. A. Weiss, et al. NATURE 316(6023):69-72, July 4, 1985.

Neutralizing antibody in Celebes black macaques recovering from infection with simian acquired immunodeficiency syndrome retrovirus type 2, by S. M. Shiigi, et al. CLINICAL IMMUNOLOGY AND IMMUNOPATHOLOGY 40(2):283-290, August 1986.

New aid in fighting AIDS? NEWSWEEK 105:85, February 18, 1985.

New AIDS forecast: a long, long siege. US NEWS & WORLD REPORT 99:14, October 14, 1985.

New A.I.D.S. guidelines and group. NURSING 16:16, February 1986.

New AIDS policy set for Boston's school workers, by C. Guilfoy. GAY COMMUNITY NEWS 13(11):1, September 28, 1985.

New AIDS research guidelines released, by C. Guilfoy. GAY COMMUNITY NEWS 12(19):1, November 24, 1984.

New AIDS risk groups identified. AMERICAN FAMILY PHYSICIAN 31:132, March 1985.

New AIDS risk: a term in jail. NEWSWEEK 106:98, October 28, 1985.

New AIDS test? THE ECONOMIST 298:82, February 22, 1986.

—. US NEWS & WORLD REPORT 98(6):48, February 18, 1985.

New AIDS test comes to light in Japan, by B. Johnstone. NEW SCIENTIST 106:8, April 18, 1985.

New AIDS viruses spark more rivalry. NEW SCIENTIST 110:20, April 3, 1986.

New aspects of AIDS, by J. Gerstoft. NORDISK MEDICIN 98(10):231-233, 1983.

New biphasic culture system for isolation of mycobacteria from blood of patients with acquired immune deficiency syndrome, by O. G. Berlin, et al. JOURNAL OF CLINICAL MICROBIOLOGY 20(3):572-574, September 1984.

New books examine the social and scientific issues surrounding AIDS. PUBLISHERS WEEKLY 228:100+, September 13, 1985.

New books put human faces on—AIDS care. ADVOCATE 452:31, August 5, 1986.

New British test for AIDS is quicker and cheaper, by O. Sattaur. NEW SCIENTIST 108:20-21, October 3, 1985.

New clues link leukemia virus to AIDS, by P. Taulbee. SCIENCE NEWS 123:324, May 21, 1983.

New complication of AIDS: thoracic myelitis caused by herpes simplex virus, by C. B. Britton, et al. NEUROLOGY 35(7):1071-1074, July 1985.

New developments in the acquired immunodeficiency syndrome: are treatment, prevention, and control possible?, by J. M. Luce. RESPIRATORY CARE 31(2):113-116, February 1986.

New directions in AIDS transmission, by J. Silberner. SCIENCE NEWS 129:101, February 15, 1986.

New disease: acquired immune deficiency of homosexuals [editorial],by A. Molins Otero. REVISTA CLINICA ESPANOLA 168(2):150-151, January 31, 1983.

New disease baffles medical community, by J. L. Marx. SCIENCE 217:618-621, August 13, 1982.

New drug boost for AIDS research. THE TIMES HIGHER EDUCATION SUPPLEMENT 675:11, October 11, 1985.

New drug joins front line against AIDS, by C. Joyce. NEW SCIENTIST 111:16, September 25, 1986.

New emphasis on psychosocial issues: AIDS studies, by N. Fain. ADVOCATE 421: 24, May 28, 1985.

New epidemic: immune deficiency, opportunistic infections, and Kaposi's sarcoma, by J. Allen, et al. AMERICAN JOURNAL OF NURSING 82:1718-1722, November 1982.

New evidence could link drugs to AIDS. RN 46:20, June 1983.

New fears that children may catch AIDS, by O. Sattaur. NEW SCIENTIST 106:4, April 18, 1985.

New federal guidelines say children with AIDS can attend school. PHI DELTA KAPPAN 67:242+, November 1985.

New findings in race for AIDS cure, by K. McAuliffe. U.S. NEWS AND WORLD REPORT 100(16):71-72, April 28, 1986.

New funds for AIDS drug centers , by D. M. Barnes. SCIENCE 233(4762):414, July 25, 1986.

New gay renaissance: a change on the wind, by T. Hopkinson. RFD 47:29, Summer 1986.

New Hampshire AIDS Conference cites discrimination, by S. Janicki. GAY COMMUNITY NEWS 13(31):3, February 22, 1986.

New Hampshire bill would ban lesbian and gay blood, by C. Guilfoy. GAY COMMUNITY NEWS 12(30):1, February 16, 1985.

New hope fighting AIDS. ALBERTA REPORT 11:40, May 7, 1984.

New hope for Californian AIDS victims?, by P. Tatchell. NEW STATESMAN 110:6, October 11, 1985.

New hope from old drug, by M. Helquist. ADVOCATE 428:30, September 3, 1985.

New HTLV-III/LAV encoded antigen detected by antibodies from AIDS patients, by J. S. Allan, et al. SCIENCE 230:810-813, November 15, 1985.

New HTLV-III/LAV protein encoded by a gene found in cytopathic retroviruses, by T. H. Lee, et al. SCIENCE 231:1546-1549, March 28, 1986.

New human retrovirus associated with acquired immunodeficiency syndrome (AIDS) or AIDS-related complex, by J. C. Chermann, et al. PROGRESS IN CLINICAL AND BIOLOGICAL RESEARCH 182:329-342, 1985.

New immune booster: both legal and inexpensive, by M. Helquist. ADVOCATE 433: 25, November 12, 1985.

New immunologic syndrome—AIDS, by W. Mazurkiewicz. PRZEGLAD DERMATOLOGICZNY 71(1):11-15, January-February 1984.

New infectious diseases and new aspects of infectious diseases. VERHANDLUNGEN DER DEUTSCHEN GESELLSCHAFT FUR INNERE MEDIZIN 20(Part 1):1-44, 1984.

New infectious diseases impact hospital planning, by P. Hawrylyshyn. HEALTH CARE 28(3):34, April 1986.

New Jersey AIDS patients often drug abusers, by S. Hartnett. NEW JERSEY NURSE 16(2):13, March-April 1986.

New Jersey prisoners file AIDS suit. GAY COMMUNITY NEWS 13(4):2, August 3, 1985.

New measures to contain AIDS. NURSING STANDARD 386:1, February 28, 1985.

New online AIDS library will be a central comprehensive source of information. COLLEAGUE ON CALL 3(5):8, October-November 1986.

New PHS grants awarded for research on AIDS. PUBLIC HEALTH REPORTS 98(3): 228, May-June 1983.

New psychopathologic findings in AIDS: case report, by E. J. Ermani, et al. JOURNAL OF CLINICAL PSYCHIATRY 46(6):240-241, June 1985.

New relatives of AIDS virus found [news],by J. L. Marx. SCIENCE 232(4747):157, April 11, 1986.

New research leads to AIDS vaccine. NEW SCIENTIST 110:17, April 17, 1986.

New safety rules for AIDS workers. NEW SCIENTIST 103:5, August 23, 1984.

New San Francisco story, by M. Helquist. ADVOCATE 429:24, September 17, 1985.

New scarlet letter, by M. Sager. WASHINGTONIAN 21:104+, January 1986.

New scarlet letter(s), pediatric AIDS, by J. A. Church, et al. PEDIATRICS 77(3):423-427, March 1986.

New strategies for AIDS therapy and prophylaxis [letter], by E. C. M. Mariman, et al. NATURE 318(6045):414, December 5-11, 1985.

New strategy to prevent the spread of AIDS among heterosexuals [editorial], by D. F. Echenberg. JAMA 254(15):2129-2130, October 18, 1985.

New study ties poopers, AIDS, by Connors. GAY COMMUNITY NEWS 13(13):1, October 12, 1985.

New terror of AIDS [special section; with editorial comment by Kevin Doyle]. MACLEAN'S 98(2):32-38, August 12, 1985.

New theories about AIDS, by J. Seligmann, et al. NEWSWEEK 103(5):50-51, January 30, 1984.

New treatment helps AIDS victims. CHEMICAL INDUSTRY 11:349, June 3, 1985.

New twist in AIDS patent fight, by C. Norman. SCIENCE 232:308-309, April 18, 1986.

New type D retrovirus isolated from macaques with an immunodeficiency syndrome, by M. D. Daniel, et al. SCIENCE 223:602-605, February 10, 1984.

New untouchables: anxiety over AIDS is verging on hysteria in some parts of the country, by E. Thomas, et al. TIME 126(12):24-26, Septemebr 23, 1985.

New untouchables of America. NEW SCIENTIST 98:927, June 30, 1983.

New victims, by E. Barnes, et al. LIFE 8:12-19, July 1985.

New viral infections and the acquired immunodeficiency syndrome, by V. M. Zhdanov, et al. SOVIET MEDICINE 10:41-46, 1985.

New York activists fight eviction of PWA's survivor, by B. Gelbert. GAY COMMUNITY NEWS 13(38):1, April 12, 1986.

New York AIDS Forum for black men/women, by C. Smith. GAY COMMUNITY NEWS 11(30):3, February 18, 1984.

New York bath owners to promote safe sex,by S. Hyde. GAY COMMUNITY NEWS 12(35):1, March 23, 1985.

New York center helps homeless AIDS patients, by P. Freiberg. ADVOCATE 435:13, December 10, 1985.

New York City grants Rights Bill to lesbians, gay men, by B. Gelbert. GAY COMMUNITY NEWS 13(37):1, April 1, 1986.

New York-Cornell becomes center for AIDS study. AMERICAN JOURNAL OF PUBLIC HEALTH 73:1193, October 1983.

New York doctor granted new lease in AIDS eviction, by P. Freiberg. ADVOCATE 4(8):10, November 27, 1984.

New York groups counter AIDS hysteria, by B. Nelson. GAY COMMUNITY NEWS 11(24):3, December 31, 1983.

New York hospital opens acute care AIDS unity, by T. L. Selby. AMERICAN NURSE 18(5):3+, May 1986.

New York jail cook dies from AIDS: not a high-risk group member. CORRECTIONS DIGEST 14(14):10, June 29, 1983.

New York locks up the "mineshaft", by Bisticas-Cocoves. GAY COMMUNITY NEWS 13(19):1, November 23, 1985.

New York officials reconsider closing baths, by P. Freiberg. ADVOCATE 433:14, November 12, 1985.

New York queers fight City Hall, by K. Westheimer. GAY COMMUNITY NEWS 13(20): 1, November 30, 1985.

New York to introduce AIDS bill, by J. Aschkenasy. THE NATIONAL UNDERWRITER (LIFE & HEALTH INSURANCE EDITION) 90:26, January 25, 1986.

New York: where intimacy is in, by G. Whitmore. ADVOCATE 3(73):22, August 4, 1983.

New York's Columbia University. ADVOCATE 3(78):19, October 13, 1983.

News analysis. Just another excuse to persecute?, by V. Scott. NURSING MIRROR 161(16):11, October 16, 1985.

Next they'll tax it: sex diseases. ECONOMIST 285:29-30, October 2, 1982.

NH bill would ban lesbian & gay blood,by C. Guilfoy. GAY COMMUNITY NEWS 12(30):1, February 16, 1985.

NIAID to fund nine new AIDS studies. PUBLIC HEALTH REPORTS 99(3):324, May-June 1984.

NIC update, by N. Sabanosh. CORRECTIONS TODAY 48(4):22+, June 1986.

Nice. . . but don't have to know, by Ehud Yonay. CALIFORNIA MAGAZINE 9:39, June 1984.

NIDA AIDS grant, by K. Callen. ADAMHA NEWS 9(21):2, December 1983.

NIDA and AIDS. ADAMHA NEWS 10(8):8, August 1984.

Nightmare coming true. BODY POLITIC 129:18, August 1986.

Nightmare of AIDS [letter], by A. Sibatani. NATURE 304(5923):206, July 21-27, 1983.

NIH Conference. Acquired immunodeficiency syndrome: epidemiologic, clinical, immunologic, and therapeutic considerations, by A. S. Fauci, et al. ANNALS OF INTERNAL MEDICINE 100(1):92-106, January 1984.

—. The acquired immunodeficiency syndrome: an update, by A. S. Fauci, et al. ANNALS OF INTERNAL MEDICINE 102(6):800-813, June 1985.

NIH scientific workshops on acquired immune deficiency syndrome. PUBLIC HEALTH REPORTS 98(4):318-319, July-August 1983.

NIH scientists report transmission of clinical AIDS infection from humans to chimpanzees, by J. Murphy. NEWS & FEATURES FROM NIH November 1984, p. 12-13.

NIJ offers a free manual on AIDS which every CJ Training Director needs. TRAINING AIDS DIGEST 11(3):1-7, March 1986.

NIJ publishes huge manual on AIDS in prisons and jails. CORRECTIONS DIGEST 17(5):1-3, February 26, 1986; also in CRIME CONTROL DIGEST 20(8):3-5, February 24, 1986.

NIMH study: gay men shun AIDS test, by J. Folkenberg. ADAMHA NEWS 11(11):2, November 1985.

9-(1,3 Dinydroxy-2-propoxymethyl)quanine for cytomegalovirus infections in patients with the acquired immunodeficiency syndrome, by M. C. Bach, et al. ANNALS OF INTERNAL MEDICINE 103(3):381-382, September 1985.

1985 update on AIDs, by J. Hardie. CANADIAN DENTAL ASSOCIATION JOURNAL 51(7):499-502, July 1985.

No AIDS for Britain's peers. DISCOVER 6:8, May 1985.

No AIDS from HB vaccine. AMERICAN JOURNAL OF NURSING 85:1268, November 1985.

No AIDS from saliva. NEWSWEEK 106:69, Decemebr 30, 1985.

No AIDS test to be required in biting of police officer. CORRECTIONS DIGEST 16(17):10, August 14, 1985; also in CRIME CONTROL DIGEST 19(33):2-3, August 19, 1985.

No cases of AIDS among nurses, by M. Allen. CANADIAN NURSE 81:13, May 1985.

No home means no home care for AIDS patients, by M. R. Traska. HOSPITALS 60(1): 69-70, January 5, 1986.

No HTLV-III antibodies after HBV vaccination, by L. Muylie, et al. NEW ENGLAND JOURNAL OF MEDICINE 314:581, February 27, 1986.

No increased incidence of AIDS in recipients of hepatitis B vaccine [letter], by J. A. Golden. NEW ENGLAND JOURNAL OF MEDICINE 308(19):1163-1164, May 12, 1983.

No lesbian blood, by S. Hyde. GAY COMMUNITY NEWS 12(27):1, January 26, 1985.

No moral panic—that's the problem, by D. Anderson. TIMES June 18, 1985, p. 12.

No more shit [editorial]. BODY POLITIC 127:8, June 1986.

No need for panic about AIDS. Acquired immune deficiency disease, now frequent among male homosexuals in the United States, is not this century's black death. The most urgent need is to understand what is going on . NATURE 302(5911):749, April 28, 1983.

No new ways of treating AIDS, by J. Maddox. NATURE 308(5955):107, March 8-14, 1984.

No sex for gays, High Court says. GUARDIAN 38(39):5, July 9, 1986.

No special hazards caused by AIDS in the hospital. Information for hospital person-nel, by A. Kümmel. KRANKENPFLEGE 39(9):312+, September 1985.

No time for secrets. OUT 3(2):4, December 1984.

No trend yet in test for HTLV-III antibody. OUT 4(2):1, December 1985.

Nondiagnosis of acquired immunodeficiency syndrome [editorial], by G. T. Hensley, et al. ARCHIVES OF PATHOLOGY AND LABORATORY MEDICINE 110(4):307-308, April 1986.

Non-Hodgkin's lymphoma in 90 homosexual men: relation to generalized lympha-denopathy and the acquired immunodeficiency syndrome, by J. L. Ziegler, et al. NEW ENGLAND JOURNAL OF MEDICINE 311(9):565-570, August 30, 1984.

Noninfectious cofactors in susceptibility to AIDS: possible contributions of semen, HLA alloantigens and lack of natural resistance, by G. M. Shearer, et al. ANNALS OF THE NEW YORK ACADEMY OF SCIENCES 437:49-57, 1984.

Nonneoplastic AIDS syndromes, by M. S. Gottlieb. SEMINARS IN ONCOLOGY 11(1): 40-46, March 1984.

Non-partisan agency slams insufficient AIDS supp, by C. Guilfoy. GAY COMMUNITY NEWS 12(35):7, March 23, 1985.

Nontyphoidal Salmonella bacteremia as an early infection in acquired immuno-deficiency syndrome, by E. J. Bottone, et al. DIAGNOSTIC MICROBIOLOGY AND INFECTIOUS DISEASE 2(3):247-250, June 1984.

Nosocomial acquired immunodeficiency syndrome and human T-cell leukaemia lymphoma virus associated disease, by D. C. Shanson. JOURNAL OF HOSPITAL INFECTION 5(1):3-6, March 1984.

"Not an easy disease to come by", by G. J. Church. TIME 126(12):27, September 23, 1985.

Not there yet, but 'on our way' in AIDs research, scientists say, by M. F. Goldsmith. JAMA 253(23):3369-3371+, by June 21, 1985.

Not a victim—a person with AIDS, by E. Jackson. BODY POLITIC 97:28, October 1983.

Notes on AIDS, by J. M. Richards. BRITISH DENTAL JOURNAL 158(6):199-201, March 23, 1985.

Notes on handling the clinical specimens from patients with AIDS or similar conditions, by T. Kawai. RINSHO BYORI 31(12):1366-1368, December 1983.

Notoriety of disease . . . famous people having diseases, by L. Klein. JOURNAL OF ENTEROSTOMAL THERAPY 12(6):191-192, November-December 1985.

Nowhere to run, nowhere to hide . . . AIDS hits India, by K. M. Pierce, et al. TIME 128(9):36, September 1, 1986.

Nucleic acid structure and expression of the human AIDS/lymphadenopathy retrovirus, by M. A. Muesing, et al. NATURE 313(6002):450-458, February 7-13, 1985.

Nucleotide sequence and expression of an AIDS-associated retrovirus (ARV-2), by R. Sanchez-Pescador, et al. SCIENCE 227(4686):484-492, February 1, 1985.

Nucleotide sequence evidence for relationship of AIDS retrovirus to lentiviruses, by I. M. Chiu, et al. NATURE 317(6035):366-368, October 26, 1985.

Nucleotide sequence of the AIDS virus, LAV, by S. Wain-Hobson, et al. CELL 40(1): 9-17, January 1985.

Nucleotide sequence of the protease-coding region in an infectious DNA of simian retrovirus (STLV) of the HTLV-I family, by J.-I. Inoue, et al. VIROLOGY 150:187-195, April 15, 1986.

Nucleotide sequence of SRV-1, a type D simian acquired immune deficiency syndrome retrovirus, by M. D. Power, et al. SCIENCE 231(4745):1567-1572, March 28, 1986.

Number of AIDS cases likely to escalate rapidly. CHEMICAL AND ENGINEERING NEWS 63:5, September 23, 1985.

Nurses and AIDS: do we know the facts?, by R. R. Caddace, et al. CALIFORNIA NURSE 82(4):4-5, May 1986.

Nurses' attitudes regarding acquired immunodeficiency syndrome (AIDS), by P. Reed, et al. NURSING FORUM 21(4):153-156, 1984.

Nurses' fear of AIDS exceeds the risks. RN 47:13-14, January 1984.

Nurses most likely to have AIDS exposure, CDC data show. HOSPITAL EMPLOYEE HEALTH 3(9):118-119, September 1984.

Nurses quit rather than treat AIDS patient. RN 46:11, August 1983.

Nurses urged to allay fears of AIDS in schools, by P. Cohen. NURSING STANDARD 418:1, October 10, 1984.

Nursing the AIDS patient, by B. Bolding, et al. RNABC NEWS 17(6):15-17, November-December 1985.

Nursing AIDS: situations vacant, by J. Sherman. NURSING TIMES 81(49):19-20, December 4-10, 1985.

Nursing care. AIDS: real solution to keep AIDS away from sensationalism, by C. Nielsen, et al. SYGEPLEJERSKEN 85(43):18-21, October 23, 1985.

Nursing care of AIDS victims . . . home care, by B. Stoller. JOURNAL OF PRACTICAL NURSING 35(4):26-30, December 1985.

Nursing care of patients suffering from acquired immunodeficiency syndrome, by C. P. Batten, et al. INFIRMIERE CANADIENNE 25(10):17-21, November 1983.

Nursing care plan for an AIDS patient. Nursing care must offer support and corrective measures in all areas—physical, psychological, social, by N. Bolash. PENNSYLVANIA NURSE 41(2):4-6, February 1986.

Nursing care plan for persons with AIDS. QRB12(10):361-365, October 1986.

Nursing diagnoses and care plans for ambulatory care patients with AIDS, by A. C. Howes. TOPICS IN CLINICAL NURSING 6(2):61-66, July 1984.

Nursing history of an AIDS patient, by E. Bages Mir, et al. REVISTA DE ENFERMERIA 8(88):20-25, November 1985.

Nursing literature on AIDS, by S. G. Fisher, et al. TOPICS IN CLINICAL NURSING 6(2): 76-82, July 1984.

Nursing management of the pediatric AIDS patient, by L. Iazzetti. ISSUES IN COMPREHENSIVE PEDIATRIC NURSING 9(2):119-129, 1986.

Nursing the patient with AIDS, by C. Batten, et al. CANADIAN NURSE 79:19-22, November 1983.

Nursing the patient with AIDS calls for special care and knowledge, by P. M. Kenny. PENNSYLVANIA NURSE 38(4):6, April 1983.

Nursing staff and AIDS: caution yes—fear no, by R. von Blarer. KRANKENPFLEGE. SOINS INFIRMIERS 79(1):23-26, January 1986.

Nutrition and the acquired immunodeficiency syndrome [letter], by R. S. Beach, et al. ANNALS OF INTERNAL MEDICINE 99(4):565-566, Octtober 1983.

Nutritional management of the AIDS patients, by R. R. Rago, et al. PHYSICIAN ASSISTANT 10(10):89-90, October 1986.

NW AIDS fund announced. NORTHWEST PASSAGE 23(13):7, August 1983.

Oat-cell carcinoma in transfusion-associated acquired immunodeficiency syndrome [letter], by R. J.\ Moser, 3d, et al. ANNALS OF INTERNAL MEDICINE 103(3):478, September 1985.

Obstacles to curing AIDS, by C. Gunderson. UTNE READER 11:15, August 1985.

Occult infections with M. intracellulare in bone-marrow biopsy specimens from patients with AIDS [letter], by R. J. Cohen, et al. NEW ENGLAND JOURNAL OF MEDICINE 308(24):1476, June 16, 1983.

Occurence of AIDS in hemophiliacs in Japan, by T. Abe, et al. SEMINARS IN THROM-
BOSIS AND HEMOSTASIS 11(4):352-356, October 1985.

Occurrence of anti-HTLV-III antibodies in Danish high-risk homosexuals in 1982-83
—seroconversion rate and risk of AIDS [letter], by B. Hoffmann, et al. AIDS RE-
SEARCH 2(1):1-3, February 1986.

Occurrence of a new microsporidan: Enterocytozoon bieneusi n.g., n. sp., in the enterocytes of a human patient with AIDS, by I. Desportes, et al. JOURNAL OF
PROTOZOOLOGY 32(2):250-254, May 1985.

Ocular effects in acquired immune deficiency syndrome, by J. S. Schuman, et al.
MOUNT SINAI JOURNAL OF MEDICINE 50(5):443-446, September-October
1983.

Ocular findings in the acquired immunodeficiency syndrome, by A. Gal, et al. BRITISH
JOURNAL OF OPTHAMOLOGY 68(4):238-241, April 1984.

Ocular manifestations of the acquired immune deficiency syndrome, by G. N. Holland.
INTERNATIONAL OPHTHALMOLOGY CLINICS 25(2):179-187, Summer 1985.

Ocular manifestations of AIDS, by S. J. Bass. JOURNAL OF THE AMERICAN OPTO-
METRIC ASSOCIATION 55(10):765-769, October 1984.

Oculomotor cranial nerve palsey associated with acquired immunodeficiency syndrome, by M. K. Jack, et al. ANNALS OF OPHTHALMOLOGY 16(5):460-462,
May 1984.

Of AIDS and abdominal pain. EMERGENCY MEDICINE 16(14):107-108+, August 15,
1984.

Of AIDS and the national blood supply. EMERGENCY MEDICINE 18(8):130+, April
30, 1986.

Of AIDS, gays and repression. NEW STATESMAN 109:3, March 1, 1985.

Officers suspended for refusing to transport inmate with AIDS. CRIME CONTROL DI-
GEST 17(42):3, October 24, 1983; also in CORRECTIONS DIGEST 14(22):8-9,
October 19, 1983.

Old cure fights AIDS, by N. Underwood. MACLEAN'S 99:52, April 28, 1986.

Old cure points to an AIDS vaccine . . . vaccinia virus—or cowpox, by M. Clark, et al.
NEWSWEEK 107(16):71, April 21, 1986.

Oligoclonal immunoglobulins in patients with the acquired immunodeficiency syndrome, by N. M. Papadopoulos, et al. CLINICAL IMMUNOLOGY AND IMMUNO-
PATHOLOGY 35(1):43-36, April 1985.

On AIDS . . . and one road to redemption . . . donate blood, by T. M. Stephany.
POINT OF VIEW 22(2):21, May 1985.

On AIDS jokes—public officials, by E. Rofes. GAY COMMUNITY NEWS 11(36):5,
March 31, 1984.

On the AIDS problem, by Lewis Thomas. DISCOVER 4:42+, May 1983.

On the AIDS trail: work continues on test, cure, vaccine, by J. Silberner. SCIENCE
NEWS 127:100, February 16, 1985.

On calling whom what, by N. Fain. ADVOCATE 3(79):20, October 27, 1983.

On HTLV-III's trail. ALBERTA REPORT 12:50, November 25, 1985.

On a Nursing AIDS Task Force: the battle for confident care, by R. B. Brock. NURS-ING MANAGEMENT 7(3):67-68, March 1986.

On Trojan horses and surrogate mothers [letter], by J. Kolins. NEW ENGLAND JOURNAL OF MEDICINE 311(1):53-54, July 5, 1984.

Oncor to offer test to detect AIDS virus. CHEMICAL AND ENGINEERING NEWS 64:6, October 6, 1986.

One against the plague . . . AIDS treatment team, by P. Goldman, et al. NEWSWEEK 108(3):38-45+, July 21, 1986.

One man connected to forty cases of AIDS in 10 cities across nation. JET 66:37, April 23, 1984.

One man's battle with AIDS, by A. S. Brodoff. PATIENT CARE 18(2):138+, January 30, 1984.

One man's fight against AIDS, by T. McGirk. SUNDAY TIMES August 11, 1985, p. 15.

Only homosexual Haitians, not all Haitians [letter], by R. Altema, et al. ANNALS OF INTERNAL MEDICINE 99(6):877-888, December 1983.

Only months to live and no place to die, by J. Seligmann. NEWSWEEK 106:26, August 12, 1985.

Only a moral revolution can contain this scourge, by I. Jakobowits. TIMES December 27, 1986, p. 20.

Ontario removes Haitians from list, by E. Jackson. BODY POLITIC 99:8, December 1983.

Ophthalmic involvement in acquired immunodeficiency syndrome, by A. G. Palestine, et al. OPHTHALMOLOGY 91(9):1092-1099, September 1984.

Ophthalmologic findings in acquired immune deficiency syndrome (AIDS), by M. Khadem, et al. ARCHIVES OF OPHTHALMOLOGY 102(2):201-206, February 1984.

Ophthalmoscopic manifestations observed in AIDS, by P. Le Hoang, et al. BULLETIN DES SOCIETES D'OPHTALMOLOGIE DE FRANCE 84(4):377-380, April 1984.

Opportunistic AIDS [letter], by J. Cohen, et al. LANCET 2(8413):1209-1210, November 24, 1984.

Opportunistic infection complicating acquired immune deficiency syndrome. Clinical features of 25 cases, by C. W. Lerner, et al. MEDICINE 63(3):155-164, May 1984.

Opportunistic infection in previously healthy women. Initial manifestations of a community-acquired cellular immunodeficiency, by H. Mauur, et al. ANNALS OF INTERNAL MEDICINE 97(4):533-539, October 1982.

Opportunistic infections and acquired cellular immune deficiency among Haitian immigrants in Montreal, by R. P. LeBlanc, et al. CANADIAN MEDICAL ASSOCIATION JOURNAL 129(11):1205-1209, December 1, 1983.

217

Opportunistic infections and impaired cell-mediated immune responses in patients with the acquired immune deficiency syndrome, by R. B. Roberts, et al. TRANS-ACTIONS OF THE AMERICAN CLINICAL AND CLIMATOLOGICAL ASSOCIATION 95:40-51, 1983.

Opportunistic infections and Kaposi's sarcoma among Haitians: evidence of a new acquired immunodeficiency state, by A. E. Pitchenik, et al. ANNALS OF INTERNAL MEDICINE 98(3):377-384, March 1983.

Opportunistic infections in acquired immune deficiency syndrome result from synergistic defects of both the natural and adaptive components of cellular immunity by F. P. Siegal, et al. JOURNAL OF CLINICAL INVESTIGATION 78(1):115-123, July 1986.

Opportunistic infections in patients with AIDS: clues to the epidemiology of AIDS and the relative virulence of pathogens, by M. J. Blaser, et al. REVIEWS OF INFECTIOUS DISEASES 8(1):21-30, January-February 1986.

Opposition to antibody test grows, by N. Fain. ADVOCATE 418:22, April 16, 1985.

Optimizing care for the AIDS patient, by A. S. Brodoff. PATIENT CARE 18(2):125-127+, January 30, 1984.

Oral candidiasis and the acquired immunodeficiency syndrome [letter], by B. Romanowski, et al. ANNALS OF INTERNAL MEDICINE 101(3):400-401, September 1984.

Oral candidiasis and AIDS [letter], by M. Joy. NEW ENGLAND JOURNAL OF MEDICINE 311(21):1378-1379, November 22, 1984.

Oral candidiasis as a marker for esophageal candidiasis in the acquired immunodeficiency syndrome, by A. Tavitian, et al. ANNALS OF INTERNAL MEDICINE 104(1):54-55, January 1986.

Oral candidiasis in high-risk patients as the initial manifestation of the acquired immunodeficiency syndrome, by R. S. Klein, et al. NEW ENGLAND JOURNAL OF MEDICINE 311(6):354-358, August 9, 1984.

Oral candidosis and AIDS [letter], by L. P. Samaranayake. BRITISH DENTAL JOURNAL 157(10):342-343, November 24, 1984.

Oral findings in people with or at high risk for AIDS: a study of 375 homosexual males, by S. Silverman, Jr., et al. JOURNAL OF THE AMERICAN DENTAL ASSOCIATION 112(2):187-192, February 1986.

Oral Kaposi's sarcoma associated with acquired immunodeficiency syndrome among homosexual males, by L. R. Eversole, et al. JOURNAL OF THE AMERICAN DENTAL ASSOCIATION 107(2):248-253, August 1983.

Oral manifestation of disseminated Mycobacterium avium intracellulare in a patient with AIDS, by F. Volpe, et al. ORAL SURGERY, ORAL MEDICINE, ORAL PATHOLOLOGY 60(6):567-570, December 1985.

Oral manifestations of tumor and opportunistic infections in the acquired imunodeficiency syndrome (AIDS): findings in 53 homosexual men with Kaposi's sarcoma, by F. Lozada, et al. ORAL SURGERY 56(5):491-494, November 1983.

Oral viral lesion (hairy leukplakia) associated with acquired immunodeficiency syndrome. JAMA 254:1694, October 4, 1985.

218

—. MMWR 34(36):549-550, September 13, 1985.

Oral viral leukoplakea—a new AIDS-associated condition, by J. S. Greenspan, et al. ADVANCES IN EXPERIMENTAL MEDICINE AND BIOLOGY 187:123-128, 1985.

Orbital Brukitt's lymphoma in a homosexual man with acquired immune deficiency, by H. L. Brooks, Jr., et al. ARCHIVES OF OPHTHALMOLOGY 102(10):1533-1537, October 1984.

Organic brain syndrome in three cases of acquired immune deficiency syndrome, by E. Kermani, et al. COMPREHENSIVE PSYCHIATRY 25(3):294-297, May-June 1984.

Organising a counseling service for problems related to the acquired immune deficiency syndrome (AIDS), by D. Miller, et al. GENITOURINARY MEDICINE 62(2): 116-122, April 1986.

Origin of AIDS: a deadly visitor from our biological past, by M. Whitby. LISTENER March 27, 1986, p. 7-8.

Origin of the human AIDS virus [letter], by R. C. Desrosiers. NATURE 319(6056): 728, Feburary 27-March 5, 1986; 319:728, February 27, 1986.

OTA critical of AIDS initiative, by C. Holden. SCIENCE 227(4691):1182-1183, March 8, 1985.

Other AIDS crisis: who pays for the treatment? WASHINGTON MONTHLY 17:25-31, January 1986.

Other factors to consider in infantile AIDS, by G. M. Shearer. NEW ENGLAND JOURNAL OF MEDICINE 311:189-191, July 19, 1984.

Otolaryngologic and head and neck manifestations of acquired immunodificiency syndrome (AIDS), by D. C. Marcusen, et al. LARYNGOSCOPE 95(4):401-405, April 1985.

Our first home care AIDS patient: Maria, by S. Brosnan. NURSING 16(9):37-39, September 1986.

Our fragile brothers, by J. P. Nieckarz. COMMONWEAL 112:404-406, July 12, 1985.

Outbreak of an acquired immunodeficiency syndrome associated with opportunistic infections and Kaposi's sarcoma in male homosexuals: an epidemic with forensic implications, by M. L. Taff, et al. AMERICAN JOURNAL OF FORENSIC MEDICINE AND PATHOLOGY 3(3):259-264, September 1982.

Outlook for AIDS bleak for remainder of year. JET 69:12, November 4, 1985.

Overview: acquired immune deficiency syndrome, by B. J. Cassens. PENNSYLVANIA MEDICINE 86(7):41-43, July 1983.

Overview of acquired immunodeficiency syndrome (AIDS)—the disease and related anesthetic considerations, by B. Sommer. AANA JOURNAL 51(4):381-384, August 1983.

Overview of clinical syndromes and immunology of AIDS, by A. S. Fauci, et al. TOPICS IN CLINICAL NURSING 6(2):12-18, July 1984.

Overview of the HTLV Symposium and reflections about the past, present, and future, by L. Gross. CANCER RESEARCH 45(Suppl. 9):4706s-4709s, September 1985.

Overview of infectious diseases and other nonmalignant conditions in the acquired immune deficiency syndrome, by D. F. Busch. FRONTIERS OF RADIATION THERAPY AND ONCOLOGY 19:52-58, 1985.

Overwhelming mycobacteriosis in an immunodeficient homosexual, by J. S. Waxman, et al. MOUNT SINAI JOURNAL OF MEDICINE 50(1):19-21, January-February 1983.

Oxford education to ward off AIDS, by M. Davie. OBSERVER June 15, 1986, p. 56.

Palm Spring Mayor protests AIDS hotel, by C. Love. ADVOCATE 4(7):12, November 13, 1984.

Panic, by O. Gillie, et al. SUNDAY TIMES February 24, 1985, p. 17-18.

Panic and prejudice-policy won't stop epidemic, by J. Jones. GUARDIAN 38(12):7, December 18, 1985.

Panic over AIDS, by M. Starr. NEWSWEEK 102:20-21, July 4, 1983.

Panorama/BBC1, by S. O'Sullivan. SPARE RIB 1(30):38, May 1983.

Paraproteinemia in patients with acquired immunodeficiency syndrome (AIDS) or lymphadenopathy syndrome (LAS), by K. Heriot, et al. CLINICAL CHEMISTRY 31(7): 1224-1226, July 1985.

Pardon my morality, by T. Stafford. CHRISTIANITY TODAY 30(9):17, June 13, 1986.

Parenterally administered acyclovir for viral retinitis associated with AIDS [letter], by J. A. Schulman, et al. ARCHIVES OF OPHTHALMOLOGY 102(12):1750, December 1984.

Parson cites AIDS/urges bar ban, by K. Orr. BODY POLITIC 97:11, October 1983.

Partial immune reconstitution in a patient with the acquired immunodeficiency syndrome, by H. C. Lane, et al. NEW ENGLAND JOURNAL OF MEDICINE 311(17): 1099-1103, October 25, 1984.

Partial restoration of impaired interleukin-2 production and Tac antigen (putative interleukin-2 receptor) expression in patients with acquired immune deficiency syndrome by isoprinosine treatment in vitro, by K. Y. Tsang, et al. JOURNAL OF CLINICAL INVESTIGATION 75(5):1538-1544, May 1985.

Parvovirus infection and the acquired immunodeficiency syndrome [letter], by M. J. Anderson, et al. ANNALS OF INTERNAL MEDICINE 102(2):275, February 1985.

Parvovirus infections: features reminiscent of AIDS, by M. E. Bloom. ANNALS OF THE NEW YORK ACADEMY OF SCIENCES 437:110-120, 1984.

Passive anal intercourse, by N. Fain. ADVOCATE 3(78):22, October 13, 1983.

Passive anal intercourse as a risk factor for AIDS in homosexual men [letter], by W. W. Darrow, et al. LANCET 2(8342):160, July 16, 1983.

Pastoral care and persons with AIDS. A means to alleviate physical, emotional, social, and spiritual suffering, by P. Murphy. AMERICAN JOURNAL OF HOSPICE CARE 3(2):38-40, March-April 1986.

Pat Buchanan's nasty nature, by P. Freiberg. ADVOCATE 3(73):18, August 4, 1983.

Patent battle of AIDS researchers, by D. Dickson. THE TIMES HIGHER EDUCATION SUPPLEMENT 673:12, September 27, 1985.

Patent dispute divides AIDS researchers [ELISA test], by C. Norman. SCIENCE 230: 640-642, November 8, 1985.

Patho-anatomical studies in patients dying of AIDS, by S. Lauland, et al. ACTA PA-THOLOGICA, MICROBIOLOGICA, ET IMMUNOLOGICA SCANDINAVICA 94(3): 201-221, May 1986.

Pathogenesis of the acquired immune deficiency syndrome (AIDS), by M. C. Heng. CUTIS 32(3):255-257, September 1983.

Pathogenesis of AIDS [letter], by J. Melov. MEDICAL JOURNAL OF AUSTRALIA 140(3):177-178, February 4, 1984.

Pathogenesis of B cell lymphoma in a patient with AIDS, by J. E. Groopman, et al. BLOOD 67(3):612-615, March 1986.

Pathogenesis of simian AIDS in rhesus macaques inoculated with the SRV-1 strain of type D retrovirus, by D. H. Maul, et al. AMERICAN JOURNAL OF VETERINARY RESEARCH 47:863-868, April 1986.

Pathogenic retrovirus—current facts and hypotheses, by E. Kazimierska. POLSKI TYGODNIK LEKARSKI 41(3):86-87, January 21, 1986.

Pathogenic retrovirus (HTLV-III) linked to AIDS, by S. Broder, et al. NEW ENGLAND JOURNAL OF MEDICINE 311(20):1292-1297, November 15, 1984.

Pathogens in children with severe combined immune deficiency disease or AIDS, by D. Lauzon, et al. CANADIAN MEDICAL ASSOCIATION JOURNAL 135(1):33-38, July 1, 1986.

Pathologic appraisal of the thymus gland in acquired immunodeficiency syndrome in children. A study of four cases and a review of the literature, by V. V. Joshi, et al. ARCHIVES OF PATHOLOGY AND LABORATORY MEDICINE 109(2):142-146, February 1985.

Pathologic features of AIDS encephalopathy in children: evidence for LAV/HTLV-III infection of brain, by L. R. Sharer, et al. HUMAN PATHOLOGY 17(3):271-284, March 1986.

Pathologic features of the lung in the acquired immune deficiency syndrome (AIDS): an autopsy study of seventeen homosexual males, by G. Nash, et al. AMERICAN JOURNAL OF CLINICAL PATHOLOGY 81(1):6-12, January 1984.

Pathologic pulmonary findings in children with the acquired immunodeficiency syn-drome: a study of ten cases, by V. V. Joshi, et al. HUMAN PATHOLOGY 16(3): 241-246, March 1985.

Pathologic-anatomic findings in acquired immunologic deficiency syndrome (AIDS), by M. Krause, et al. VASA 13(2):99-106, 1984.

Pathology of an epizootic of acquired immunodeficienycy in rhesus macaques, by K. G. Osborn, et al. AMERICAN JOURNAL OF PATHOLOGY 114(1):94-103, January 1984.

Pathology of suspected acquired immune deficiency syndrome in children: a study of eight cases, by V. V. Joshi, et al. PEDIATRIC PATHOLOGY 2(1):71-87, 1984.

Pathophysiologic aspects of lymphokines, by D. T. Boumpas, et al. CLINICAL IMMUNOLOGY REVIEWS 4(2):201-240, 1985.

Pathophysiology and clinical aspects of acquired immunologic deficiency syndrome (AIDS), by F. D. Goebel. OFFENTLICHE GESUNDHEITSWESEN 48(5):225-227, May 1986.

Patient with a mild form of the acquired immunodeficiency syndrome (AIDS), by P. Reiss, et al. NEDERLANDS TIJDSCHRIFT VOOR GENEESKUNDE 127(19): 824-825, May 7, 1983.

Patient with opportunistic infections due to acquired immunodeficiency syndrome, by C. S. de Graaff, et al. NEDERLANDS TIJDSCHRIFT VOOR GENEESKUNDE 128(12):549-553, March 24, 1984.

Patients at risk for AIDS-related opportunistic infection. Clinical manifestations and impaired gamma interferon production, by H. W. Murray, et al. NEW ENGLAND JOURNAL OF MEDICINE 313(24):1504-1510, December 12, 1985.

Patients' concerns about AIDS [letter], by B. Roberson, et al. JOURNAL OF THE AMERICAN DENTAL ASSOCIATION 112(2):162, 164, February 1986.

Patients of doctor with AIDS symptoms tested, by L. Famiglietti. AIR FORCE TIMES 46:3, January 20, 1986.

Patients with acquired immunodeficiency syndrome (AIDS) have peripheral blood lymphocytes expressing plasma-cell differentiation antigens, by G. J. Ruiz-Argüelles, et al. REVISTA DE INVESTIGACION CLINICA 36(2):99-101, April-June 1984.

PBS runs anti-black, anti-gay AIDS show, by B. Gelbert. GAY COMMUNITY NEWS 13(37):3, April 1, 1986.

Pediatric acquired immunodeficiency syndrome, by A. J. Ammann, et al. ANNALS OF THE NEW YORK ACADEMY OF SCIENCES 437:340-349, 1984.

Pediatric AIDS, by A. Rubinstein. CURRENT PROBLEMS IN PEDIATRICS 16(7): 361-409, July 1986.

Pediatric AIDS: a disease spectrum causally associated with HTLV-III infection, by W. P. Parks, et al. CANCER RESEARCH 45(Suppl. 9):4659s-4661s, September 1985.

Peer review: face to face with AIDS phobia, by C. Cox. NURSING TIMES 81(15):22, April 10-16, 1985.

Pentagon AIDS test that sparked furor. US NEWS & WORLD REPORT 99:12, September 9, 1985.

Pentagon delays policy on military blood donors, by Bisticas-Cocoves. GAY COMMUNITY NEWS 13(4):1, August 3, 1985.

Pentagon orders mass HTLV-III screening, by Bisticas-Cocoves. GAY COMMUNITY NEWS 13(18):1, November 16, 1985.

Pentagon reviews policy on tests for AIDS virus, by S. B. Young. AIR FORCE TIMES 47:8, October 13, 1986.

Pentamidine-induced hypoglycemia in patients with the acquired immune deficiency syndrome, by C. M. Stahl-Bayliss, et al. CLINICAL PHARMACOLOGY AND THERAPEUTICS 39(3):271-275, March 1986.

Pentamidine isethionate approved for P. Carinii pneumonia. FDA DRUG BULLETIN 14(3):25-26, December 1984.

Pentamidine methanesulfonate to be distributed by CDC. JAMA 251(20):2641, May 25, 1985; also in MMWR 33(17):225-226, May 4, 1984.

Pentamidine treatment of Pneumocystis carinii pneumonia in the acquired immuno-deficiency syndrome. Association with acute renal failure and myoglobinuria, by J. W. Sensakovic, et al. ARCHIVES OF INTERNAL MEDICINE 145(12):2247, December 1985.

People of color and AIDS: who's taking action, by Bisticas-Cocoves. GAY COMMUNITY NEWS 13(24):3, December 28, 1985.

People with AIDS honored at 70 vigils worldwide, by Bisticas-Cocoves. GAY COMMUNITY NEWS 13(45):1, June 7, 1986.

People with AIDS make presence felt, by N. Fain. ADVOCATE 3(72):11, July 21, 1983.

Percutaneous needle lung aspiration for diagnosing pneumonitis in the patient with acquired immunodeficiency syndrome (AIDS), by J. M. Wallace, et al. AMERICAN REVIEW OF RESPIRATORY DISEASE 131(3):389-392, March 1985.

Performing safe phlebotomy on AIDS patients, by S. A. Diffley. MLO 15(11):75-76, November 1983.

Perhaps his death will help us to realize, by C. Jackson. GAY COMMUNITY NEWS 13(47):5, June 21, 1986.

Perinatal AIDS. AMERICAN FAMILY PHYSICIAN 33:364+, February 1986.

Peripheral neuropathy of the inflammatory polyradiculoneuritis-type in immune disorders, evoking the acquired immunodeficiency syndrome [letter], by H. Dehen, et al. PRESSE MEDICALE 14(4):226, February 2, 1985.

Perivasculitis of the retinal vessels as an important sign in children with AIDS-related complex, by P. Kestelyn, et al. AMERICAN JOURNAL OF OPHTHALMOLOGY 100(4):614-1615, October 15, 1985.

Persistence of Pneumocystis carinii in lung tissue of acquired immunodeficiency syndrome patients treated for pneumocystis pneumonia, by J. H. Shelhamer, et al. AMERICAN REVIEW OF RESPIRATORY DISEASE 130(6):1161-1165, December 1984.

Persistence of Pneumosystis carinii pneumonia in the acquired immunodeficiency syndrome. Evaluation of therapy by follow-up transbronchial lung biopsy, by L. J. deLorenzo, et al. CHEST 88(1):79-83, July 1985.

223

Persistence of public health problems: SF, STD, and AIDS, by A. Yankauer. AMERI-CAN JOURNAL OF PUBLIC HEALTH 76:494-495, May 1986.

Persistent generalized adenopathies in subjects at high risk of AIDS. Diagnostic and prognostic value of lymph node lesion syndromes. Apropos of 8 cases, by D. Canioni, et al. ARCHIVES D'ANATOMIE ET DE CYTOLOGIE PATHOLOGIQUES 33(3):129-139, 1985.

Persistent generalized lymphadenopathy: immunological and mycological investi-gations, by J. Torssander, et al. ACTA DERMATO-VENEREOLOGICA 65(6): 515-520, 1985.

Persistent generalized lymphadenopathy: pre-AIDS. First description of a case ob-served in Italy, by G. B. Gabrielli, et al. MINERVA MEDICA 75(44):2653-2658, November 17, 1984.

Persistent infection of chimpanzees with human T-lymphotropic virus type III/lympha-denopathy-associated virus: a potential model for acquired immunodeficiency syndrome, by P. N. Fultz, et al. JOURNAL OF VIROLOGY 58(1):116-124, April 1986.

Persistent infection with human T-lymphotropic virus type III/lymphadenopathy-associated virus in apparently healthy homosexual men, by H. W. Jaffe, et al. ANNALS OF INTERNAL MEDICINE 102(5):627-628, May 1985.

Persistent lymphadenopathy in patients at risk of contracting acquired immune defi-ciency syndrome, by J. P. Clauvel, et al. EUROPEAN JOURNAL OF CLINICAL MICROBIOLOGY 3(1):72, February 1984.

Persistent noncytopathic infection of normal human T lymphocytes with AIDS-associated retrovirus, by J. A. Hoxie, et al. SCIENCE 229:1400-1402, Septem-ber 27, 1985.

Person behind the disease, by A. C. Crovella. NURSING 15(9):42, September 1985.

Personal experience with AIDS. Courageous patient shares his ordeal through news-paper, by L. M. Keen. AMERICAN JOURNAL OF HOSPICE CARE 3(2):10-16, March-April 1986.

Personal you: gay cancer isn't just gay anymore, by M. Horosko. DANCE MAGAZINE 57:72, February 1983.

Personal you update. DANCE MAGAZINE 58:88, February 1984.

Perspective on AIDS cases among health care workers, by R. S. Gordon. ANNALS OF THE NEW YORK ACADEMY OF SCIENCES 437:420, 1984.

Perspectives. Responses to the AIDS crisis. WASHINGTON REPORT ON MEDI-CINE AND HEALTH 39(41):Suppl. 4, October 21, 1985.

Perspectives on the future of AIDS, by T. C. Quinn. JAMA 253(2):247-249, January 1985.

Perspectives on the immunotherapy of AIDS, by J. W. Hadden. ANNALS OF THE NEW YORK ACADEMY OF SCIENCES 437:76-87, 1984.

Phagocytic and fungicidal activity of monocytes from patients with acquired immuno-deficiency syndrome [letter], by R. G. Washburn, et al. JOURNAL OF INFEC-TIOUS DISEASES 151(3):565-566, March 1985.

Phallusy of waiting for science to cure AIDS, by K. Barton. RFD 47:20, Summer 1986.

Pharyngeal obstruction by Kaposi's sarcoma in a homosexual male with acquired immune deficiency syndrome, by C. A. Patow, et al. OTOLARYNGOLOGY AND HEAD AND NECK SURGERY 92(6):713-716, December 1984.

Phenotypic and functional correlations in circulating lymphocytes of prodromal homosexuals and patients with AIDS, by P. H. Tsang, et al. JOURNAL OF CLINICAL AND LABORATORY IMMUNOLOGY 17(1):7-11, May 1985.

Phlegmonous gastritis associated with the acquired immunodeficiency syndrome/ pre-acquired immunodeficiency syndrome, by R. E. Mittleman, et al. ARCHIVES OF PATHOLOGY AND LABORATORY MEDICINE 109(8):765-767, August 1985.

Phone Company fires Boston PWA, by J. Kiely. GAY COMMUNITY NEWS 14(4):1, August 3, 1986.

PHS invites industry collaboration on AIDS vaccine, by D. M. Barnes. SCIENCE 233: 1034-1035, September 5, 1986.

PHS issues guidelines on AIDS testing and follow-up for positives. MLO 17(3):25-27, March 1985.

PHS projects dramatic rise in AIDS cases, by D. Walter. ADVOCATE 451:22, July 22, 1986.

PHS steps up activities and increases grant support to combat acquired immune deficiency syndrome. PUBLIC HEALTH REPORTS 97:589, November-December 1982.

Physician knowledge and concerns about AIDS, by E. Barrett-Connor. WESTERN JOURNAL OF MEDICINE 140(4):652-653, April 1984.

Physician surveillance and the AIDS crisis [editorial], by D. W. Fisher. HOSPITAL PRACTICE 20(9):8, September 15, 1985.

Physicians should report cases of acquired immune deficiency syndrome [editorial], by D. P. Drotman. ARCHIVES OF INTERNAL MEDICINE 143(12):2247, December 1983.

Physicians urge mandatory AIDS testing, by V. Kimble. AIR FORCE TIMES 47:8+, November 24, 1986.

Picking plays in AIDS research, by S. J. Smiurda. VENTURE 7:20, August 1985.

Pickle family's fool, by R. Hurwitt. CALIFORNIA 10:32+, February 1985.

Pigs provide clues about AIDS epidemic. SCIENCE DIGEST 91:30, August 1983.

Pilot study of surrogate tests to prevent transmission of acquired immune deficiency syndrome by transfusion, by T. L. Simon, et al. TRANSFUSION 24(5):373-378, September-October 1984.

Pinning down the psychosocial dimensions of AIDS, by S. Feinblum. NURSING AND HEALTH CARE 7(5):254-256, May 1986.

Pity the poor patient. NEW SCIENTIST 106:2, April 25, 1985.

Plague and panic, by R. Porter. NEW SOCIETY December 12, 1986, p. 11-13.

Plague in the shadows, by F. Bentayou. CLEVELAND MAGAZINE 14:90+, November 1985.

Plague on all their homes? THE ECONOMIST 297:27-28+, November 2, 1985.

Plague on homosexuals? THE ECONOMIST 294:16-17, March 2, 1985.

Plague years (I), by D. Black. ROLLING STONE March 28, 1985, p. 48-50+.

— (II), by D. Black. ROLLING STONE April 25, 1985, p. 35-36+.

Plagued by AIDS scare, by D. J. Dent. BLACK ENTERPRISE 14:24, December 1983.

Planning for the impact—AIDS, by I. Goldstone. RNABC NEWS 17(6):20, November-December 1985.

Planning for the neurologically impaired AIDS patient, by E. Barker. JOURNAL OF NEUROSCIENCE NURSING 18(5):241, October 1986.

Planning more research on AIDS, by J. Maddox. NATURE 303(5916):377, June 2, 1983.

Plans underway for blood test, by C. Guilfoy. GAY COMMUNITY NEWS 12(36):7, March 30, 1985.

Plasma products withdrawn after donor dies of AIDS. AMERICAN FAMILY PHYSICIAN 28:18, December 1983.

Plasmacytoma and the acquired immunodeficiency syndrome, by A. M. Israel, et al. ANNALS OF INTERNAL MEDICINE 99(5):635-636, November 1983.

Plasmapheresis increases T4 lymphocytes in a patient with AIDS, by R. H. Tomar, et al. AMERICAN JOURNAL OF CLINICAL PATHOLOGY 81(4):518-521, April 1984.

Playing gay, by H. Johnson. US 3:55+, November 18, 1985.

Pneumocystis carinii infection in a homosexual adult subject with immunodeficiency : apropos of a case, by F. L. Goncales Júnior, et al. REVISTA PAULISTA DE MEDICINA 101(4):160-164, July-August 1983.

Pneumocystis carinii: a misunderstood opportunist, by L. L. Pifer. EUROPEAN JOURNAL OF CLINICAL MICROBIOLOGY 3(3):169-173, June 1984.

Pneumocystis carinii pneumonia, by C. B. Wofsy. FRONTIERS OF RADIATION THERAPY AND ONCOLOGY 19:74-81, 1985.

Pneumocystis carinii pneumonia and disseminated cytomegalovirus infection in previously healthy bisexual man, by G. F. Ragalie, et al. WISCONSIN MEDICAL JOURNAL 82(11):10-14, November 1983.

Pneumocystis carinii pneumonia: a comparison between patients with the acquired immunodeficiency syndrome and patients with other immunodeficiencies, by J. A. Kovacs, et al. ANNALS OF INTERNAL MEDICINE 100(5):663-6672, May 1984.

Pneumocystis carinii pneumonia in homosexual males with AIDS, by L. Bergmann, et al. PRAXIS UND KLINIK DER PNEUMOLOGIE 37(Suppl. 1):1035-1038, October 1983.

Pneumocystis carinii pneumonia in the patient with AIDS, by J. R. Catterall, et al. CHEST 88(5):758-762, November 1985.

Pneumocystis carinii pneumonia treated with alpha-difluoromethylornithine. A prospective study among patients with the acquired immunodeficiency syndrome, by J. A. Golden, et al. WESTERN JOURNAL OF MEDICINE 141(5):613-623, November 1984.

Pneumocystis pneumonia and disseminated toxoplasmosis in a male homosexual, by W. R. Gransden, et al. BRITISH MEDICAL JOURNAL 286(6378):1614, May 21, 1983.

Pneumocystis pneumonia as an expression of acquired immune deficiency (AIDS) in homosexual men, by P. Stark, et al. PRAXIS UND KLINIK DER PNEUMOLOGIE 38(1):26-28, January 1984.

Pneumocystis with normal chest X-ray film and arterial oxygen tension. Early diagnosis in a patient with the acquired immune deficiency syndrome, by J. L. Goodman, et al. ARCHIVES OF INTERNAL MEDICINE 143(10):1981-1982, October 1983.

Pneumonia due to Pneumocystis carinii in AIDS patients, by V. G. Pereira, et al. REVISTA DO HOSPITAL DAS CLINICAS; FACULDADE DE MEDICINA DA UNIVERSIDADE DE SAO PAULO 39(3):123-125, May-June 1984.

Pneumonia in the acquired immune deficiency syndrome [editorial], by N. M. Johnson. BRITISH MEDICAL JOURNAL 290(678):1299-1301, May 4, 1985.

Pneumonia in AIDS patients. AMERICAN FAMILY PHYSICIAN 33:266, January 1986.

Pneumosystis carinii pneumonia in the acquired immunodeficiency syndrome (AIDS). Diagnosis with bronchial brushings, biopsy, and bronchoalveolar lavage, by B. Hartman, et al. CHEST 87(5):603-607, May 1985.

Pneumosystis carinii pneumonia in the acquired immune deficiency syndrome: response to inadvertent steroid therapy, by d. K. MacFadden, et al. CANADIAN MEDICAL ASSOCIATION JOURNAL 132(10):1161-1163, May 15, 1985.

Podiatric implications of acquired immunodeficiency syndrome, by C. Abramson. JOURNAL OF THE AMERICAN PODIATRIC MEDICAL ASSOCIATION 76(3):124-136, March 1986.

Pointer to AIDS diagnosis found. CHEMICAL INDUSTRY 8:276, April 16, 1984.

Poland—out of sight, out of mind, by Darski, et al. BODY POLITIC 12:21, April 1986.

Police, court officials arraign AIDS victim in Rhode Island jail cell. CORRECTIONS DIGEST 16(26):5, December 18, 1985.

—. CRIME CONTROL DIGEST 20(1):3-4, January 6, 1986.

Political consequences of AIDS, by Fowler, et al. SOCIALIST WORKER 76:5, August 1983.

Political medicine [editorial]. GUARDIAN 37(42):22, August 21, 1985.

Political posturing over AIDS, by L. Bush. ADVOCATE 3(74):20, August 18, 1983.

Politics and science clash on African AIDS, by C. Norman. SCIENCE 230:1140+, December 6, 1985.

Politics and test of AIDS, by S. Norman. RFD 44:53, Fall 1985.

Politics of AIDS, by F. Barnes. THE NEW REPUBLIC 193:11-12+, November 4, 1985.

—, by L. Van Gelder. MS 11(11):103, May 1983.

—, by Payne, et al. SCIENCE FOR THE PEOPLE 16(5):17, September 1984.

Politics of AIDS in prison, by E. Mead. GAY COMMUNITY NEWS 13(25):5, January 11, 1986.

Politics of AIDS—a tale of two states [Texas and Montana], by A. Trafford, et al. US NEWS & WORLD REPORT 99(21):70-71, November 18, 1985.

Politics of disease, by R. Kaye. ADVOCATE 441:52, March 4, 1986.

Politics of an epidemic, by K. Kelley. GUARDIAN 35(32):1, May 11, 1983.

Politics of a plague, by C. Krauthammer. THE NEW REPUBLIC 189:18-21, August 1, 1983.

Pols, actors, art crowd help gays fight AIDS, by H. Hanson. CHICAGO 34:18, July 1985.

Polymicrobial cholangitis and Kaposi's sarcoma in blood product transfusion-related acquired immune deficiency syndrome, by f. R. Cockerill, 3d, et al. AMERICAN JOURNAL OF MEDICINE 80(6):1237-1241, June 1986.

Positive direct antiglobulin test associated with hyperglobulinemia in acquired immunodeficiency syndrome (AIDS), by P. T. Toy, et al. AMERICAN JOURNAL OF HEMATOLOGY 19(2):145-150, June 1985.

Possible AIDS cure, by K. Scanlon. MACLEAN'S 99:46, March 24, 1986.

Possible AIDS remedy tested, by L. Goldsmith. GAY COMMUNITY NEWS 11(3):1, July 30, 1983.

Possible AIDS transmission is concern to nurses. AMERICAN FAMILY PHYSICIAN 28:17, July 1983.

Possible cause of acquired immune deficiency syndrome (AIDS) and other new diseases,by R. de Long. MEDICAL HYPOTHESES 13(4):395-397, April 1984.

Possible cure for crytosporidiosis . . . spiramycin. EMERGENCY MEDICINE 16(14): 115-116, August 15, 1984.

Possible genetic susceptibility to the acquired immunodeficiency syndrome in hemophiliacs [letter], by L. Jacob, et al. ANNALS OF INTERNAL MEDICINE 104(1): 130, January 1986.

Possible origin of human AIDS [letter], by P. K. Lewin. CANADIAN MEDICAL ASSOCIATION JOURNAL 132(10):1110, May 15, 1985.

—,by I. D. Mackie, et al. CANADIAN MEDICAL ASSOCIATION JOURNAL 133(6):547-548, September 15, 1985.

Possible risk of steroid administration in patients at risk for AIDS [letter], by R. W. Shafer, et al. LANCET 1(8434):934-935, April 20, 1985.

Possible role of a new lymphotropic retrovirus (LAV) in the pathogeny of AIDS and AIDS-related diseases, by F. Brun-Vezinet, et al. PROGRESS IN MEDICAL VIROLOGY 32:189-194, 1985.

Possible transfusion-associated acquired immune deficiency syndrome (AIDS)—California. MMWR 31(48):652-654, December 10, 1982.

Possible transmission of a human lymphotropic retrovirus (LAV) from mother to infant with AIDS [letter], by E. Vilmer, et al. LANCET 2(8396):229-230, July 28, 1984.

Possible viral interactions in the acquired immunodeficiency syndrome (AIDS), by M. S. Hirsch, et al. REVIEWS OF INFECTIOUS DISEASES 6(5):726-731, September-October 1984.

Possible viral link to AIDS, by L. Goldsmith. GAY COMMUNITY NEWS 11(9):1, September 17, 1983.

Post-transcriptional regulation accounts for the transactivation of the human T-lymphotrophic virus type III, by C. A. Rosen, et al. NATURE 319:555-559, February 13, 1986.

Post-transfusion AIDS outside of hemophilia: facts, questions and commentary, by B. Habibi. REVUE FRANCAISE DE TRANSFUSION ET IMMUNOHEMATOLOGIE 27(4):497-507, September 1984.

Postnatal transmission of AIDS-associated retrovirus from mother to infant, by J. B. Ziegler, et al. LANCET 1(8434):896-898, April 20, 1985.

Potential check on heterosexual transmission of AIDS [letter], by A. Comfort. JOURNAL OF THE ROYAL SOCIETY OF MEDICINE 78(11):969-970, November 1985.

Potential for transmission of AIDS-associated retrovirus from bisexual men in San Francisco to their female sexual contacts, by W. Winkelstein, Jr., et al. JAMA 255:901, February 21, 1986.

Potential liability for transfusion-associated AIDS, by P. J. Miller, et al. JAMA 253(23):3419-3424, June 21, 1985.

Poverty's harvest: AIDS, by J. Murphy. GUARDIAN 38(15):1, January 15, 1986.

Power to shut bathhouses voted by House, by Bisticas-Cocoves. GAY COMMUNITY NEWS 13(14):1, October 19, 1985.

Practitioner and AIDS, by M. B. Gregg. JOURNAL OF THE MEDICAL ASSOCIATION OF GEORGIA 73(8):555-556, August 1984.

Pre-AIDS in a child of a drug-addict. Clinical and laboratory description, by D. Pavesio, et al. MINERVA PEDATRICA 37(1-2):73-74, January 31, 1985.

Pre-AIDS patients will get experimental drug, by S. Burke. OUT 3(4):2, February 1985.

Preaching to the infected, by M. Jones. SUNDAY TIMES December 14, 1986, p. 25.

Precautions against acquired immunodeficiency syndrome [editorial]. LANCET 1(8317):164, January 22, 1983.

Precautions against transmittable disease, By K. S. Kawala. ILLINOIS MEDICAL JOURNAL 166(6):387, December 1984.

Precautions for the home care of patients with AIDS. CANADIAN MEDICAL ASSOCIATION JOURNAL 134(1):51+, January 1, 1986.

Precautions for patients hopitalized with acquired immunodeficiency syndrome [editorial],by T. C. Quinn. INFECTION CONTROL 4(2):79-80, March-April 1983.

Precautions in care of patients with the acquired immunodeficiency syndrome [letter],by D. W. Blayney. ANNALS OF INTERNAL MEDICINE 101(2):275, August 1984.

Precautions prevent transmission of HTLV-III virus, by J. Prescott. TEXAS HOSPITALS 41(11):16-17, April 1986.

Precautions recommended in treating patients with AIDS [letter],by J. R. Masci, et al. NEW ENGLAND JOURNAL OF MEDICINE 308(3):156, January 20, 1983.

Precipitable immune complexes in healthy homosexual men, acquired immune deficiency syndrome and the related lymphadenopathy syndrome, by H. H. Euler, et al. CLINICAL AND EXPERIMENTAL IMMUNOLOGY 59(2):267-275, February 1985.

Preclinical determination of AIDS disease by a series of tests [letter], by R. B. Bhalla, et al. CLINICAL CHEMISTRY 32(7):1426-1427, July 1986.

Precoccious thymic involution manifest by epithelial injury in the acquired immune deficiency syndrome, by T. A. Seemayer, et al. HUMAN PATHOLOGY 15(5):469-474, May 1984.

Preferences of homosexual men with AIDS for life-sustaining treatment, by R. Steinbrook, et al. NEW ENGLAND JOURNAL OF MEDICINE 314:457-460, February 13, 1986.

Preliminary clinical observations with recombinant interleukin-2 in patients with AIDS or LAS, by P. Kern, et al. BLUT 50(1):1-6, 1985.

Preliminary results on clinical and immunological effects of thymopentin in AIDS, by N. Clumeck, et al. INTERNATIONAL JOURNAL OF CLINICAL PHARMACOLOGICAL RESEARCH 4(6):459-463, 1984.

Preparing for the worst in Halifax, by R. Metcalf. BODY POLITIC 118:19, September 1985.

Presence of AIDS victims poses no risk to others on campuses, committee says, by L. Biemiller. CHRONICLE OF HIGHER EDUCATION 31:25-26, December 11, 1985.

Presence of antibodies to human lymphoma-leukemia virus (HTLV-I) in Germans with symptoms of the acquired immunodeficiency syndrome (AIDS), by M. Born, et al. JOURNAL OF MEDICAL VIROLOGY 15(1):57-63, January 1985.

Presence of antibodies to the human T-cell leukemia virus HTLV I in German patients with symptoms of AIDS, by D. Wernicke, et al. HAMATOLOGIE UND BLUT-TRANSFUSION 29:338-341, 1985.

Presence of immunoglobulin D in endocrine disorders and diseases of immunoregulation, including the acquired immunodeficiency syndrome, by N. M. Papadopoulos, et al. CLINICAL IMMUNOLOGY AND IMMUNOPATHOLOGY 32(2):248-252,
August 1984.

Presence of ultrastructural markers of AIDS in rectal biopsies at the early stage of the
disease [letter], by C. Leport, et al. GASTROENTEROLOGIE CLINIQUE ET BI-
OLOGIQUE 8(12):983-984, December 1984.

Presence of viral antibodies to the human lymphoma-leukemia virus in patients with
acquired immune deficiency syndrome, by M. Born, et al. EUROPEAN
JOURNAL OF CLINICAL MICROBIOLOGY 3(1):77-78, February 1984.

President's 1987 budget request. ADAMHA NEWS 12(3):1+, March 1986.

Prevalence, clinical manifestations, and immunology of herpesvirus infections in the
acquired immunodeficiency syndrome, by G. V. Quinnan, Jr., et al. ANNALS OF
THE NEW YORK ACADEMY OF SCIENCES 437:200-206, 1984.

Prevalence of AIDS-associated retrovirus and antibodies among male homosexuals at
risk for AIDS in Greenwich Village, by D. Casareale, et al. AIDS RESEARCH 1(5):
407-421, 1984-1985.

Prevalence of antibodies against HTLV-III in various regions in Switzerland, by J.
Schüpbach, et al. SCHWEIZERISCHE MEDIZINISCHE WOCHENSCHRIFT
115(30):1048-1054, July 27, 1985.

Prevalence of antibodies to AIDS-associated retrovirus in single men in San Francisco
[letter], by R. E. Anderson, et al. LANCET 1(8422):217, January 26, 1985.

Prevalence of antibodies to HTLV-III in AIDS risk groups in West Germany, by V. Erfle,
et al. CANCER RESEARCH 45(Suppl. 9):4627s-4629s, September 1985.

Prevalence of antibodies to lymphadenopathy-associated retrovirus in African patients with AIDS, by F. Brun-Vézinet, et al. SCIENCE 226(4673):453-456, October 26, 1984.

Prevalence of antibody to human T-lymphotropic virus type III in AIDS and AIDS-risk
patients in Britain,by R. Cheingsong-Popov, et al. LANCET 2(8401):477-480,
September 1, 1984.

Prevalence of antibody to LAV/HTLV-III among homosexual men in Seattle, by A. C.
Collier, et al. AMERICAN JOURNAL OF PUBLIC HEALTH 76:564-565, May
1986.

Prevalence of HTLV-III antibodies in homosexual men in Johannesburg [letter], by R.
Sher, et al. SOUTH AFRICAN MEDICAL JOURNAL 67(13):484, March 30, 1985.

Prevalence of HTLV-III antibody in American blood donors, by J. B. Schoor, et al.
NEW ENGLAND JOURNAL OF MEDICINE 313:384, August 8, 1985.

Prevalence of HTLV-III infection among New Haven, Connecticut, parenteral drug
abusers in 1982-1983, by R. D'Aquila, et al. NEW ENGLAND JOURNAL OF
MEDICINE 314:117-118, January 9, 1986.

Prevalence of HTLV-III infection in London. AMERICAN FAMILY PHYSICIAN 33:306,
February 1986.

Prevalence of HTLV-III/LAV antibodies among intravenous drug users attending treatment programs in California: a preliminary report, by N. Levy, et al. NEW ENGLAND JOURNAL OF MEDICINE 314:446, February 13, 1986.

Prevalence of HTLV-III/LAV in household contacts of patients with confirmed AIDS and controls in Kinshasa, Zaire, by J. M. Mann, et al. JAMA 256(6):721-724, August 8, 1986.

Prevalence of infection caused by AIDS and hepatitis B viruses in jailed people, by P. Crovari, et al. BOLLETTINO DELL ISTITUTO SIEROTERAPICO MILANESE 64(5):367-370, 1985.

Prevalence of Kaposi's sarcoma among patients with AIDS [letter], by H. W. Haverkos, et al. NEW ENGLAND JOURNAL OF MEDICINE 312(23):1518, June 6,1985.

Prevalence of neurologic abnormalities in AIDS patients. AMERICAN FAMILY PHYSICIAN 31:158, January 1985.

Preventing the acquired immunodeficiency syndrome [letter],by L. A. Hassell. NEW ENGLAND JOURNAL OF MEDICINE 309(22):1395, December 1, 1983.

Preventing AIDS transmission: should blood donors be screened? , by W. A. Check. JAMA 249(5):567-570, February 4, 1983.

Preventing the spread of AIDS [letter], by R. F. Wykoff. JAMA 255(13):1706-1707, April 4, 1986.

Prevention of acquired immune deficiency syndrome (AIDS): report of inter-agency recommendations. CONNECTICUT MEDICINE 47(6):361-362, June 1983; also in JAMA 249 (12)1544-1555, March 25, 1983 and MMWR 32(8):101-103, March 4, 1983.

Prevention of acquired immunodeficiency syndrome [letter], by A. E. Pitchenick, et al. ANNALS OF INTERNAL MEDICINE 98(4):558-559, April 1983.

Prevention of AIDS [letter]. LANCET 2(8468):1362-1363, December 14, 1985.

Prevention of AIDS by modifying sexual behavior, by D. C. William. ANNALS OF THE NEW YORK ACADEMY OF SCIENCES 437:283-285, 1984.

Prevention of HTLV-III infection [letter],by P. R. Gustafson. JAMA 256(3):346-347, July 18, 1986.

Prevention of in-hospital transmission of the acquired immune deficiency syndrome virus (HTLV III): current USA policy, by F. S. Rhame. JOURNAL OF HOSPITAL INFECTION 6(Suppl. C):53-66, December 1985.

Preventive measures against HTLV-III/LAV infections among hemophiliacs and their relatives, by S. A. Evensen, et al. TIDSSKRIFT FOR DEN NORSKE LAEGEFORENING 106(1):19-21, January 10, 1986.

Price of AIDS, by S. Meyer. MIAMI /SOUTH FLORIDA MAGAZINE January 26, 1986.

Priest urges bishops: support work of Christ, by Peter Hebblethwaite. NATIONAL CATHOLIC REPORTER 23:7, November 14, 1986.

Priests AIDS deaths: shame, fear, compassion. NATIONAL CATHOLIC REPORTER 23:23-26, December 12, 1986.

Primary Addison's disease in a patient with the acquired immunodeficiency syndrome by E E. Guenthner, et al. ANNALS OF INTERNAL MEDICINE 100(6):847-848, June 1984.

Primary lymph node pathology in AIDS and AIDS-related lymphadenopathy, by E. P. Ewing, Jr., et al. ARCHIVES OF PATHOLOGY AND LABORATORY MEDICINE 109(11):977-981, November 1985.

Primary lymphoma of the brain associated with AIDS. A study of one case, by M. J. Payan, et al. ACTA NEUROPATHOLOGICA 64(1):78-80, 1984.

Primary lymphoma of the nervous system associated with acquired immune-deficiency syndrome [letter],by W. D. Snider, et al. NEW ENGLAND JOURNAL OF MEDICINE 308(1):45, January 6, 1983.

Primary malignant lymphoma of the brain in acquired immune deficiency syndrome [letter], by C. V. Reyes. ACTA CYTOLOGICA 29(1):85-86, January-February 1985.

Prime time for instant monogamy, by A. Duncan. TIMES December 1, 1986, p. 15.

Principal muco-cutaneous aspects encountered in AIDS, by O. Picard, et al. REVUE FRANCAISE DE TRANSFUSION ET IMMUNOHEMATOLOGIE 27(4):427-436, September 1984.

Prisoner with AIDS: double isolation, by E. Bubbenmayer. GAY COMMUNITY NEWS 13(25):5, January 11, 1986.

Privacy provision signed into law. OUT 3(10):1, August 1985.

Pro and con: should AIDS victims be isolated? [interview]. U.S. NEWS & WORLD REPORT 99(14):50, September 30, 1985.

Probable cause of AIDS identified. BIOSCIENCE 34:413, July-August 1984.

Problem of Kaposi's sarcoma in AIDS, by P. A. Volberding. FRONTIERS OF RADIATION THERAPY AND ONCOLOGY 19:91-98, 1985.

Problems in the therapy of AIDS-associated malignancies, by R. E. Wittes, et al. ANNALS OF THE NEW YORK ACADEMY OF SCIENCES 437:454-460, 1984.

Problems raised by the treatment of Kaposi's sarcoma in subjects with AIDS, by H. Félix, et al. BULLETIN DE LA SOCIETE DE PATHOLOGIE EXOTIQUE ET DE SES FILLIALES 77(4, Part 2):592-598, 1984.

Problems with Hepatitis B and HTLV III infections in hospital, by D. C. Shanson. JOURNAL OF STERILE SERVICE MANAGEMENT? 3(3):29-30, October 1985.

Prodromal acquired immune deficiency syndrome in Australian homosexual men, by C. I. Smith, et al. MEDICAL JOURNAL OF AUSTRALIA 1(12):561-563, June 11, 1983.

Prodromal syndromes in AIDS, by U. Mathur-Wagh, et al. ANNALS OF THE NEW YORK ACADEMY OF SCIENCES 437:184-191, 1984.

Prodrome, Kaposi sarcoma, and infections associated with acquired immunodeficiency syndrome: radiologic findings in 39 patients, by C. A. Hill, et al. RADIOLOGY 149(2):383-399, November 1983.

Professional demands, human frailties. Doctors respond to AIDS, by C. Wiebe. NEW PHYSICIAN 35(1):14-17+, January-February 1986.

Prognosis of Pneumocystis carinii pneumonia in the acquired immunodeficiency syndrome [letter], by M. J. Rosen, et al. ANNALS OF INTERNAL MEDICINE 101(2);276, August 1984.

Prognostic value of histopathology in persistent generalized lymphadenopathy in homosexual men [letter], by R. Fernandez, et al. NEW ENGLAND JOURNAL OF MEDICINE 309(3):185-186, July 21, 1983.

Prognostically significant classification of immune changes in AIDS with Kaposi's sarcoma, by J. Taylor, et al. BLOOD 67(3):666-671, March 1986.

Progress at last. THE ECONOMIST 291:40, April 28, 1984.

Progress, but bleak prospects. BODY POLITIC 115:23, June 1985.

Progress on AIDS. FDA DRUG BULLETIN 15(3):27-32, October 1985.

Progress toward the 1990 objectives for sexually transmitted diseases: good news and bad, by W. C. Parra, et al. PUBLIC HEALTH REPORTS 100(3):261-269, May-June 1985.

Progressive encephalopathy in children with acquired immune deficiency syndrome, by L. G. Epstein, et al. ANNALS OF NEUROLOGY 17(5):488-496, May 1985.

Progressive multifocal leukoencephalopathy in acquired immune deficiency syndrome, by L. W. Blum, et al. ARCHIVES OF NEUROLOGY 42(2):137-139, February 1985.

— [letter], by J. Bedri, et al. NEW ENGLAND JOURNAL OF MEDICINE 309(8):492-493, August 25, 1983.

Progressive multifocal leukoencephalopathy in a case of acquired immune deficiency syndrome, by J. D. Speelman, et al. CLINICAL NEUROLOGY AND NEUROSURGERY 87(1):27-33, 1985.

Progressive multifocal leukoencephalopathy in a patient with acquired immune deficiency syndrome, by C. Bernick, et al. ARCHIVES OF NEUROLOGY 41(7):780-782, July 1984.

—, by M. Morente Gallego, et al. MEDICINA CLINICA 83(16):680-682, November 17, 1984.

Progressive multifocal leukoencephalopathy occurring with the acquired immune deficiency syndrome, by J. D. England, et al. SOUTHERN MEDICAL JOURNAL 77(8):1041-1043, August 1984.

Proliferation of accessory cells in LAS and AIDS [letter], by H. Müller, et al. DEUTSCHE MEDIZINISCHE WOCHENSCHRIFT 111(7):278, February 14, 1986.

Prolonged incubation period of AIDS in intravenous drug abusers: epidemiological evidence in prison inmates, by J. P. Hanrahan, et al. JOURNAL OF INFECTIOUS DISEASES 150(2):263-266, August 1984.

Promise of AIDS, by R. Teitelman. FORBES 134:302+, November 19, 1984.

Promising results halt trial of anti-AIDS drug, by D. M. Barnes. SCIENCE 234:15-16, October 3, 1986.

Promising treatment, by N. Underwood. MACLEAN'S 99:58, October 13, 1986.

Prophylactic lover, by R. Bebout. BODY POLITIC 126:25, May 1986.

Prophylaxis of Pneumocystis carinii infection in AIDS with pyrimethamine-sulfadoxine [letter], by M. S. Gottlieb, et al. LANCET 2(8399):398-399, August 18, 1984.

Proposals for the prevention and control of AIDS by the Public Health Department, by G. Jantzen. OFFENTLICHE GESUNDHEITSWESEN 45(10):544-545, October 1983.

Proposed government AIDS list draws fire, by S. Kulieke. ADVOCATE 404:14, October 2,1 984.

Prospective evaluation of health-care workers exposed via parenteral or mucous-membrane routes to blood and body fluids of patients with acquired immuno-deficiency syndrome. JAMA 251(16):2071+, April 27, 1984; also in MMWR 33(13):181-182, April 6, 1984.

Prospective observations of viral and immunologic abnormalities in homosexual males, by M. Lange, et al. ANNALS OF THE NEW YORK ACADEMY OF SCI-ENCES 437:350-363, 1984.

Prospective study of the ophthalmologic findings in the acquired immune deficiency syndrome, by W. R. Freeman, et al. AMERICAN JOURNAL OF OPHTHALMOLO-GY 97(2):133-142, February 1984.

Prospective study of the ophthalmologic findings in the acquired immune deficien-cy syndrome in Africa, by P. Kestelyn, et al. AMERICAN JOURNAL OF OPH-THALMOLOGY 100(2):230-238, August 15, 1985.

Prospects for and pathways toward a vaccine for AIDS, by D. P. Francis, et al. NEW ENGLAND JOURNAL OF MEDICINE 313(25):1586-1590, December 19, 1985.

Prospects for treatment of human retrovirus-associated diseases, by D. P. Bolognesi, et al. CANCER RESEARCH 45(Suppl. 9):4700s-4705s, September 1985.

Prospects of therapy for infections with human T-lymphotropic virus type III, by M. S. Hirsch, et al. ANNALS OF INTERNAL MEDICINE 103(5):750-755, November 1985.

Prostitutes taking the heat for the AIDS, by A. Phibbs. GAY COMMUNITY NEWS 13(36):3, March 29, 1986.

Protect yourself against AIDS, CDC urges. RN 46:11, February 1983.

Protecting against A.I.D.S. NURSING 14:22, December 1984.

Protecting the health care worker . . . AIDS, by A. Beaufoy, et al. RNABC NEWS 17(6):18-19, November-December 1985.

Protecting New Yorkers' health: an interview with NY Health Commissioner Dr. David Axelrod. EMPIRE STATE REPORT 11:9-10+, August 1985.

Protecting ourselves against AIDS, by R. Rodale. PREVENTION 37:17-18+, Decem-ber 1985.

Protection money , by L. Gubernick. FORBES 136:216, November 4, 1985.

Protection of T cells against infectivity and cytopathic effect of GTLV-III in vitro, by H. Mitsuya, et al. INTERNATIONAL SYMPOSIUM OF THE PRINCESS TAKAMATSU CANCER RESEARCH FUND 15:277-288, 1984.

Proviral DNA of a retrovirus, human T-cell leukemia virus, in two patients with AIDS, by E. P. Gelmann, et al. SCIENCE 220(4599):862-865, May 20, 1983.

Provisional Public Health Service inter-agency recommendations for screening donated blood and plasma for antibody to the virus causing acquired immunodeficiency syndrome. MMWR 34(1):1-5, January 11, 1985.

Pseudo-AIDS [letter],by D. A. Walker, et al. LANCET 2(8345):344, August 6, 1983.

Pseudo-AIDS syndrome following from fear of AIDS, by D. Miller, et al. BRITISH JOURNAL OF PSYCHIATRY 146:550-551, May 1985.

Pseudomembranous necrotizing bronchial aspergillosis. A variant of invasive aspergillosis in a patient with hemophilia and acquired immune deficiency syndrome, by N. K. Pervez, et al. AMERICAN REVIEW OF RESPIRATORY DISEASE 131(6): 961-963, June 1985.

Psoriasis in acquired immunodeficiency syndrome—new aspects for an immunopathogenesis of psoriasis, by G. K. Steigleder, et al. ZEITSCHRIFT FUR HAUTKRANKHEITEN 60(24):1913-1914, December 15, 1985.

Psychiatric aspects of AIDS, by R. Zumbrunnen, et al. SCHWEIZERISCHE RUNDSCHAU FUER MEDIZIN PRAXIS 73(43):1311-1312, October 23, 1984.

—, by S. E. Nichols, Jr. PSCHOSOMATICS 24(12):1083-1089, December 1983.

Psychiatric problems of AIDS inpatients at the New York Hospital: preliminary report, by S. W. Perry, et al. PUBLIC HEALTH REPORTS 99(2):200-205, 1984.

Psychiatric staff response to acquired immune deficiency syndrome, by M. A. Cummings, et al. AMERICAN JOURNAL OF PSYCHIATRY 143:682, May 1986.

Psychic channel on AIDS, by J Ferguson. RFD 45:48, Winter 1985.

Psycho nursing care of AIDS victims, by M. Fiske. CHART 83(5):+, May-June 1986.

Psychological factors associated with AIDS under study. PUBLIC HEALTH REPORTS 100(3):345, May-June 1985.

Psychological impact of AIDS on gay men, by S. F. Morin, et al. AMERICAN PSYCHOLOGIST 39(11):1288-1293, November 1984.

Psychological impact of AIDS on primary care physicians [letter],by L. McKusick, et al. WESTERN JOURNAL OF MEDICINE 144(6):751-752, June 1986.

Psychological support and counseling for patients with acquired immune deficiency syndrome (AIDS), by D. Miller, et al. GENITOURINARY MEDICINE 61(4):273-278, August 1985.

Psychological themes in patients with acquired immune deficiency syndrome [letter], by L. R. Hays, et al. AMERICAN JOURNAL OF PSYCHIATRY 143(4):551, April 1986.

Psychopathology complicating acquired immune deficiency syndrome (AIDS), by H. G. Nurnberg, et al. AMERICAN JOURNAL OF PSYCHIATRY 141(1):95-96, January 1984.

236

Psychosocial and ethical issues of AIDS health care programs, by D. G. Ostrow, et al. QRB. QUALITY REVIEW BULLETIN 12(8):284-294, August 1986.

Psychosocial and neuropsychiatric sequelae of the acquired immunodeficiency syndrome and related disorders, by J. C. Holland, et al. ANNALS OF INTERNAL MEDICINE 103(5):760-764, November 1985.

Psychosocial aspects of AIDS and AIDS-related complex: a pilot study, by J. N. Donlou, et al. JOURNAL OF PSYCHOSOCIAL ONCOLOGY 3(2):39-55, Summer 1985.

Psychosocial aspects of hospice care for AIDS patients. Addressing these issues is a key aspect of treatment, by K. Schoen. AMERICAN JOURNAL OF HOSPICE CARE 3(2):32-34, March-April 1986.

Psychosocial care team for patients with AIDS in a municipal hospital [letter], by F. Rosner, et al. JAMA 23(16):2361, April 26, 1985.

Psychosocial impact of acquired immune deficiency syndrome [letter], by H. Holtz, et al. JAMA 250(2):167, July 8, 1983.

Psychosocial impact of the acquired immunodeficiency syndrome, by M. Forstein. SEMINARS IN ONCOLOGY 11(1):77-82, March 1984.

Psychosocial impact of AIDS, by D. R. Rubinow. TOPICS IN CLINICAL NURSING 6(2): 26-30, July 1984.

Psychosocial issues for people with AIDS, by d. W. Smith, et al. JOURNAL OF THE MEDICAL ASSOCIATION OF GEORGIA 73(8):535-536, August 1984.

Psychosocial reactions of persons with the acquired immunodeficiency syndrome, by S. E. Nichols. ANNALS OF INTERNAL MEDICINE 103(5):765-767, November 1, 1985.

Psychosocial research is essential to understanding and treating AIDS, by T. J. Coates, et al. AMERICAN PSYCHOLOGIST 39(11):1309-1314, November 1984.

Public attitudes toward the control of AIDS: the homosexual's plight, by P. Ottenberg. TRANSACTIONS AND STUDIES OF THE COLLEGE OF PHYSICIANS OF PHILADELPHIA 8(2):113-119, June 1986.

Public education on AIDS: not only the media's responsiblity, by W. Check. HASTINGS CENTER REPORT 15(4):27-31, August 1985.

Public funding increased to halt spread of AIDS, by E. F. Kuntz. CITY AND STATE HEALTH FINANCES 2(7):2+, September 1985.

Public health and AIDS, by J. Foster, et al. CARING 5(6):4-11+, June 1986.

Public health implications of HIV infection, by A. B. Williams. NURSE PRACTITIONER 11(10):8-10+, October 1986.

Public Health Service plan for the prevention and control of acquired immune deficiency syndrome (AIDS), by J. O. Mason. PUBLIC HEALTH REPORT 100:453-455, September-October 1985.

Public Health Service; program announcement; alternate testing sites to perform HTLV-III antibody testing. FEDERAL REGISTER 50(48):9909-9910, March 12, 1985.

Public Health Service sets new AIDS guidelines, by D. Walter. ADVOCATE 436:24, December 24, 1985.

Public Health Service's number one priority [editorial],by E. N. Brandt, Jr. PUBLIC HEALTH REPORTS 98(4):306-307, July-August 1983.

Public response and public health: scientific, social and political interdigitations. Special session, by R. Enlow. ANNALS OF THE NEW YORK ACADEMY OF SCIENCES 437:290-311, 1984.

Pulling away the blanket, by M. Johnson. DISABILITY RAG 7(5):22, September 1986.

Pulmonary cell populations in the immunosuppressed patient. Bronchoalveolar lavage findings during episodes of pneumonitis, by D. A. White, et al. CHEST 88(3): 352-359, September 1985.

Pulmonary complications of the acquired immunodeficiency syndrome. Report of a National Heart, Lung, and Blood Institute workshop, by J. F. Murray, et al. NEW ENGLAND JOURNAL OF MEDICINE 310(25):1682-1688, June 21, 1984.

Pulmonary complications of the acquired immunodeficiency syndrome: a clinicopathologic study of 70 cases, by A. Marchevsky, et al. HUMAN PATHOLOGY 16(7): 659-670 July 1985.

Pulmonary complications of AIDS. AMERICAN FAMILY PHYSICIAN 31:215, March 1985.

Pulmonary complications of AIDS [letter], by J. R. Masci, et al. NEW ENGLAND JOURNAL OF MEDICINE 311(18):1182-1183, November 1, 1984.

Pulmonary complications of AIDS. Evaluating the tests [editorial], by J. Glassroth. CHEST 87(5):562-563, May 1985.

Pulmonary complications of AIDS: radiologic features, by B. A. Cohen, et al. AJR 143(1):115-122, July 1984.

Pulmonary cruptosporidiosis in acquired immune deficiency syndrome, by E. M. Brady, et al. JAMA 252:89-90, July 6, 1984.

Pulmonary disease in the acquired immune deficiency syndrome, by M. S. Gottlieb. CHEST 86(Suppl 3):29S-31S, September 1984.

Pulmonary involvement in the acquired immunodeficiency syndrome, by P. C. Hopewell, et al. CHEST 87(1):104-112, January 1985.

Pulmonary involvement in AIDS. Postmortem study of 50 cases, by E. Lampoureux, et al. ARCHIVES D'ANATOMIE ET DE CYTOLOGIE PATHOLOGIQUES 34(1): 12-16, 1986.

Pulmonary Kaposi's sarcoma in the acquired immune deficiency syndrome. Clinical, radiographic, and pathologic manifestations, by G. U. Meduri, et al. AMERICAN JOURNAL OF MEDICINE 81(1):11-18, July 1986.

Pulmonary manifestations of the acquired immunodeficiency syndrome (AIDS), by C. M. Wollschlager, et al. CHEST 85(2):197-202, February 1984.

—, by H. C. Hu, et al. CHUNG-HUA CHIEH HO HO HU HSI HSI CHI PING TSA CHIH 8(6):364-366, December 1985.

Pursuing the 'gay plague,' by S. Riley. MACLEAN'S 95:20d, November 22, 1982.

Pursuit of a cure (AIDS), by P. Ohlendorf. MACLEAN'S 98:36-37, August 12, 1985.

Putting AIDS in perspective, by B. Foley. REBEL 69:11, April 1985.

Putting rhetoric aside, by N. Lynch. BODY POLITIC 127:33, June 1986.

Puzzling case of the nun with AIDS. RN 47:19, January 1984.

PWAs demand treatment, by D. Larventz. BODY POLITIC 126:14, May 1986.

PWAs, PWARC: organize for their lives, by K. Westheimer. GAY COMMUNITY NEWS 13(45):3, June 7, 1986.

PX protein of HTLV-I is a transcriptional activator of its long terminal repeats, by B. K. Felber, et al. SCIENCE 229:675-679, August 16, 1985.

Pyogenic otorhinologic infections in acquired immune deficiency syndrome, by M. D. Poole, et al. ARCHIVES OF OTO-RHINO-LARYNGOLOGY 110(2):130-131, February 1984.

Pyrexia of undetermined origin, diarrhoea, and primary cerebral lymphoma associated with acquired immunodeficiency, by C. R. Shiach, et al. BRITISH MEDICAL JOURNAL 288(6415):449-450, February 11, 1984.

Qualitative analysis of immune function in patients with the acquired immunodeficiency syndrome. Evidence for a selective defect in soluble antigen recognition, by H. C. Lane, et al. NEW ENGLAND JOURNAL OF MEDICINE 313(2):79-84, July 11, 1985.

Quandry of advice, by R. Bebout. BODY POLITIC 126:26, May 1986.

Quantitation of and neutralizing antibodies to AIDS-retroviruses; a novel system using HTLV-I carrying MT-4 cells, by S. Harada, et al. TANPAKUSHITSU KAKUSAN KOSO 30(13):1394-1407, December 1985.

Quantitation of beta 2-microglobulin and other immune characteristics in a prospective study of men at risk for acquired immune deficiency syndrome, by S. Zolla-Pazner, et al. JAMA 251(22):2951-2955, June 8, 1984.

Quantitative analysis of AIDS-related virus-carrying cells by plaque-forming assay using an HTLV-I-positive MT-4 cell line, by S. Harada, et al. GANN 76(6):432-435, June 1985.

Quantitative changes in T helper or T suppressor/cytotoxic lymphocyte subsets that distinguish acquired immune deficiency syndrome from other immune subset disorders, by J. L. Fahey, et al. AMERICAN JOURNAL OF MEDICINE 76(1):95-100, January 1984.

Quarantine and AIDS, by A. Novick. CONNECTICUT MEDICINE 49(2):81-83, February 1985.

Quarantine corner. PROCESSED WORLD 15:10, Winter 1985.

Quarantine is no way to fight AIDS, by C. Guilfoy. GAY COMMUNITY NEWS 13(21):8, Decemebr 7, 1985.

Quarantine of prostitutes with AIDS rumored, by K. Westheimer. GAY COMMUNITY NEWS 13(21):1, Decemebr 7, 1985.

239

Queer across the nation. GAY COMMUNITY NEWS 11(50):9, July 7, 1984.

Queers demand AIDS &, by S. Hyde. GAY COMMUNITY NEWS 12(33):6, March 9, 1985.

Queers go after Buckley, picket National Review, by B. Gelbert. GAY COMMUNITY NEWS 13(42):1, May 17, 1986.

Question of possible relationship between hepatitis B vaccine and AIDS [letter], by L. B. Taubman,e t al. AMERICAN JOURNAL OF MEDICINE 76(4):A59, April 1984.

Questions and answers. CORPORATE SECURITY June 1986, p. 5.

Questions and answers about AIDS . . . patient education aid. PATIENT CARE 18(1): 187-188, January 15, 1984.

Questions from Israel, by M. Helquist. ADVOCATE 446:21, May 13, 1986.

Quick-bibs: AIDS, by B. Ott. AMERICAN LIBRARIES 16:681, November 1985.

Racial and other characteristics of human T cell leukemia/lymphoma (HTLV-I) and AIDS (HTLV-III) in Trinidad, by C. Bartholomew, et al. BRITISH MEDICAL JOUR-NAL 290(6477):1243-1246, April 27, 1985.

Racing to sell an AIDS test to blood banks, by E. t. Smith, et al. BUSINESS WEEK February 18, 1985, p. 136.

Radiation therapy of Kaposi's sarcoma in AIDS. Memorial Sloan-Kettering experi-ence, by L. Z. Nisce, et al. FRONTIERS OF RADIATION THERAPY AND ONCOL-OGY 19:133-137, 1985.

Radiographic features in patients with pulmonary manifestations of the acquired im-mune deficiency syndrome, by C. W. Heron, et al. CLINICAL RADIOLOGY 36(6): 583-588, November 1985.

Radiographic findings in acquired immune deficiency syndrome, by W. T. Miller, et al. APPLIED RADIOLOGY 14(3):86-8, May-June 1985.

Radiographic immune deficiency syndrome (AIDS) and pre-AIDS, by A. E. Pitchenik, et al. AMERICAN REVIEW OF RESPIRATORY DISEASE 131(3):393-396, March 1985.

Radioimmunoassay and enzyme-linked immunoassay of antibodies to the core pro-tein (P24) of human T-lymphotropic virus (HTLVIII), by A. R. Neurath, et al. JOUR-NAL OF VIROLOGICAL METHODS 11(1):75-86, May 1985.

Radiologic-pathologic correlation conference: SUNY Upstate Medical Center. Pro-gressive lung disease in a homosexual man, by E. G. Theros, et al. AJR 140(5): 897-902, May 1983.

Radiotherapy for AIDS-related Kaposi's sarcoma. AMERICAN FAMILY PHYSICIAN 31:245-246, April 1985.

Raised serum neopterin levels and imbalances of T-lymphocyte subsets in viral dis-eases, acquired immune deficiency and related lymphadenopathy syndromes, by P. Kern, et al. BIOMEDICINE AND PHARMACOTHERAPY 38(8):407-411, 1984.

Rapid detection of immunoreactive interferon-alpha in AIDS [letter], by S. R. Abbott, et al. LANCET 1(8376):564, March 10, 1984.

240

Rapid spread of HTLV-III infection among drug addicts in Italy [letter], by G. Angarano, et al. LANCET 2(8467):1302, December 7, 1985.

Rating crisis coverage/AIDS/media, by N. Fain. ADVOCATE 3(77):24, September 29, 1983.

Ray of hope in the fight against AIDS . . . an experimental drug called AZT prolongs the life of patients, by J. Levine, et al. TIME 128(13):60-61, September 29, 1986.

Reaching out to someone with AIDS, by G. Whitmore. NEW YORK TIMES MAGA- ZINE May 19, 1985, p. 68-71+.

Reactions and counter-reactions to transfusion-associated-AIDS [news], by M. F. Goldsmith. JAMA 251(2):177-179, January 13, 1984.

Reactions of psychiatric staff to an AIDS patient, by R. B. Rosse. AMERICAN JOUR- NAL OF PSYCHIATRY 142(4):523, April 1985.

Reactivity of E. coli-derived trans-activating protein of human T lymphotropic virus type III with sera from patients with acquired immune deficiency syndrome, by A. D. Barone, et al. JOURNAL OF IMMUNOLOGY 137(2):669-673, July 1, 1986.

Reagan doubles fiscal '84 AIDS funds, by L. Bush. ADVOCATE 3(78):20, October 13, 1983.

Reagan—1984 Health Emergency Bill, by B. Nelson. GAY COMMUNITY NEWS 11(2):1, July 23, 1983.

Reagan seeks $50M AIDS cut, by G. Gottlieb. GAY COMMUNITY NEWS 13(31):1, February 15, 1986.

Real epidemic: fear and despair, by J. Leo. TIME 122:56-58, July 4, 1983.

'Reasonable' discrimination against homosexuals [letter],by H. Warter. HOSPITAL PRACTICE 18(12):16+, December 1983.

Reasons behind blood donor screening, by R. W. Miller. FDA CONSUMER 19(9):31- 34, November 1985.

Recent developments: public health and employment issues generated by the AIDS crisis, by M. J. Lazzo, et al. WASHBURN LAW JOURNAL 25(3):505-535, 1986.

Recent progress in research on AIDS (acquired immune deficiency syndrome), by A. Pana, et al. RECENTI PROGRESSI IN MEDICINA 74(8):879-887, August 1983.

Recombinant alpha-2 interferon therapy for Kaposi's sarcoma associated with the ac- quired immunodeficiency syndrome, by J. E. Groopman, et al. ANNALS OF IN- TERNAL MEDICINE 100(5):671-676, May 1984.

Recombinant interferon alpha in the treatment of acquired immune deficiency syn- drome-related Kaposi's sarcoma, by P. A. Volberding, et al. SEMINARS IN ON- COLOGY 12(4, Suppl. 5):2-6, December 1985.

Recombinant polypeptide from the endonuclease region of the acquired immune de- ficiency syndrome retrovirus polymerase (pol) gene detects serum antibodies in most infected individuals, by K. s. Steimer, et al JOURNALOF VIROLOGY 58(1): 9-16, April 1986.

Recommendations: diagnosis of AIDS used by the Centers for Disease Control. EUROPEAN JOURNAL OF CANCER AND CLINICAL ONCOLOGY 20(2):169-173, February 1984.

Recommendations for assisting in the prevention of perinatal transmissions of HTLV-III/LAV and acquired immunodeficiency syndrome. JAMA 255:25-27+, January 3, 1986; also in MMWR 34(48):721-726+, December 6, 1985.

Recommendations for preventing possible HTLV-III/LAV virus from tears. JAMA 254(11):1429, September 20, 1985.

Recommendations for preventing possible transmission of human T-lymphotropic virus type III/lymphadenopathy-associated virus from tears. MMWR 34(34):533-534, August 30, 1985.

Recommendations for preventing transmission of infection with human T-lymphotropic virus type III/lymphadenopathy-associated virus during invasive procedures. ANNALS OF INTERNAL MEDICINE 104(6):824-825, June 1986; also in PENNSYLVANIA NURSE 41(7):3, July 1986.

Recommendations for providing dialysis treatment to patients infected with human T-lymphotropic virus type III/lymphadenopathy-associated virus. ANNALS OF INTERNAL MEDICINE 105(4):558-559, October 1986; also in MMWR 35(23): 376-378+, June 13, 1986.

Recommendations on preventing AIDS transmissions released. TEXAS HOSPITALS 42(1):20-21, June 1986.

Recommended guidelines for dealing with AIDS in the schools from the National Education Association. JOURNAL OF SCHOOL HEALTH 56(4):129-130, April 1986.

Recommended precautions for patients undergoing hemodialysis who have AIDS or non-A, non-B hepatitis, by M. S. Favero. INFECTION CONTROL 6(8):301-305, August 1985.

Recovery from AIDS, by J. Bolen. RFD 45:43, Winter 1985.

Recovery of AIDS-associated retroviruses from patients with AIDS or AIDS-related conditions and from clinically healthy individuals, by J. A. Levy, et al. JOURNAL OF INFECTIOUS DISEASES 152(4):734-738, October 1985.

Recovery of herpes viruses from cerebrospinal fluid of immunodeficient homosexual men, by R. D. Dix, et al. ANNALS OF NEUROLOGY 18(5):611-614, November 1985.

Recreational drugs: relationship to AIDS, by J. J. Goedert. ANNALS OF THE NEW YORK ACADEMY OF SCIENCES 437:192-199, 1984.

Rectal epithelium in the acquired immunodeficiency syndrome [letter], by D. C. Snover. ANNALS OF INTERNAL MEDICINE 102(2):278-279, February 1985.

Rectal insemination modifies immune responses in rabbits, by J. M. Richards, et al. SCIENCE 224:390-392, April 27, 1984.

Recurrent infectious diseases and AIDS, by F. di Nola. MINERVA MEDICA 75(47-48): 2847-2848, Decembr 15, 1984.

Recurrent Salmonella typhimurium bacteremia associated with the acquired immuno-deficiency syndrome, by J. B. Glaser, et al. ANNALS OF INTERNAL MEDICINE 102(2):189-193, February 1985.

Red blood's not good enough. BODY POLITIC 119:25, October 1985.

Red-cell alloantibody response in AIDS [letter],by G. Ramsey, et al. LANCET 2(8349):575, September 3, 1983.

Red Cross backs off donor policy, by E. Jackson. BODY POLITIC 93:11, May 1983.

Red Cross new blood donation guidlines, by L. Goldsmith. GAY COMMUNITY NEWS 10(37):1, April 9, 1983.

Red Cross/resisting AIDS panic, by E. Jackson. BODY POLITIC 91:17, March 1983.

Red Cross to educate public on AIDS: goal to dispel myths, by J. Cassell. PENNSYL-VANIA NURSE 41(3):17, March 1986.

Red Cross to public: fight AIDS with facts, by L. Checco. PENNSYLVANIA NURSE 41(2):7-8, February 1986.

Reduced ecto-5"-nucleotidase activity and enhanced OKT10 and HLA-DR expression on CD8 (T suppressor/cytotoxic) lymphocytes in the acquired immune deficiency syndrome: evidence of CD8 cell immaturity, by J. F. Salazar-Gonzalez, et al. JOURNAL OF IMMUNOLOGY 135(3):1778-1785, September 1985.

Reduced la-positive Langerhans' cells in AIDS [letter]. NEW ENGLAND JOURNAL OF MEDICINE 311(13):857-858, Septemebr 27, 1984.

Reduced Langerhans' cell la antigen and ATPase activity in patients with the acquired immunodeficiency syndrome, by D. V. Belsito, et al. NEW ENGLAND JOURNAL OF MEDICINE 310(20):1279-1282, May 17, 1984.

Reducing psychological complications for the critically ill AIDS patient, by J. D. Durham, et al. DIMENSIONS OF CRITICAL CARE NURSING 3(5):300-306, September-October 1984.

Reducing the risk of acquiring AIDS . . . the condom,by M. S. Tillis. AAOHN JOUR-NAL 34(9):432-434, September 1986.

Reducing the risk of job related disease, by R. Zack. LAW AND ORDER 33(2):59-60, February 1985.

Reflections on AIDS, by C. Levasseur. CANADIAN NURSE 82(3):23-25+, March 1986.

Refusal to treat: abandonment and AIDS, by P. A. Plumeri. JOURNAL OF CLINICAL GASTROENTEROLOGY 6(3):281-284, June 1984.

Regression of Kaposi's sarcoma in AIDS after treatment with dapsone [letter], by A. Poulsen, et al. LANCET 1(8376):560, March 10, 1984.

Relation between sexual practices and T-cell subsets in homosexually active men, by R. Detels, et al. LANCET 1(8325):609-611, March 19, 1983.

Relationship of AIDS to other retroviruses [letter], by S. Wain-Hobson, et al. NATURE 313(6005):743, February 28-March 6, 1985.

Relationship of mitogen reactivity to type D retrovirus infection in Celebes black macaques (Macaca nigra), by B. J. Wilson, et al. LABORATORY ANIMALS 36(3): 237-239, June 1986.

Religion—moralizing and AIDS, by K. Gordon. GAY COMMUNITY NEWS 11(22):6, December 17, 1983.

Religious leaders declare AIDS not God's punishment, by P. Freiberg. ADVOCATE 417:18, April 2, 1985.

"Remember who you are" . . . working with people with AIDS, by C. Morrison. JEN 12(5):254-255, September-October 1986.

Remission without drugs/drugs without remission, by M. Helquist. ADVOCATE 431: 21, October 15, 1985.

Renal disease and the acquired immunodeficiency syndrome [letter], by S. J. Bennett, et al. ANNALS OF INTERNAL MEDICINE 102(2):274-275, February 1985.

Renal disease in patients with AIDS: a clinicopathologic study, by M. H. Gardenswartz, et al. CLINICAL NEPHROLOGY 21(4):197-204, April 1984.

Renal ultrasound in acquired immune deficiency syndrome, by R. M. Schaffer, et al. RADIOLOGY 153(2):511-513, November 1984.

Repairing the T-cell defect in AIDS [letter], by D. Zagury, et al. LANCET 2(8452):449, August 24, 1985.

Replication of Epstein-Barr virus within the epithelial cells of oral "hairy" leukoplakia, an AIDS-associated lesion, by J. S. Greenspan, et al. NEW ENGLAND JOURNAL OF MEDICINE 313(25):1564-1571, December 19, 1985.

Replicative and cytopathic potential of HTLV-III/LAV with *sor* gene deletions, by J. Sodroski, et al. SCIENCE 231:1549-1553, March 28, 1986.

Report from the First International Congress on AIDS held at Atlanta: the American society threatened by sexually transmitted disease numbering more than 25, by C. Ikegami. KANGOGAKU ZASSHI 49(9):1074-1076, September 1985.

Report from the PHLS Communicable Disease Surveillance Centre. BRITISH MEDICAL JOURNAL 292(6533):1447-1448, May 31, 1986.

Report of a WHO meeting on AIDS. INTERNATIONAL NURSING REVIEW 32(3):80-83, May-June 1985.

Report on acquired immunodeficiency syndrome, by E. Rodríguez Domingo. MEDICINA CLINICA 82(11):491-493, March 24, 1984.

Reported changes in the sexual behavior of men at risk for AIDS, San Francisco, 1982-84—the AIDS Behavioral Research Project, by L. McKusick, et al. PUBLIC HEALTH REPORTS 100(6):622-629, November-December 1985.

Request for proposals: NSA soliciting bids to produce three videotapes on AIDS. CRIME CONTROL DIGEST 20(43):10, October27, 1986.

Requiem for an AIDS victim, by D. K. Ciannella. WITNESS 68(9):10-11, September 1985.

Research center urges privacy for AIDS subjects, by P. Frieberg. ADVOCATE 409: 87, December 11, 1984.

Research developments in AIDS [editorial], by J. A. Armstrong. MEDICAL JOURNAL OF AUSTRALIA 141(9):556-557, October 27, 1984.

Research on AIDS. FDA DRUG BULLETIN 12(3):21-23, December 1982.

Research reported at press seminar. ADAMHA NEWS 11(8):1, August 1985.

Researcher: tools exist to battle AIDS' spread, by G. Willis. AIR FORCE TIMES 47:8+, November 24, 1986.

Researchers clone genes of AIDs-linked virus. BIOSCIENCE 34:685, December 1984.

Researchers discover new AIDS virus gene. CHEMICAL AND ENGINEERING NEWS 64:6, June 2, 1986.

Researchers discuss safety of AIDS testing, by L. Goldsmith. GAY COMMUNITY NEWS 12(3):3, July 28, 1984.

Researchers find that AIDS patients have defects in T and B cells, by P. Randall. NEWS & FEATURES FROM NIH November 1983, p. 8.

Researchers tackle AIDS. HIGH TECHNOLOGY 5:8, May 1985.

Reserves to start AIDS tests Sept. 1, by P. Dalton. AIR FORCE TIMES 47:30, August 25, 1986.

Respiratory cryptosporidiosis in the acquired immune deficiency syndrome. Use of modified cold Kinyoun and Hemacolor stains for rapid diagnoses, by P. Ma, et al. JAMA 252(10):1298-1301, September 14, 1984.

Responding to AIDS in prisons: the team approach, by J. J. Maffucci. CORREC-TIONS TODAY 45:68+, December 1983.

Responding to, learning from AIDS: for starters: principles and theologies, by J. B. Nelson. CHRISTIANITY AND CRISIS 46:176-181, May 19, 1986.

Responding to the psychological crisis of AIDS, by S. F. Morin, et al. PUBLIC HEALTH REPORTS 99(1):4-9, January-February 1984.

Response of hospital infection control programs to the AIDS epidemic [editorial],by W. Schaffner. INFECTION 13(5):201-202, September-October 1985.

Response to AIDS, by J. Robinson. GAY COMMUNITY NEWS 11(11):13, October 3, 1983.

— [editorial],by J. R. Bove. TRANSFUSION 25(1):1-2, January-February 1985.

—, by T. Dollar. FUNDAMENTALIST JOURNAL 4(10):74, November 1985.

Results of a Gallup poll on acquired immunodeficiency syndrome—New York City, United States, 1985. MMWR 34(33):513-514, August 23,1 985.

Results of human T-lymphotropic virus type III test kits reported from blood collection centers—United States, April 22 to May 19, 1985. JAMA 254:741, August 9, 1985.

Retinal cotton-wool patches in acquired immunodeficiency syndrome [letter]. NEW ENGLAND JOURNAL OF MEDICINE 307(27):1704-1705, December 30, 1982.

Retinal lesions of the acquired immune deficiency syndrome, by A. H. Friedman. TRANSACTIONS OF THE AMERICAN OPHTHALMOLOGICAL SOCIETY 82: 447-491, 1984.

245

Retinal manifestations of acquired immunodeficiency syndrome (AIDS). Report of a
case, by G. Buckman, et al. ANNALS OF OPHTHALMOLOGY 16(12):1136-
1138, December 1984.

Retinal manifestations of the acquired immune deficiency syndrome (AIDS): cytomegalovirus, candida albicans, cryptococcus, toxoplasmosis and Pneumocystis
carinii, by J. S. Schuman, et al. TRANSACTIONS OF THE OPHTHALMOLOGI-
CAL SOCIETIES OF THE UNITED KINGDOM 103(Part 2):177-190, 1983.

Retirement evaluation due AIDS-stricken sailor, by P. Smith. AIR FORCE TIMES 44:
12, March 5, 1984.

Retroperitoneal fibromatosis and acquired immunodeficiency syndrome in macques.
Pathologic observations and transmission studies, by W. E. Giddens, Jr., et al.
AMERICAN JOURNAL OF PATHOLOGY 119(2):253-263, May 1985.

Retroperitoneal nodal aplasia, asplenia, chylous effusion and lymphatic dysplasia: an
acquired immunodeficiency syndrome?, by L. Carini, et al. LYMPHOLOGY 18(1):
31-36, March 1985.

Retrovaccine. SCIENTIFIC AMERICAN 253:62, August 1985.

Retrovirus and malignant lymphoma in homosexual men, by A. M. Levine, et al. JAMA
254:1921-1925, October 11, 1985.

Retrovirus associated with AIDS. AMERICAN FAMILY PHYSICIAN 31:249, March
1985.

Retrovirus-induced acquired immunodeficiencies, by M. Bendinelli, et al. AD-
VANCES IN CANCER RESEARACH 45:125-181, 1985.

Retrovirus-like particles in salivary glands, prostate and testes of AIDS patients, by G.
Lecatsas, et al. PROCEEDINGS OF THE SOCIETY FOR EXPERIMENTAL BIOL-
OGY AND MEDICINE 178(4):653-655, April 1985.

Retrovirus linked to simian AIDS. CHEMICAL AND ENGINEERING NEWS 62:6, March
5, 1984.

Retrovirus resembling HTLV in macrophages of patients with AIDS [letter], by F.
Gyorkey, et al. LANCET 1(8420):106, January 12, 1985.

Retroviruses, AIDS and systemic lupus erythematosus [editorial],by A. Schattner.
HAREFUAH 109(9):251-253, November 1985.

Retroviruses and acquired immunodeficiency syndrome (AIDS), by J. C. Chermann,
et al. BULLETIN DE L'ACADEMIE NATIONALE DE MEDECINE 168(1-2):288-
295, January-February 1984.

Retroviruses and human disease [editorial], by R. A. Weinberg. HOSPITAL PRAC-
TICE 18(7):13+, July 1983.

Retroviruses associated with leukemia and ablative syndromes in animals and in human beings, by M. Essex, et al. CANCER RESEARCH 45(Suppl. 9):4534s-
4538s, September 1985.

Retroviruses in Kaposi-sarcoma cells in AIDS [letter], by F. Gyorkey, et al. NEW ENG-
LAND JOURNAL OF MEDICINE 311(18):1183-1184, November 1, 1984.

Retroviruses linked with AIDS, by R. Weiss. NATURE 309(5963):12-13, May 3,
1984.

Rev. Jerry Falwell/AIDS God's judgment, by Zeh, et al. ADVOCATE 3(74):15, August 18, 1983.

Review of a support group for patients with AIDS, by D. A. Newmark. TOPICS IN CLINICAL NURSING 6(2):38-44, July 1984.

Revised definition of persons who should refrain from donating blood and plasma. JAMA 254(14):1886, October 11, 1985.

Revision of case definition of acquired immunodeficiency syndrome for national reporting—United States. ANNALS OF INTERNAL MEDICINE 103(3):402-403, September 1985.

—. JAMA 254(5):599-600, August 2, 1985.

—. MMWR 34(25):373-375, June 28, 1985.

Ride for wellness: positive radicalism, by T. Barrus. GAY COMMUNITY NEWS 13(16): 6, November 2, 1985.

Rights before responsibility, by J. O'Sullivan. TIMES October 12, 1985, p. 8.

Rising prevalence of human T-lymphotropic virus type III (HTLV-III) infection in homosexual men in London, by C. A. Carne, et al. LANCET 1(8440):1261-1262, June 1, 1985.

Risk factor analysis among men referred for possible acquired immune deficiency syndrome, by G. R. Newell, et al. PREVENTIVE MEDICINE 14(1):81-91, January 1985.

Risk factors in pediatric AIDS [letter],by J. H. Joncas, et al. CANADIAN MEDICAL ASSOCIATION JOURNAL 132(6):614-615, March 15, 1985.

Risk of AIDS after hepatitis vaccination [letter]. JAMA 253(20):296-2961, May 24-31, 1985.

Risk of AIDS in recipients of hepatitis B vaccine [letter], by G. Papaevangelou, et al. NEW ENGLAND JOURNAL OF MEDICINE 312(6):376-377, February 7, 1985.

Risk of AIDS to health care workers [editorial], by A. M. Geddes. BRITISH MEDICAL JOURNAL 292(6522):711-722, March 15, 1986.

Risk of AIDS with artificial insemination, by J. Morgan, et al. NEW ENGLAND JOURNAL OF MEDICINE 314:386, February 6, 1986.

Risk of HTLV-III/LAV transmission to household contacts [letter]. NEW ENGLAND JOURNAL OF MEDICINE 315(4):257-259, July 24, 1986.

Risk of nosocomial infection with human T-cell lymphotropic virus III (HTLV-III), by M. S. Hirsch, et al. NEW ENGLAND JOURNAL OF MEDICINE 312(1):1-4, January 3, 1985.

Risk of nosocomial infection with human T-cell lymphotropic virus type III/lymphadenopathy-associated virus in a large cohort of intensively exposed health care workers,by D. K. Henderson, et al. ANNALS OF INTERNAL MEDICINE 104(5):644-647, May 1986.

Risk of seroconversion for acquired immunodeficiency syndrome (AIDS) in San Francisco health workers, by A. Moss, et al. JOURNAL OF OCCUPATIONAL MEDICINE 28(9):821-824, September 1986.

Risk of transferring AIDS or hepatitis via immune globulin, by M. A. Kane, et al. JAMA 252:1057, August 24, 1984.

Risk of transmission of HTLV-III by needle stick [letter], by C. E. DuBeau. NEW ENGLAND JOURNAL OF MEDICINE 312(17):1128-1129, April 25, 1985.

Risk reduction for the acquired immunodeficiency syndrome among intravenous drug users, by D. C. Des Jarlais, et al. ANNALS OF INTERNAL MEDICINE 103(5):755-759, November 1985.

Risks of transmission of the HTLV-III and hepatitis B virus in the hospital, by D. Shanson. INFECTION CONTROL 7(2):128-132, February 1986.

Risks with danazol in the acquired immunodeficiency syndrome [letter], by . E Metroka, et al. ANNALS OF INTERNAL MEDICINE 101(4)564-565, October 1984.

Ritodrine-responsive bullous pemphigoid in a patient with AIDS-related complex [letter],by P. M. Levy, et al. BRITISH JOURNAL OF DERMATOLOGY 114(5):635-636, May 1986.

Rivalry to defeat AIDS, by J. Carey. US NEWS & WORLD REPORT 100(1):67-68, January 13, 1986.

RN gives supportive care to patients dying of AIDS, by C. Donovan. AMERICAN NURSE 17(10):1+, November-December 1985.

Rock Hudson. PEOPLE WEEKLY 24:108+, December 23-30, 1985.

—, by G. Gottlieb. GAY COMMUNITY NEWS 14(7), August 24, 1986.

Rock Hudson AIDS case sends a message. U.S. NEWS & WORLD REPORT 99:12, August 5, 1985.

Rock Hudson and the war against AIDS, by J. Barber. MACLEAN'S 98:44, August 5, 1985.

Rock Hudson: the great gay hope, by S. Bronski. GAY COMMUNITY NEWS 13(7):7, August 24, 1985.

Rock Hudson has AIDS. ADVOCATE 427:22, August 20, 1985.

Rock Hudson: legacy of hope, by J. Adler. NEWSWEEK 106:36, October 14, 1985.

Rock Hudson: on camera and off, by J. Yarbrough. PEOPLE 24:34-41, August 12, 1985.

Role of bronchial brush biopsy in AIDS with Pneumocystis carinii pneumonia [letter], by T. K. Sarkar, et al. CHEST 87(4):553-554, April 1985.

Role of Epstein-Barr virus in acquired immune deficiency syndrome, by D. T. Purtilo, et al. ADVANCES IN EXPERIMENTAL MEDICINE AND BIOLOGY 187:53-65, 1985.

Role of hepatitis B virus in acquired immunodeficiency syndrome, y R. T. Ravenholt. LANCET 2(8355):885-886, October 15, 1983.

Role of interferon in AIDS, by O. t. Preble, et al. ANNALS OF THE NEW YORK ACADEMY OF SCIENCES 437:65-75, 1984.

Role of mononuclear phagocytes in HTLV-III/LAV infection, by S. Gartner, et al. SCI-ENCE 233(4760):215-219, July 11, 1986.

Role of a national organization in the AIDS issue, by C. J. Carman. SCANDINAVIAN JOURNAL OF HAEMATOLOGY. SUPPLEMENTUM 40:461-467, 1984.

Role of surgery in the prognosis of AIDS and related syndromes. Case reports, by F. Badellino, et al. MINERVA MEDICA 77(9-10):March 10, 1986.

Roy Cohn: a queer-baiter dies, by M. Bronski. GAY COMMUNITY NEWS 14(5):3, August 10, 1986.

Royal Alexandra develops AIDS infection control protocol, by S. I. Hnatko. DIMEN-SIONS IN HEALTH SERVICE 62(8):25-28, September 1985.

Royal College of Nursing. AIDS and the media. NURSING STANDARD 385:4, February 21, 1985.

—. Food for thought; facing reality. NURSING STANDARD 448:4, May 22, 1986.

—. Put to the test. NURSING STANDARD 379:4, January 10, 1985.

—. The real victims; rewarding cuts. NURSING STANDARD 418:4, October 10, 1984.

Rx for AIDS: a grim race against the clock, by J. Carey. U.S. NEWS & WORLD RE-PORT 99(14):48-49, September 30, 1985.

Safe blood for transfusion. MEDICAL LETTER ON DRUGS AND THERAPEUTICS 25(646):93-95, October 14, 1983.

Safe handling of laboratory samples from AIDS patients, by J. G. Roberts. IMLS GAZ-ETTE 29(11):564-566, November 1985.

Safe method for identifying cryptosporidium cysts in the faeces of patients with sus-pected AIDS, or those infected with other serious concomitant pathogens [let-ter], by J. E. Williams, et al. JOURNAL OF CLINICAL PATHOLOGY 38(11):1313-1314, November 1985.

Safe sex: guidelines that could save your life, by M. Helquist. ADVOCATE 426:36, August 6, 1985.

Safe sex: warm, approaching hot, by K. Bowling. OUT 4(8):8, June 1986.

Safety cabinets and AIDS, by R. P. Clark. NATURE 315:626, June 20, 1985.

Safety in the forensic immunology laboratory, by W. W. Bond. CRIME LABORATORY DIGEST 13(1):15-24, January 1986.

Safety of hepatitis B vaccine confirmed. FDA DRUG BULLETIN 15(2):14-15, August 1985.

SAG union fears kiss of AIDS. ADVERTISING AGE 56:1+, November 4, 1985.

St. Martin's book to probe the AIDS mystery, by J. Davis. PUBLISHERS WEEKLY 223:30, April 29, 1983.

Salmonella infections in patients with acquired immunodeficiency syndrome, by S. Profeta, et al. ARCHIVES OF INTERNAL MEDICINE 145(4):670-672, April 1985.

—, by J. L. Jacobs, et al. ANNALS OF INTERNAL MEDICINE 102(2):186-188, February 1985.

Salmonella septicemia in acquired immunodeficiency syndrome [letter], by D. Fassin, et al. PRESSE MEDICALE 14(16):894, April 20, 1985.

Salmonella typhimurium aenteritis and bacteremia in the acquired immunodeficiency syndrome, by P. D. Smith, et al. ANNALS OF INTERNAL MEDICINE 102(2):207-209, February 1985.

San Francisco AIDS antibody testing program, by M. Helquist. ADVOCATE 424:14, July 9, 1985.

San Francisco AIDS vigil in 12th week, by S. Poggi. GAY COMMUNITY NEWS 13(27): 1, January 25, 1986.

San Francisco AIDS vigilers stand firm in 8th month, by Bisticas-Cocoves. GAY COMMUNITY NEWS 13(48):1, June 28, 1986.

San Francisco General Hospital's AIDS/ARC care plan. CALIFORNIA NURSE 82(4): 13, May 1986.

San Francisco Judge closes gay baths, sex clubs, by R. O'Loughlin. ADVOCATE 4(7):8, November 13, 1984.

San Francisco man files $5 million AIDS insurance suit, by M. Helquist. ADVOCATE 442:23, March 18, 1986.

San Francisco nurses provide AIDS care, by T. L. Selby. AMERICAN NURSE 18(2): 1+, February 1986.

San Francisco recoils. ECONOMIST August 23, 1986, p. 32-33.

San Francisco sex regulations tightened up, by C. Guilfoy. GAY COMMUNITY NEWS 12(25):1, January 12, 1985.

San Francisco solution: debate continues, by S. Kulieke. ADVOCATE 41:9, March 5, 1985.

San Francisco vigil for AIDS funds enters fourth week, by K. Westheimer. GAY COMMUNITY NEWS 13(20):1, November 30, 1985.

San Francisco's AIDS toll nears thousand, by I. Anderson. NEW SCIENTIST 102:8, April 12, 1984.

Scare hits women not gay men alone, by V. Groocock. NEW STATESMAN 110:12-13, August 30, 1985.

Scarlet letters and public risks, by W. Hampton Sides. CONNECTICUT MAGAZINE 47:68+, March 1984.

Scholars face AIDS test [West Germany]. THE TIMES HIGHER EDUCATION SUP-PLEMENT 684:8, December 13, 1985.

School attendance of children and adolescents with human T lyphotropic virus III/lymphadenopathy-associated virus infection, by the American Academy of Pediatrics. Committee on School Health, Committee on Infectious Diseases. PEDIA-TRICS 77(3):430-432, March 1986.

School Boards ignore medical advice on AIDS. OUT 4(3):1, January 1986.

School law, by D. A. Splitt. EXECUTIVE EDUCATOR 8(3):12, March 1986.

School ordered to admit New Jersey girl with AIDS. JET 69:26, November 25, 1985.

Schools await decision. BODY POLITIC 120:29, November 1985.

Schools flunk on AIDS instruction, by L. Fraser. MOTHER JONES 11(4):8, June 1986.

Schools try to abate fears about AIDS kids. JET 69:6, September 30, 1985.

Science base underlying research on acquired immune deficiency syndrome, by S. Taube, et al. PUBLIC HEALTH REPORTS 98(6):559-565, November-December 1983.

Scientific speculation continues in Atlanta, by Bistecas-Cocoves. GAY COMMUNITY NEWS 12(43):3, May 18, 1985.

Scientist allays fears about AIDS; claims fewer than 10 cases have been recorded in USSR. CURRENT DIGEST OF THE SOVIET PRESS 37:16+, December 25, 1985.

Scientist attacks AIDS slur on Africa, by O. Sattaur. NEW SCIENTIST 108:15-16, November 28, 1985.

Scientists honored for achievements in cancer research, by S. D. Levine. NEWS & FEATURES FROM NIH August 1984, p. 12-13.

Scism over the scourge, by C. Longley. TIMES December 23, 1986, p. 12.

Scourge spreads panic: as AIDS reaches around the globe, governments are galvanized into action, by M. S. Serrill, et al. TIME 126(17):50-52, October 28, 1985.

Scrapie-associated fibrils and AIDS encephalopathy [letter],by P. H. Gibson. LANCET 2(8455):612-613, September 14, 1985.

—, by P. N. Goldwater, et al. LANCET 2(8467):1300, December 7, 1985.

"Screaming room" reveals agony of AIDS, by L. Mohn. NEW DIRECTIONS FOR WOMEN September 1986, p. 4.

Screening blood donations for AIDS, by F. Peterson. FDA CONSUMER 19(4):5-11, May 1985.

Screening blood: public health and medical uncertainty, by C. Levine, et al. HASTINGS CENTER REPORT 15(4):8-11, August 1985.

Screening donated blood and plasma for HTLV-III antibody. Facing more than one crisis?, by M. T. Osterholm, et al. NEW ENGLAND JOURNAL OF MEDICINE 312(18):1185-1189, May 2, 1985.

Screening for acquired immune deficiency syndrome with dinitrochlorobenzene [letter],by W. A. McLeod, et al. CANADIAN MEDICAL ASSOCIATION JOURNAL 130(2):100-101, January 15, 1984.

Screening for acquired immunodeficiency syndrome [letter],by N. M. Arnott. CANADIAN MEDICAL ASSOCIATION JOURNAL 129(5):412, September 1, 1983.

Screening for AIDS. MEDICAL LETTER ON DRUGS AND THERAPEUTICS 27(684): 29-30, March 29, 1985.

Screening for AIDS or for gays?, by T. Ensign. GUARDIAN 37(44):5, September 11, 1985.

Screening for antibody to HTLV-III in blood donors of Liguria. BOLLETTINO DELL ISTITUTO SIEROTERAPICO MILANESE 64(5):363-366, 1985.

Screening for HIV antibodies, by N. P. Guarda, et al. NURSING 16(11):28-29, November 1986.

Screening for HTLV-III antibodies—a government blunder?, by C. S. Bryan. JOURNAL OF THE SOUTH CAROLINA MEDICAL ASSOCIATION 81(4):242-244, April 1985.

Screening for HTLV-III antibodies: the relation between prevalence and positive predictive value and its social consequences [letter]. JAMA 253(23):3395-3398, June 21, 1985.

Screening for risk of acquired immune-deficiency syndrome [letter],by F. Greenberg, et al. NEW ENGLAND JOURNAL OF MEDICINE 307(24):1521-1522, December 9, 1982.

Screening of all donors for preventing transmission of AIDS via blood, semen, tissues. LAKARTIDNINGEN 82(20):1881, May 15, 1985.

Screening test for HTLV-III (AIDS agent) antibodies. Specificity, sensitivity, and applications, by S. H. Weiss, et al. JAMA 253(2):221-225, January 11, 1985.

Screening tests for blood donors presumed to have transmitted the acquired immunodeficiency syndrome, by J. S. McDougal, et al. BLOOD 65(3):772-775, March 1985.

Scrofula followed by AIDS [letter],by A. Marchiando. EAR, NOSE, AND THROAT JOURNAL 63(3):197-198, March 1984.

Search for an AIDS vaccine, by W. Dowdle. PUBLIC HEALTH REPORTS 101(3):232-233, May-June 1986.

Searching for AZT (azidothymidine): monthly search hint, by R. L. Stander. NLM TECH BULLETIN 210:15-17, October 1986.

Searching for cases of AIDS in Britain, by S. Connor, et al. NEW SCIENTIST 98:361, May 12, 1983.

Searching for the cause of the acquired immune deficiency syndrome, by R. D. Leavitt. EUROPEAN JOURNAL OF CLINICAL MICROBIOLOGY 3(1):79-84, February 1984.

Searching for the cause of AIDS: is HTLV the culprit?, by R. Bock. BIOSCIENCE 33: 619-620, November 1983.

Seattle AIDS Action Committee, by G. Bakan. NORTHWEST PASSAGE 24(2):7, September 1983.

Seborrheic dermatitis and acquired immunodeficiency syndrome [letter],by R. B. Skinner, Jr., et al. JOURNAL OF THE AMERICAN ACADEMY OF DERMATOLOGY 14(1):147-148, January 1986.

Seborrheic dermatitis and butterfly rash in AIDS [letter], by B. A. Eisenstat, et al. NEW ENGLAND JOURNAL OF MEDICINE 311(3):189, July 19, 1984.

Seborrheic dermatitis may signify AIDS in high-risk groups, by B. M. Mathes. AMERICAN FAMILY PHYSICIAN 33:263, March 1986.

Seborrheic-like dermatitis of acquired immunodeficiency syndrome. A clinicopathologic study, by F. F. Soeprono, et al. JOURNAL OF THE AMERICAN ACADEMY OF DERMATOLOGY 14(2, Part 1):242-248, February 1986.

SecDef decides to test active members for AIDS, by P. Smith. AIR FORCE TIMES 46:3, October 28, 1985.

SecDef issues guidelines for AIDS testing, by P. Smith. AIR FORCE TIMES 46:10, November 4, 1985.

Second virus linked to AIDS cancer, by O. Sattaur, et al. NEW SCIENTIST 106:8, April 11, 1985.

Secondary pulmonary alveolar proteinosis occurring in two patients with acquired immune deficiency syndrome, by F. L. Ruben, et al. AMERICAN JOURNAL OF MEDICINE 80(6):1187-1190, June 1986.

Secondary syphilis masquerading as AIDS in a young gay male, by R. A. Smego, Jr., et al. NORTH CAROLINA MEDICAL JOURNAL 45(4):253-254, April 1984.

Selective cytotoxicity of AIDS virus infection towards HTLV-I-transformed cell lines, by Y. Koyanagi, et al. INTERNATIONAL JOURNAL OF CANCER 36(4):445-451, October 15, 1985.

Selective defects in cytomegalovirus-and mitogen-induced lymphocyte proliferation and interferon release in patients with acquired immunodeficiency syndrome, by J. S. Epstein, et al. JOURNAL OF INFECTIOUS DISEASES 152(4):727-733, October 1985.

Selective tropism of lymphadenopathy associated virus (LAV) for helper-inducer T lymphocytes, by D. Klatzmann, et al. SCIENCE 225(4657):59-63, July 6, 1984.

Self-reported behavioral change among gay and bisexual men—San Francisco. MMWR 34(40):613-615, October 11, 1985.

Semen and AIDS [letter],by G. M. Shearer, et al. NATURE 308(5956):230, March 15-21, 1984.

—, by R. E. Rewell. NATURE 309(5967):394, May 31-June 6, 1984.

Semen polyamines in AIDS pathogenesis [letter], by J. D. Williamson. NATURE 310(5973):103, July 12-18, 1984.

Seminal lymphocytes, plasma and AIDS, by G. P. Olsen, et al. NATURE 309:116-117, May 10, 1984.

Seminar discusses 'AIDS: issues in the workplace,' by N. P. Guarda, et al. FLORIDA NURSE 35(2):5, February 1986.

Senate approves $22m for AIDS, by Bisticas-Cocoves. GAY COMMUNITY NEWS 13(16):1, November 2, 1985.

Senate votes to expand anti-AIDS drug trials, by D. M. Barnes. SCIENCE 233:1382, September 26, 1986.

Sense of power in San Francisco, by K. Kelley. GUARDIAN 37(46):10, September 25, 1985.

Sensible summer sex , by Bronski, et al. GAY COMMUNITY NEWS 12(40):4, April 27, 1985.

Sequence homology and morphologic similarity of HTLV-III and visna virus, a pathogenic lentivirus, by M. A. Gonda, et al. SCIENCE 227:173-177, January 11, 1985.

Sequence homology of the simian retrovirus genome with human T-cell leukemia virus type I, by T. Watanabe, et al. VIROLOGY 144:59-65, July 15, 1985.

Sera from patients with the acquired immunodeficiency syndrome inhibit production of interleukin-2 by normal lymphocytes, by J. P. Siegel, et al. JOURNAL OF CLINICAL INVESTIGATION 75(6):1957-1964, June 1985.

Serodiagnosis of Pneumosystis carinii [letter] by L. L. Pifer. CHEST 87(5):698-700, May 1985.

Seroepidemiologic screening for antibodies to LAV/HTLV-III in Sri Lanka, 1908-1982, by R. A. Miller, et al. NEW ENGLAND JOURNAL OF MEDICINE 313:1352-1353, November 21, 1985.

Seroepidemiological evidence for HTLV-III infection as the primary etiologic factor for acquired immunodeficiency syndrome, by M. G. Sarngadharan, et al. PROGRESS IN CLINICAL AND BIOLOGICAL RESEARCH 182:309-327, 1985.

Seroepidemiological studies of HTLV-III antibody prevalence among selected groups of heterosexual Africans, by N. Clumeck, et al. JAMA 254:2599-2603, November 8, 1985.

Seroepidemiological studies of human T-lymphotropic retrovirus type III in acquired immunodeficiency syndrome, by B. Safai, et al. LANCET 1(8392):1438-1440, June 30, 1984.

Seroepidemiology of HTLV-III antibodies in a remote population of eastern Zaire, by R. J. Biggar, et al. BRITISH MEDICAL JOURNAL 290(6471):808-810, March 16, 1985.

Sero-epidemiology of HTLV-III antibody in southern Africa, by S. F. Lyons, et al. SOUTH AFRICAN MEDICAL JOURNAL 67(24):961-962, June 15, 1985.

Seroepidemiology of HTLV-III (LAV) in the Federal Republic of Germany, by G. Hunsmann, et al. KLINISCHE WOCHENSCHRIFT 63(5):233-235, March 1, 1985.

Seroepidemiology of human T-cell leukemia virus in the French West Indies: antibodies in blood donors and patients with lymphoproliferative diseases who do not have AIDS, by A. Calender, et al. ANNALS OF THE NEW YORK ACADEMY OF SCIENCES 437:175-176, 1984.

Seroepidemiology of human T-lymphotropic virus type III among homosexual men with the acquired immunodeficiency syndrome or generalized lymphadenopathy and among asymptomatic controls in Boston, by J. E. Groopman, et al. ANNALS OF INTERNAL MEDICINE 102(3):334-337, March 1985.

Serologic identification and characterization of a macaque T-lymphotropic retrovirus closely related to HTLV-III, by P. J. Kanki, et al. SCIENCE 228(4704):1199-1201, June 7, 1985.

Serological analysis of a subgroup of human T-lymphotropic retroviruses (HTLV-III) associated with AIDS, by J. Schüpbach, et al. SCIENCE 224(4648):503-505, May 4, 1984.

Serological characterization of HTLV-III infection in AIDS and related disorders, by J. E. Groopman, et al. JOURNAL OF INFECTIOUS DISEASES 153(4):736-742, April 1986.

Serological characterization of human T-cell leukemia (lymphotropic) virus, type I (HTLV-I) small envelope protein, by M. J. Newman,e t al. VIROLOGY 150:106-116, April 15, 1986.

Serological markers as indicators of sexual orientation in AIDS virus-infected men [letter], by J. J. Potterat, et al. JAMA 256(6):712, August 8, 1986.

Serotherapy for AIDS and pre-AIDS syndrome [letter], by H. F. Sewell, et al. NATURE 320(6058):113-114, March 13-19, 1986.

Serotypes of Cryptococcus neoformans in patients with AIDS [letter], by M. G. Rinaldi, et al. JOURNAL OF INFECTIOUS DISEASES 153(3):642, March 1986.

Serum angiotensin converting enzyme in the acquired immunodeficiency syndrome or related syndromes [letter], by D. Vittecoq, et al. PRESSE MEDICALE 15(16): 758-759, April 19, 1986.

Serum beta 2-microglobulin and interferon in homosexual males: relationship to clinical findings and serologic status to the human T lymphotropic virus (HTLV-III), by L. H. Calabrese, et al. AIDS RESEARCH 1(6):423-438, 1984-1985.

Serum immunoglobulin elevations in the acquired immunodeficiency syndrome (AIDS): IgG, IgA, IgM, and IgD, by Q. Chess, et al. DIAGNOSTIC IMMUNOLOGY 2(3):148-153, 1984.

Serum interferon and clinical manifestations of infection with human T-lymphotropic virus type III, by J. Abb. MEDICAL MICROBIOLOGY AND IMMUNOLOGY 174(4): 205-210, 1985.

Serum lactate dehydrogenase levels in adults and children with acquired immune deficiency syndrome (AIDS) and AIDS-related complex: possible indicator of B cell lymphoproliferation and disease activity. Effect of intravenous gammaglobulin on enzyme levels, by B. A. Silverman, et al. AMERICAN JOURNAL OF MEDICINE 78(5):728-736, May 1985.

Serum marker may identify potential AIDS victims. AMERICAN JOURNAL OF NURSING 84:177, February 1984.

Serum suppression of lymphocyte activation in vitro in acquired immunodeficiency disease, by S. Cunningham-Rundles, et al. JOURNAL OF CLINICAL IMMUNOLOGY 3(2):156-165, Apr8il 1983.

Service groups say: "Don't take the test". BODY POLITIC 112:19, March 1985.

Services report 30 cases of AIDS, by P. Smith. AIR FORCE TIMES 44:26, May 14, 1984.

Several NIH Institutes involved in tracking down cause of AIDS, by J. McCarthy. NEWS & FEATURES FROM NIH April 1983, p 12-13.

Severe acquired immune deficiency syndrome in male homosexuals: diminished capacity to make interferon-alpha in vitro associated with severe opportunistic infections, by C. Lopez, et al. JOURNAL OF INFECTIOUS DISEASES 148(6): 962-966, December 1983.

Severe combined immunodeficiency associated with absent T4+ helper cells, by K. M. Edwards, et al. JOURNAL OF PEDIATRICS 105(1):70-72, July 1984.

Severe diarrhea in a patient with AIDS [letter], by J. M. Guerin, et al. JAMA 256(5): 591, August 1, 1986.

Severe digestive complications of AIDS in a group of patients from Zaire, by C. Jonas, et al. ACTA GASTROENTEROLOGICA BELGICA 47(4):396-402, July-August 1984.

Severe hyponatremia after colonoscopy preparation in a patient with the acquired immune deficiency syndrome, by J. M. Salik, et al. AMERICAN JOURNAL OF GASTROENTEROLOGY 80(3):177-179, March 1985.

Severe neutropenia during pentamidine treatment of immunodeficiency syndrome—New York City. JAMA 251(10):1253-1254, March 9, 1984; also in MMWR 33(6): 65-67, February 17, 1984.

Sex and germs, by K. Hale-Wehmann. SCIENCE FOR THE PEOPLE 18(4):26, July 1986.

Sex ban in baths proposed in D.C., by J. Ryan. GAY COMMUNITY NEWS 12(346):3, March 30, 1985.

Sex for the second millennium, by M. Pye. OBSERVER October 29, 1985, p. 41.

Sex in the age of AIDS, by L. Giteck.. ADVOCATE 450:42, July 8, 1986.

—, Part 2, by L. Giteck. ADVOCATE 451:28, July 22, 1986.

Sex scolding ignores fact: gays have changed. OUT 3(12):4, October 1985.

Sex transmits AIDS. THE ECONOMIST 300:14, July 5, 1986.

Sexual slander, by D. Rist. ADVOCATE 446:42, May 13, 1986.

Sharing of needles among users of intravenous drugs, by J. L. Black, et al. NEW ENGLAND JOURNAL OF MEDICINE 314:446, February 13, 1986.

Sharper tests for AIDS, by O. Sattaur. NEW SCIENTIST 106:23, May 2, 1985.

'Sheet sign' [letter], by F. Adams. JAMA 251(7):891, February 17, 1984.

Shigella flexneri bacteraemia in a patient with acquired immune deficiency syndrome, by Y. Glupczynski, et al. ACTA CLINICA BELGICA 40(6):388-390, 1985.

Short-term results with suramin for AIDS-related conditions [letter], by D. Rouvoy, et al. LANCET 1(8433):878-879, April 13, 1985.

Should actors take AIDS test before filming a kiss? JET 68:60-61, September 9, 1985.

Should AIDS victims be isolated? [interviews with R. Restak and C. Levine]. US NEWS & WORLD REPORT 99:50, September 30, 1985.

Should the bathhouses be closed?, by P. Freiberg. ADVOCATE 41:8, March 5, 1985.

Should corneal transplant donors be screened for human T-cell lymphotropic virus type III antibody? [editorial], by C. E. Margo. ARCHIVES OF OPHTHALMOLOGY 103(11):1643, November 1985.

Should I take the test? OUT 4(1):3, November 1985.

Should nurses be told if a patient has AIDS? RN 48:10, November 1985.

Should nursing homes take AIDS patients?, by R. B. Gebhardt. NURSING HOMES 35(2):13-15, March-April 1986.

Should pregnant women care for AIDS patients? [letter], by P. Solenberger. INFECTION CONTROL 6(5):180, May 1985.

Should the risk of acquired immunodeficiency syndrome deter hepatitis B vaccination? A decision analysis, by H. S. Sacks, et al. JAMA 252(24):3375-3377, December 28, 1984.

Side effects of substitution therapy, by L. M. Aledort. SCANDINAVIAN JOURNAL OF HAEMATOLOGY. SUPPLEMENTUM 40:331-333, 1984.

Significance of AIDS to dentists and dental practice, by D. R. Davis, et al. JOURNAL OF PROSTHETIC DENTISTRY 52(5):736-738, November 1984.

Significance of altered nutritional status in acquired immune deficiency syndrome (AIDS), by R. T. Chlebowski. NUTRITION AND CANCER 7(1-2):85-91, 1985.

Significance of non-A, non-B hepatitis, cytomegalovirus and the acquired immune deficiency syndrome in transfusion practice, by W. L. Bayer, et al. CLINICS IN HAEMATOLOGY 13(1):253-269, February 1984.

Signs of omission: press coverage of AIDS has left some things unsaid, by J. Alter. NEWSWEEK 106(13):25, Septemebr 23, 1985.

Simian AIDS: evidence for a retrovirus etiology, by M. Gardner, et al. FRONTIERS OF RADIATION THERAPY AND ONCOLOGY 19:26-32, 1985; also in HEMATOLOGICAL ONCOLOGY 2(3):259-268, July-September 1984.

Simian AIDS: isolation of a type D retrovirus and transmission of the disease, by P. A. Marx, et al. SCIENCE 223(4640):1083-1086, March 9, 1984.

Simian models of acquired immunodeficiency syndrome (AIDS): a review, by N. W. King. VETERINARY PATHOLOGY 23(4):345-353, July 1986.

Similarities between AIDS and PCM [letter], by R. H. Gray. AMERICAN JOURNAL OF PUBLIC HEALTH 73(11):1332, November 1983.

Simple method for determination of antibodies to AIDS associated virus (HTLV-III), by G. Biberfeld, et al. LAKARTIDNINGEN 81(39):3482-3483, September 26, 1984.

Simultaneous occurrence of Pneumocystis carinii pneumonia, cytomegalovirus infection, Kaposi's sarcoma, and B-immunoblastic sarcoma in a homosexual man, by R. L. Brukes, et al. JAMA 253(23):3425-3428, June 21, 1985.

Sinusitis caused by Legionella pneumophila in a patient with the acquired immune deficiency syndrome, by G. Schlanger, et al. AMERICAN JOURNAL OF MEDICINE 77(5):957-960, November 1984.

600 rally/march for AIDS fund, by L. Goldsmith. GAY COMMUNITY NEWS 10(49):1, July 2, 1983.

Skin disease in homosexual patients with acquired immune deficiency syndrome (AIDS) and lesser forms of human T cell leukaemia virus (HTLV III) disease, by C. F. Farthing, et al. CLINICAL AND EXPERIMENTAL DERMATOLOGY 10(1):3-12, January 1985.

Slow, insidious natures of the HTLV's, by J. L. Marx. SCIENCE 231:50-51, January 31, 1986.

Slow progress on AIDS vaccines. NEW SCIENTIST 111:17, September 11, 1986.

Small AIDS, by M. Nemeth. ALBERTA REPORT 12:48, July 8, 1985.

Small and rurals await impending AIDS crisis, by D. Burda. HOSPITALS 60(3):71-73, February 5, 1986.

Small bowel lymphoma associated with AIDS, by P. E. Collier. JOURNAL OF SURGERY AND ONCOLOGY 32(2):131-133, June 1986.

Small intestinal lymphoma in three patients with acquired immune deficiency syndrome, by J. J. Steinberg, et al. AMERICAN JOURNAL OF GASTROENTEROLOGY 80(1):21026, January 1985.

Small noncleaved B cell Burkitt-like lymphoma with chromosome t(8;14) translocation and Epstein-Barr virus nuclear-associated antigen in a homosexual man with acquired immune deficiency syndrome, by J. M. Petersen, et al. AMERICAN JOURNAL OF MEDICINE 78(1):141-148, January 1985.

Social aspects of the AIDS problem. The best possibility lies in reality-oriented actions, by R. Osterwalder. KRANKENPFLEGE. SOINS INFIRMIERS 79(5):43-45, May 1986.

Social consequences of the acquired immunodeficiency syndrome, by B. J. Cassens. ANNALS OF INTERNAL MEDICINE 103(5):768-771, November 1985.

Social disease [editorial]. NATION 241(7):195, September 14, 1985.

Social meaning of AIDS, by P. Conrad. SOCIAL POLICY 17(1):51, Summer 1986.

Social networks and the spread of infectious diseases: the AIDS example, by A. S. Klovdahl. SOCIAL SCIENCE & MEDICINE 21(11):1203-1216, 1985.

Social work and AIDS, by A-L. Furstenberg, et al. SOCIAL WORK IN HEALTH CARE 9(4):45-62, 1984.

Society's survival first, then victims' rights: AIDS plague, by Richard Restak. HUMAN EVENTS 45:18+, October 5, 1985.

Sodomy and the Supreme Court, by D. Robinson, Jr. COMMENTARY 82:57-61, October 1986.

Soluble factors inhibitory for T-cell-dependent immune responses in patients with the acquired immune deficiency syndrome and its prodromes, by J. Laurence, et al. ANNALS OF THE NEW YORK ACADEMY OF SCIENCES 437:518-525, 1984.

Soluble suppressor factors in patients with acquired immune deficiency syndrome and its prodrome. Elaboration in vitro by T lymphocyte-adherent cell interactions, by J. Laurence, et al. JOURNAL OF CLINICAL INVESTIGATION 72(6):2072-2081, December 1983.

Some complications of the therapy of classic hemophilia, by O. D. Ratnoff. JOURNAL OF LABORATORY AND CLINICAL MEDICINE 103(5):653-659, May 1984.

Some problems in the prediction of future numbers of cases of the acquired immuno-deficiency syndrome in the UK, by M. McEvoy, et al. LANCET 2(8454):541-542, September 7, 1985.

Some questions and answers about AIDS. PENNSYLVANIA NURSE 41(2):9+, February 1986.

Some sex out of danger?, by K. Popert. BODY POLITIC 123:15, February 1986.

Sound policies and expert advice are your best protection against AIDS, by K. McCormick. AMERICAN SCHOOL BOARD JOURNAL 173(5):36-37, May 1986.

Soviet offer on AIDS, by V. Rich. NATURE 317:659, October 24, 1985.

Soviets admit AIDS cases, by V. Rich. NATURE 318(6046):502, December 12, 1985.

Speaking VD, by P. Masters. GAY INFORMATION JOURNAL OF GAY STUDIES 12:19, Summer 1982.

Special challenge of AIDS: providing facts, calming fears. PUBLIC HEALTH RE-PORTS 99(1):99-100, January-February 1984.

Special pathologico-anatomical aspects of AIDS—acquired immune deficiency syn-drome, By G. R. Krueger, et al. ZEITSCHRIFT FUR HAUTKRANKHEITEN 59(8):507-522, April 15, 1984.

Special report: AIDS testing. CITIZEN AIRMAN 37:8, Winter 1985-1986.

Special report: infection-control guidelines for patients with the acquired immunodefi-ciency syndrome (AIDS), by J. E. Conte, Jr., et al. HOSPITAL TOPICS 62(2):44-48, March-April 1984.

Specific antibodies against human T cell leukemia virus found in AIDS patients,by K. Nagy, et al. ORVOSI HETILAP 125(26):1557-1560, June 24, 1984.

Specific gastrointestinal manifestations of a generalized cytomegalovirus infection in a patient with acquired immune deficiency syndrome, by A. Krämer, et al. DEUTSCHE MEDIZINISCHE WOCHENSCHRIFT 110(12):462-468, March 22, 1985.

Specific translocations characterize Burkitt's-like lymphoma of homosexual men with the aquired immunodeficiency syndrome, by R. S. Chaganti, et al. BLOOD 61(6):126-1268, June 1983.

Specificity of lyphocytotoxic antibodies in AIDS and pre-AIDS patients, by V. Wicher, et al. AIDS RESEARCH 1(2):139-148, 1983-1984.

Spectrum of central nervous system complications in homosexual men with acquired immune deficiency syndrome [letter], by S. D. Pitlik, et al. JOURNAL OF INFEC-TIOUS DISEASES 148(4):771-772, October 1983.

Spectrum of Kaposi's sarcoma in the epidemic of AIDS, by B. Safai, et al. CANCER RESEARCH 45(Suppl. 9):4646s-4648s, September 1985.

Spectrum of liver disease in the acquired immunodeficiency syndrome, by S. C. Gordon, et al. JOURNAL OF HEPATOLOGY 2(3):475-484, 1986.

Spectrum of morphologic changes of lymph nodes from patients with AIDS or AIDS-related complexes, by P. Rácz, et al. PROGRESS IN ALLERGY 37:81-181, 1986.

Spectrum of pulmonary diseases associated with the acquired immune deficiency syndrome, by D. E. Stover, et al. AMERICAN JOURNAL OF MEDICINE 78(3): 429-437, March 1985.

Spectrum of renal abnormalities in acquired immune-deficiency syndrome, by N. D. Vaziri, et al. JOURNAL OF THE NATIONAL MEDICAL ASSOCIATION 77(5):369-375, May 1985.

Speculations on the viral etiology of acquired immune deficiency syndrome and Kaposi's sarcoma, by M. A. Conant. JOURNAL OF INVESTIGATIVE DERMATOLOGY 83(Supl. 1):57s-62s, July 1984.

Sperm wary: Aussie AIDS puts Calgary insemination on hold, by K. Diotte, et al. ALBERTA REPORT 12:35, August 12, 1985.

Spermatozoa and immune dysregulation in homosexual men [letter]. JAMA 252(9): 1130, September 7, 1984.

Spinal cord degeneration in AIDS, by L. Goldstick, et al. NEUROLOGY 35(1):103-106, January 1985.

Spontaneous and interferon resistant natural killer cell energy in AIDS, by W. M. Mitchell, et al. AIDS RESEARCH 1(3):221-229, 1983-1984.

Spontaneous colonic perforation secondary to cytomegalovirus in a patient with acquired immune deficiency syndrome, by H. B. Kram, et al. CRITICAL CARE MEDICINE 12(5):469-471, May 1984.

Spontaneous regression of Kaposi's sarcoma in patients with AIDS [letter], by F. X. Real, et al. NEW ENGLAND JOURNAL OF MEDICINE 313(26):1659, December 26, 1985.

Spontaneous resolution of cryptosporidiosis in a child with acquired immunodeficiency syndrome [letter], by C. D. Berkowitz, et al. AMERICAN JOURNAL OF DISEASES OF CHILDREN 189(10):967, October 1985.

Spontaneous rupture of the spleen due to acquired immunodeficiency syndrome in an intravenous drug abuser, by H. G. Mirchandani, et al. ARCHIVES OF PATHOLOGY AND LABORATORY MEDICINE 109(12):1114-1116, December 1985.

Spontaneously healing Kaposi's sarcoma in AIDS [letter], by M. Janier, et al. NEW ENGLAND JOURNAL OF MEDICINE 312(25):1638-1639, June 20, 1985.

Sporadic, endemic and AIDS-related Kaposi's sarcoma. Different clinical course variants of the tumor demonstrated by 3 typical cases, by H. Rasokat, et al. ZEITSCHRIFT FUR HAUTKRANKHEITEN 60(1-2):109-115, January 1985.

Spread of AIDS sparks new health concern, by J. L. Marx. SCIENCE 219:42-43, January 7, 1983.

Spreading alarm about AIDS, by J. Seligmann, et al. NEWSWEEK 107(25):68, June 23, 1986.

Spreading of AIDS panic: Edmonton reports its fourth victim as public fear mounts, by L. Cohen. ALBERTA REPORT 12:52, November 4, 1985.

Squamous-cell carcinoma, Kaposi's sarcoma and Burkitt's lymphoma are consequences of impaired immune surveillance of ubiquitous viruses in acquired immune deficiency syndrome, allograft recipients and tropical African patients, by D. T. Purtilo, et al. IARC SCIENTIFIC PUBLICATIONS 63:749-770, 1984.

Squamous cell carcinoma of the epiglottis in a homosexual man at risk for AIDS [letter], by M. M. Alhashimi, et al. JAMA 253(16):2366, April 26, 1985.

SSI benefits approved AIDS patients, by P. Byron. GAY COMMUNITY NEWS 10(44):1, May 29, 1983.

Standing up for life, by Friends, et al. RFD 35:15, Summer 1983.

Star-studded gala raises $1 mil. for AIDS research. JET 69:56, October 7, 1985.

Start of a plague mentality, by L. Morrow. TIME 126(12):92, September 23, 1985.

Startling AIDS-related discovery [modified hemoglobin blood substitute; work of C. Hsia], by M. McDonald. MACLEAN'S 98:42-43, July 15, 1985.

State plans to trace sex, needle partners. OUT 4(5):1, April 1986.

State proposes $1.8M for AIDS, by C. Guilfoy. GAY COMMUNITY NEWS 12(42):1, May 11, 1985.

State regulators to probe impact of AIDS on insurance underwriting, by J. Diamond. THE NATIONAL UNDERWRITER 89:1+, December 28, 1985.

State seeking sites for antibody testing. OUT 3(6):3, April 1985.

Statement on the development of guidelines for the prevention of AIDS transmission in the workplace, by J. O. Mason. PUBLIC HEALTH REPORTS 101(1):6-8, January-Febraury 1986.

Status report on the acquired immunodeficiency syndrome: human T-cell lymphotropic virus type III testing. JAMA 254:1342-1345, September 13, 1985.

—, by AMA Council on Scientific Affairs. CONNECTICUT MEDICINE 49(10):667-670, October 1985; also in JAMA 254(10):1342-1345, September 13, 1985.

Stevens: keep AIDS-positive civilians home,by A. Laurent. AIR FORCE TIMES 46: 58, June 2, 1986.

Stigmatizing the victim [editorial]. NATION 242(14):505, April 12, 1986.

Still in the waiting room, by R. Joyce. BODY POLITIC 127:13, June 1986.

Stimulation of cellular function by thymopentin (TP-5) in three AIDS patients [letter], by F. Mascart-Lemone, et al. LANCET 2(8352):735-736, September 24, 1983.

Stop the LaRouche panic!, by P. Drucker. AGAINST THE CURRENT 455:17, September 16, 1985.

Stopping the AIDS epidemic, by P. Kawata. PUBLIC WELFARE 44(3):35, Summer 1986.

Story of the year: the AIDS trauma touched everyone, by David Black, et al. ROLLING STONE p. 121+, December 19, 1985, January 2, 1986.

Straight talk about AIDS. AMERICAN JOURNAL OF NURSING 83:1170, August 1983.

Strategic plan for the management of patients with AIDS, by S. Malik-Nitto, et al. NURSING MANAGEMENT 17(6):46+, June 1986.

Strategies for an AIDS vaccine, by D. M. Barnes. SCIENCE 233:1149-1150+, September 12, 1986.

Streptococcus bovis bacteremia and acquired immunodeficiency syndrome [letter], by J. B. Glaser, et al. ANNALS OF INTERNAL MEDICINE 99(6):878, December 1983.

Streptococcus pneumoniae infections and bacteremia in patients with acquired immune deficiency syndrome, with report of a pneumococcal vaccine failure, by M. S. Simberkoff, et al. AMERICAN REVIEW OF RESPIRATORY DISEASE 130(6): 1174-1176, December 1984.

Stress management on the job, by C. Dunphy. WASHINGTON NURSE 15(2):9, February 1985.

Strong new candidate for AIDS agent [news], by J. L. Marx. SCIENCE 224(4648): 475-477, May 4, 1984.

Structural analysis of p19 and p24 core polypeptides of primate lymphotropic retroviruses (PLRV), by E. Jurkiewicz, et al. VIROLOGY 150:291-298, April 15, 1986.

Structure and function of human leukemia and AIDS viruses, by W. A. Haseltine, et al. INTERNATIONAL SYMPOSIUM OF THE PRINCESS TAKAMATSU CANCER RESEARCH FUND 15:187-196, 1984.

Structures resembling scrapie-associated fibrils in AIDS encephalopathy [letter],by P. N. Goldwater, et al. LANCET 2(8452):447-448, August 24, 1985.

Struggle looms over AIDS tests, by L. J. Lyons. THE NATIONAL UNDERWRITER 90:1+, March 1, 1986.

Struggling to save the next generation, by T. Prentice. TIMES October 28, 1986, p. 14.

Students run Stanford AIDS education project, by G. Koskovich. ADVOCATE 455: 17, September 16, 1985.

Studies further speculation on AIDS, by L. Goldsmith. GAY COMMUNITY NEWS 10(43):3, May 21, 1983.

Studies in homosexual patients with and without lymphadenopathy. Relationships to the acquired immune deficiency syndrome,by R. D. deShazo, et al. ARCHIVES OF INTERNAL MEDICINE 144(6):1153-1158, June 1984.

Studies of the putative transforming protein of the type I human T-cell leukemia virus, by D. J. Slamon, et al. SCIENCE 228:1427-1430, June 21, 1985.

Studies show no link between swine fever/AIDS, by M. Kelquist. ADVOCATE 432: 23, October 29, 1985.

Study proves condoms block AIDS virus, by M. Helquist. ADVOCATE 438:20, January 21, 1986.

Subacute encephalitis in acquired immune deficiency syndrome: a postmortem study, by S. L. Nielsen, et al. AMERICAN JOURNAL OF CLINICAL PATHOLOGY 82(6):678-682, December 1984.

Subcellular localization of the product of the long open reading frame of human T-cell leukemia virus type, by I. W. C. Goh, et al. SCIENCE 227:1227-1228, March 8, 1985.

Subcutaneous fibromatosis associated with an acquired immune deficiency syndrome in pig-tailed macaques, by C. C. Tsai, et al. AMERICAN JOURNAL OF PATHOLOGY 120(1):30-37, July 1985.

Subunit vaccines against exogenous retroviruses: overview and perspectives, by G. Hunsmann. CANCER RESEARCH 45(Suppl. 9):4691s-4693s, September 1985.

Success quotients: dealing with AIDS, by P. Kerschner. JOURNAL OF THE AMERICAN HEALTH CARE ASSOCIATION 11(8):44, December 1985.

Successful treatment of lethal protozoal infections with the ornithine decarboxylase inhibitor, alpha-difluoromethylornithine, by A. Sjoerdsma, et al. TRANSACTIONS OF THE ASSOCIATION OF AMERICAN PHYSICIANS 97:70-79, 1984.

Successful treatment of Pneumocystis carinii pneumonia with trimethoprim-sulfamethoxazole in hypersensitive AIDS patients, by R. B. Gibbons, et al. JAMA 253:1259-1260, March 1,1985.

Such were some of you: a Christian response to homosexuals, by M. Braun. FUNDA-MENTALIST JOURNAL 4(3):22-24, March 1985.

Suicide AIDS related. OUT 2(10):3, September 1984.

Sulphadiazine desensitisation in AIDS patients [letter], by E. t. Bell, et al. LANCET 1(8421):163, January 19, 1985.

Summary: recommendations for preventing transmission of infection with HTLV-III/LAV in the workplace. JAMA 254:3023-3024+, December 6, 1985.

Summer reading on AIDS, by N. Fain. ADVOCATE 3(75):15, September 1, 1983.

Supergerms: the new health menace, by J. Mann. US NEWS AND WORLD REPORT 94:35-36, February 28, 1983.

Support for DNCB research, by M. Helquist. ADVOCATE 446:21, May 13, 1986.

Suppressor function of T lymphocytes in the acquired immunodeficiency syndrome as assessed by allogeneic mixed lymphocyte culture, by R. Y. Lin, et al. JOUR-NAL OF CLINICAL AND LABORATORY IMMUNOLOGY 16(2):69-73, Feburary 1985.

Suppressor T cells and the immune response to tumors, by S. Schatten, et al. CRC CRITICAL REVIEWS IN IMMUNOLOGY 4(4):335-379, 1984.

Suramin drug is disappointing in AIDS. NEW SCIENTIST 107:30, September 26, 1985.

Suramin protection of T cells in vitro against infectivity and cytopathic effect of HTLV-III, by H. Mitsuya, et al. SCIENCE 226:172-174, October 12, 1984.

Suramin therapy in patients with LAS/AIDS (letter), by W. Busch, et al. DEUTSCHE MEDIZINISCHE WOCHENSCHRIFT 110(40)1552, October 4, 1985.

Suramin treatment for AIDS [letter], by w. Busch, et al. LANCET 2(8466):1247, November 30, 1985.

Sure fire blood test for AIDS sought, by N. Fain. ADVOCATE 8(78):23, October 13, 1983.

Surgeon and HTLV-III infection [editorial], by C. D. Forbes. BRITISH JOURNAL OF SURGERY 73(3):168-169, March 1986.

Surgical abdomen in the acquired immunodeficiency syndrome. Apropos of 4 cases, by A. Olivier, et al. CHIRURGIE 111(1):69-75, 1985.

Surgical biopsy for persistent generalized lymphadenopathy, by H. J. Rashleigh-Belcher, et al. BRITISH JOURNAL OF SURGERY 73(3):183-185, March 1986.

Surgical considerations in the diagnosis and management of AIDS, by M. T. Lotze. AIDS RESEARCH 2(2):141-148, Spring 1986.

Surgical perspective on AIDS. AMERICAN FAMILY PHYSICIAN 29:265, June 1984.

Surprising action for the AIDS virus, by J. L. Marx. SCIENCE 231:798, February 21, 1986.

Surveillance and control of infectious diseases: progress toward the 1990 objectives, by W. R. Dowdle. PUBLIC HEALTH REPORTS 98(3):210-218, May-June 1983.

Surveillance of the acquired immune deficiency syndrome in the United Kingdom, Jan. '82-July 1983. BRITISH MEDICAL JOURNAL 287:407-408, August 6, 1983.

Surveillance of AIDS in Britain: September 1983. BRITISH MEDICAL JOURNAL 287(6401):1284, October 29, 1983.

Survey: Bay Area men reduce AIDS risk, by S. Hyde. GAY COMMUNITY NEWS 12(18):3, November 17, 1984.

Survey of hospital personnel on the understanding of the acquired immunodeficiency syndrome, by W. M. Valenti, et al. AMERICAN JOURNAL OF INFECTION CONTROL 14(2):60-63, April 1986.

Survey of the prevalence of AIDS-associated virus (LAV) infection in Japan, by H. Tsuchie, et al. JOURNAL OF INFECTION 10(3):272-276, May 1985.

Survey search: four studies of employers' responses to AIDS. HEALTH COST MANAGEMENT 3(1):7-15+, January-February 1986.

"Survival kit". OUT 4(6):1, May 1986.

Survival of HIV in the common bedbug [letter],by S. F. Lyons, et al. LANCET 2(8497):45, July 5, 1986.

Suspected AIDS: an approach that helps patients, whatever the diagnosis, by J. T. Wheeler. CONSULTANT 25(18):102-103+, December 1985.

Sydney AIDS Project. Sydney AIDS study group. MEDICAL JOURNAL OF AUS-
TRALIA 141(9):569-573, October 27, 1984.

Symposium on HTLV. Bethesda, Maryland, December 6 & 7, 1984. CANCER RE-
SEARCH 45(Suppl. 9):4520s-4711s, September 1985.

Symposium on infections in the compromised host. The acquired immunodeficiency
syndrome, by D. J. LaCamera, et al. NURSING CLINICS OF NORTH AMERICA
20(1):241-256, March 1985.

Syndrome of unexplained generalized lymphadenopathy in young men in New York
City. Is it related to the acquired immune deficiency syndrome?, by B. Miller, et al.
JAMA 251(2):242-246, January 13, 1984.

Synthesis of kappa light chains by cell lines containing an 8;22 chromosomal translocation derived from a male homosexual with Burkitt's lymphoma, by I. Magrath,
et al. SCIENCE 222:1094-1098, December 9, 1983.

T and B cell reactions in AIDS and AIDS risk groups, by J. Kekow, et al. IMMUNITÄT
UND INFEKTION 13(1):26-28, February 1985.

T-cell imbalances in blood and lymph nodes from patients with acquired immune deficiency syndrome or AIDS-related complex, by C. E. Grossi, et al. ALABAMA
JOURNAL OF MEDICAL SCIENCES 22(2):160-163, April 1985.

T-cell lymphoma associated with immunologic evidence of retrovirus infection in a low-
land gorilla, by A. W. Prowten, et al. JOURNAL OF THE AMERICAN VETERIN-
ARY MEDICAL ASSOCIATION 187:1280-1282, December 1, 1985.

T cell malignancies and human T cell leukemia (lymphotropic) retroviruses (HTLV), by
P. S. Sarin, et al. PROGRESS IN CLINICAL AND BIOLOGICAL RESEARCH 184:
445-456, 1985.

T cell malignancies and human T cell leukemia virus, by R. C. Gallo, et al. SEMINARS
IN ONCOLOGY 11(1):12-17, March 1984.

T cell proliferation and ablation. A biologic spectrum of abnormalities induced by the
human T cell lymphotropic virus group, by S. Broder. PROGRESS IN ALLERGY
37:224-243, 1986.

T cell ratios in AIDS [letter], by A. J. Pinching. BRITISH MEDICAL JOURNAL
287(6406):1716-1717, December 3, 1983.

T cell surface antigen expression on lymphocytes of patients with AIDS during in vitro
mitogen stimulation, y C. G. Munn, et al. CANCER IMMUNOLOGY AND IMMUNO-
THERAPY 18(3):141-148, 1984.

T-cells and sympathy, by R. Massa. VILLAGE VOICE 30:110, April 23, 1985.

T-lymphocyte subpopulations in hemophiliacs and other groups at risk for the acquired immunodeficiency syndrome (AIDS), by T. Gallart. MEDICINA CLINICA
83(12):492-496, October 20, 1984.

T-lymphocyte subset phenotypes: a multisite evaluation of normal subjects and
patients with AIDS, by M. F. La Via, et al. DIAGNOSTIC IMMUNOLOGY 3(2):75-
82, 1985.

T4 lymphocyte in AIDS [editorial], by R. S. Kalish, et al. NEW ENGLAND JOURNAL
OF MEDICINE 313(2):112-113, July 11, 1985.

Tabloid terror from not-so-United Kingdom, by N. DeJongh. ADVOCATE 417:43, April 2, 1985.

Take no risks in AIDs care, by A. Fong, et al. RN 47:104, April 1984.

Take the test!, by B. Voeller. ADVOCATE 419:5, April 30, 1985.

Taking aim with an empty gun, by K. Popart. BODY POLITIC 116:14, July 1985.

Taking control—women, sex and AIDS, by C. Patton. GAY COMMUNITY NEWS 11(9):5, September 17, 1983.

Taking a sexual history, by R. A. Gremminger. WISCONSIN MEDICAL JOURNAL 82(11):20-24, November 1983.

Taking the test: what for?, by J. Aynsley. BODY POLITIC 121:17, December 1985.

Talcosis in AIDS victims? [letter] by D. Brauner, et al. AMERICAN JOURNAL OF CLINI-CAL PATHOLOGY 81(1):145, January 1984.

Talking about AIDS, by Andrew, et al. GAY COMMUNITY NEWS 10(47):6, June 18, 1983.

Tapeworms for lunch, by G. Halak. CHANGING MEN 14:15, Spring 1985.

Task Force to meet president aide, by S. Hyde. GAY COMMUNITY NEWS 10(47):1, June 18, 1983.

Tattoo trouble: fear of AIDS prompts a call for regulations, by B. Henker. ALBERTA REPORT 13:52-53, April 14, 1986.

Taxonomy over treatment?, by J. Beldekas. GAY COMMUNITY NEWS 12(30):7, February 16, 1985.

Ten thousand join AIDS vigil, by M. Cocoves. GAY COMMUNITY NEWS 12(26):1, June 8,   1985.

Tenth annual Eastern Claims Conference: AIDS—only the tip of the iceberg? by A. G. Clarke. BEST'S REVIEW 86:131-132, April 1986.

Test centers: shifting funds, by D. Walter. ADVOCATE 420:13, May 14, 1985.

Test insurance applicants for signs of AIDS? [interviews with S. Rish and J. Corcoran]. US NEWS & WORLD REPORT 99:71, November 25, 1985.

Test shows AIDS bug well established here. BODY POLITIC 111:14, February 1985.

Test with no right answers, by S. Burke. OUT 3(5):1, March 1985.

Test your knowledge of AIDS: a self-quiz, by F. R. Velazquez. MLO 18(8):40-42+, August 1986.

Testicular cancer in homosexual men with cellular immune deficiency: report of 2 cases, by C. J. Logothetis, et al. JOURNAL OF UROLOGY 133(3):484-486, March 1985.

Testicular toxoplasmosis in two men with the acquired immunodeficiency syndrome (AIDS), by M. Nistal, et al. ARCHIVES OF PATHOLOGY AND LABORATORY MEDICINE 110(8):744-746, August 1986.

Testing donors for AIDS. AMERICAN FAMILY PHYSICIAN 32:251, August 1985.

—, by A. Finlayson. MACLEAN'S 98:49, May 27, 1985.

Testing donors of organs, tissues, and semen for antibody to human T-lymphotropic virus type III/lymphadenopathy-associated virus. JAMA 253:3391, June 21, 1985.

Testing of donor blood for AIDS agents, by A. Novick, et al. JAMA 253:3463-3465, June 21, 1985.

Tests show virus common, long-established/Africa. BODY POLITIC 114:21, May 1985.

Tetanus prophylaxis in AIDS patients, by R. T. Chen, et al. JAMA 255:1061, February 28, 1986.

Texas attorney activist dies of AIDS, by H. Hod. ADVOCATE 3(86):11, January 24, 1984.

Texas attorney dies of AIDS. GAY COMMUNITY NEWS 11(25):3, January 14, 1984.

Texas backs off from "incorrigibles" quarantine, by Bisticas-Cocoves. GAY COMMUNITY NEWS 13(28):1, February 1, 1986.

Texas health official drops AIDS quarantine sup., by D. Walter. ADVOCATE 440:15, February 18, 1986.

Texas health officials seek quarantine, by S. Conn. GAY COMMUNITY NEWS 13(26): 1, January 18, 1986.

Texas set to approve AIDS quarantine rule, by D. Walter. ADVOCATE 438:15, January 21, 1986.

Theatre [review of plays The Normal Heart and As Is], by J. C. Thorpe. THE CRISIS 92:13+, October 1985.

Theater as therapy: "AIDS/US" creates drama, by S. McDonald. ADVOCATE 450:39, July 8, 1986.

Theatre in the plague years, by R. Hardy. BODY POLITIC 116:34, July 1985.

Theatre of AIDS, by K. Plummer. NEW SOCIETY June 28, 1985, p. 476-477.

Therapeutic approaches to patients with AIDS, by H. C. Lane, et al. CANCER RESEARCH 45(Suppl. 9):4674s-4676s, September 1985.

Therapy of Kaposi's sarcoma in AIDS, by P. Volberding. SEMINARS IN ONCOLOGY 11(1):60-70, March 1984.

Thirteenth annual UCLA symposium. Abstracts: acquired immune deficiency syndrome. JOURNAL OF CELLULAR BIOCHEMISTRY 8A(Suppl):1-23, 1984.

Thirty-eight-year-old male with bilateral pulmonary infiltrates and the septic picture of fatal development [clinical conference]. REVISTA CLINICA ESPAÑOLA 177(9):459-467, December 1985.

Thirty-nine-year-old man with thrombocytopenia, cough, fever, and shaking chills [clinical conference]. NEW YORK STATE JOURNAL OF MEDICINE 85(1):27-33, January 1985.

Thirty seconds that could shake the country, by H. Hawkins. GUARDIAN November 11, 1986, p. 26.

Thirty-two-year-old AIDs patient with progressive pulmonary infiltrates [clinical conference], by A. White, et al. INDIANA MEDICINE 78(10):884-890, October 1985.

This century's catastrophe? (4). No isolation of AIDS patients in the hospital, by B. A. Ostby. SYKEPLEIEN 73(7A):28-30+, April 1986.

— (5). Fear of meeting AIDS patients, by T. Sorhus. SYKEPLEIEN 73(9):20-25, May 23, 1986.

— (6). World's first AIDS unit, by S. B. Roll. SYKEPLEIEN 73(11):16-18, June 20, 1986.

This seeing the sick endears them, by M. Lynch. BODY POLITIC 91:36, March 1983.

Thoracic manifestations of the acquired immune deficiency syndrome, by H. I. Pass, et al. JOURNAL OF THORACIC AND CARDIOVASCULAR SURGERY 88(5, Part 1):654-658, November 1984.

Thousands demand AIDS funding. BODY POLITIC 95:19, July 1983.

Thousands demand more AIDS funding, by B. Nelson. GAY COMMUNITY NEWS 10(42):1, May 14, 1983.

Threat of AIDS widening to the general public [interview with J. Curran]. US NEWS & WORLD REPORT 99:66, August 5, 1985.

Three cases of AIDS-related psychiatric disorders, by J. R. Rundell, et al. AMERICAN JOURNAL OF PSYCHIATRY 143:777-778, June 1986.

Three fungal infections in an AIDS patient, by G. P. Holmes, et al. JOURNAL OF THE KENTUCKY MEDICAL ASSOCIATION 84(5):225-226, May 1986.

Three-year incidence of AIDS in five cohorts of HTLV-III infected risk group members, by J. J. Goedert, et al. SCIENCE 231:992-995, February 28, 1986.

Thymic dysplasia in acquired immunodeficiency syndome [letter], by R. Elfie, et al. NEW ENGLAND JOURNAL OF MEDICINE 308(14):841-842, April 7, 1983.

Thymopentin treatment in AIDS and pre-AIDS patients, by N. Clumeck, et al. SURVEY OF IMMUNOLOGICAL RESEARCH 4(Suppl. 1):58-62, 1985.

Thymosin in the early diagnosis and treatment of high risk homosexuals and hemophiliacs with AIDS-like immune dysfunction, by P. H. Naylor, et al. ANNALS OF THE NEW YORK ACADEMY OF SCIENCES 437:88-99, 1984.

Thymosin in the staging and treatment of HTLV-III positive homosexuals and hemophiliacs with AIDS-related immune dysfunction, by A. L. Goldstein, et al. ADVANCES IN EXPERIMENTAL MEDICINE AND BIOLOGY 187:129-140, 1985.

Thymus fragment transplantation in the acquired immunodeficiency syndrome [letter], by N. Ciobanu, et al. ANNALS OF INTERNAL MEDICINE 103(3):479, September 1985.

Thymus in AIDS [letter], by K. Welch. AMERICAN JOURNAL OF CLINICAL PATHOLOGY 85(4):531, April 1986.

Thymus involution in the acquired immunodeficiency syndrome, by W. W. Grody, et al. AMERICAN JOURNAL OF CLINICAL PATHOLOGY 84(1):85-95, July 1985.

Thymus protein offers a clue to AIDS vaccine. NEW SCIENTIST 110:20, May 29, 1986.

Time for honest talk on AIDS, by M. Adler. TIMES July 8, 1986, p. 10.

Times poll: public support for quarantine tattoo, by M. Daniels. ADVOCATE 438:15, January 21, 1986.

Tinea faciale mimicking seborrheic dermatitis in a patient with AIDS, by C. Perniciaro, et al. NEW ENGLAND JOURNAL OF MEDICINE 314:315-316, January 30, 1986.

Tinseltown and St. Petersburg, by D. Altman. BODY POLITIC 123:25, February 1986.

Tissue culture isolation of Toxoplasma from blood of a patient with AIDS, by J. M. Hofflin, et al. ARCHIVES OF INTERNAL MEDICINE 145(5):925-926, May 1985.

To let nurses work in ignorance is despicable says College. Nurses not told patients had AIDS. NURSING STANDARD 380:1, January 17, 1985.

To stop AIDS, by M. Larkin. HEALTH 17:64, December 1985.

Too close for comfort: gays afraid of gays w/AIDS, by C. Guilfoy. GAY COMMUNITY NEWS 13(13):8, October 12, 1985.

Too little aid for AIDS, by J. Randal. TECHNOLOGY REVIEW 87(6):10-13+, August-September 1984.

Top AIDS researcher testify, by M. Helquist. ADVOCATE 429:18, September 17, 1985.

Toronto to get hospice for AIDS patients. CANADIAN NURSE 82:15, March 1986.

Tough AIDS-funding fight predicted, by D. Walter. ADVOCATE 413:8, February 5, 1985.

Tough new problems for institutions: inmates with AIDS. CRIMINAL JUSTICE NEWS-LETTER 16(17):1-2, September 3, 1985.

Toughers virus of all: can a drug or vaccine be found to vanquish AIDS? TIME 128(18):76-77, November 3, 1986.

Toxic shock research lessons—AIDS, by C. Patton. GAY COMMUNITY NEWS 11(32):3, March 3, 1984.

Toxoplasma encephalitis in acquired immunodeficiency syndrome by A. Vital, et al. ANNALS OF PATHOLOGY 4(1):80-82, January-March 1984.

Toxoplasma encephalitis in Haitian adults with acquired immunodeficiency syndrome: a clinical-pathologic-CT correlation, by M. J. Post, et al. AJR 140(5):861-868, May 1983.

Toxoplasmic encephalitis in patients with acquired immune deficiency syndrome, by B. J. Luft, et al. JAMA 252(7):913-917, August 17, 1984.

Toxoplasmosis. Immunohistochemical study of a case of acquired toxoplasmosis in a patient with AIDS and of a case of congenital toxoplasmosis, by C. Herbert, et al. REVUE MEDICALE DE LA SUISSE ROMANDE 105(1):89-100, January 1985.

Toxoplasmosis and AIDS. AMERICAN FAMILY PHYSICIAN 31:345, February 1985.

Toxoplasmosis diagnosis and immunodeficiency [editorial]. LANCET 1(8377):605-606, March 17, 1984.

Toxoplasmosis encephalitis in patients with AIDS, by W. Enzensberger, et al. DEUTSCHE MEDIZINISCHE WOCHENSCHRIFT 110(3):83-87, January 18, 1985.

Toxoplasmosis in immunosuppression and AIDS, by B. Velimirovic. INFECTION 12(5):315-317, September-October 1984.

Toxoplasmosis presenting as panhypopituitarism in a patient with the acquired immune deficiency syndrome, by S. A. Milligan, et al. AMERICAN JOURNAL OF MEDICINE 77(4):760-764, October 1984.

Tracing the origin of AIDS. NEW SCIENTIST 105:20, February 28, 1985.

—, by J. Seligmann. NEWSWEEK 103:101-102, May 7, 1984.

Trade-off mars AIDS report, by K. Orr. BODY POLITIC 127:17, June 1986.

Trailing AIDS in Central Africa, by P. Newmark. NATURE 315(6017):273, May 23-29, 1985.

Trans-acting transcriptional regulation of human T-cell leukemia virus type III long terminal repeat, by J. Sodroski, et al. SCIENCE 227:171-173, January 11, 1985.

Trans-activator gene of HTLV-II induces IL-2 receptor and IL-2 cellular gene expression, by W. C. Greene, et al. SCIENCE 232:877-880, May 16, 1986.

Trans-activator gene of human T-lymphotropic virus type III (HTLV-III), by S. K. Arva, et al. SCIENCE 229:69-73, July 5, 1985.

Transactivation induced by human T-lymphotropic virus type III (HTLV-III) maps to a viral sequence encoding 58 amino acids and lacks tissue specificity, by L. J. Seigel, et al. VIROLOGY 148:226-231, January 15, 1986.

Transamerica Occidental using controversial blood test to detect the presence of AIDS virus, by L. Kocolowski. THE NATIONAL UNDERWRITER 89:6, October 19, 1985.

Transcription of novel open reading frames of AIDS retrovirus during infection of lymphocytes, by A. B. Rabson, et al. SCIENCE 229(4720):1388-1390, September 27, 1985.

Transcriptional activator protein encoded by the *x-lor* region of the human T-cell leukemia virus, by J. Sodroski, et al. SCIENCE 228:1430-1434, June 21, 1985.

Transfer of AIDS patient—inhumane, by R. Oloughlin. ADVOCATE 3(82):10, December 8, 1983.

Transfusion-associated acquired immune deficiency syndrome in infants, by J. A. Church, et al. JOURNAL OF PEDIATRICS 105(5):731-737, November 1984.

Transfusion-associated acquired immunodeficiency syndrome: evidence for persistent infection in blood donors, by P. M. Feorino, et al. NEW ENGLAND JOURNAL OF MEDICINE 312:1293-1296, May 16, 1985.

Transfusion-associated acquired immunodeficiency syndrome in a twin infant, by F. Cox, et al. PEDIATRIC INFECTIOUS DISEASE 4(1):106-108, January-February 1985.

Transfusion-associated acquired immunodeficiency syndrome in the United States, by T. A. Peterman, et al. JAMA 254:2913-2917, November 22-29, 1985.

Transfusion associated AIDS, by J. E. Menitove. JOURNAL OF CLINICAL APHERE-SIS 2(4):423-426, 1985.

—, by H. A. Perkins. AMERICAN JOURNAL OF HEMATOLOGY 19(3):307-313, July 1985.

—, by H. A. Perkins. FRONTIERS OF RADIATION THERAPY AND ONCOLOGY 19:23-25, 1985.

— [editorial], by S. Bar-Shani. HAREFUAH 108(5):264-266, March 1, 1985.

Transfusion-associated AIDS—a cause for concern [editorial], by J. R. Bove. NEW ENGLAND JOURNAL OF MEDICINE 310(2):115-116, January 12, 1984.

Transfusion-associated AIDS: serologic evidence of human T-cell leukemia virus in-fection of donors, by H. W. Jaffe, et al. SCIENCE 223(4642):1309-1312, March 23, 1984.

Transfusion-associated cytomegalovirus infection and acquired immune deficiency syndrome in an infant, by K. Shannon, et al. JOURNAL OF PEDIATRICS 103(6): 859-863, December 1983.

Transfusion induced acquired immunodeficiency syndrome (AIDS) with Kaposi's sar-coma in a patient with congenital factor V deficiency, by E. Vélez-García, et al. AIDS RESEARCH 1(6):401-406, 1984-1985.

Transfusion-induced AIDS in four premature babies [letter], by J. F. O'Duffy, et al. LANCET 2(8415):1346, December 8, 1984.

Transfusion-related acquired immunodeficiency syndrome and directed donations: would the national blood supply be safer with directed donations? by J. Umlas. HUMAN PATHOLOGY 17(2):108-110, February 1986.

Transglutaminase: co-factor in aetiology of AIDS? [letter], by R. J. Ablin. LANCET 1(8432):813-814, April 6, 1985.

Transient antibody to lymphadenopathy-associated virus/human T-lymphocyte virus type III and T-lymphocyte abnormalities in the wife of a man who developed the acquired immunodeficiency syndrome, by H. Burger, et al. ANNALS OF INTER-NAL MEDICINE 103(4):545-547, October 1985.

Transient immunoglobulin and antibody production. Occurrence in two patients with common vairied immunodeficiency, by C. C. Zielinski, et al. ARCHIVES OF IN-TERNAL MEDICINE 143(10):1937-1940, October 1983.

Transmissible lymphoma and simian acquired immunodeficiency syndrome in rhesus monkeys, by G. B. Baskin, et al. JNC I77(1):127-139, July 1986.

271

Transmission experiments with human T-lymphotropic retroviruses and human AIDS tissue [letter], by D. C. Gajdusek, et al. LANCET 1(8391):1415-1416, June 23, 1984.

Transmission of the acquired immunodeficiency syndrome through heterosexual activity, by M. M. Lederman. ANNALS OF INTERNAL MEDICINE 104(1):115-117, January 1986.

Transmission of AIDS [letter], by G. A. Ahronheim. NATURE 313(6003):534, February 14-20, 1985.

Transmission of AIDS, and blood donors, by D. G. Penington. MEDICAL JOURNAL OF AUSTRALIA 142(3):213, February 4, 1985.

Transmission of AIDS: the case against casual contagion, by M. A. Sande. NEW ENGLAND JOURNAL OF MEDICINE 314:380-382, February 6, 1986.

Transmission of AIDS virus at renal transplantation [letter], by C. A. Prompt, et al. LANCET 2(8456):672, September 21, 1985.

Transmission of hepatitis B and AIDS, by R. A. Garibaldi. INFECTION CONTROL 7(2 Supl):132-134, February 1986.

Transmission of hepatitis B without transmission of AIDS by accidental needlestick [letter], by J. L. Gerberding, et al. NEW ENGLAND JOURNAL OF MEDICINE 312(1):56-57, January 3, 1985.

Transmission of HTLV-III [letter], by H. S. Kant. JAMA 254(14):1901, October 11, 1985.

Transmission of HTLV-III infection from human plasma to chimpanzees: an animal model for AIDS, by H. J. Alter, et al. SCIENCE 226:549-552, November 2, 1984.

Transmission of human T-cell leukemia virus type I to an S+L- cat kidney cell line, by H. Hoshino, et al. VIROLOGY 147:223-236, November 1985.

Transmission of human T-cell lymphotropic virus type III (HTLV-III) by artificial insemination by donor, by G. J. Stewart, et al. LANCET 2(8455):581-585, September 14, 1985.

Transmission of lymphotropic retroviruses (HTLV-I and LAV/HTLV-III) by blood transfusion and blood products, by C. J. Melief, et al. VOX SANGUINIS 50(1):1-11, 1986.

Transmission of simian acquired immunodeficiency syndrome (SAIDS) with blood or filtered plasma, by M. Gravell, et al. SCIENCE 223(4631):74-76, January 6, 1984.

Transmission of simian acquired immunodeficiency syndrome (SAIDS) with type D retrovirus isolated from saliva or urine, by M. Gravell, et al. PROCEEDINGS OF THE SOCIETY FOR EXPERIMENTAL BIOLOGY AND MEDICINE 177(3):491-494, December 1984.

Transmission of simian AIDS with type D retrovirus isolate [letter], by M. Gravell, et al. LANCET 1(8372):334-335, February 11, 1984.

Transplacental transmission of HTLV-III virus [letter], by N. Lapointe, et al. NEW ENGLAND JOURNAL OF MEDICINE 312(20):1125-1126, May 16, 1985.

Transplacental transmission of human immunodeficiency virus [letter], by H. di Maria, et al. LANCET 2(8500):215-216, July 26, 1986.

Treating victims of AIDS poses challenge to psychiatrists. Part 1, by K. Hausman. PSYCHIATRIC NEWS 18(15):1+, August 5, 1983.

Treatment of the acquired immune deficiency syndrome, by S. Gupta, et al. JOURNAL OF CLINICAL IMMUNOLOGY 6(3):183-193, May 1986.

Treatment of acquired immunodeficiency syndrome-related Kaposi's sarcoma with lymphoblastoid interferon, by A. Rios, et al. JOURNAL OF CLINICAL ONCOLOGY 3(4):506-512, April 1985.

Treatment of dental patients with acquired immune deficiency syndrome (AIDS), by E. M. Moskowitz. NEW YORK JOURNAL OF DENTISTRY 54(3):119-120, March 1984.

Treatment of immunodeficiency with interleukin-2: initial exploration, by R. Mertelsmann, et al. JOURNAL OF BIOLOGICAL RESPONSE MODIFIERS 3(5):483-490, October 1984.

Treatment of infections in patients with the acquired immunodeficiency syndrome, by D. Armstrong, et al. ANNALS OF INTERNAL MEDICINE 103():738-743, November 1985.

Treatment of infectious complications of acquired immunodeficiency syndrome, by M. M. Furio, et al. CLINICAL PHARMACY 4(5):539-554, September-October 1985.

Treatment of Kaposi's sarcoma and thrombocytopenia with vincristine in patients with the acquired immunodeficiency syndrome, by D. M. Mintzer, et al. ANNALS OF INTERNAL MEDICINE 102(2):200-202, February 1985.

Treatment of opportunistic infections in AIDS, by S. Staszewski, et al. MUENCHENER MEDIZINISCHE WOCHENSCHRIFT 125(39):841-844, September 30, 1983.

Treatment of Pneumosystis carinii pneumonia in the acquired immunodeficiency syndrome, by C. B. Small, et al. ARCHIVES OF INTERNAL MEDICINE 145(5):837-840, May 1985.

Treatment of serious cytomegalovirus infections with 9-(1,3-dihydroxy-2-propoxy-methyl)guanine in patients with AIDS and other immunodeficiencies, by the Collaborative DHPG Treatment Study Group. NEW ENGLAND JOURNAL OF MEDICINE 314(13):801-805, March 27, 1986.

'Trojan Horse' leukocytes in AIDS [letter], by D. J. Anderson, et al. NEW ENGLAND JOURNAL OF MEDICINE 309(16):984-985, October 20, 1983.

Truth about AIDS: an optimistic review, by S. G. Rainsford. CONTEMPORARY REVIEW 248:256-261, May 1986.

Trying to head off AIDS, by S. Deaton. ALBERTA REPORT 12:32-33, September 16, 1985.

Trying to live with the AIDS plague, by P. Blauner. NEW YORK 18:51-52, June 17, 1985.

Trying to lock out AIDS, by J. Adler, et al. NEWSWEEK 106(12):65, September 16, 1985.

Tuberculin testing for persons with positive serologic studies for HTLV-III, by A. E. Pitchenik, et al. NEW ENGLAND JOURNAL OF MEDICINE 314:447, February 13, 1986.

Tuberculosis as a manifestation of the acquired immunodeficiency syndrome (AIDS), by G. Sunderam, et al. JAMA 256(3):362-366, July 18, 1986.

Tuberculosis, atypical mycobacteriosis, and the acquired immunodeficiency syndrome among Haitian and non-Haitian patients in south Florida, by A. E. Pitchenik, et al. ANNALS OF INTERNAL MEDICINE 101(5):641-645, November 1984.

Tuberculosis—United States, 1985—and possible impact of human T-lymphotropic virus type III/lymphadenopathy-associated virus infection. JAMA 255:1010+, February 28, 1986.

Tuberculous brain abscess and Toxoplasma encephalitis in a patient with the acquired immunodeficiency syndrome, by M. A. Fischl, et al. JAMA 253(23):3428-3430, June 21, 1985.

Tubuloreticular structures in peripheral blood cells from patients with AIDS-associated Kaposi's sarcoma, by P. Schenk, et al. ARCHIVES OF DERMATOLOGICAL RESEARCH 278(3):249-251, 1986.

Tumor infiltrates in acquired immunodeficiency syndrome [letter], by A. J. Cochran, et al. LANCET 1(8321):416, February 19, 1983.

Tumorlike proliferation of 'granular histiocytes' in a lymph node, by D. Dharkar, et al. ULTRASTRUCTURAL PATHOLOGY 7(4):339-343, 1984.

TV news and Aids: how bad reporting scared America, by Edwin Diamond. TV GUIDE 31:4+, October 22, 1983.

TV show hides main victims, by S. Garvey. IN THESE TIMES 8(32):21, August 22, 1984.

$12 million cut in Reagan's AIDS budget, by D. Walter. ADVOCATE 416:16, March 19, 1985.

Twenty questions about AIDS in the workplace, by F. E. Kuzmits, et al. BUSINESS HORIZONS 29:36-42, July-August 1986.

Two AIDS studies issued. ADVOCATE 423:26, June 25, 1985.

Two British blood tests launched [news], by M. Clarke. NATURE 316(6028):474, August 8-14, 1985.

Two cases of AIDS with florid Mycobacterium avium-intracellalare infection in the T-cell areas of the spleen [letter], by B. Seshi. HUMAN PATHOLOGY 16(9):964-965, September 1985.

Two elements in the bovine leukemia virus long terminal repeat that regulate gene expression, by D. Derse, et al. SCIENCE 231:1437-1440, March 21, 1986.

Two steps closer to stopping AIDS. SCIENCE DIGEST 93:19, April 1985.

Type D retrovirus in prodromal AIDS? [letter], by T. F. Warner, et al. LANCET 1(8381):860, April 14, 1984.

UC sets guide on AIDS. CALIFORNIA NURSE 79(2):1+, July-August 1983.

UCLA psychological study of AIDS, by D. K. Wellisch. FRONTIERS OF RADIATION THERAPY AND ONCOLOGY 19:155-158, 1985.

UK case of AIDS in an intravenous drug abuser [letter], by S. J. Winterton, et al. LANCET 1(8439):1223, May 25, 1985.

UK money for AIDS, by M. Clarke. NATURE 318(6045):401, December 5, 1985.

Ultrastructural and immunoelectron microscopic studies of cells with abnormal cytoplasmic inclusions in patients with AIDS, by M. Kostianovsky, et al. AIDS RESEARCH 1(3):181-196, 1983-1984.

Ultrastructural aspects of a cutaneous biopsy in acquired immune deficiency syndrome (AIDS), by P. Bruneval, et al. ANNALS OF PATHOLOGY 4(4):305-307, September-November 1984.

Ultrastructural comparison of the retroviruses associated with human and simian acquired immunodeficiency syndromes, by R. J. Munn, et al. LABORATORY INVESTIGATION 53(2):194-199, August 1985.

Ultrastructural demonstration of retrovirus antigens with immuno-gold staining in prodromal acquired immune deficiency syndrome, by W. W. Feremans, et al. JOURNAL OF CLINICAL PATHOLOGY 37(12):399-1403, December 1984.

Ultrastructural markers in acquired immune deficiency syndrome [letter], by J. M. Orenstein, et al. ARCHIVES OF PATHOLOGY AND LABORATORY MEDICINE 108(11):845-849, November 1984.

Ultrastructural markers in AIDS [letter]. LANCET 2(8344):284, July 30, 1983.

Ultrastructural markers in LAV-HTLV III virus infection: study of the rectal mucosa in 16 patients, by P. Bruneval, et al. GASTROENTEROLOGIE CLINIQUE ET BIOLOGIQUE 10(4):328-333, April 1986.

Ultrastructural markers of AIDS [letter], by G. S. Sidhu, et al. LANCET 1(8331):990-991, April 30, 1983.

Ultrastructural markers of lymph nodes in patients with acquired immune deficiency syndrome and in homosexual males with unexplained persistent lymphadenopathy. A quantitative study, by R. M. Onerheim, et al. AMERICAN JOURNAL OF CLINICAL PATHOLOGY 82(3):380-388, September 1984.

Ultrastuctural morphology and histogenesis of Kaposi sarcoma in AIDS, by H. J. Leu. VASA 13(2):107-113, 1984.

Ultrastructure of AIDS lymph nodes [letter]. NEW ENGLAND JOURNAL OF MEDICINE 309(19):1188-1190, November 10, 1983.

Ultrastructure of Kaposi's sarcoma in acquired immune deficiency syndrome (AIDS), by P. Schenk, et al. ARCHIVES OF OTORHINOLARYNGOLOGY 242(3):305-313, 1985.

Unborn babies and the AIDS virus, by W. Cooper. GUARDIAN February 4, 1986, p. 10.

Uncertainty surrounds anti-viral drug plan, by K. Westheimer. GAY COMMUNITY NEWS 14(11):1, September 28, 1986.

Unconventional vaccines: immunization with anti-idiotype antibody against viral diseases, by H. Koprowski. CANCER RESEARCH 45(Suppl. 9):4689s-4690s, September 1985.

Understanding the acquired immune deficiency syndrome, by P. Jemison-Smith. NITA 7(2):114-116, March-April 1984.

Understanding AIDS, by J. Pipher. RNAO NEWS 1(1):5-7+, Winter 1986.

—, by K. Scholl. CANADIAN NURSE 79(10):16-18, November 1983.

Understanding the gay reality, by J. S. Spong. CHRISTIAN CENTURY 103(3):62-63, January 22, 1986.

Unexplained immunodeficiency in children. A surveillance report, by P. A. Thomas, et al. JAMA 252(5):639-644, August 3, 1984.

Unexplained persistent lymphadenopathy in homosexual men and the acquired immune deficiency syndrome, by J. W. Gold, et al. MEDICINE 64(3):203-213, May 1985.

Unidentified virus-like particles in the intestine of patients with the acquired immunodeficiency syndrome, by F. W. Chandler, et al. ANNALS OF INTERNAL MEDICINE 100(6):851-853, June 1984.

Unilateral cytomegalovirus retinochoroiditis and bilateral cytoid bodies in a bisexual man with the acquired immunodeficiency syndrome, by M. M. Rodrigues, et al. OPHTHALMOLOGY 9(Suppl. 1):1577-1582, January 1984.

Unilateral cytomegalovirus retinochoroiditis and bilateral immunodeficiency syndrome, by M. M. Rodrigues, et al. OPHTHALMOLOGY 90(12):1577-1582, December 1983.

Unique pattern of HTLV-III (AIDS-related) antigen recognition by sera from African children in Uganda (1972), by C. Saxinger, et al. CANCER RESEARCH 45(Suppl. 9):4624s-4626s, September 1985.

United employee reinstated, by C. Guilfoy. GAY COMMUNITY NEWS 12(30):3, February 16, 1985.

United not friendly to workers with AIDS, by C. Guilfoy. GAY COMMUNITY NEWS 12(21):1, December 8, 1984.

United takes AIDS testing stance. OUT 4(5):3, March 1986.

Unknown disease creates fear: AIDS—a professional challenge, by G. Causse, et al. SYKEPLEIEN 71(10):11-15, June 5, 1984.

Unleashing bias [editorial]. NATION 243(1):3, July 5, 1986.

Unmasking AIDS, by T. M. Graf. HOME HEALTHCARE NURSE 2(1):44-47, January-February 1984.

Unregulated production of virus and/or sperm specific anti-idiotypic antibodies as a cause of AIDS, by S. Hsia, et al. LANCET 1(8338):1212-1214, June 2, 1984.

Untouchable disease, by J. G. Deedy. TABLET 239:872-873, August 24, 1985.

Unusual acquired immune deficiency syndrome —AIDS, by Z. Hollán, et al. ORVOSI HETILAP 125(7):375-382, February 12, 1984.

Unusual and newly recognized patterns of nontuberculous mycobacterial infection with emphasis on the immunocompromised host, by A. C. Chester, et al. PATHOLOGY ANNUAL 21(Part 1):251-270, 1986.

276

Unusual CT presentation of cerebral toxoplasmosis, by W. Cohen, et al. JOURNAL OF COMPUTER ASSISTED TOMOFRAPHY 9(2):384-386, March-April 1985.

Unusual cytoplasmic body in lymphoid cells of homosexual men with unexplained lymphadenopathy. A preliminary report, by E. P. Ewing, Jr., et al. NEW ENGLAND JOURNAL OF MEDICINE 308(14):819-822, April 7, 1983.

Unusual diseases in homosexual men. AMERICAN FAMILY PHYSICIAN 26:249, September 1982.

Unusual pulmonary infection in a puzzling presentation of AIDS [letter], by J. M. Tourani, et al. LANCET 1(8435):989, April 27, 1985.

Unusual virus produced by cultured cells from a patient with AIDS, by A. Karpas. MOLECULAR BIOLOGY AND MEDICINE 1(4):457-459, November 1983.

Update. SCIENCE 5:13, April 1984.

Update: acquired immunodeficiency syndrome (AIDS) among patients with hemophilia—United States. MMWR 32(47):613-615, December 2, 1983.

Update: acquired immunodeficiency syndrome (AIDS) in persons with hemophilia. MMWR 33(42):589-591, October 26, 1984.

Update: acquired immunodeficiency syndrome (AIDS)—United States. MMWR 32(30):389-391, August 5, 1983; also in subsequent issues.

Update: acquired immunodeficiency syndrome—Europe. JAMA 253:1106+, February 2, 1985; also in subsequent issues.

—. MMWR 33(43):607-609, November 2, 1984; also in subsequent issues.

Update: acquired immunodeficiency syndrome—Europe, by the Centers for Disease Control. CONNECTICUT MEDICINE 49(5):317-319, May 1985.

Update: acquired immunodeficiency syndrome in the San Francisco Cohort Study, 1978-1985. MMWR 34(38):573-575, September 27, 1985.

Update: acquired immunodeficiency syndrome—United States. JAMA 253:3386-3387+, June 21, 1985.

—. JAMA 255:593-594+, February 7, 1986.

—. MMWR 34(18):245-248, May 10, 1985.

Update: evaluation of human T-lymphotropic virus type III/lymphadenopathy-associated virus infection in health-care personnel—United States. MMWR 34(38):575-578, September 27, 1985; also in CONNECTICUT MEDICINE 49(11):772, November 1985.

Update on acquired immune deficiency syndrome [letter], by L. Scarpinato. JOURNAL OF THE AMERICAN OSTEOPATHIC ASSOCIATION 82(7):452-454, March 1983.

Update on acquired immune deficiency syndrome (AIDS) among patients with hemophilia A. CONNECTICUT MEDICINE 47(3):169-170, March 1983.

—. MMWR 31(48):644-646+, December 10, 1982.

Update on AIDS. MEDICAL BULLETIN OF THE U.S. ARMY, EUROPE 43(2):12, February 1986.

Update on AIDS, by E. Marshall. ARIZONA NURSE 37(2):1+, March-April 1984.

—, by H. Glenister. NURSING TIMES 81(23):4-6, June 5-11, 1985.

—, by P. Kenny. PENNSYLVANIA NURSE 40(7):4, July 1985.

—, by W. M. Valenti. INFECTION CONTROL 6(2):85-86, February   1985.

Update on AIDS: critical review, by A. Modiano, et al. GIORNALE DI CLINICA MEDICA 66(7-8):239-251, July-August 1985.

Update on AIDS information for health care personnel. CANADIAN MEDICAL AS-SOCIATION JOURNAL 134(3):251, February 1, 1986.

Update on AIDS—virology, immunology, epidemiology, by G. Biberfeld, et al. LAK-ARTIDNINGEN 81(26-27):2595-2599, June 27, 1984.

Update: prospective evaluation of health-care workers exposed via the parenteral or mucous-membrane route to blood or body fluids from patients with acquired immunodeficiency syndrome—United States. MMWR 34(7):101-103, February 22, 1985.

Update: revised Public Health Service definition of persons who should refrain from donating blood and plasma—United States. MMWR 34(35):547-548, September 6, 1985.

Update: treatment of cryptosporidiosis in patients with acquired immunodeficiency syndrome (AIDS). MMWR 33(9):117-119, March 9, 1984.

Upper airway obstruction secondary to acquired immunodeficiency syndrome-related Kaposi's sarcoma, by J. E. Greenberg, et al. CHEST 88(4):638-640, October 1985.

Urinary excretion of modified nucleosides in patients with acquired immune deficiency syndrome (AIDS) and individuals at high risk of AIDS, by A. Fischbein, et al. CANCER DETECTION AND PREVENTION 8(1-2):271-277, 1985.

Urinary neopterin and biopterin levels in patients with AIDS and AIDS-related complex [letter], by J. P. Abita, et al. LANCET 2(8445):51-52, July 6, 1985.

Urinary neopterin in the diagnosis of acquired immune deficiency syndrome, by D. Fuchs, et al. EUROPEAN JOURNAL OF CLINICAL MICROBIOLOGY 3(1):70-71, February 1984.

Urinary neopterin, a useful marker for AIDS?, [letter], by M. Perna, et al. LANCET 1(8436):1048, May 4, 1985.

United States administration's parsimony criticized [news], by S. Budiansky. NATURE 313(6005):725, February 28-March 6, 1985.

United States AIDS cases pass the 20,000 mark, by Bisticas-Cocoves. GAY COM-MUNITY NEWS 13(43):1, May 24, 1986.

United States blood-bank tests established [news], by T. Beardsley. NATURE 316(6028):474, August 8-14, 1985.

United States cities fight HTLV-3 test plan, by M. Cocoves. GAY COMMUNITY NEWS 12(40):1, April 27, 1985.

United States French studies link leukemia virus to AIDS [news]. HOSPITAL PRACTICE 18(7):33+, July 1983.

United States funds AIDS education, by N. Fain. ADVOCATE 422:26, June 11, 1985.

United States Government AIDS research, by C. Shively. DELAWARE ALTERNATIVE PRESS 6(1):9, 1983.

United States licenses blood test for AIDS, by C. Joyce, et al. NEW SCIENTIST 105:3-4, March 7, 1985.

United States Mayor Panel calls—end antigay, by L. Bush. ADVOCATE 3(88):8, February 21, 1984.

United States mayors are told "don't quarantine," by D. Walter. ADVOCATE 441: 22, March 4, 1986.

United States mayors increase research funds, by L. Bush. ADVOCATE 3(72):11, July 21, 1983.

United States memo claims AIDS phobia is not illegal, by J. Kiely. GAY COMMUNITY NEWS 13(49):1, June 29, 1986.

United States new right linked to New Zealand homophobes, by S. Poggi. GAY COMMUNITY NEWS 13(10):1, September 21, 1985.

United States policy on AIDS hit, by Bisticas-Cocoves. GAY COMMUNITY NEWS 13(3):3, July 27, 1985.

United States prepares for AIDS blood test. NEW SCIENTIST 105:3, January 17, 1985.

United States troops and AIDS , by T. Beardsley. NATURE 316(6030):668, August 22-28, 1985.

Use of AIDS antibody test may provide more answers , by C. Marwick. JAMA 253(12):1694-1695+, March 22-29, 1985.

Use of beta-2 microglobulin in the diagnosis of AIDS, suspected AIDS, and pre-clinical AIDS, by S. Zolla-Pazner, et al. ANNALS OF THE NEW YORK ACADEMY OF SCIENCES 437:526-529, 1984.

Use of interleukin-2 in patients with acquired immunodeficiency syndrome, by H. C. Lane, et al. JOURNAL OF BIOLOGICAL RESPONSE MODIFIERS 3(5):512-516, October 1984.

Use of the transbronchial biopsy for diagnosis of opportunistic pulmonary infections in acquired immunodeficiency syndrome (AIDS), by W. Blumfeld, et al. AMERICAN JOURNAL OF CLINICAL PATHOLOGY 8(1):1-5, January 1984.

Useless "plague politics". BODY POLITIC 124:26, March 1986.

Uses of epidemiology in the development of health policy, by W. H. Foege. PUBLIC HEALTH REPORTS 99(3):233-236, May-June 1984.

Vaccine against AIDS is on the way. US NEWS & WORLD REPORT 96:12, May 7, 1984.

Vaccine for simian AIDS developed. CHEMICAL AND ENGINEERING NEWS 64:5, September 8, 1986.

Vacuolar myelopathy in patients with the acquired immunodeficiency syndrome [letter], by R. D. Kimbrough. NEW ENGLAND JOURNAL OF MEDICINE 313(13): 827, September 26, 1985.

Vacuolar myelopathy pathologically resembling subacute combined degeneration in patients with the acquired immunodeficiency syndrome, by C. K. Petito, et al. NEW ENGLAND JOURNAL OF MEDICINE 312(14):874-879, April 4, 1985.

Value of the cytological examination of the bronchoalveolar lavage fluid in patients with acquired immunodeficiency syndrome and related syndromes, by P. Fouret, et al. ANNALS OF PATHOLOGY 6(1):45-52, 1986.

Value of digestive endoscopic examination in acquired immunodeficiency syndrome (45 cases), by J. Cosnes, et al. ANNALES DE GASTROENTEROLOGIE ET D'HEPATOLOGIE 22(3):123-128, May-June 1986.

Value of electroencephalography in AIDS [letter], by W. Enzensberger, et al. LANCET 1(8436):1047-1048, May 4, 1985.

Value of haematological screening for AIDS in an at risk population, by J. N. Weber, et al. GENITOURINARY MEDICINE 61(5):325-329, October 1985.

Value of lymph node biopsy in unexplained lymphadenopathy in homosexual men, by R. K. Brynes, et al. JAMA 250(10):1313-1317, September 9, 1983.

Vampire trade?, by D. Cottle. ARENA 75:38, 1986.

Vancouver AIDS study ranks risk of sex acts, by K. Popert. BODY POLITIC 113:8, April 1985.

Vancouver Lymphadenopathy-AIDS Study: 1. Persistent generalized lympha-denopathy, by M. T. Schechter, et al. CANADIAN MEDICAL ASSOCIATION JOURNAL 132(11):1273-1279, June 1, 1985.

—: 2. Seroepidemiology of HTLV-III antibody, by E. Jeffries, et al. CANADIAN MEDICAL ASSOCIATION JOURNAL 132(12):1373-1377, June 15, 1985.

—: 3. Relation of HTLV-III seropositivity, immune status and lymphadenopathy, by W. J. Boyko, et al. CANADIAN MEDICAL ASSOCIATION JOURNAL 133(1):28-32, July 1, 1985.

—: 4. Effects of exposure factors, cofactors and HTLV-III seropositivity on number of helper T cells, by M. T. Schechter, et al. CANADIAN MEDICAL ASSOCIATION JOURNAL 133(4):286-292, August 15, 1985.

Variables affecting T-lymphocyte subsets in a volunteer blood donor population by J. D. Lifson, et al. CLINICAL IMMUNOLOGY AND IMMUNOPATHOLOGY 36(2):151-160, August 1985.

Variably acid-fast bacteria in vivo in a case of reactive lymph node hyperplasia occurring in a young male homosexual, by A. R. Cantwell, Jr. GROWTH 46(4:331-336, Winter 1982.

Vascular tumors produced by NIH/3T3 cells transfected with human AIDS Kaposi's sarcoma DNA, by S. C. Lo, et al. AMERICAN JOURNAL OF PATHOLOGY 118(1): 7-13, January 1985.

Vasculitis in a suspected AIDS patient, by R. A. Berg, et al. SOUTHERN MEDICAL JOURNAL 79(7):914-915, July 1986.

Venereophobia [letter]. BRITISH JOURNAL OF HOSPITAL MEDICINE 32(3):155, September 1984.

Victimizing the victim. WOMANEWS 6(9):14, October 1985.

Vie Douce, by D. Janoff. BODY POLITIC 118:21, September 1985.

Vigil—a profile of gay courage, by M. Hippler. ADVOCATE 444:42, April 15, 1986.

Vinblastine therapy fo Kaposi's sarcoma in the acquired immunodeficiency syndrome, by P. A. Volberding, et al. ANNALS OF INTERNAL MEDICINE 103(3):335-338, Septembr 1985.

Vincristine and Kaposi's sarcoma in the acquired immunodeficiency syndrome [letter], by E. Rieber, et al. ANNALS OF INTERNAL MEDICINE 101(6):876, December 1984.

Viral AIDS suspect stripped of alibi, by D. Franklin. SCIENCE NEWS 126:6, July 7, 1984.

Viral cancers: AIDS virus at the centre, by J. Palca. NATURE 319:170, January 16, 1986.

Viral culprit in simian AIDS, by D. Franklin. BIOSCIENCE 34:292, May 1984.

Viral etiologies of AIDS: facts and hypotheses, by F. Brun-Vézinet, et al. REVUE FRANCAISE DE TRANSFUSION ET IMMUNO-HEMATOLOGIE 27(4):445-454, September 1984.

Viral fugitive captured in monkey AIDS. SCIENCE NEWS 125:170, March 17, 1984.

Viral infections and cell-mediated immunity in immunodeficient homosexual men with Kaposi's sarcoma treated with human lymphoblastoid interferon, by W. R. Frederick, et al. JOURNAL OF INFECTIOUS DISEASES 152(1):162-170, July1 985.

Viral type particles in the germinal centers during a lymphadenopathic syndrome related to AIDS, by A. Le Tourneau, et al. ANNALS OF PATHOLOGY 592):137-142, 1985.

Virologic, immunologic, and epidemiologic associations with AIDS among gay males in a low incidence area, by C. Rinaldo, et al. ANNALS OF THE NEW YORK ACADEMY OF SCIENCES 437:544-548, 1984.

Virologic studies in a case of transfusion-associated AIDS [letter], by D. J. Salberg. NEW ENGLAND JOURNAL OF MEDICINE 312(13):857-858, March 28, 1985.

—, by J. E. Groopman, et al. NEW ENGLAND JOURNAL OF MEDICINE 311(22): 1419-1422, November 29, 1984.

Virological diagnosis of HTLV-III infections, by J. Suni, et al. DUODECIM 102(7):423-428, 1986.

281

Virologists discount fear of AIDS in hepatitis B vaccine. NEW SCIENTIST 108:21, November 7, 1985.

Virology of AIDS: taxonomy, molecular biology, and pathogenicity, by J. T. Griffith. JOURNAL OF MEDICAL TECHNOLOGY 3(3):149-151+, March 1986.

Virus as a Rosetta stone: AIDS cases increase, but new research shows some signs of hope, by C. Wallis. TIME 124(19):91, November 5, 1984.

Virus by any other name . . . would still cause AIDS, by J. L. Marx. SCIENCE 227(4693): 1449-1451, March 22, 1985.

Virus clones multiply [news], by T. Beardsley. NATURE 311(5983):195, September 20-26, 1984.

Virus envelope protein of HTLV-III represents major target antigen for antibodies in AIDS patients, by F. Barin, et al. SCIENCE 228(4703):1094-1096, May 31, 1985.

Virus identified as possible cause of simian AIDS, by R. Cowen. RESEARCH RE-SOURCES REPORTER 8(4):1-6, April 1984.

Virus in Edinburgh, by M. Kohn. NEW SOCIETY May 2, 196, p. 11-13.

Virus isolation studies in simian AIDS [letter], by P. A. Marx, et al. LANCET 1(8373): 403, February 18, 1984.

Virus-like particles in AIDS-related lymphadenopathy [letter], by J. H. Humphrey. LANCET 2(8403):643, September 15, 1984.

'Virus-like particles' in lymphocytes in AIDS are normal organelles, not viruses [letter], by T. Gardiner, et al. LANCET 2(8356):963-964, October 22,1 983.

Virus-like particles in lymphocytes of seven cases of AIDS in Black Africans [letter], by W. Feremans, et al. LANCET 2(8340):52-53, July 2, 1983.

Virus-like rods in a lymphoid line from an infant with AIDS [letter], by T. G. Burrage, et al. NEW ENGLAND JOURNAL OF MEDICINE 310(22):1461-1461, May 31, 1984.

Virus linked to AIDS: variant of cancer virus may be cause. CHEMICAL AND ENGI-NEERING NEWS 62:4, April 23, 1984.

Virus-neutralizing activity, serologic heterogeneity, and retrovirus isolation from homosexual men in the Los Angeles area, by S. Rasheed, et al. VIROLOGY 150(1):1-9, April 15, 1986.

Viruses and cancer: the Japanese connection [adult T-cell leukemia and HTLV-I], by G. Vines. NEW SCIENTIST 107:36-37+, July 11, 1985.

Viruses linked to AIDS. FDA CONSUMER 18:5-6, October 1984.

Vital clue to AIDS, by B. D. Johnson. MACLEAN'S 96:54, May 23, 1983.

Vitamin C in the treatment of acquired immune deficiency syndrome (AIDS), by R. F. Cathcart, 3d. MEDICAL HYPOTHESES 14(4):423-433, August 1984.

VNA of Akron, Ohio. AIDS and the VNA, by P. Mahovich, et al. CARING 5(6):62-68, June 1986.

Vocal gay presence at Atlanta Conference, by J. Beldekas. GAY COMMUNITY NEWS 12(43):3, May 18, 1985.

Volatile nitrites. Use and adverse effects related to the current epidemic of the acquired immune deficiency syndrome, by G. R. Newell, et al. AMERICAN JOURNAL OF MEDICINE 78(5):811-816, May 1985.

Volunteers needed for AIDS study. OUT 3(6):1, April 1985.

Wake up—AIDS hysteria will change your life, by S. Schulman. WOMANEWS 7(1):1, December 1985.

Waking up to AIDS, by R. Bazell. THE NEW REPUBLIC 192:17-19, May 13, 1985.

Walter Reed staging classification for HTLV-III/LAV infection, by R. R. Redfield, et al. NEW ENGLAND JOURNAL OF MEDICINE 314:131-132, January 9, 1986.

Wandering the woods in a season of death, by A. Troxier. RFD 45:39, Winter 1985.

Warrior, by J. Howard. ESQUIRE 102:270-272+, December 1984.

Was it your son who spoke to me, by Okin, et al. BODY POLITIC 93:4, May 1983.

Way we are, by W. M. Hoffman. VOGUE 175:174-175+, July 1985.

Welcome but inadequate cash to fight AIDS, by M. Sargent. NURSING STANDARD 417:1, October 3, 1985.

Welcome the grand alliance, by N. Fain. ADVOCATE 3(77):22, September 29, 1983.

Welcome news. THE ECONOMIST September 27, 1986, p. 86+.

West Germany moves to register HTLV-3 positive test, by E. Gill. ADVOCATE 432: 25, October 29, 1985.

What about poppers, by N. Fain. ADVOCATE 3(79):20, October 27, 1983.

What (and why) you should know about . . . AIDS, by E. Copage. ESSENCE 14:51, July 1983.

What answers for AIDS?, by D. Gergen. US NEWS & WORLD REPORT 99:78, September 23, 1985.

What are we doing about AIDS? [letter]. NEW ENGLAND JOURNAL OF MEDICINE 312(11):726-727, March 14, 1985.

What are we going to do about AIDS and HTLV-III/LAV infection? [editorial], by T. C. Merigan. NEW ENGLAND JOURNAL OF MEDICINE 311(20):1311-1333, November 15, 1984.

What can I do to avoid getting AIDS, doctor?, by A. S. Brodoff. PATIENT CARE 18(2): 153-154+, January 30, 1984.

What can we do on AIDS?, by J. Laurance. NEW SOCIETY October 18, 1985, p. 103-105.

What Delaware's physicians should know about HTLV-III antibody testing, by P. R. Silverman, et al. DELAWARE MEDICAL JOURNAL 57(5):331-332, May 1985.

What does the dermatologist need to know about the new disease AIDS?, by N. Sönnichsen, et al. DERMATOLOGISCHE MONATSSCHRIFT 170(3):153-159, 1984.

What every laboratorian should know about AIDS part 1, by S. L. Haber. MLO 17(11):
32-38, November 1985.

— part 2, by S. L. Haber. MLO 17(12):55-59, December 1985.

What every Ohio physician should know about AIDS, by S. Porter. OHIO STATE
MEDICAL JOURNAL 81(10):704-705+, October 1985.

What the experts know about AIDS. FDA CONSUMER 17(7):15-19, September
1983.

What hope for AIDS? NATURE 316(6030):663-664, August 22-28, 1985.

What impact has the public health scare of A.I.D.S. had on your housekeeping
department and how have you addressed it? EXECUTIVE HOUSEKEEPING
TODAY 7(3):12-13, March 1986.

What is the role of cytomegalovirus in AIDS?, by W. L. Drew, et al. ANNALS OF THE
NEW YORK ACADEMY OF SCIENCES 437:320-324, 1984.

What is role of factor VIII therapy in inducing helper suppressor ratio reversals in
hemophiliacs? [news], by T. Hager. JAMA 249(24):3277, June 24, 1983.

What is this disease called AIDS?, by D. Meers. KENTUCKY NURSE 31(6):31-32, November-December 1983.

What nurses think about gay AIDS victims. RN 48:10, July 1985.

What our readers said about resuscitating a patient with AIDS. NURSING LIFE 6(5):
23-25, September-October 1986.

What proportion of HTLV-III antibody positives will proceed to AIDS? [letter], by A. R.
Moss. LANCET 2(8448):223-224, July 27, 1985.

What should a doctor tell a patient? [hemophiliac boy and AIDS antibody test], by P.
Klass. DISCOVER 6:20-21, October 1985.

What should employers do when AIDS strikes the work force?, by M. Braxton. RISK
MANAGEMENT 33:64+, February 1986.

What state officials should know about AIDS, by S. H. King. STATE GOVERNMENT
NEWS 28(9):8-10, September 1985.

What we know about AIDS part 1, by J. A. Bennett. AMERICAN JOURNAL OF NURS-
ING 86(9):1016-1021, September 1986.

What we know about AIDS, by J. Seale. NEW SCIENTIST 107:29-30, August 1,
1985.

What we're doing about AIDS, by W. Mayer. DEFENSE 86(1):30-32, January-February 1986.

What you can do to stop the AIDS panic, by J. A. McCutchan. RN 49(10):18-21,
October 1986.

What you should know about AIDS, by K. McCoy. SEVENTEEN 44:24+, November
1985.

What's in a name? by C. Norman. SCIENCE 230:641, November 8, 1985.

—, by M. Helquist. ADVOCATE 426:32, August 6, 1985.

What's new: acquired immunodeficiency syndrome (AIDS) and Kaposi's sarcoma, by H. L. Lucia. TEXAS MEDICINE 79(6):39-40, June 1983.

When aid does not come to the rescue, by D. Hacket. NEW SCIENTIST 98:237, April 28, 1983.

When is AIDS communicable? [letter], by H. H. Neumann. JAMA 251(12):1553, March 23-30, 1984.

When is AIDS not AIDS? [letter], by R. D. Maw, et al. LANCET 2(8409):986, October 27, 1984.

When should the acquired immunodeficiency syndrome be considered in children (AIDS)?, by A. Getlík. CESKOSLOVENSKA PEDIATRIE 89(8):485-4867, August 1984.

When will prevention of HTLV-III infection be possible?, by R. Tedder, et al. VACCINE 2(3):171-172, September 1984.

When will we have an AIDS vaccine?, by N. Heneson. NEW SCIENTIST 109:20, March 27, 1986.

Where can an AIDS patient turn for care?, by S. A. DiTullio. AMERICAN JOURNAL OF HOSPICE CARE 3(2):4, March-April 1986.

Where is the AIDS virus harbored? SCIENCE 232:1197, June 6, 1986.

Where now with AIDS? [editorial]. NATURE 313(6000):254, January 24-30, 1985.

Whipple-like disease in AIDS [letter], by C. D. Kooijman, et al. HISTOPATHOLOGY 8(4):705-708, July 1984.

Whitewash, by Peter Collier, et al. CALIFORNIA MAGAZINE 8:52+, July 1983.

Who decides what AIDS protection is enough? RN 48:10, October, 1985.

Whose blood can now be safe?, by T. Beardsley. NATURE 303(5913):102, May 12-18, 1983.

Why an AIDS vaccine is a long time coming. NEW SCIENTIST 109:39, January 2, 1986.

Why the AIDS virus is not like HTLVs-I or II. NEW SCIENTIST 105:4, February 7, 1985.

Why can't they find the agent causing AIDS? THE ECONOMIST 288:77, September 3, 1983.

Why is a lefty so different?, by S. Begley. NEWSWEEK 100:62-63, August 30, 1982.

Why this young hunk risked playing an AIDS victim: taking a role others nervously avioded, Aidan Quinn was out to prove something to Hollywood—and to himself, by Michael Leahy. TV GUIDE 34:34+, April 26, 1986.

Widening the definition of AIDS? [letter], by J. M. Guerin, et al. LANCET 1(8392): 1464-1465, June 30, 1984.

Widening scourge: lethal new ailment claims another group of victims, by J. E. Bishop. WALL STREET JOURNAL 200:1+, December 10, 1982.

Widespread cytomegalovirus gastroenterocolitis in a patient with acquired immuno-deficiency syndrome, by A. B. Knapp, et al. GASTROENTEROLOGY 85(6): 1399-1402, December 1983.

Widows story: life after lover died of AIDS, by B. Hillard. ADVOCATE 421:5, May 28, 1985.

Will an AIDS vaccine bankrupt the company that makes it?, by D. M. Barnes. SCIENCE 233:1035, September 5, 1986.

Will New York close the baths?, by L. Bush. VILLAGE VOICE 29:24+, December 18, 1984.

Winning smiles as the AIDS patent battle continues. NEW SCIENTIST 112:20, October 2, 1986.

Wisconsin cares about AIDS. OUT 4(2):12, December 1985.

Wisconsin ranks in middle on AIDS, by W. Handy. OUT 4(5):6, March 1986.

Wisdom of the despised, by A. Lumsden. NEW STATESMAN November 14, 1986, p. 14.

Women and AIDS, by A. G. Fettner. HEALTH 18(11):61-66, November 1986.

—, by M. Clark, et al. NEWSWEEK 108(2):60-61, July 14, 1986.

Women of the year, by L. Van Gelder. MS. 14:31-34+, January 1986.

Women susceptible to AIDS, too? AMERICAN JOURNAL OF NURSING 83:1199, August 1983.

Women's Studies Conference: sex & culture, by B. Duren. GAY COMMUNITY NEWS 12(39):7, April 20, 1985.

Workers and AIDS—Uncle Sam speaks [Public Health Service guidelines]. US NEWS & WORLD REPORT 99:14, November 25, 1985.

Workers who get AIDS: combating coworkers' fears, by B. McCormick. HOSPITALS 60(13):110, July 5, 1986.

Working with AIDS, by M. B. Pfeiffer. EMPIRE STATE REPORT 12:44-67, October 1986.

World AIDS developments. BODY POLITIC 130:19, September 1986.

World Health Organization workshop: conclusions and recommendations on acquired immunodeficiency syndrome. JAMA 253(23):3385-3386, June 21, 1985; also in MMWR 34(19):275-276, May 17, 1985.

Worst fears made flesh, by J. Sunderland. CHARTIST 105:5, Juy 1985.

Wrong AIDS customers. FDA CONSUMER 17:1, December 1983-January 1984.

Wrong without remedy, by D. M. Freedman. AMERICAN BAR ASSOCIATION JOURNAL 72:36-40, June 1, 1986.

x gene is essential for HTLV replication, by I. S. Y. Chen, et al. SCIENCE 229:54-58, July 5, 1985.

X-linked factor in acquired immunodeficiency syndrome? [letter], by M. F. Lyon, et al. LANCET 1(8327):768, April 2, 1983.

You won't get AIDS from hepatitis vaccine. RN 48:11, April 1985.

You're not likely to get AIDS from patients. RN 48:12-13, June 1985.

Young victims. TIME 120:79, December 27, 1982.

Youngest victims of AIDS, by M. Dobbin, et al. U.S. NEWS & WORLD REPORT 101(3): 71-72, July 7, 1986.

Your money or your life—David Groat, by L. Goldsmith. GAY COMMUNITY NEWS 10(33):3, March 12, 1983.

Your role as AIDS educator, by C. Hanks, et al. OHIO NURSES REVIEW 61(5):12-13, May 1986.

Your role in the diagnosis and management of AIDS, by R. D. Smith. PATHOLOGIST 37(9):609-611, September 1983.

Zoo sex, by R. Emmett Tyrrell Jr. AMERICAN SPECTATOR 18:8, November 1985.

PERIODICAL LITERATURE

SUBJECT INDEX

ADVERTISING
AIDS fear poses crisis for some, market for others, by P. Winters. ADVERTISING
AGE 57:1+, February 3, 1986.

AIDS—GENERAL
ABC of sexually transmitted diseases. Acquired immune deficiency syndrome,
by I. Weller. BRITISH MEDICAL JOURNAL 288(6411):136-137, January 14,
1984.

Acid-labile alpha interferon [letter]. NEW ENGLAND JOURNAL OF MEDICINE
310(14):922-924, April 5, 1984.

Acquired-cell immune deficiency syndrome, by J. F. Heidelman, et al. ORAL
SURGERY 55(5):452-453, May 1983.

Acquired cellular immunodeficiency syndrome [editorial], by F. Andreu-Kern, et
al. MEDICINA CLINICA 80(12):532-534, April 9, 1983.

Acquired immune deficiency disease after three years. The unsolved riddle, by
H. L. Ioachim. LABORATORY INVESTIGATION 51(1):1-6, July 1984.

Acquired immune deficiency syndrome. Commentary. Council on Scientific
Affairs. JAMA 252(15):2037-2043, October 19, 1984.

Acquired immune deficiency syndrome. A contemporary overview, by K.
Crossley. MINNESOTA MEDICINE 69(1):29-30, January 1986.

Acquired immune deficiency syndrome. A deadly new disease, by F. A. Khan, et
al. POSTGRADUATE MEDICINE 74(2):180-185+, August 1983.

Acquired immune deficiency syndrome. A dynamic clinico-biological situation, by
X. Estivill, et al. SANGRE 28(6):753-769, 1983.

Acquired immune deficiency syndrome. The ever-broadening clinical spectrum
[editorial], by A. S. Fauci. JAMA 249(17):2375-2376, May 6, 1983.

Acquired immune deficiency syndrome. Introduction, by J. E. Groopman.
SEMINARS IN ONCOLOGY 11(1):3, March 1984.

Acquired immune deficiency syndrome. Light microscopic, ultrastructural and
immunocytochemical studies of one case, by S. R. Allegra, et al. JOURNAL
OF SUBMICROSCOPIC CYTOLOGY 16(3):561-568, July 1984.

Acquired immune deficiency syndrome. Medical challenge of the 80's, by C. B. Daul, et al. POSTGRADUATE MEDICINE 76(1):167-174+, July 1984.

Acquired immune deficiency syndrome. A proderomal form, by A. G. Dalgleish, et al. MEDICAL JOURNAL OF AUSTRALIA 1(12):558-560, June 11, 1983.

Acquired immune deficiency syndrome. A review, by S. H. Landesman, et al. ARCHIVES OF INTERNAL MEDICINE 143(12):2307-2309, December 1983.

Acquired immune deficiency syndrome. An update 1984, by S. R. Porter, et al. BRITISH DENTAL JOURNAL 157(11):387-391, December 8, 1984.

Acquired immune deficiency syndrome (AIDS)—a case report, by R. Tamir, et al. HAREFUAH 105(11):360-361, December 1, 1983.

Acquired immune deficiency syndrome (AIDS): number one priority, by E. D. Glover. HEALTH VALUES 8(2):3-12, March-April 1984.

Acquired immune deficiency syndrome (AIDS): of concern to us all [editorial], by D. N. Lawrence. JOURNAL OF THE FLORIDA MEDICAL ASSOCIATION 70(2):101- 102, February 1983.

Acquired immune deficiency syndrome: the facts, by D. G. Penington, et al. QUEENSLAND NURSE 4(1):17-24, January-February 1985.

Acquired immune deficiency syndrome: implications and directions, by W. A. Andes. AUAA JOURNAL 5(3):8-10, January-March 1985.

Acquired immune deficiency syndrome: an international health problem of increasing importance, by C. B. Oofsy, et al. KLINISCHE WOCHENSCHRIFT 62(11):512-522, June 1, 1984.

Acquired immune deficiency syndrome—a new, thus far unexplained syndrome with a severe course, by J. Sejda, et al. VNITRNI LEKARSTVI 29(11):1107-1113, November 1983.

Acquired immune deficiency syndrome—an overview, by J. A. Gracie, et al. SCOTTISH MEDICAL JOURNAL 30(1):1-7, January 1985.

Acquired immune deficiency syndrome part 1, by A. J. Pinching. MIDWIFE, HEALTH VISITOR AND COMMUNITY NURSE 22(5):142-146+, May 1986.

Acquired immune deficiency syndrome—recommendations of the working party [letter]. JOURNAL OF HOSPITAL INFECTION 7(3):295-296, May 1986.

—, by R. E. Warren, et al. JOURNAL OF HOSPITAL INFECTION 7(3):306-307, May 1986.

Acquired immune deficiency syndrome: a review, by K. C. Davis. RESPIRATORY THERAPY 14(5):15-16+, September-October 1984.

Acquired immune deficiency syndrome: review, by C. Scully, et al. BRITISH DENTAL JOURNAL 161(2):53-60, July 19, 1986.

Acquired immune deficiency syndrome—update, by A. Hasner, et al. HARE-FUAH 108(9):448-453, May 1, 1985.

Acquired immune deficiency syndrome: an update and interpretation, by C. B. Daul, et al. ANNALS OF ALLERGY 51(3):351-361, September 1983.

Acquired immunodeficiency, by A. González-Angulo, et al. GACETA MEDICA DE MEXICO 121(1-2):1-17, January-February 1985.

—, by O. A. Strand. TIDSSKRIFT FOR DEN NORSKE LAEGEFORENING 103(11):895-897, April 20, 1983.

Acquired immunodeficiency (AIDS), by H. G. Thiele. IMMUNITAT UND INFEK-TION 11(5):177-180, September 1983.

Acquired immunodeficiency and related syndromes, by J. Debold. PATHO-LOGY, RESEARCH AND PRACTICE 179(1):124-126, September 1984.

Acquired immunodeficiency syndrome [letter]. ANNALS OF INTERNAL MEDICINE99(5):734-736, November 1983.

Acquired immunodeficiency syndrome, by H. Masur. PROGRESS IN CLINICAL AND BIOLOGICAL RESEARCH 182:271-276, 1985.

—, by H. Minkoff. JOURNAL OF NURSE-MIDWIFERY 31(4):189-193, July-August 1986.

—, by J. M. Orenstein. HUMAN PATHOLOGY 16(12):1285-1286, December 1985.

—, by J. Racouchot. PRESSE MEDICALE 14(5):287, February 9, 1985.

—, by K. Crossley. MINNESOTA MEDICINE 69(4):211-213, April 1986.

— (a review of the literature), by E. N. Sidorenko. VRACHEBNOE DELO 10:104-110, October 1985.

— [editorial], by M. S. Hutt. TROPICAL DOCTOR 15(1):1, January 1985.

—, by S. A. Danner, et al. NEDERLANDS TIJDSCHRIFT VOOR GENEESKUNDE 127(19):830-832, May 7, 1983.

—, by V. Gong. AMERICAN JOURNAL OF EMERGENCY MEDICINE 2(4):336-346, July 1984.

—, by V. Suvakovic. SRPSKI ARHIV ZA CELOKUPNO LEKARSTVO 112(11-12):1205-1215, November-December 1984.

—, by Y. Ueda. NIPPON RINSHO 41(9):2185-2190, September 1983.

Acquired immunodeficiency syndrome (AIDS). REVISTA DE ENFERMERIA 8(81):55-59, April 1985.

—, by C. Bogdan, et al. FORTSCHRITTE DER MEDIZEN 103(35):817-821, September 19, 1985.

—, by F. Cambazard. SOINS. GYNECOLOGIE, OBSTETRIQUE, PUERICUL-TURE, PEDIATRIE 56:21-26, January 1986.

290

—, by F. S. Rosen. JOURNAL OF CLINICAL INVESTIGATION 75(1):1-3, January 1985.

—, by G. Levi. AMB 31(9-10):173-187, September-October 1985.

—, by J. Besner, et al. AARN NEWSLETTER 42(2):25-27, February 1986.

—, by J. Frottier. SOINS 930:53-56, May 1984.

—, by M. Dicato. BULLETIN DE LA SOCIETE DES SCIENCES MEDICALES DU GRAND-DUCHE DE LUXEMBOURG 121(2):5-6, 1984.

—, by O. W. van Assendelft. NEDERLANDS TIJDSCHRIFT VOOR GENEES-KUNDE 127(19):826-30, May 7, 1983.

—, by P. Jansa. ACTA UNIVERSITATIS PALACKIANAE OLOMUCENSIS FACULTATIS MEDICAE 108:193-195, 1985.

Acquired immunodeficiency syndrome (AIDS). A 2-year review, by M. Vogt, et al. DEUTSCHE MEDIZINISCHE WOCHENSCHRIFT 108(50):1927-1933, December 16, 1983.

Acquired immunodeficiency syndrome (AIDS). An Update after 4 years, by M. Vogt, et al. SCHWEIZERISCHE MEDIZINISCHE WOCHENSCHRIFT 115(19):665-671, May 11, 1985.

Acquired immunodeficiency syndrome (AIDS)—a current or future problem?, by Z. Kuratowska. POLSKI TYGODNIK LEKARSKI 39(36):1189-1192, September 3, 1984.

Acquired immunodeficiency syndrome (AIDS): an epidemiologic and clinical overview, by K. G. Castro, et al. JOURNAL OF THE MEDICAL ASSOCIATION OF GEORGIA 78(8):537-542, August 1984.

Acquired immunodeficiency syndrome 'AIDS': limits of the unknown, by W. Rozenbaum. ANNALES DE MEDECINE INTERNE 135(1):3-6, 1984.

Acquired immunodeficiency syndrome (AIDS): new reports, by W. Mazurkiewicz. PRZEGLAD DERMATOLOGICZNY 71(5):423-429, September-October 1984.

Acquired immunodeficiency syndrome (AIDS): an update, by A. S. Fauci, et al. INTERNATIONAL ARCHIVES OF ALLERGY AND APPLIED IMMUNOLOGY 77(1-2):81-88, 1985.

Acquired immunodeficiency syndrome (AIDS)—an update, by L. Robinson. CRITICAL CARE NURSE 4(5):75-83, September-October 1984.

Acquired immunodeficiency syndrome—an assessment of the present situation in the world: memorandum from a WHO meeting. BULLETIN OF THE WORLD HEALTH ORGANIZATION 62(3):419-432, 1984.

Acquired immunodeficiency syndrome: current and future trends, by W. M. Morgan, et al. PUBLIC HEALTH REPORTS 101(5):459-465, September-October 1986.

Acquired immunodeficiency syndrome: current status, by V. Quagliarello. YALE JOURNAL OF BIOLOGY AND MEDICINE 55(5-6):443-452, September-December 1982.

Acquired immuno-deficiency syndrome: a fatal but preventable disease, by N. Clumeck. ACTA CLINICA BELGICA 38(3):145-147, 1983.

Acquired immunodeficiency syndrome in the adult. Its value in tropical medicine, by J. P. Coulaud, et al. MEDECINE TROPICALE 44(1):9-15, January-March 1984.

Acquired immunodeficiency syndrome in a small community, by S. S. Lee, et al. IOWA MEDICINE 75(8):351-352, August 1985.

Acquired immunodeficiency syndrome; neuroradiologic findings, by W. M. Kelly, et al. RADIOLOGY 149(2):485-491, November 1983.

Acquired immunodeficiency syndrome—a new virus infection? VOPROSY VIRUSOLOGII 28(4):124-126, July-August 1983.

Acquired immunodeficiency syndrome: an overview, by R. L. Baker, et al. INDIANA MEDICINE 78(6):459-465, June 1985.

Acquired immunodeficiency syndrome: an update, by M. W. Moon. JEN 12(5):291-296, September-October 1986.

—, by W. A. Stein, et al. PHYSICIAN ASSISTANT 10(1):23-24+, January 1986.

Acts of humor, acts of courage, by M. Bronski. GAY COMMUNITY NEWS 12(49):10, June 29, 1985.

Acute HTLV III infection [letter], by K. R. Romeril. NEW ZEALAND MEDICAL JOURNAL 98(779):401, May 22, 1985.

Addressing the AIDS crisis, by D. Collum. SOJOURNERS 15(2):6, February 1986.

Addressing the AIDS threat [interview with C. E. Koop]. CHRISTIANITY TODAY 29(7):52, November 22, 1985.

Advance against AIDS, by A. Steacy. MACLEAN'S 99:36, June 16, 1986.

Advocates for better health care, by P. Freiberg. ADVOCATE 3(72):13, July 21, 1983.

AFRAIDS. THE NEW REPUBLIC 193:7-8+, Octoebr 14, 1985.

After AIDS: a walk on the mild side, by N. Meredith. PSYCHOLOGY TODAY 18:60-61, January 1984.

After Amerika, AIDS, by A. Cockburn. IN THESE TIMES 10(31):17, August 6, 1986.

Aid to A.I.D.S. [editorial], by B. W. Otridge. IRISH MEDICAL JOURNAL 76(9): 373-374, September 1983.

AIDophobia [letter], by E. Freed. MEDICAL JOURNAL OF AUSTRALIA 2(10): 479, November 12, 1983.

AIDS [editorial]. AMERICAN FAMILY PHYSICIAN 28(1):111, July 1983.

—. LANCET 2(8497):51, July 5, 1986.

— [letter]. MEDICAL JOURNAL OF AUSTRALIA 2(12):601-602, December 10-24, 1983.

— [letter]. NATURE 319(6056):716, February 27-March 5, 1986.

— [special section]. NEWSWEEK 106:20-24+, August 12, 1985.

—. RIVISTA DELL INFERMIERE 3(1):51-53, March 1984.

—. SCIENCE NEWS 127:328, May 25, 1985.

—, by A. Rosser. POLICE JOURNAL 49(3):258-262, 1986.

—, by B. Dixon. WORLD HEALTH August 1983, p. 10-13.

—, by B. Hanczyk. PROFESSIONAL MEDICAL ASSISTANT 17(4):14-15, July-August 1984.

—, by B. Ott. AMERICAN LIBRARIES 16:681, November 1985.

—, by B. Ridgway. LAMP 42(2):7-9, March 1985.

—, by B. Stoller. JOURNAL OF PRACTICAL NURSING 35(4):26-31, December 1985.

—, by C. Dunphy. WASHINGTON NURSE 14(6):9, September 1984.

— [special section], by J. Langone. DISCOVER 6:28-33+, December 1985.

—[letter], by J. P. Krajeski. NORTH CAROLINA MEDICAL JOURNAL 44(8):525, August 1983.

—, by M. F. Silverman. EMERGENCY: JOURNAL OF EMERGENCY SERVICES 18(5):44-46, May 1986.

—, by M. Morichau-Beauchant. GASTROENTEROLOGIE CLINIQUE ET BIOLO-GIQUE 9(4):323-326, April 1985.

—, by R. A. Kiel. CORRECTIONS TODAY 48:68-70, February 1986.

—, by R. Augusta. JOURNAL OF PRACTICAL NURSING 33(8):48-51, September-October 1983.

—, by R. Wells, et al. INTERNATIONAL NURSING REVIEW 32(3):76-79, May-June 1985.

—, by T. Lizuka. KANGO 35(11):92-93, October 1983.

—, by W. F. Batchelor. AMERICAN PSYCHOLOGIST 39(11):1277-1278, November 1984.

AIDS. Epidemic or Hysteria? by S. Gesenhues. ZFA 59(33):1865-1869, November 30, 1983.

AIDS: academy looks for strategy, by J. Palca. NATURE 319:441, February 6, 1986.

AIDS: acquired immune deficiency syndrome, by A. Ramirez. NEW ZEALAND NURSING JOURNAL 78(7):July 1985.

—, by J. A. Johson. CONGRESSIONAL RESEARCH SERVICE REVIEW 4(10): 19-21, November 1983.

—, by J. Cohen. IMPRINT 31(4):50, November 1984.

—, by P. A. Miles. JEN 9(5):254-258, September-October 1983.

AIDS: acquired immunodeficiency syndrome. FLASH-INFORMATIONS 3:6-8, May-June 1985.

—, by G. Altay. MIKROBIYOLOJI BULTENI 19(4):238-251, October 1985.

—, by J. P. Soulier. REVUE FRANCAISE DE TRANSFUSION ET IMMUNO-HEMATOLOGIE 26(5):437-445, November 1983.

—, by K. O. Habermehl. INTERNIST 26(2):113-120, February 1985.

—, by M. Spoljar, et al. LIJECNICKI VJESNIK 106(1):21-24, January 1984.

—, by N. J. Gilmore, et al. CANADIAN MEDICAL ASSOCIATION JOURNAL 128(11):1281-1284, June 1, 1983.

—, by R. Piffer. RIVISTA DELL INFERMIERE 4(4):207-217, December 1985.

—, by W. Dowdle. SERVIR 34(3):151-157, May-June 1986.

AIDS: act now, don't pay later [editorial]. BRITISH MEDICAL JOURNAL 293 (6543):348, August 9, 1986.

AIDS action: a policy of gestures. BODY POLITIC 96:21, September 1983.

AIDS alarm, by F. Orr. ALBERTA REPORT 12:35, May 20, 1985.

AIDS alert. CORRECTIONS DIGEST 17(4):3, February 12, 1986.

AIDS alert [letter], by S. Ashman, et al. JOURNAL OF THE AMERICAN DENTAL ASSOCIATION 111(5):712, November 1985.

AIDS: the American nightmare, by D. Thompson. TIMES August 12, 1985, p. 8.

AIDS and all of us, by J. Zeh. GUARDIAN 38(31):20, May 7, 1986.

AIDS and ecology/wellfounded fears, by R. Summerbell. BODY POLITIC 94:6, June 1983.

AIDS and the electromyographer, by D. B. Karam. ARCHIVES OF PHYSICAL MEDICINE AND REHABILITATION 67(7):491, July 1986.

AIDS and the general population, by M. F. Silverman. FRONTIERS OF RADIA-TION THERAPY AND ONCOLOGY 19:168-171, 1985.

AIDS and heat, by G. Weissmann. HOSPITAL PRACTICE 18(10):136-137+, October 1983.

AIDS and us, by E. Ropes. GAY COMMUNITY NEWS 10(47):5, June 18, 1983.

AIDS, arms control, and the future, by A. Hammond. ISSUES IN SCIENCE AND TECHNOLOGY 2:2, Winter 1986.

AIDS as crisis and opportunity, by K. L. Vaux. CHRISTIAN CENTURY 102:910-911, October 16, 1985.

AIDS as metaphor, by B. Teixiea. BODY POLITIC 96:40, September 1983.

AIDS: attacking the problem, by D. Steele. SOLDIERS 41(1):6-11, January 1986.

AIDS: bad news, good news. NATURE 311:206, September 20, 1984.

AIDS: a balance of sorrows, by L. L. Curtin. NURSING MANAGEMENT 17(3):7-8, March 1986.

AIDS beyond the hospital. 1. What we know about AIDS, by J. A. Bennett. AMERICAN JOURNAL OF NURSING 86(9):1015-1021, September 1986.

AIDS bibliography, by J. P. Martin. CALIFORNIA NURSE 82(4):17, May 1986.

AIDS: boys and girls come out to play?, by C. Clementson. NURSING TIMES 82(7):19-20, February 12-18, 1986.

AIDS breakthrough, by D. Silburt. MACLEAN'S 97:56, May 7, 1984.

—, by Kate Nolan. PLAYBOY 31:59+, May 1984.

—, by M. Clark, et al. NEWSWEEK 106(20):88, November 11, 1985.

AIDS casts a longer shadow [news], by J. Maddox. NATURE 312(5990):97, No-vember 8-14, 1984.

AIDS: the challenge to science and medicine, by M. Krim. HASTINGS CENTER REPORT 15(Suppl. 2-7), August 1985.

—, by M. Krim. QRB 12(8):278-283, August 1986.

AIDS, a complex syndrome, by A. Locke. MASSACHUSETTS NURSE 54(7):1+, August 1985.

AIDS conflict, by J. Adler, et al. NEWSWEEK 106(13):18-24, September 23, 1985.

AIDS connection, by G. Kolata. SCIENCE 226:958, November 23,1 984.

AIDS contact [letter]. NATURE 304(5928):678, August 25-31, 1983.

AIDS: could you be at risk, by D. Apuzzo-Berger. RN 46:67-68+, February 1983.

AIDS crisis action. CHRISTIAN CENTURY 102:1056, November 20, 1985.

AIDS crisis update. ADVOCATE 443:20, April 1, 1986; also in volumes 444, 445, 447, 448, 450, 452, 455.

AIDS: current achievement, future problems [editorial], by L. H. Calabrese. CLEVELAND CLINIC QUARTERLY 52(2):217-218, Summer 1985.

AIDS: current status and present-day knowledge, by M. Vogt, et al. THERA-PEUTISCHE UMSCHAU 42(11):798-804, November 1985.

AIDS debate: must we wait until all answers are at hand?, by S. B. Roll. SYKE-PLEIEN 73(12):20+, July 4, 1986.

AIDS declared public enemy no. 1. AMERICAN JOURNAL OF NURSING 83:988, July 1983.

AIDS dilemma. TIME 122:54, October 24,1 983.

AIDS: double exposure, by E. Jackson. BODY POLITIC 121:15, December 1985.

AIDS elephant, by R. D. Smith. THE SCIENCES 24:8+, March-April 1984.

AIDS epidemic. US NEWS AND WORLD REPORT 94:56, June 6, 1983.

—, by J. Seligmann. NEWSWEEK 101:74-79, April 18, 1983.

—, by S. H. Landesman, et al. NEW ENGLAND JOURNAL OF MEDICINE 312(8): 521-525, February 21, 1985.

—, by S. L. Hellman. AAOHN JOURNAL 34(6):285-290, June 1986.

AIDS epidemic: continental drift [news], by J. E. Groopman, et al. NATURE 307(5948):211-212, January 19-25, 1984.

AIDS epidemic continues, moving beyond high-risk groups, by R. M. Baum. CHEMICAL AND ENGINEERING NEWS 63:19-22+, April 1, 1985.

AIDS epidemic: multidisciplinary trouble, by J. E. Osborn. NEW ENGLAND JOURNAL OF MEDICINE 314(12):779-782, March 20, 1986.

AIDS—the epidemic of the decade and the medical mystery of the century, by D. E. Stover. RESPIRATORY CARE 29(1):19-20, January 1984.

AIDS epidemic: an overview of the science, by J. E. Osborn. ISSUES IN SCIENCE AND TECHNOLOGY 2:40-55, Winter 1986.

AIDS extra. A model for the world's struggle, by A. Brummer. GUARDIAN November 6, 1985, p. 23.

AIDS—facts and fiction, by M. Karlovac. MEDICINSKI PREGLED 38(9-10):429-433, 1985.

AIDS: fatal, incurable and spreading. PEOPLE WEEKLY 23:42-49, June 17, 1985.

AIDS fears. CHRISTIAN CENTURY 103(10):290, March 19-26, 1986.

Aids for AIDS, by P. DAvid. NATURE 303:743, June 30, 1983.

AIDS forum—it hasn't gone away, by M. Perigard. GAY COMMUNITY NEWS 11(36):3, March 31, 1984.

AIDS: a fresh lead. THE ECONOMIST 287:94-95, May 28, 1983.

AIDS—from the clinical viewpoint, by H. D. Pohle. OFFENTLICHE GESUNDHEIT-SWESEN 47(8):349-352, August 1985.

AIDS from west to east?, by M. Khurana. NURSING JOURNAL OF INDIA 77(8): 207+, August 1986.

AIDS—a further development, by T. Aoki, et al. GAN TO KAGAKU RYOHO 13(5): 1791-1797, May 1986.

AIDS: the good news. SCIENTIFIC AMERICAN 255:55, November 1986.

AIDS group urges monitoring,by C. Guilfoy. GAY COMMUNITY NEWS 12(9):6, September 15, 1983.

AIDS: a growing threat, by C. Wallis, et al. TIME 126(6):40-45+, August 12, 1985.

AIDS: the health crisis of the 80's, by P. Alexander. NATIONAL NOW TIMES 18(8):4, February 1986.

AIDS horror story worsens, by M. Stanton Evans. HUMAN EVENTS 45:7, November 30, 1985.

AIDS: how do we continue in the interim?, by J. Huisman. NEDERLANDS TIJD-SCHRIFT VOOR GENEESKUNDE 129(31):1459-1462, August 3, 1985.

AIDS: how a problem became a priority, by B. J. Stiles. FOUNDATION NEWS 27(2):48-56, March-April 1986.

AIDS: the human element, by J. Aberth. PERSONNEL JOURNAL 65(8):119-123, August 1986.

AIDS IDs: protection or hysteria?, by J. Shevach. NEW AGE May 1986, p. 12.

AIDS an illness with many questionmarks, by N. Albrecht-van Lent, et al. TIJD-SCHRIFT VOOR ZIEKENVERPLEGING 36(21):666-668, October 18, 1983.

AIDS in the east: now it's official. NEW SCIENTIST 109:25, March 6, 1986.

AIDS in perspective. CANADIAN NURSE 80:16, May 1984.

—, by N. Fain. ADVOCATE 3(98):20, July 10, 1984.

—, by A. Nichols. JOURNAL OF NEPHROLOGY NURSING 2(3):101-104, May-June 1985.

AIDS is all of us, by J. Carpenter. NORTHWEST PASSAGE 24(4):6, November 1983.

AIDS is getting to us, by J. Adams. LESBIAN CONTRADICTION 16:20, Summer 1986.

AIDS is here, by D. Fallowell. TIMES July 27, 1983, p. 8.

AIDS: is it the body turned against itself?, by M. Helquist. ADVOCATE 435:23, December 10, 1985.

AIDS: 'it's just a matter of time,' by R. Streitmatter. QUILL 72:22-25+, May 1984.

AIDS journal, by M. Helquist. ADVOCATE 3(79):26, October 27, 1983.

AIDS: a killer confined, by L. A. Engelhard, et al. TODAY'S OR NURSE 5(10):26-30+, December 1983.

AIDS: the latest facts, by B. Weinhouse. LADIES' HOME JOURNAL 100:100+, November 1983.

AIDS: legacy of the '60s?, by J. G. Fuller. SCIENCE DIGEST 91:84-86+, December 1983.

AIDS: a lethal mystery story, by M. Clark. NEWSWEEK 100:63-64, December 27, 1982.

AIDS mecca of the world, by A. Jetter. MOTHER JONES 10(3):6+, April 1985.

AIDS: a medical conundrum, by R. E. Stahl, et al. JOURNAL OF CUTANEOUS PATHOLOGY 10(6):550-558, December 1983.

AIDS: a medical time bomb, by M. Stanton Evans. HUMAN EVENTS 44:7, July 14, 1984.

AIDS—mobilizing to put on the pressure. BODY POLITIC 116:27, July 1985.

AIDS: more troubling questions, by M. Weiss. LUTHERAN FORUM 120(1):5, 1986.

AIDS—mysteries and hidden dangers, by J. Rechy. ADVOCATE 3(83):31, December 22, 1983.

AIDS mystery: new clues, by J. Seligmann. NEWSWEEK 101:94, May 16, 1983.

AIDS myths, by T. Barrett. CALIFORNIA NURSE 82(4):5, May 1986.

AIDS, nature, and the nature of AIDS. NATIONAL REVIEW 37:18, November 1, 1985.

AIDS—the need for an integrated approach, by J. K. van Wijngaarden. NEDERLANDS TIJDSCHRIFT VOOR GENEESKUNDE 128(22):1061-1062, June 2, 1984.

AIDS neglect, by R. Kaye. NATION 236(20):627, May 21, 1983.

AIDS: a new disease, by M. A. Conant. FRONTIERS OF RADIATION THERAPY AND ONCOLOGY 19:1-7, 1985.

—, by R. Schuppli. SCHWEIZERISCHE MONATSSCHRIFT FÜR ZAHNMEDIZIN 94(9):840-842, September 1984.

—. A nurse speaks, by F. Mignot. SOINS 469-470:31-32, January 1986.

AIDS: a new disease's deadly odyssey, by R. M. Henig. THE NEW YORK TIMES MAGAZINE February 6, 1983, p. 28-30+.

AIDS—a new immunodeficiency syndrome,by W. H. Hitzig. SCHWEIZERISCHE RUNDSCHAU FUR MEDIZIN PRAXIS 73(8):217-220, February 21, 1984.

AIDS news update. ADVOCATE 3(75):10, September 1, 1983.

—. ADVOCATE 3(80):14, November 10, 1983.

—, by C. Heim. ADVOCATE 3(82):12, December 8, 1983.

—. ADVOCATE 3(85):12, January 10, 1984.

AIDS news update—8000 LA marchers, by S. Anderson. ADVOCATE 3(71):8, July 7, 1983.

AIDS—a nightmare in our time. ORSTERREICHISCHE KRANKENPFLEGEZEIT-SCHRIFT 38(11):271-272, November 1985.

AIDS—nightmares, by M. Perigard. GAY COMMUNITY NEWS 11(30):5, February 18, 1984.

AIDS—no relief in sight, by S. Lawrence. SCIENCE NEWS 122:202-203, September 25, 1982.

AIDS no threat in central service, by D. Dildine. HPN 7(10):1+, October 1983.

AIDS: no time for apathy, by W. Greaves. JOURNAL OF THE NATIONAL MEDICAL ASSOCIATION 78(2):97-98, February 1986.

AIDS not an opportunistic infection [letter], by A. Ellrodt, et al. LANCET 2(8351): 680, September 17, 1983.

AIDS notes, by S. Hyde. GAY COMMUNITY NEWS 10(50):2, July 9, 1983.

—. GAY COMMUNITY NEWS 11(3):2, July 30, 1983.

AIDS: an old disease under a new name? RN 47:19, March 1984.

AIDS on the front line. EMERGENCY MEDICINE 18(1):24-28+, January 15, 1986.

AIDS on stage, by G. Weales. COMMONWEAL 112:406-407, July 12, 1985.

AIDS: one answer, many questions. SCIENCE DIGEST 93:44, January 1985.

AIDS: one man's story, by P. Morrisroe. NEW YORK 18:28-35, August 19, 1985.

AIDS or acquired immunodeficiency syndrome, by J. Leikola. REVUE DE L'INFIRMIERE 33(16):37-40, October 1983.

AIDS or not AIDS? Comments on the acquired immune deficiency syndrome, by J. E. Ollé Goig. MEDICINA CLINICA 83(6):244-248, July 14, 1984.

AIDS outcome: a first follow-up [letter], by B. E. Rivin, et al. NEW ENGLAND JOURNAL OF MEDICINE 311(13):857, September 27, 1984.

AIDS part 1, by R. Wells. INTERNATIONAL NURSING REVIEW 32(3/261):76-77, May-June 1985.

— part 2, by P. Nuttall. INTERNATIONAL NURSING REVIEW 32(3/261):78-79+, May-June 1985.

AIDS: planning for the impact, by I. Goldstone. RNABC NEWS 17(6):20, November-December 1985.

AIDS: the portrait of a victim, by K. S. Edwards. OHIO STATE MEDICAL JOURNAL 81(10):706+, October 1985.

AIDS—practical guidelines, by N. I. Abdou. JOURNAL OF THE KANSAS MEDICAL SOCIETY 85(3):32-84+, March 1984.

AIDS priority [letter], by L. Montagnier. NATURE 310(5977):46, August 9-15, 1984.

AIDS prognosis is grim, by D. Walter. ADVOCATE 421:8, May 28, 1985.

AIDS: a programmer of action, by M. Adler. TIMES September 6, 1985, p. 12.

AIDS: progress at last. THE ECONOMIST 291:40, April 28, 1984.

AIDS progress report, by A. Hecht. FDA CONSUMER 20:33-35, February 1986.

AIDS: prologue. ISSUES IN SCIENCE AND TECHNOLOGY 2:39, Winter 1986.

AIDS: protecting two publics, by D. Franklin. SCIENCE 6:16-17, December 1985.

AIDS: the public reacts. PUBLIC OPINION 8:35-37, December 1985-January 1986.

—. HASTINGS CENTER REPORT 15(4):23-26, August 1985.

AIDS: putting an alternative to the test, by R. Kotsch. EAST WEST JOURNAL 16(9):52, September 1986.

AIDS: putting the puzzle together, by J. B. Peter, et al. DIAGNOSTIC MEDICINE 7(2):56-60+, February 1984.

AIDS question, by W. F. Buckley. NATIONAL REVIEW 37:63, October 18, 1985.

AIDS: a rational approach. AMERICAN FAMILY PHYSICIAN 30:298, November 1984.

AIDS—report of a site visit. ADAMHA NEWS 11(20):1+, October 1985.

AIDS repository [letter], by R. A. Kaslow. SCIENCE 229(4708):8, July 5, 1985.

AIDS: responding to the crisis. Will the needs be met?, by J. Cassidy. HEALTH PROGRESS 67(4):53-56, May 1986.

AIDS—a review, by J. Cohen. BRITISH JOURNAL OF HOSPITAL MEDICINE 31(4):250-254+, April 1984.

AIDS: the risk to you, by W. F. Taylor. SURGICAL TECHNOLOGIST 18(4):17-20, July-August 1986.

AIDS—selective disease or public epidemic, by R. Baumgarten, et al. ZEITSCHRIFT FUR ARZTLICHE FORTBILDUNG 79(18):761-762, 1985.

AIDS: sharing out the spoils. NEW SCIENTIST 108:14, October 10, 1985.

AIDS—should we care, by B. Miller. SPARE RIB 141:28, April 1984.

AIDS show adapted, by S. Hachem. ADVOCATE 450:36, July 6, 1986.

AIDS: Sifting for facts about a puzzling disease, by D. H. Murphy. AMERICAN PHARMACY NS23(10):18-22, October 1983.

AIDS: some unsettling questions, by R. Bier. BEST'S REVIEW 86:16+, January 1986.

AIDS—something new under the sun [editorial], by S. G. Baum. LUNG 161(4): 193-194, 1983.

AIDS: special report, by J. Langone. DISCOVER 6:28-33+, December 1985.

AIDS: spreading mystery disease, by R. Thompson. EDITORIAL RESEARCH REPORTS pp. 599-616, August 9, 1985.

AIDS: a spreading scourge, by C. Wallis. TIME 126:50-51, August 5, 1985.

AIDS—still no concensus, by M. Hamilton. OCCUPATIONAL HEALTH 38(3):76, March 1986.

AIDS strikes a star, by D. Gelman. NEWSWEEK 106:68-69, August 5, 1985.

AIDS survival study, by S. Poggi. GAY COMMUNITY NEWS 13(46):2, June 14, 1986.

AIDS: 'This is not a little problem,' by A. W. Rogers. TEXAS HOSPITALS 41(11): 10-11, April 1986.

AIDS: the tip of the iceberg, by M. Helquist. ADVOCATE 427:32, June 20, 1985.

AIDS to the rescue?, by M. Beauchamp. FORBES 136:72+, November 18, 1985.

AIDS: too few facts, by A. J. Fugh-Berman. OFF OUR BACKS 13(10):12+, November 11, 1983.

AIDS update. AMERICAN FAMILY PHYSICIAN 30:322+, September 1984.

—. FDA DRUG BULLETIN 13(2):9-11, August 1983.

—. SCIENCE NEWS 128:40, July 20, 1985.

—. SCIENTIFIC AMERICAN 252:70, April 1985.

—. US NEWS & WORLD REPORT 98:48, February 18, 1985.

—, by B. Olson, et al. PRARIE ROSE 54(4):16, October-December 1983.

—, by L. M. Aledort. HOSPITAL PRACTICE 18(9):159-165+, September 1983.

—, by V. Gong, et al. MARYLAND MEDICAL JOURNAL 35(5):361-371, May 1986.

AIDS update: HTLV-III/LAV infection, by B. J. Cassens. PENNSYLVANIA MEDICINE 89(1):24-26, January 1986.

AIDS update: little to cheer about, by S. Hyde. GAY COMMUNITY NEWS 12(20): 3, December 1, 1984.

AIDS: an update on what we know now, by D. Anderson. RN 49(3):49-54+, March 1986.

AIDS update Part 2, by W. M. Valenti. INFECTION CONTROL 6(10):421-423, October 1985.

AIDS versus prodromal AIDS [letter]. UGESKRIFT FOR LAEGER 146(9):673-674, February 27, 1984.

AIDS: waiting for cure or treatment, by J. Silberner. SCIENCE NEWS 128:229, October 12, 1985.

AIDS watch. NURSING 14:15+, July 1984.

AIDS—what is it?, by I. Goldstone. RNABC NEWS 17(6):12-15, November - December 1985.

AIDS: what is it? Who is at risk? How can it be prevented?, by W. R. Dowdle. PUBLIC WELFARE 44(3):14-19, Summer1986.

AIDS: what is now known: part 3, clinical aspects, by P. A. Selwyn. HOSPITAL PRACTICE 21(9):119-131+, September 15, 1986.

AIDS: what is our response, by H. C. McGehee, Jr. WITNESS 68(8):4, August 1985.

AIDS: what is to be done? HARPER'S 271:39-52, October 1985.

AIDS: what you should know; interview by Sally Armstrong, by C. Tsoukas. CANADIAN LIVING 11:53-55, January 1986.

AIDS; the widening gyre, by J. E. Groopman, et al. NATURE 303:575-576, June 16, 1983.

AIDS: a world with no hiding place, by T. Prentice. TIMES November 19, 1986, p. 16.

Alert on AIDS. FDA CONSUMER 17:2, June 1983.

All about AIDS. GAY COMMUNITY NEWS 10(31):11, February 26, 1983; also in USA TODAY 112:16+, October 1983.

All so young, by T. Fennell. ALBERTA REPORT 12:48, November 25, 1985.

All who come to its doors, by T. J. Druhot. HEALTH PROGRESS 67(4):80, May 1986.

Americans stop talks about AIDS discovery, by S. Connor. NEW SCIENTIST 110:30, May 15, 1986.

Analysis of the interferon system in African patients with acquired immunodeficiency syndrome, by K. Huygen, et al. EUROPEAN JOURNAL OF CLINICAL MICROBIOLOGY 4(3):304-309, June 9185.

Another look at the acquired immunodeficiency syndrome, by M. L. Santaella. BOLETIN—ASOCIACION MEDICA DE PUERTO RICO 76(6):249-251, June 1984.

Answering the AIDS alarm, by J. Lang. RESTAURANT BUSINESS 84:108-109+, December 10, 1985.

Apropos the series: threatening advice on AIDS?, by C. Allmedal, et al. SYKEPLEIEN 73(11):36-37, June 20, 1986.

ARC (the AIDS-related complex [letter], by G. J. Ruiz-Argüelles, et al. REVISTA DE INVESTIGACION CLINICA 36(3):307-308, July-September 1984.

ARCW seeks input. OUT 4(4):5, February 2, 1986.

Aspects of the acquired immunodeficiency syndrome (AIDS), by V. Persaud. WEST INDIAN MEDICAL JOURNAL 32(3):119-121, September 1983.

Assault on AIDS and smoking, by D. McKie. LANCET 2(8468):1371, December 14, 1985.

Asymptomatic acquired immunological deficiencies. Nosologic and therapeutic problems, by J. P. Revillard. PRESSE MEDICALE 13(32):1933-1935, September 22, 1984.

At risk, by P. Wilsher, et al. SUNDAY TIMES November 2, 1986, p. 25.

Attrition, not conquest, of disease [news]. NATURE 309(5963):1-2, May 3-9, 1984.

Band-aids. THE ECONOMIST 288:22+, August 13-19, 1983.

Bandaids for AIDS. CULTURAL SURVIVAL QUARTERLY 3:19, Fall 1984.

Battling AIDS: more misery, less mystery, by C. Wallis, et al. TIME 125(17):68, April 29, 1985.

Bensons bomb, by S. Kulieke. ADVOCATE 3(73):18, August 4, 1983.

Bidirectionality of AIDS questioned. SCIENCE NEWS 129:11, January 4, 1986.

Body heat, by B. Thomson. EAST WEST JOURNAL 16(1):42, January 1986.

Boston forum calls for radical confrontation, by N. Wechsler. GAY COMMUNITY NEWS 13(24):2, Decemebr 28, 1985.

Boston shows pride, by L. Goldsmith. GAY COMMUNITY NEWS 10(49):1, July 2, 1983.

Breakthrough against a modern plague (AIDS), by P. Ohlendorf. MACLEAN'S 98:47-48, February 4, 1985.

Can contact tracing help fight AIDS? OUT 4(8);1, June 1986.

Can we help AIDS?, by A. Brown. SPECTATOR January 19, 1985, p. 16.

Can we talk?, by J. Bodis. BODY POLITIC 111:47, February 1985.

Capitol report, by L. Bush. ADVOCATE 3(72):18, July 21, 1983 and subsequent issues

Carl Wittman: an activist's life, by M. Bronski. GAY COMMUNITY NEWS 13(31):7, February 15, 1986.

Case 46-1984 [a 63-year-old man with respiratory failure after an unmaintained remission of acute myelogenous leukemia], by R. E. Scully, et al. NEW ENGLAND JOURNAL OF MEDICINE 311:1303-1310, November 15, 1984.

Case history—triumph over AIDS, by F. Cantaloupe. EAST WEST JOURNAL 14(2):46, February 1984.

Catalyst for change, by R. Berkowitz. GAY COMMUNITY NEWS 11(15):5, October 29, 1983.

Century's catastrophe? (2) How contagious—no infection with AIDS virus?, by O. Nilsen. SYKEPLEIEN 73(6):6-11+, March 21, 1986.

Challenge of the acquired immunodeficiency syndrome, by M. M. Heckler. ANNALS OF INTERNAL MEDICINE 103(5):655-656, November 1985.

Challenge of AIDS, by D. Coleman. OHIO NURSES REVIEW 61(6):11-12, June 1986.

Challenge of AIDS in a free society, by M. Arias-Klein. LAW ENFORCEMENT NEWS 12(1):8+, January 6, 1986.

Chance of a lifetime, by N. Deutsch. GAY COMMUNITY NEWS 13(41):11, May 3, 1986.

Channeled reading of AIDS, by J. Harvey. RFD 47:23, Summer 1986.

Code forbids AIDS bids, by N. Irwin. BODY POLITIC 124:17, March 1986.

Cofactor in AIDS? SCIENCE NEWS 128:77, August 3, 1985.

Combating AIDS. THE ECONOMIST 298:13-14, February 1, 1986.

Coming of AIDS: it didn't start with homosexuals, and it won't end with them, by J. F. Grutsch, et al. AMERICAN SPECTATOR 19(3):12-15, March 1986.

Coming to terms with AIDS, by J. Laurance. NEW SOCIETY November 14, 1986, p. 9-11.

Comment—need for bridge building, by Horowitz, et al. NACLA'S REPORT ON THE AMERICAS 18(2):2, March 1984.

Common bond of suffering, by W. A. Henry, III. TIME 125:85, May 13, 1985.

Complexing AIDS, by J. Silberner. SCIENCE NEWS 128:267, October 26, 1985.

Conspectus. Acquired immune deficiency syndrome, by D. R. Howard. COMPREHENSIVE THERAPY 9(8):3-5, August 1983.

Containing AIDS. THE ECONOMIST 296:13-14, August 10, 1985.

Continuing fight for all our lives, by L. Kessler. GAY COMMUNITY NEWS 11(20):5, December 3, 1983.

Coping with AIDS, by A. Moreton. NURSING MIRROR 161(1):49-51, July 3, 1985.

Coping with AIDS: crucial considerations, by W. V. Soughton. DIMENSIONS IN HEALTH SERVICE 61(9):19-20, September 1984.

Coping with the tragedy of AIDS, by M. Helquist. MS. 12:22, February 1984.

Countering AIDS . THE ECONOMIST 294:84-85, January 19, 1985.

Cream City boosts AIDS support efforts, by S. Burke. OUT 3(2):6, December 1984.

Cry of the normal heart, by D. Smith. NEW YORK 18:42-46, June 3, 1985.

Cycle for life. GAY COMMUNITY NEWS 13(42):7, May 17, 1986.

Cycle for life to visit Madison. OUT 4(8):5, June 1986.

Damage control. TIME 126:25, November 4, 1985.

David's story. READERS DIGEST (CANADA) 127:50-55, August 1985.

Dealing with AIDS, by C. Hays. NATIONAL CATHOLIC REGISTER 63:1+, March 16, 1986.

Deconstructing a syndrome. GAY COMMUNITY NEWS 13:30, Fall 1983.

Dedicated soldier: in war against AIDS, Samuel Broder serves as general and private, by M. Chase. WALL STREET JOURNAL 208:1+, October 17, 1986.

Detection of terminal deoxynucleotidyl transferase [letter],by R. D. Barr, et al. BLOOD 66(4):1006-1007, October 1985.

Different view of AIDS,by C. R. Tennison, Jr. NORTH CAROLINA MEDICAL JOURNAL 44(7):457-458, July 1983.

Do not go gently, by W. Blumenfeld. GAY COMMUNITY NEWS 11(16):8, November 5, 1983.

Double agent. SCIENTIFIC AMERICAN 251:66+, July 1984.

Early data about AIDS infections, by M. Helquist. ADVOCATE 424:26, July 9, 1985.

Eastern AIDS, by V. Rich. NATURE 308(5955):105, March 8, 1984.

Emotional hearings on AIDS held in S.F., by M. Helquist. ADVOCATE 426:15, August 6, 1985.

Endemic acquired immunodeficiency syndrome [letter], by W. M. Valenti, et al. ANNALS OF INTERNAL MEDICINE 101(3):399-400, September 1984.

Epidemic or Hysteria? by S. Gesenhues. ZFA 59(33):1865-1869, November 30, 1983.

Epidemic's unsung heroes, by C. Norman. SCIENCE 230:1020, November 29, 1985.

Everything you need to know about AIDS, by C. L. Carney. PARENTS 61(4): 105-108+, April 1986.

Exchange on AIDS, by J. Lieberson. THE NEW YORK REVIEW OF BOOKS 30:43-45, October 13, 1983.

Facing a common enemy, by E. Jackson. BODY POLITIC 116:13, July 1985.

Facing a fatal disease, by B. Levin. MACLEAN'S 99:48-49, January 6, 1986.

Facing it: a novel of AIDS, by J. Andriote. ADVOCATE 423:43, June 25, 1985.

Facts about acquired immune deficiency syndrome (AIDS). WISCONSIN MEDICAL JOURNAL 82(11):15-18, November 1983.

Facts about acquired immune deficiency syndrome, by the AIDS Task Force. HEALTHRIGHT 4:27-29, May 1985.

Facts about AIDS. NEW ZEALAND NURSING JOURNAL 77(4):1-4, April 1984.

—. PLASTIC SURGICAL NURSING 3(3):73-75, Fall 1983.

—, by J. Nelson. ESSENCE 16:56+, August 1985.

Facts about AIDS: a detention training program, by L. D. Carlin. TRAINING AIDS DIGEST 10(11):1+, November 1985.

Facts that stay concealed, by D. Anderson. TIMES August 19, 1986, p. 10.

Fighting for our lives, by C. Sorrel. OFF OUR BACKS 13:10, November 1983.

Fighting for their lives, by B. Egerton. OUT 3(1):1, November 1984.

Fighting off AIDS. NEW SCIENTIST 108:13, October 31, 1985.

Fighting off a killer called Slim, by T. Prentice. TIMES October 27, 1986, p 14.

Fighting a scourge: gains against AIDS have come rapidly, but a cure is distant; need for effective therapies is urgent as cases rise, by M. Case. WALL STREETJOURNAL 206:1+, August 5, 1985.

Figure it out, by A. Lumsden. NEW STATESMAN November 7, 1986, p. 8-9.

Fires, by M. Totke. BODY POLITIC 128:31, July 1986.

First AIDS, by J. McQuaid. THE NEW REPUBLIC 189:16, August 1, 1983.

—, by J. Melville. GUARDIAN September 24, 1986, p. 11.

Fresh lead. THE ECONOMIST 287:94-95, May 28-June 3, 1983.

Friends gone with the wind, by A. Kantrowitz. ADVOCATE 454:43, September 2, 1986.

From the editor's desk. ADVOCATE 449:5, June 24, 1986.

From New York, by S. Jacoby. PRESENT TENSE 13:45-47, Winter 1986.

Future shock [New York City], by L. Glynn. MACLEAN'S 98:52, November 18, 1985.

Germ of doubt, by A. Veitch. GUARDIAN December 20, 1985, p. 15.

GLCS and the HTLV-III, by Varnum, et al. GAY COMMUNITY NEWS 13(16):5, November 2, 1985.

Good news, bad news: 21 views on AIDS. UTNE READER 17:70, August 1986.

Greetings—with a brief look back [editorial], by T. F. Zuck. TRANSFUSION 23(6): 459, November-December 1983.

Guardian angel, by P. Morrisroe. NEW YORK 18:46-49+, December 9, 1985.

Health, by N. Fain. ADVOCATE 3(72):20, July 21, 1983; also in subsequent issues.

Health-AIDS—the gold rush, by N. Fain. ADVOCATE 3(74):22, August 18, 1983.

Health—creative responses from all, by N. Fain. ADVOCATE 3(81):22, November 24, 1983.

Health—two kinds of answers to AIDS, by N. Fain. ADVOCATE 3(76):16, September 15, 1983.

Heckler stand on AIDS hit. GAY COMMUNITY NEWS 12(43):3, May 18, 1985.

Helping AIDS victims. CHRISTIANITY TODAY 30(2):59, February 7, 1986.

Helping battle AIDS, by J. Fierman. FORTUNE 111:57-58, April 15, 1985.

Helping gay AIDS patients in crisis, by D. J. Lopez, et al. SOCIAL CASEWORK 65(7):387-394, 1984.

Helquist report, by M. Helquist. ADVOCATE 445:21, April 29, 1986; also in 447:21, 448:21, 452:21, 455:21.

Holistic health: one approach to AIDS. OUT 4(6):3, May 1986.

Holistic hyperbole, by R. Trow. BODY POLITIC 93:38, May 1983.

Hollywood faces AIDS, by S. Rosenthal. US 3:27+, October 7, 1985.

Hospitals may be AIDS victims too. MEDICAL WORLD NEWS 26(23):92-93, December 9, 1985.

How AIDS threatens all of us, by T. Stuttaford. SPECTATOR November 15, 1986, p. 9-11.

How America nurtured AIDS. NEW SCIENTIST 110:25, May 29, 1986.

How dangerous is AIDS?, by G. Jörgensen. KRANKENPFLEGE JOURNAL 24(6):12-14+, June 1, 1986.

How fast we forget, by F. S. Welch. PHOENIX 21:192, January 1986.

Hudson and AIDS—in retrospect, by M. Bronski. GAY COMMUNITY NEWS 13(13):3, October 12, 1985.

Hug an AIDS victim—he is safe. NEW SCIENTIST 109:15, February 13, 1986.

Hunting down AIDS, by B. Henker, et al. ALBERTA REPORT 12:39-40, March 18, 1985.

Hunting for the hidden killers, by W. Isaacson. TIME 122:50-55, July 4, 1983.

Hygeia's comments, by D. Sage. I KNOW YOU KNOW 1(5):9, April 1985.

Idiotypes and AIDS [letter], by J. Gheuens. LANCET 2(8393):41, July 7, 1984.

Immunodeficiency syndrome, by W. A. Blattner, et al. ANNALS OF INTERNAL MEDICINE 103(5):665-670, November 1985.

In pursuit of AIDS. NEW SCIENTIST 105:2, February 7, 1985.

INA Board acts on AIDS recommendations. CHART 83(5):3, May-June 1986.

Indiscriminate killer, by J. Barber. MACLEAN'S 98:38, August 12, 1985.

Industry worry: is AIDS in the red bag?, by T. Naber. WASTE AGE 16(10):48-49, October 1985.

Inevitable love, by M. Bronski. GAY COMMUNITY NEWS 13(41):11, May 3, 1986.

Informed consent/choices about AIDS, by L. Fishman. GAY COMMUNITY NEWS 10(42):8, May 14, 1983.

Interview [M. Krim], by B. Lawren. OMNI 8:76-78+, November 1985.

Interview with Bobbi Campbell, by R. Evans. NORTHWEST PASSAGE 24(2):7, September 1983.

Investing in hope on AIDS, by D. Dorfman. NEW YORK 18:21, September 9, 1985.

Iron, ferritin, and AIDS [letter], by I. Kushner. LANCET 1(8377):633, March 17, 1984.

Is this any way to run a movement? 6 leaders, by L. Giteck. ADVOCATE 448:42, June 10, 1986.

Is your organization ready for AIDS? TRAINING 23:87-88, March 1986.

Jumping guns? by S. Budiansky. NATURE 309:106, May 10, 1984.

Keeping AIDS at bay, by R. McKie, et al. OBSERVER November 9, 1986, p. 11.

Know the enemy. THE ECONOMIST 300:74-75, July 5, 1986.

Knowing the face of the enemy, by C. Wallis, et al. TIME 123(18):66-67, April 30, 1984.

Knowing Ron. P. L. Spechko. JAMA 253:985, February 15, 1985.

Kramer v. cruising; "The Normal Heart" [play review]. THE ECONOMIST 299:104, April 5, 1986.

Last minute withdrawal, by Armstrong, et al. BODY POLITIC 121:37, December 1985.

Last weeks of an AIDS sufferer at Berkeley: a friend remembers, by L. Biemiller. THE CHRONICLE OF HIGHER EDUCATION 31:1+, December 4, 1985.

Leading edge. FINANCIAL WORLD 154:47, May 15-28, 1985.

Learning from AIDS, by J. Wilson. GAY COMMUNITY NEWS 11(5):6, August 13, 1983.

Letter from Commissioner Young, by F. E. Young. FDA DRUG BULLETIN 3:26, October 1985.

Little knowledge, dangerous thing [editorial]. BODY POLITIC 121:8, December 1985.

Living and dying day-by-day, by M. Bronski. GAY COMMUNITY NEWS 45:9, June 7, 1986.

Living as we do, by A. O'Connor. BODY POLITIC 123:31, February 1986.

Living with AIDS, by C. Maves. ADVOCATE 421:30, May 28, 1985.

— [editorial], by L. Watson. MEDICAL JOURNAL OF AUSTRALIA 141(9):559 - 560, October 27, 1984.

—, by M. Herron. WHOLE EARTH REVIEW 48:34-53, Fall 1985.

Living with AIDS: when the system fails, by R. Cecchi. AMERICAN JOURNAL OF NURSING 86(1):45+, January 1986.

Looking for rhyme and reason, by J. Aynsley. BODY POLITIC 124:14, March 1986.

Louise Hay—can she really help people?, by G. DeStefano. ADVOCATE 452: 50, August 5, 1986.

Love in a chilling climate, by J. Sherman, et al. TIMES November 5, 1986, p. 14.

Lurking killer without a cure, by A. Veitch. GUARDIAN November 2, 1983, p. 13.

Making sense of AIDS, by M. Amis. OBSERVER June 23, 1985, p. 17-18.

Making sure you don't miss AIDS, by A. S. Brodoff. PATIENT CARE 18(1):166-167+, January 15, 1984.

Man who may shut the tabs, by B. Averill. VILLAGE VOICE 30:36, January 22, 1985.

Mark Halberstadt. GAY COMMUNITY NEWS 12(5):6, August 11, 1984.

MASN to expand, hires coordinators. OUT 4(6):5, May 1986.

Meanwhile at the NCI, by N. Fain. ADVOCATE 3(78):23, October 13, 1983.

Medical response to AIDS epidemics [letter],by B. S. Bender, et al. NEW ENGLAND JOURNAL OF MEDICINE 310(6):389, February 9, 1984.

Medicine's fearsome new public enemy (acquired immune deficiency syndrome), by D. Grady, et al. READERS DIGEST 123:145-146+, October 1983.

Meeting the AIDS challenge in Illinois. CHART 83(5):4-5, May-June 1986.

Menace of AIDS, by L. Cohen. ALBERTA REPORT 11:39, September 10, 1984.

Modern life, by C. Ratcliff. ARTFORUM 24:8, January 1986.

More AIDS, more questions. SCIENCE NEWS 127:173, March 16, 1985.

Mother cares . . . and so does Zelda!, by M. Daniels. ADVOCATE 448:50, June 10, 1986.

Moving target. SCIENTIFIC AMERICAN 253:85, October 1985.

My personal experience with AIDS, by A. J. Ferrara. AMERICAN PSYCHOLO-GIST 39(11):1285-1287, November 1984.

Mystery of AIDS [most asked questions and answers], by B. Rensberger. SCIENCE DIGEST 94:40-41+, January 1986.

Nationwide AIDS report/checking up, by E. Jackson. BODY POLITIC 95:12, July 1983.

Nature's deadly experiment, by S. DeGarmo. SCIENCE DIGEST 91:6, December 1983.

New aid in fighting AIDS? NEWSWEEK 105:85, February 18, 1985.

New AIDS forecast: a long, long siege. US NEWS & WORLD REPORT 99:14, October 14, 1985.

New AIDS guidelines and group. NURSING 16:16, February 1986.

New aspects of AIDS, by J. Gerstoft. NORDISK MEDICIN 98(10):231-233, 1983.

New disease: acquired immune deficiency of homosexuals [editorial],by A. Molins Otero. REVISTA CLINICA ESPANOLA 168(2):150-151, January 31, 1983.

New disease baffles medical community, by J. L. Marx. SCIENCE 217:618-621, August 13, 1982.

New hope fighting AIDS. ALBERTA REPORT 11:40, May 7, 1984.

New hope for Californian AIDS victims?, by P. Tatchell. NEW STATESMAN 110:6, October 11, 1985.

New San Francisco story, by M. Helquist. ADVOCATE 429:24, September 17, 1985.

New scarlet letter, by M. Sager. WASHINGTONIAN 21:104+, January 1986.

New study ties poopers, AIDS, by Connors. GAY COMMUNITY NEWS 13(13):1, October 12, 1985.

New theories about AIDS, by J. Seligmann, et al. NEWSWEEK 103(5):50-51, January 30, 1984.

New victims, by E. Barnes, et al. LIFE 8:12-19, July 1985.

Nice. . . but don't have to know, by Ehud Yonay. CALIFORNIA MAGAZINE 9:39, June 1984.

NIDA and AIDS. ADAMHA NEWS 10(8):8, August 1984.

Nightmare coming true. BODY POLITIC 129:18, August 1986.

Nightmare of AIDS [letter], by A. Sibatani. NATURE 304(5923):206, July 21-27, 1983.

1985 update on AIDS, by J. Hardie. CANADIAN DENTAL ASSOCIATION JOURNAL 51(7):499-502, July 1985.

No more shit [editorial]. BODY POLITIC 127:8, June 1986.

Obstacles to curing AIDS, by C. Gunderson. UTNE READER 11:15, August 1985.

On AIDS . . . and one road to redemption . . . donate blood, by T. M. Stephany. POINT OF VIEW 22(2):21, May 1985.

On the AIDS problem, by Lewis Thomas. DISCOVER 4:42+, May 1983.

On calling whom what, by N. Fain. ADVOCATE 3(79):20, October 27, 1983.

One man's battle with AIDS, by A. S. Brodoff. PATIENT CARE 18(2):138+, January 30, 1984.

One man's fight against AIDS, by T. McGirk. SUNDAY TIMES August 11, 1985, p. 15.

Our fragile brothers, by J. P. Nieckarz. COMMONWEAL 112:404-406, July 12, 1985.

Outlook for AIDS bleak for remainder of year. JET 69:12, November 4, 1985.

Overview: acquired immune deficiency syndrome, by B. J. Cassens. PENNSYL-VANIA MEDICINE 86(7):41-43, July 1983.

Oxford education to ward off AIDS, by M. Davie. OBSERVER June 15, 1986, p. 56.

Panorama/BBC1, by S. O'Sullivan. SPARE RIB 1(30):38, May 1983.

Pat Buchanan's nasty nature, by P. Freiberg. ADVOCATE 3(73):18, August 4, 1983.

Patient with a mild form of the acquired immunodeficiency syndrome (AIDS), by P. Reiss, et al. NEDERLANDS TIJDSCHRIFT VOOR GENEESKUNDE 127(19):824-825, May 7, 1983.

People with AIDS make presence felt, by N. Fain. ADVOCATE 3(72):11, July 21, 1983.

Person behind the disease, by A. C. Crovella. NURSING 15(9):42, September 1985.

Personal you update. DANCE MAGAZINE 58:88, February 1984.

Perspective on AIDS cases among health care workers, by R. S. Gordon. ANNALS OF THE NEW YORK ACADEMY OF SCIENCES 437:420, 1984.

Perspectives. Responses to the AIDS crisis. WASHINGTON REPORT ON MEDI-CINE AND HEALTH 39(41):Suppl. 4, October 21, 1985.

Phallacy of waiting for science to cure AIDS, by K. Barton. RFD 47:20, Summer 1986.

Pickle family's fool, by R. Hurwitt. CALIFORNIA 10:32+, February 1985.

Pity the poor patient. NEW SCIENTIST 106:2, April 25, 1985.

Progress at last. THE ECONOMIST 291:40, April 28, 1984.

Progress, but bleak prospects. BODY POLITIC 115:23, June 1985.

Progress on AIDS. FDA DRUG BULLETIN 15(3):27-32, October 1985.

Promise of AIDS, by R. Teitelman. FORBES 134:302+, November 19, 1984.

Pulling away the blanket, by M. Johnson. DISABILITY RAG 7(5):22, September 1986.

Putting rhetoric aside, by N. Lynch. BODY POLITIC 127:33, June 1986.

PWAs demand treatment, by D. Larventz. BODY POLITIC 126:14, May 1986.

PWAs, PWARC: organize for their lives, by K. Westheimer. GAY COMMUNITY NEWS 13(45):3, June 7, 1986.

Recovery from AIDS, by J. Bolen. RFD 45:43, Winter 1985.

Reflections on AIDS, by C. Levasseur. CANADIAN NURSE 82(3):23-25+, March 1986.

Report on acquired immunodeficiency syndrome, by E. Rodríguez Domingo. MEDICINA CLINICA 82(11):491-493, March 24, 1984.

Response to AIDS, by J. Robinson. GAY COMMUNITY NEWS 11(11):13, October 3, 1983.

— [editorial], by J. R. Bove. TRANSFUSION 25(1):1-2, January-February 1985.

—, by T. Dollar. FUNDAMENTALIST JOURNAL 4(10):74, November 1985.

Rights before responsibility, by J. O'Sullivan. TIMES October 12, 1985, p. 8.

Rivalry to defeat AIDS, by J. Carey. US NEWS & WORLD REPORT 100(1):67-68, January 13, 1986.

Safety cabinets and AIDS, by R. P. Clark. NATURE 315:626, June 20, 1985.

San Francisco recoils. ECONOMIST August 23, 1986, p. 32-33.

San Francisco solution: debate continues, by S. Kulieke. ADVOCATE 41:9, March 5, 1985.

Scarlet letters and public risks, by W. Hampton Sides. CONNECTICUT MAGA- ZINE 47:68+, March 1984.

"Screaming room" reveals agony of AIDS, by L. Mohn. NEW DIRECTIONS FOR WOMEN September 1986, p. 4.

Sense of power in San Francisco, by K. Kelley. GUARDIAN 37(46):10, September 25, 1985.

'Sheet sign' [letter], by F. Adams. JAMA 251(7):891, February 17, 1984.

Some questions and answers about AIDS. PENNSYLVANIA NURSE 41(2):9+, February 1986.

Standing up for life, by Friends, et al. RFD 35:15, Summer 1983.

Still in the waiting room, by R. Joyce. BODY POLITIC 127:13, June 1986.

Story of the year: the AIDS trauma touched everyone, by David Black, et al. ROLLING STONE p. 121+, December 19, 1985, January 2, 1986.

Studies further speculation on AIDS, by L. Goldsmith. GAY COMMUNITY NEWS 10(43):3, May 21, 1983.

Success quotients: dealing with AIDS, by P. Kerschner. JOURNAL OF THE AMERICAN HEALTH CARE ASSOCIATION 11(8):44, December 1985.

"Survival kit". OUT 4(6):1, May 1986.

Taking aim with an empty gun, by K. Popart. BODY POLITIC 116:14, July 1985.

Taking the test: what for?, by J. Aynsley. BODY POLITIC 121:17, December 1985.

Talking about AIDS, by Andrew, et al. GAY COMMUNITY NEWS 10(47):6, June 18, 1983.

Tapeworms for lunch, by G. Halak. CHANGING MEN 14:15, Spring 1985.

Taxonomy over treatment?, by J. Beldekas. GAY COMMUNITY NEWS 12(30):7, February 16, 1985.

Theatre [review of plays The Normal Heart and As Is], by J. C. Thorpe. THE CRISIS 92:13+, October 1985.

Theatre in the plague years, by R. Hardy. BODY POLITIC 116:34, July 1985.

Theatre of AIDS, by K. Plummer. NEW SOCIETY June 28, 1985, p. 476-477.

Thirty seconds that could shake the country, by H. Hawkins. GUARDIAN November 11, 1986, p. 26.

This seeing the sick endears them, by M. Lynch. BODY POLITIC 91:36, March 1983.

Tinseltown and St. Petersburg, by D. Altman. BODY POLITIC 123:25, February 1986.

To stop AIDS, by M. Larkin. HEALTH 17:64, December 1985.

Toxic shock research lessons—AIDS, by C. Patton. GAY COMMUNITY NEWS 11(32):3, March 3, 1984.

Trade-off mars AIDS report, by K. Orr. BODY POLITIC 127:17, June 1986.

Truth about AIDS: an optimistic review, by S. G. Rainsford. CONTEMPORARY REVIEW 248:256-261, May 1986.

Unusual acquired immune deficiency syndrome —AIDS, by Z. Hollán, et al. ORVOSI HETILAP 125(7):375-382, February 12, 1984.

Update on AIDS. MEDICAL BULLETIN OF THE U.S. ARMY, EUROPE 43(2):12, February 1986.

—, by E. Marshall. ARIZONA NURSE 37(2):1+, March-April 1984.

—, by H. Glenister. NURSING TIMES 81(23):4-6, June 5-11, 1985.

—, by P. Kenny. PENNSYLVANIA NURSE 40(7):4, July 1985.

—, by W. M. Valenti. INFECTION CONTROL 6(2):85-86, February 1985.

Update on AIDS: critical review, by A. Modiano, et al. GIORNALE DI CLINICA MEDICA 66(7-8):239-251, July-August 1985.

Update on AIDS—virology, immunology, epidemiology, by G. Biberfeld, et al. LAKARTIDNINGEN 81(26-27):2595-2599, June 27, 1984.

Vie Douce, by D. Janoff. BODY POLITIC 118:21, September 1985.

Waking up to AIDS, by R. Bazell. THE NEW REPUBLIC 192:17-19, May 13, 1985.

Warrior, by J. Howard. ESQUIRE 102:270-272+, December 1984.

Was it your son who spoke to me, by Okin, et al. BODY POLITIC 93:4, May 1983.

Way we are, by W. M. Hoffman. VOGUE 175:174-175+, July 1985.

Welcome the grand alliance, by N. Fain. ADVOCATE 3(77):22, September 29, 1983.

Welcome news. THE ECONOMIST September 27, 1986, p. 86+.

What about poppers, by N. Fain. ADVOCATE 3(79):20, October 27, 1983.

What answers for AIDS?, by D. Gergen. US NEWS & WORLD REPORT 99:78, September 23, 1985.

What are we doing about AIDS? [letter]. NEW ENGLAND JOURNAL OF MEDI-CINE 312(11):726-727, March 14, 1985.

What are we going to do about AIDS and HTLV-III/LAV infection? [editorial], by T. C. Merigan. NEW ENGLAND JOURNAL OF MEDICINE 311(20):1311-1333, November 15, 1984.

What can we do on AIDS?, by J. Laurance. NEW SOCIETY October 18, 1985, p. 103-105.

What the experts know about AIDS. FDA CONSUMER 17(7):15-19, September 1983.

What hope for AIDS? NATURE 316(6030):663-664, August 22-28, 1985.

What we know about AIDS, by J. Seale. NEW SCIENTIST 107:29-30, August 1, 1985.

What we know about AIDS part 1, by J. A. Bennett. AMERICAN JOURNAL OF NURSING 86(9):1016-1021, September 1986.

What we're doing about AIDS, by W. Mayer. DEFENSE 86(1):30-32, January-February 1986.

What's in a name? by C. Norman. SCIENCE 230:641, November 8, 1985.

—, by M. Helquist. ADVOCATE 426:32, August 6, 1985.

Where now with AIDS? [editorial]. NATURE 313(6000):254, January 24-30, 1985.

Whitewash, by Peter Collier, et al. CALIFORNIA MAGAZINE 8:52+, July 1983.

Why is a lefty so different?, by S. Begley. NEWSWEEK 100:62-63, August 30, 1982.

Why this young hunk risked playing an AIDS victim: taking a role others nervously avioded, Aidan Quinn was out to prove something to Hollywood—and to himself, by Michael Leahy. TV GUIDE 34:34+, April 26, 1986.

Widening the definition of AIDS? [letter], by J. M. Guerin, et al. LANCET 1(8392): 1464-1465, June 30, 1984.

Working with AIDS, by M. B. Pfeiffer. EMPIRE STATE REPORT 12:44-67, October 1986.

Worst fears made flesh, by J. Sunderland. CHARTIST 105:5, Juy 1985.

Wrong AIDS customers. FDA CONSUMER 17:1, December 1983-January 1984.

Wrong without remedy, by D. M. Freedman. AMERICAN BAR ASSOCIATION JOURNAL 72:36-40, June 1, 1986.

AFRICA
Africa's latest torment: AIDS. U.S. NEWS & WORLD REPORT 99:8, December 23, 1985.

AIDS: African connection [editorial], by I. Braveny. EUROPEAN JOURNAL OF CLINICAL MICROBIOLOGY 2(6):521-522, December 1983.

AIDS: the African connection [letter], by P. Jenkins, et al. BRITISH MEDICAL JOURNAL 290(6477):1284-1285, April 27, 1985.

—, by P. Jones. BRITISH MEDICAL JOURNAL 291(6489):216, July 20, 1985.

AIDS—an African disease?, by K. M. De Cock. ADVANCES IN EXPERIMENTAL MEDICINE AND BIOLOGY 187:1-12, 1985.

AIDS' African genesis argued at symposium, by M. Helquist. ADVOCATE 437:20, January 7, 1986.

AFRICA

AIDS could cause new havoc in starving Africa. NEW SCIENTIST 111:24, July 3, 1986.

AIDS: a deadly silence in Africa, by A. Stewart. TIMES November 8, 1985, p. 14.

AIDS—its implications for South African homosexuals and the mediating role of the medical practitioner, by G. Isaacs, et al. SOUTH AFRICAN MEDICAL JOURNAL 68(5):327-330, August 31, 1985.

AIDS: an old disease from Africa? [letter], by C. J. Lacey, et al. BRITISH MEDICAL JOURNAL 289(6443):496, August 25, 1984.

—, by K. M. De Cock. BRITISH MEDI CAL JOURNAL 289(6440):306-308, August 4, 1984.

— [letter], by K. M. De Cock. BRITISH MEDICAL JOURNAL 289(6456):1454-1455, November 24, 1984.

—, by R. Colebunders, et al. BRITISH MEDICAL JOURNAL 289(6447):765, September 22, 1984.

AIDS problem in Africa, by R. J. Biggar. LANCET 1(8472):79-83, January 11, 1986.

AIDS that Africa could do without, by A. Veitch. GUARDIAN October 31, 1984, p. 13.

Politics and science clash on African AIDS, by C. Norman. SCIENCE 230:1140+, December 6, 1985.

ARABIA

AIDS in Arabia. NEW SCIENTIST 109:23, January 30, 1986.

ARGENTINA

Acquired immunodeficiency syndrome (AIDS) with Kaposi's sarcoma in homosexuals in Argentina [letter], by M. E. Estevez, et al. MEDICINA 43(4):477, 1983.

AUSTRALIA

Acquired immune deficiency syndrome. Report of the NHMRC Working Party. MEDICAL JOURNAL OF AUSTRALIA 141(9):561-568, October 27, 1984.

AIDS guide offsets hysteria [Australia], by L. Garcia. THE TIMES EDUCATIONAL SUPPLEMENT 3609:11, August 30, 1985.

AIDS in Australia, by S. Hyde. GAY COMMUNITY NEWS 12(22):2, December 15, 1984.

Sydney AIDS Project. Sydney AIDS study group. MEDICAL JOURNAL OF AUSTRALIA 141(9):569-573, October 27, 1984.

CANADA

> Acquired immunodeficiency syndrome (AIDS)—Canada. MMWR 32(48):635-636, December 9, 1983.

> AIDS comes to Halifax, by S. MacPhee. ATLANTIC INSIGHT 7:6, November 1985.

> Canadian gay health groups, by T. Stroll. ADVOCATE 3(77):9, September 29, 1983.

> Halifax: getting together to battle AIDS, by D. Henderson. BODY POLITIC 109:14, December 1984.

> Preparing for the worst in Halifax, by R. Metcalf. BODY POLITIC 118:19, September 1985.

EUROPE

> Acquired immunodeficiency syndrome (AIDS)—Europe. JAMA 250(24): 3278, December 23-30, 1983. Also in: MMWR 32(46):610-611, November 25, 1983.

> AIDS: plan for European centre agreed [news]. NATURE 305(5937):751, October 27-November 2, 1983.

> Clinical and epidemiological survey of acquired immune deficiency syndrome in Europe, by M. P. Glauser, et al. EUROPEAN JOURNAL OF CLINICAL MICROBIOLOGY 3(1):55-58, February 1984.

> Europeans confer—increase slows. BODY POLITIC 1(1):17, March 1984.

FRANCE

> Acquired immunologic deficiency syndrome. Recommendations of group of French physicians and hemophilia specialists. REVUE FRANCAISE DE TRANSFUSION ET IMMUNO-HAEMATOLOGIE 28(3):273-274, June 1985.

> AIDS exiles in Paris, by M. Clark, et al. NEWSWEEK 106(6):71, August 5, 1985.

> AIDS: French sue over who was first, by C. Joyce, et al. NEW SCIENTIST 108:3, December 19-26, 1985.

> France packs AIDs kit. NEW SCIENTIST 104:5, December 6, 1984.

> French believe AIDS discovery is theirs, by A. Lloyd. NEW SCIENTIST 102: 6, April 26, 1984.

GERMANY

> Acquired immune deficiency syndrome: current status. Position of the German Association for the Control of Virus Diseases and the Virology Section of the German Society for Hygiene and Microbiology, by F. Deinhardt, et al. DEUTSCHE MEDIZINISCHE WOCHENSCHRIFT 110(7): 274-276, February 15, 1985.

> AIDS 1976 in Cologne? [letter], by A. Konrads, et al. DEUTSCHEMEDIZI-NISCHE WOCHENSCHRIFT 108(35):1336, September 2, 1983.

GREAT BRITAIN

AIDS guidance for heads [Great Britain], by J. Meikle. THE TIMES EDUCA-TIONAL SUPPLEMENT 3639:10, March 28, 1986.

AIDS: London scare ends [news], by M. Chown. NATURE 310(5979):614, August 23-29, 1984.

AIDS: London's last chance, by K. Conlon, et al. ILLUSTRATED LONDON NEWS 274:26-30, December 1986.

American AIDS team in talks with British PWAs, by A. Lumsden. NEW STATESMAN 109:5, May 24, 1985.

British AIDS [news], by H. Barnes. NATURE 312(5995):583, December 13-19, 1984.

British AIDS; paper prophylaxis backfires, by H. Barnes. NATURE 312:583, December 13, 1984.

British relief for AIDS victims is threatened, by S. Yanchinski. NEW SCI-ENTIST 98:361, May 12, 1983.

Letter from London, by N. DeJongh. ADVOCATE 450:28, July 8, 1986.

No AIDS for Britain's peers. DISCOVER 6:8, May 1985.

Surveillance of the acquired immune deficiency syndrome in the United King-dom, Jan. '82-July 1983. BRITISH MEDICAL JOURNAL 287:407-408, August 6, 1983.

Surveillance of AIDS in Britain: September 1983. BRITISH MEDICAL JOUR-NAL 287(6401):1284, October 29, 1983.

HAITI

Acquired immune deficiency syndrome: specific aspects of the disease in Haiti, by J. M. Guerin, et al. ANNALS OF THE NEW YORK ACADEMY OF SCIENCES 437:254-263, 1984.

AIDS: the Haitian connection, by H. M. Smith. MD 27(12):46-52, December 1983.

AIDS: The Haitian Factor, by Alfredo S. Lanier. CHICAGO 33:120+, August 1984.

Haitian Ambassador deplores AIDS connection [letter], by S. Sherman. NEW ENGLAND JOURNAL OF MEDICINE 309(11):668-669, September 15, 1983.

Haiti—AIDS stigma, by M. Cooley. NACLA'S REPORT ON THE AMERICAS 17(5):47, September 1983.

Haiti and the acquired immunodeficiency syndrome [letter]. ANNALS OF INTERNAL MEDICINE 99(4):565, October 1983.

Haiti and the acquired immunodeficiency syndrome, by J. R. Leonidas, et al. ANNALS OF INTERNAL MEDICINE 98(6):1020-1021, June 1983.

HAITI
>Haiti and the stigma of AIDS [letter],by R. S. Greco. LANCET 2(8348):515-516, August 27, 1983.

>Mystery immune disorder; the Haitian connection. ECONOMIST 286:77, January 29, 1983.

INDIA
>India against AIDS, by K. S. Jayaraman. NATURE 318(6043):201, November 21, 1985.

ISRAEL
>Questions from Israel, by M. Helquist. ADVOCATE 446:21, May 13, 1986.

NEW ZEALAND
>AIDS—New Zealand's position. NEW ZEALAND HOSPITAL 37(8):11, September 1985.

POLAND
>Poland—out of sight, out of mind, by Darski, et al. BODY POLITIC 12:21, April 1986.

SWEDEN
>AIDS: what Sweden is doing to meet the peril of a disease that has already claimed 20,000 victims worldwide, by M. Jeffries. SWEDEN NOW 19(6): 22-25, 1985.

UNITED STATES
>Acquired immune deficiency syndrome. Health and Public Policy Committee, American College of Physicians; and The Infectious Diseases Society of America. ANNALS OF INTERNAL MEDICINE 104(4):575-581, April 1986.

>Acquired immunodeficiency syndrome (AIDS) update—United States. JAMA 250(3):335-336, July 15, 1983. Also in: MMWR 32(24):309-311, June 24, 1983.

>Acquired immunodeficiency syndrome: a San Francisco perspective, by J. M. Luce, et al. INTENSIVE CARE MEDICINE 11(4):172-173, 1985.

>AIDS concerns in Iowa: an interview with Laverne Wintermeyer. IOWA MEDICINE 75(8):346-347, August 1985.

USSR
>AIDS: Moscow's new weapon in its secret war of smears, by I. Elliot. TIMES October 31, 1986, p. 20.

>Soviet offer on AIDS, by V. Rich. NATURE 317:659, October 24, 1985.

>Soviets admit AIDS cases, by V. Rich. NATURE 318(6046):502, December 12, 1985.

AIDS—HAITIANS
Haitian connection. THE ECONOMIST 286:77, January 29-February 4, 1983.

Haitian liason for AIDS group, by C. Guilfoy. GAY COMMUNITY NEWS 12(34):1, March 16, 1985.

Haitians and AIDS. AMERICAN FAMILY PHYSICIAN 31:241, June 1985.

AIDS—HOTLINES
AIDS action line. BOSTON MAGAZINE 77:33, December 1985.

AIDS support organizations and information services. QRB 12(8):304-305, August 1986.

Feds open hotline on AIDS. CORRECTIONS DIGEST 14(15):8, July 13, 1983; also in CRIME CONTROL DIGEST 17(28):6, July 18, 1983.

Helping out the hot line, by N. Fain. ADVOCATE 3(77):23, September 29, 1983.

ANESTHESIA
Acquired immune deficiency syndrome: a brief review and anesthetic implications, by J. Layon. CURRENT REVIEWS FOR RECOVERY ROOM NURSES 8(9):67-72, 1986.

Acquired immunodeficiency syndrome: an overview for anesthesiologists, by E. R. Greene, Jr. ANESTHESIA AND ANALGESIA 65(10):1054-1058, October 1986.

AIDS and the anaesthetist, by A. s. Cordero, et al. CANADIAN ANAESTHETISTS SOCIETY JOURNAL 32(1):45-48, January 1985.

Overview of acquired immunodeficiency syndrome (AIDS)—the disease and related anesthetic considerations, by B. Sommer. AANA JOURNAL 51(4): 381-384, August 1983.

ANIMAL STUDIES
Acquired immune deficiency syndrome of macaque monkeys, by N. L. Letkin, et al. ANNALS OF THE NEW YORK ACADEMY OF SCIENCES 437:121-130, 1984.

Acquired immunodeficiency syndrome in a colony of macaque monkeys, by N. L. Letvin, et al. PROCEEDINGS OF THE NATIONAL ACADEMY OF SCIENCES USA 80(9):2718-2722, May 1983.

AIDS animal model. AMERICAN FAMILY PHYSICIAN 27:247, May 1983.

AIDS in monkeys. AMERICAN FAMILY PHYSICIAN 33:372, February 1986.

AIDS in monkeys and men [letter]. LANCET 1(8333):1097-1098, May 14, 1983.

AIDS-infected chimps. AMERICAN FAMILY PHYSICIAN 30:343, October 1984.

AIDS virus: equine similarities? by J. Silberner. SCIENCE NEWS 129:84, February 8, 1986.

Animal models of AIDS, by J. F. Manser. RESEARCH RESOURCES REPORTER 7(6):1-4, June 1983.

—, by N. L. Letvin, et al. SEMINARS IN ONCOLOGY 11(1):18-28, March 1984.

Antibodies to simian T-lymphotropic retovirus type III in African green monkeys and recognition of STLV-III viral proteins by AIDS and related sera, by P. J. Kanki, et al. LANCET 1(8441):1330-1332, June 8, 1985.

Apes and AIDS, by C. Holden. SCIENCE 222:596+, November 11, 1983.

Bovine leukemia virus-related antigens in lmphocyte cultures infected with AIDS-associated viruses, by L. Thiry, et al. SCIENCE 227(4693):1482-1484, March 22, 1985.

Californians give AIDS to monkeys, by I. Anderson. NEW SCIENTIST 101:7, March 8, 1984.

Characterization of exogenous type D retrovirus from a fibroma of a macaque with simian AIDS and fibromatosis, by K. Stromber, et al. SCIENCE 224(4646): 289-292, April 20, 1984.

Chimps infected with AIDS-linked virus, by D. Franklin. SCIENCE NEWS 126: 261, October 27, 1984.

Clinical and pathologic features of an acquired immune deficiency syndrome (AIDS) in macaque monkeys, by N. L. Letvin, et al. ADVANCES IN VETERINARY SCIENCE AND COMPARATIVE MEDICINE 28:237-265, 1984.

Clinical features of simian acquired immunodeficiency syndrome (SAIDS) in rhesus monkeys, by R. V. Henrckson, et al. LABORATORY ANIMAL SCIENCE 34(2):140-145, April 1984.

Comparative pathology of cardiac neoplasms in humans and in laboratory rodents: a review, by C. Hoch-Ligeti, et al. JOURNAL OF THE NATIONAL CANCER INSTITUTE 76(1):127-142, January 1986.

Comparative ultrastructural study of virions in human pre-AIDS and simian AIDS, by T. F. Warner, et al. ULTRASTRUCTURAL PATHOLOGY 7(4):251-258, 1984.

Could AIDS agent be a new variant of African swine fever virus? [letter], by J. Teas. LANCET 1(8330):923, April 23, 1983.

Disease-specific and tissue-specific production of unintegrated feline leukaemia virus variant DNA in feline AIDS, by J. I. Mullins, et al. NATURE 319:333-336, January 23, 1986.

Distribution of type D retrovirus sequences in tissues of macaques with simian acquired immune deficiency and retroperitoneal fibromatosis, by M. L. Bryant, et al. VIROLOGY 150(1):149-160, April 15, 1986.

Do these primates have AIDS?, by C. Macek. JAMA 249(13):1696-1697, April 1, 1983.

Epidemic of acquired immunodeficiency in rhesus monkeys, by R. V. Henrickson, et al. LANCET 1(8321):388-390, February 19, 1983.

Equine infectious anemia virus *gag* and *pol* genes: relatedness to visna and AIDS virus, by R. M. Stephens, et al. SCIENCE 231:589-594, February 7, 1986.

Experimental transmission of macaque AIDS by means of inoculation of macaque lymphoma tissue, by N. L. Letvin, et al. LANCET 2(8350):599-602, September 10, 1983.

Experimental transmission of simian acquired immunodeficiency syndrome (SAIDS) and Kaposi-like skin lesions, by W. T. London,e t al. LANCET 2(8355):869-873, October 15, 1983.

FeLV-induced feline acquired immune deficiency syndrome. A model for human AIDS, by W. D. Hardy, Jr., et al. PROGRESS IN ALLERGY 37:353-376, 1986.

First chimp infected with AIDS virus. SCIENCE NEWS 126:121, August 25, 1984.

Hematogenous hexamitiasis in a macaque monkey with an immunodeficiency syndrome [letter], by N. L. Letvin, et al. JOURNAL OF INFECTIOUS DISEASES 149(5):828, May 1984.

Histopathologic changes in macaques with an acquired immunodeficiency syndrome (AIDS), by W. King, et al. AMERICAN JOURNAL OF PATHOLOGY 113(3):382-388, December 1983.

Human T-cell leukemia virus type I is a member of the African subtype of simian viruses (STLV), by T. Watanabe, et al. VIROLOGY 148:385-388, January 30, 1986.

Immune defects in simian acquired immunodeficiency syndrome, by D. H. Maul, et al. VETERINARY IMMUNOLOGY AND IMMUNOPATHOLOGY 8(3):201-214, February 1985.

Immunologic alterations in monkeys with simian acquired immunodeficiency syndrome (SAIDS), by D. B. Budzko, et al. PROCEEDINGS OF THE SOCIETY FOR EXPERIMENTAL BIOLOGY AND MEDICINE 179(2):227-231, June 1985.

Immunopathologic evaluation of lymph nodes from monkey and man with acquired immune deficiency syndrome and related conditions, by P. R. Meyer, et al. HEMATOLOGICAL ONCOLOGY 3(3):199-210, July-September 1985.

Induction of AIDS-like disease in macaque monkeys with T-cell tropic retrovirus STLV-III, by N. L. Letvin, et al. SCIENCE 230(4721):71-73, October 4, 1985.

Induction of immunodeficiency in mice by injection with syngeneic splenocytes immune to semi-allogeneic hybrid cells, by B. S. Kim. CELLULAR IMMUNOLOGY 88(1):222-227, October 1, 1984.

Infection of chimpanzees by human T-lymphotropic retoviruses in brain and other tissues from AIDS patients [letter], by D. C. Gajdusek, et al. LANCET 1(8419):55-56, January 5, 1985.

Infection of chimpanzees with lymphadenopathy-associated virus [letter], by D. P. Francis, et al. LANCET 2(8414):1276-1277, December 1, 1984.

Isolation of T-lymphotropic retrovirus related to HTLV-III/LAV from wild-caught African Green monkeys, by P. J. Kanki, et al. SCIENCE 230:951-954, November 22, 1985.

Lymphoma in macaques: association with virus of human T lymphotrophic family, by T. Homma, et al. SCIENCE 225:716-718, August 17, 1984.

Malignant rabbit fibroma syndrome. A possible model for acquired immunodeficiency syndrome (AIDS), by D. S. Strayer, et al. AMERICAN JOURNAL OF PATHOLOGY 120(1):170-171, July 1985.

Mason-Pfizer monkey virus and simian AIDS [letter], by D. L. Fine. LANCET 1(8372):335, February 11, 1984.

Monkey AIDS, by T. Gauntt. OMNI 6:22, April 1984.

Monkey business in AIDS research. NEW SCIENTIST 97:747, March 17, 1983.

Monkey puzzle. TIME 123:60, March 12, 1984.

Monkeys possible source of human AIDS [African green monkeys; research by Max Essex, et al.], by J. Silberner. SCIENCE NEWS 127:245, April 20, 1985.

Monkeys too: relentless immunity disease, by J. A. Miller. SCIENCE NEWS 123:151, March 5, 1983.

Morphologic changes in lymph nodes of macaques with an immunodeficiency syndrome, by L. V. Chalifoux, et al. LABORATORY INVESTIGATION 51(1):22-26, July 1984.

Morphology of the retroviruses associated with AIDS and SAIDS, by G. Lecatsas, et al. PROCEEDINGS OF THE SOCIETY FOR EXPERIMENTAL BIOLOGY AND MEDICINE 177(3):495-498, December 1984.

Natural resistance to parental T-lymphocyte-induced immunosuppression in F1 hybrid mice: implications for acquired immune deficiency syndrome (AIDS),by G. M. Shearer. IMMUNOLOGICAL REVIEWS 73:115-126, 1983.

Neutralizing antibody in Celebes black macaques recovering from infection with simian acquired immunodeficiency syndrome retrovirus type 2, by S. M. Shiigi, et al. CLINICAL IMMUNOLOGY AND IMMUNOPATHOLOGY 40(2): 283-290, August 1986.

New type D retrovirus isolated from macaques with an immunodeficiency syndrome, by M. D. Daniel, et al. SCIENCE 223:602-605, February 10, 1984.

Nucleotide sequence of the protease-coding region in an infectious DNA of simian retrovirus (STLV) of the HTLV-I family, by J.-I. Inoue, et al. VIROLOGY 150:187-195, April 15, 1986.

Nucleotide sequence of SRV-1, a type D simian acquired immune deficiency syndrome retrovirus, by M. D. Power, et al. SCIENCE 231(4745):1567-1572, March 28, 1986.

Relationship of mitogen reactivity to type D retrovirus infection in Celebes black macaques (Macaca nigra), by B. J. Wilson, et al. LABORATORY ANIMALS 36(3):237-239, June 1986.

Retroperitoneal fibromatosis and acquired immunodeficiency syndrome in macaques. Pathologic observations and transmission studies, by W. E. Giddens, Jr., et al. AMERICAN JOURNAL OF PATHOLOGY 119(2):253-263, May 1985.

Retrovirus linked to simian AIDS. CHEMICAL AND ENGINEERING NEWS 62:6, March 5, 1984.

Retroviruses associated with leukemia and ablative syndromes in animals and in human beings, by M. Essex, et al. CANCER RESEARCH 45(Suppl. 9): 4534s-4538s, September 1985.

Sequence homology of the simian retrovirus genome with human T-cell leukemia virus type I, by T. Watanabe, et al. VIROLOGY 144:59-65, July 15, 1985.

Serologic identification and characterization of a macaque T-lymphotropic retrovirus closely related to HTLV-III, by P. J. Kanki, et al. SCIENCE 228(4704): 1199-1201, June 7, 1985.

Simian AIDS: isolation of a type D retrovirus and transmission of the disease, by P. A. Marx, et al. SCIENCE 223(4640):1083-1086, March 9, 1984.

Simian models of acquired immunodeficiency syndrome (AIDS): a review, by N. W. King. VETERINARY PATHOLOGY 23(4):345-353, July 1986.

Studies show no link between swine fever/AIDS, by M. Kelquist. ADVOCATE 432:23, October 29, 1985.

Transmissible lymphoma and simian acquired immunodeficiency syndrome in rhesus monkeys, by G. B. Baskin, et al. JNC I77(1):127-139, July 1986.

Ultrastructural comparison of the retroviruses associated with human and simian acquired immunodeficiency syndromes, by R. J. Munn, et al. LABORATORY INVESTIGATION 53(2):194-199, August 1985.

Viral fugitive captured in monkey AIDS. SCIENCE NEWS 125:170, March 17, 1984.

Virus isolation studies in simian AIDS [letter], by P. A. Marx, et al. LANCET 1(8373):403, February 18, 1984.

AFRICA
   African swine fever and AIDS [letter], by C. V. Martins, et al. LANCET 1(8496):1504-1505, June 28, 1986.

   African swine fever virus and AIDS [letter], by J. Beldekas, et al. LANCET 1(8480):564-565, March 8, 1986.

   African swine fever virus antibody not found in AIDS patients [letter], by J. Colaert, et al. LANCET 1(83333):1098, May 14, 1983.

HAITI
AIDS hunt homes in on Haitian pigs, by O. Sattaur. NEW SCIENTIST 98:199, April 28, 1983.

ANIMAL STUDIES—ETIOLOGY
Simian AIDS: evidence for a retrovirus etiology, by M. Gardner, et al. FRONTIERS OF RADIATION THERAPY AND ONCOLOGY 19:26-32, 1985; also in HEMATOLOGICAL ONCOLOGY 2(3):259-268, July-September 1984.

ANIMAL STUDIES—GENETICS
Two elements in the bovine leukemia virus long terminal repeat that regulate gene expression, by D. Derse, et al. SCIENCE 231:1437-1440, March 21, 1986.

ANIMAL STUDIES—PATHOLOGY
Pathogenesis of simian AIDS in rhesus macaques inoculated with the SRV-1 strain of type D retrovirus, by D. H. Maul, et al. AMERICAN JOURNAL OF VETERINARY RESEARCH 47:863-868, April 1986.

Pathology of an epizootic of acquired immunodeficienycy in rhesus macaques, by K. G. Osborn, et al. AMERICAN JOURNAL OF PATHOLOGY 114(1):94-103, January 1984.

T-cell lymphoma associated with immunologic evidence of retrovirus infection in a low-land gorilla, by A. W. Prowten, et al. JOURNAL OF THE AMERICAN VETERINARY MEDICAL ASSOCIATION 187:1280-1282, December 1, 1985.

ANIMAL STUDIES—RESEARCH—TRANSMISSION
Transmission of HTLV-III infection from human plasma to chimpanzees: an animal model for AIDS, by H. J. Alter, et al. SCIENCE 226:549-552, November 2, 1984.

Transmission of human T-cell leukemia virus type I to an S+L- cat kidney cell line, by H. Hoshino, et al. VIROLOGY 147:223-236, November 1985.

ANIMAL STUDIES—SECONDARY LESIONS
Subcutaneous fibromatosis associated with an acquired immune deficiency syndrome in pig-tailed macaques, by C. C. Tsai, et al. AMERICAN JOURNAL OF PATHOLOGY 120(1):30-37, July 1985.

ANIMAL STUDIES—TRANSMISSION
Transmission of simian AIDS with type D retrovirus isolate [letter], by M. Gravell, et al. LANCET 1(8372):334-335, February 11, 1984.

ANIMAL STUDIES—TRANSMISSION—BLOOD TRANSFUSIONS
Transmission of simian acquired immunodeficiency syndrome (SAIDS) with blood or filtered plasma, by M. Gravell, et al. SCIENCE 223(4631):74-76, January 6, 1984.

ANIMAL STUDIES—TRANSMISSION—SALIVA
Transmission of simian acquired immunodeficiency syndrome (SAIDS) with type D retrovirus isolated from saliva or urine, by M. Gravell, et al. PROCEEDINGS OF THE SOCIETY FOR EXPERIMENTAL BIOLOGY AND MEDICINE 177(3): 491-494, December 1984.

Persistent infection of chimpanzees with human T-lymphotropic virus type III/lymphadenopathy-associated virus: a potential model for acquired immunodeficiency syndrome, by P. N. Fultz, et al. JOURNAL OF VIROLOGY 58(1):116-124, April 1986.

Viral culprit in simian AIDS, by D. Franklin. BIOSCIENCE 34:292, May 1984.

ATTITUDES

Abetting the hysteria of AIDS, by E. E. Bartlett. PATIENT EDUCATION AND COUNSELING 8(2):111-113, June 1986.

Abolishing the myths about AIDS, by P. Holmes. NURSING TIMES 80(49):19, December 5-11, 1984.

Accusations and a new drug, by N. Fain. ADVOCATE 416:22, March 19, 1985.

AHA says fear of AIDS goes too far. RN 47:13, March 1984.

AIDS: administrators fear the fear itself, by E. LeBourdais. HEALTH CARE 28(3):14-16, April 1986.

AIDS and homosexual panic [letter], by M. Rapaport, et al. AMERICAN JOURNAL OF PSYCHIATRY 142(12):1516, December 1985.

AIDS and hysterria a problem of health education, by N. J. Flumara. HEALTH VALUES 7(6):3, November-December 1983.

AIDS and a plague mentality, by R. Fisher. NEW SOCIETY 71(1157):322-325, February 28, 1985.

AIDS anxiety. TIME 124:59, December 24, 1984.

—, by M. Daly. NEW YORK 16:24-29, June 20, 1983.

AIDS—an epidemic of hysteria, by Ardill. SPARE RIB 153:13, April 1985.

AIDS extra. Fighting bigotry as well as an epidemic, by A. Veitch. GUARDIAN November 5, 1985, p. 11.

AIDS: the facts behind the fears [interview with B Starrett], by J. Kluger. MCCALL'S 111:66, April 1984.

AIDS: the facts, the fears, the future, by D. Fallowell. TIMES March 6, 1985, p. 10.

AIDS: facts not fear, by C. Weinstein. CALIFORNIA PRISONER 14(3):12, April 1985.

AIDS: fear and loathing. EMERGENCY MEDICINE 15(18):157-161, October 30, 1983.

AIDS fear is leading to safer sex, expert says [views of Dr. L. Edwards]. JET 68:5, September 2, 1985.

AIDS fear may cause less kissing under the mistletoe. JET 69:25, December 23, 1985.

AIDS fear puts panic in open-mouth kissing for actors, actresses. JET 69:59, November 18, 1985.

AIDS: from fear to fightback, by K. Kelley. GUARDIAN 37(31):1, May 8, 1985.

AIDS has both sexes running scared, by E. Cantarow. MADEMOISELLE 90:158-159+, February 1984.

AIDS: Hollywood jitters, by E. Salholz. NEWSWEEK 106:73, August 26, 1985.

AIDS: how we kept the kids in school and averted a panic, by P. J. Hagerty, et al. EXECUTIVE EDUCATOR 8(1):28-30, January 1986.

AIDS hysteria. NEWSWEEK 101:42, May 30, 1983.

AIDS hysteria [letter], by J. C. Katz. CANADIAN MEDICAL ASSOCIATION JOURNAL 134(6):573+, March 15, 1986.

AIDS hysteria and the common cup: take and drink, by R. W. Hovda. WORSHIP 60(1):67-73, January 1986.

AIDS hysteria: a contagious side effect, by M. Korcok. CANADIAN MEDICAL AS-SOCIATION JOURNAL 133(12):1241-1248, December 15, 1985.

AIDS hysteria: a housekeeper's nightmare, by M. Polito. EXECUTIVE HOUSE-KEEPING TODAY 7(3):10, March 1986.

AIDS hysteria: how it began and what nurses can do [editorial], by P. N. Palmer. AORN JOURNAL 43(2):418+, February 1986.

AIDS hysteria strikes New York City, by P. Freiberg. ADVOCATE 431:13, October 15, 1985.

AIDS in the mind of America, by G. Keenan. SCIENCE FOR THE PEOPLE 18(2):31, March 1986.

AIDS: Its victims are this century's lepers, by B. Kenkelen. NATIONAL CATHOLIC REPORTER 20:6-7, July 6, 1984.

AIDS—misplaced and better-placed hysteria, by R. Smith. MEDICAL JOURNAL OF AUSTRALIA 143(1):35, July 8, 1985.

AIDS: a narrow line between complacency and alarmism, by J. Wilkinson. LISTENER February 14, 1985, p. 5-6.

AIDS panic, by D. Viza. NATURE 317(6035):281, September 26-October 2, 1985.

AIDS panic: AIDS-induced psychogenic states [letter], by G. O'Brien, et al. BRITISH JOURNAL OF PSYCHIATRY 147:91, July 1985.

AIDS: panic and public policy, by J. Stryker. HEALTHSPAN 2(10):3-15, November-December 1985.

AIDS panic: are you safe?, by S. Horwitz. HARPER'S BAZAAR 116:28+, August 1983.

AIDS: a plague of fear, by D. Grady, et al. READER'S DIGEST 123:152-156, October 1983.

—. DISCOVER 4:74+, July 1983.

AIDS: a plague on all their houses? THE ECONOMIST 297:27-28, November 2, 1985.

AIDS: prejudice and progress, by J. Levine, et al. TIME 128(10):68, September 8, 1986.

AIDS: safeguards, not panic [editorial]. BRITISH DENTAL JOURNAL 158(6): 195, March 23, 1985.

AIDS: sense not fear [editorial], by M. W. Adler, et al. BRITISH MEDICAL JOURNAL 288(6425):1177-1178, April 21, 1984.

AIDS—solution: a difficult fight against prejudice, by C. Almedal. SYKEPLEIEN 73(10):24-25+, June 6, 1986.

AIDS: trust not fear, by J. Imhoff. CATHOLIC WORKER 52:1+, September 1985.

AIDS: turmoil in the medical profession, by K. Weiss. NEW PHYSICIAN 32(6):13-17, June 1983.

AIDS "unreasonable anxiety" ambiguous research. BODY POLITIC 110:18, January 1985.

AIDS victims, modern pariahs [editorial], by D. Scott. POSTGRADUATE MEDI-CINE 78(5):21+, October 1985.

AIDS victims pose threat to health in life, death. JET 67:37, January 28, 1985.

Anatomy of a panic, by R. McKie, et al. OBSERVER February 24, 1985, p. 11.

As fear of AIDS spreads, people change ways they live and work. WALL STREET JOURNAL 206:35, October 10, 1985.

Attitudes toward AIDS, herpes II, and toxic shock syndrome, by L. Simkins, et al. PSYCHOLOGICAL REPORTS 55(3):7790786, December 1984.

Backlash builds against AIDS. U.S. NEWS & WORLD REPORT 99:9, November 4, 1985.

Behind the AIDS hysteria [editorial]. GUARDIAN 35(39):26, July 13, 1983.

Behind spreading fear of two modern "plagues" . . . acquired immune deficiency syndrome and Alzheimer's disease, by A. Trafford, et al. US NEWS & WORLD REPORT 99(7):46-47, August 12, 1985.

Case of nerves. SCIENTIFIC AMERICAN 254:65, March 1986.

Compassion for AIDS victims, by N. Mallovy. HOMEMAKERS' MAGAZINE 21:38+, March 1986.

Dateline: San Francisco: a crisis of mounting AIDS hysteria, by D. Kline. MACLEAN'S 96:6-8, August 1, 1983.

Defuse AIDS panic!, by H. Cole. RFD 45:34, Winter 1985.

Dissenter in the AIDS capital of the world [Belle Glade, Fla.; views of Mark Whiteside]. DISCOVER 6:48, December 1985.

Don't shy away from a friend, by W. Handy. OUT 4(2):7, December 1985.

Effect of death fear on decadence of the 1970s, by M. Bronski. ADVOCATE 437:8, January 7, 1986.

Epidemic of fear (AIDS), by J. Barber. MACLEAN'S 98:61+, September 23, 1985.

Failure to thrive due to fear of AIDS [letter], by W. L. Henley. LANCET 2(8498): 112-113, July 12, 1986.

Faith, hope and bigotry, by O. Sattaur. NEW SCIENTIST 106:45, May 16, 1985.

Fear and healing in the AIDS crisis, by L. Hancock. CHRISTIANITY AND CRISIS 45:255-258, June 24, 1985.

Fear and loathing in the workplace: what managers can do about AIDS, by I. Pave. BUSINESS WEEK November 25, 1985, p. 126.

Fear and loathing . . . lack of compassion in dealing with AIDS victims, by J. Neuberer. NURSING TIMES 82(6):22, February 5-11, 1986.

Fear in San Francisco, by Nora Gallagher. CALIFORNIA MAGAZINE 11:93+, March 1,1986.

Fear of AIDS, by M. P. Rowe, et al. HARVARD BUSINESS REVIEW 64(4):28-30+, July-August 1986.

Fear of AIDS and gonorrhea rates in homosexual men [letter],by F. N. Judson. LANCET 2(8342):159-160, July 16, 1983.

Fear of AIDS causes crisis in blood banks across nation. JET 69:28-29, December 16, 1985.

Fear of AIDS: illness as a metaphor, by E. M. Gjersten SYKEPLEIEN 72(18):16-17+, October 21, 1985.

Fear of AIDS infects the nation. U.S. NEWS & WORLD REPORT 94:13, June 27, 1983.

Fear of dying. THE ECONOMIST 296:29-30, September 14, 1985.

Fears/frustrations stymie patients, by P. Byron. GAY COMMUNITY NEWS 11(10):3, September 24, 1983.

Fighting the backlash/AIDS network, by P. Albert. GUILD NOTES 9(3):12, Summer 1985.

Frightened,suffering and resented, by D. France. GUARDIAN 36(21):6, February 29, 1984.

Furor over an AIDS announcement, by c. Wallis, et al. TIME 126(19):77, November 11, 1985.

Further anxieties about AIDS, by J. Maddox. NATURE 319:9, January 2, 1986.

Gays must not take the rap for straight fears, by S. Anderson. ADVOCATE 444:9, April 15, 1986.

Green door to peace of mind, by M. Dynes, et al. TIMES November 17, 1986, p. 14.

Guidance on AIDS in bid to quell fears, by S. Ellis. NURSING STANDARD 311:3, September 1, 1983.

Hate, fear and Rock Hudson, by J. Brady. ADVERTISING AGE 56:39, August 15, 1985.

Haven for AIDS outcasts. LIFE 7:78-82, January 1984.

How to explain the fears, by C. Phillips. CHATELAINE 59:40, November 1986.

How to reduce the AIDS hysteria in central service, by S. Romey. HOSPITAL TOPICS 61(6):34, November-December 1983.

In fear of AIDS, by T. Allis. D MAGAZINE 12:136+, October 1985.

Inadequate reaction to AIDS, by B. Tivey. BODY POLITIC 124:17, March 1986.

Incidents dramatize level of fear. LAW ENFORCEMENT NEWS 12(1):1+, January 6, 1986.

Infected by the AIDS panic, by N. von Hoffman. SPECTATOR September 28, 1985, p. 9-10.

Is this brochure "vile and disgusting"? OUT 4(3):5, January 1986.

Just be a friend. NURSING 16(8):71 August 1986.

Justice, compassion needed in treating AIDS patients, by J. M. Cox. HEALTH PROGRESS 67(4):34-37, May 1986.

Learning to talk about an unspeakable disease, by R. Summerbell. BODY POLITIC 126:37, May 1986.

Let's face it—we're frightened about AIDS, by M. J. Carpenter. LAW ENFORCE- MENT NEWS 12(1):8, January 6, 1986.

Malign neglect, by D. Altman. VILLAGE VOICE 30:181, April 2, 1985.

Mind set for the fight against AIDS, by P. Tatchell. GUARDIAN September 5, 1986, p. 17.

Minority access: still shut out. MEDIAFILE 5(4):8, November 1984.

Neither sensationalism nor balanced discussion has resulted in a good strategy on AIDS, by D. Borley. NURSING STANDARD 387:5, March 7, 1985.

New terror of AIDS [special section; with editorial comment by Kevin Doyle]. MACLEAN'S 98(2):32-38, August 12, 1985.

New untouchables: anxiety over AIDS is verging on hysteria in some parts of the country, by E. Thomas, et al. TIME 126(12):24-26, Septemebr 23, 1985.

New untouchables of America. NEW SCIENTIST 98:927, June 30, 1983.

New York groups counter AIDS hysteria, by B. Nelson. GAY COMMUNITY NEWS 11(24):3, December 31, 1983.

No moral panic—that's the problem, by D. Anderson. TIMES June 18, 1985, p. 12.

No need for panic about AIDS. Acquired immune deficiency disease, now frequent among male homosexuals in the United States, is not this century's black death. The most urgent need is to understand what is going on . NATURE 302(5911):749, April 28, 1983.

Not a victim—a person with AIDS, by E. Jackson. BODY POLITIC 97:28, October 1983.

Panic, by O. Gillie, et al. SUNDAY TIMES February 24, 1985, p. 17-18.

Panic and prejudice-policy won't stop epidemic, by J. Jones. GUARDIAN 38(12): 7, December 18, 1985.

Panic over AIDS, by M. Starr. NEWSWEEK 102:20-21, July 4, 1983.

Patients' concerns about AIDS [letter], by B. Roberson, et al. JOURNAL OF THE AMERICAN DENTAL ASSOCIATION 112(2):162, 164, February 1986.

Peer review: face to face with AIDS phobia, by C. Cox. NURSING TIMES 81(15): 22, April 10-16, 1985.

Plague and panic, by R. Porter. NEW SOCIETY December 12, 1986, p. 11-13.

Plagued by AIDS scare, by D. J. Dent. BLACK ENTERPRISE 14:24, December 1983.

Public attitudes toward the control of AIDS: the homosexual's plight, by P. Ottenberg. TRANSACTIONS AND STUDIES OF THE COLLEGE OF PHYSICIANS OF PHILADELPHIA 8(2):113-119, June 1986.

Putting AIDS in perspective, by B. Foley. REBEL 69:11, April 1985.

Reactions of psychiatric staff to an AIDS patient, by R. B. Rosse. AMERICAN JOURNAL OF PSYCHIATRY 142(4):523, April 1985.

Real epidemic: fear and despair, by J. Leo. TIME 122:56-58, July 4, 1983.

Red Cross/resisting AIDS panic, by E. Jackson. BODY POLITIC 91:17, March 1983.

Results of a Gallup poll on acquired immunodeficiency syndrome—New York City, United States, 1985. MMWR 34(33):513-514, August 23,1 985.

SAG union fears kiss of AIDS. ADVERTISING AGE 56:1+, November 4, 1985.

Scare hits women not gay men alone, by V. Groocock. NEW STATESMAN 110: 12-13, August 30, 1985.

Spreading alarm about AIDS, by J. Seligmann, et al. NEWSWEEK 107(25):68, June 23, 1986.

Start of a plague mentality, by L. Morrow. TIME 126(12):92, September 23, 1985.

Stigmatizing the victim [editorial]. NATION 242(14):505, April 12, 1986.

Too close for comfort: gays afraid of gays w/AIDS, by C. Guilfoy. GAY COM-MUNITY NEWS 13(13):8, October 12, 1985.

United States Mayor Panel calls—end antigay, by L. Bush. ADVOCATE 3(88):8, February 21, 1984.

United States memo claims AIDS phobia is not illegal, by J. Kiely. GAY COM-MUNITY NEWS 13(49):1, June 29, 1986.

Unknown disease creates fear: AIDS—a professional challenge, by G. Causse, et al. SYKEPLEIEN 71(10):11-15, June 5, 1984.

Unleashing bias [editorial]. NATION 243(1):3. July 5, 1986.

Untouchable disease, by J. G. Deedy. TABLET 239:872-873, August 24, 1985.

Wake up—AIDS hysteria will change your life, by S. Schulman. WOMANEWS 7(1):1, December 1985.

What our readers said about resuscitating a patient with AIDS. NURSING LIFE 6(5):23-25, September-October 1986.

What you can do to stop the AIDS panic, by J. A. McCutchan. RN 49(10):18-21, October 1986.

Wisconsin cares about AIDS. OUT 4(2):12, December 1985.

Wisconsin ranks in middle on AIDS, by W. Handy. OUT 4(5):6, March 1986.

Wisdom of the despised, by A. Lumsden. NEW STATESMAN November 14, 1986, p. 14.

AFRICA
　　Scientist attacks AIDS slur on Africa, by O. Sattaur. NEW SCIENTIST 108:15-16, November 28, 1985.

CANADA
　　Alberta's AIDS menace: doctors seek solutions as the non-homosexual public begins to panic, by S. Weatherbe. ALBERTA REPORT 12:46-51, November 25, 1985.

ATTITUDES

CANADA
Spreading of AIDS panic: Edmonton reports its fourth victim as public fear
mounts, by L. Cohen. ALBERTA REPORT 12:52, November 4, 1985.

UNITED STATES
AIDS fear cited in Atlanta bathhouse bust, by S. Poggi. GAY COMMUNITY
NEWS 12(31):1, February 23, 1985.

Hawaii report. A lesson in AIDS hysteria, by C. Ikegami. JOSANPU ZASSHI
37(10):860-863, October 1983.

Miami: cycles of fear, by M. E. Schoonover. CHRISTIANITY AND CRISIS
46(8):174-175, May 19, 1986.

ATTITUDES—HOSPITALS
Managing AIDS and AIDS hysteria in hospitals. HOSPITAL SECURITY AND
SAFETY MANAGEMENT 4(8):5-12, Decembe 1983.

ATTITUDES—NURSES
What nurses think about gay AIDS victims. RN 48:10, July 1985.

BACTERIOLOGY
Opportunistic AIDS [letter], by J. Cohen, et al. LANCET 2(8413):1209-1210, November 24, 1984.

Opportunistic infection complicating acquired immune deficiency syndrome.
Clinical features of 25 cases, by C. W. Lerner, et al. MEDICINE 63(3):155-
164, May 1984.

Opportunistic infections and impaired cell-mediated immune responses in
patients with the acquired immune deficiency syndrome, by R. B. Roberts, et
al. TRANSACTIONS OF THE AMERICAN CLINICAL AND CLIMATOLOGICAL
ASSOCIATION 95:40-51, 1983.

Opportunistic infections in acquired immune deficiency syndrome result from
synergistic defects of both the natural and adaptive components of cellular
immunity by F. P. Siegal, et al. JOURNAL OF CLINICAL INVESTIGATION
78(1):115-123, July 1986.

CANADA
Opportunistic infections and acquired cellular immune deficiency among
Haitian immigrants in Montreal, by R. P. LeBlanc, et al. CANADIAN MEDI-
CAL ASSOCIATION JOURNAL 129(11):1205-1209, December 1, 1983.

HAITI
Opportunistic infections and acquired cellular immune deficiency among
Haitian immigrants in Montreal, by R. P. LeBlanc, et al. CANADIAN MEDI-
CAL ASSOCIATION JOURNAL 129(11):1205-1209, December 1, 1983.

BACTERIOLOGY—WOMEN
Opportunistic infection in previously healthy women. Initial manifestations of a
community-acquired cellular immunodeficiency, by H. Mauur, et al. ANNALS
OF INTERNAL MEDICINE 97(4):533-539, October 1982.

BIBLIOGRAPHIES
see: LITERATURE

334

Black community organizes to fight AIDS, by S. Poggi. GAY COMMUNITY NEWS 14(11):3, September 28, 1986.

Black gay man battles United for job, by C. Smith. GAY COMMUNITY NEWS 12(23):3, December 22, 1984.

Black gays—clinic—DC AIDS Forum, by U. Vaid. GAY COMMUNITY NEWS 11(12):3, October 7, 1983.

BLOOD

'Acquired immunodeficiency 'of blood stored overnight [letter], by B. J. Weiblen, et al. NEW ENGLAND JOURNAL OF MEDICINE 809(13):793, September 29, 1983.

AIDS and the blood, by L. Goldsmith. GAY COMMUNITY NEWS 10(27):3, January 29, 1983.

AIDS and the use of blood components and derivatives: the Canadian perspective [editorial], by J. B. Derrick. CANADIAN MEDICAL ASSOCIATION JOURNAL 131(1):20-22 July 1, 1984.

AIDS: a reminder on preventing the spread of blood-borne viruses while teaching blood glucose self-monitoring, by L. C. Mullen, et al. DIABETES EDUCATOR Suppl. 12:186-187, May 1986.

AIDS: in the blood. SCIENTIFIC AMERICAN 251:89+, September 1984.

Beta 2-microglobulin and the acquired immunodeficiency syndrome in a low-incidence area [letter]. JAMA 253(1):43-44, January 4, 1985.

Beta-2-microglobulin in acquired immune deficiency syndrome, by P. Francioli, et al. ANTIBIOTICS AND CHEMOTHERAPY 32:147-152, 1983.

Beta2m: there in the beginning, by D. R. Zimmerman. MOSAIC 15(2):10-15, 1984.

Case for heat-treated blood products [letter], by G. F. Pierce. LANCET 1(8426): 451, February 23, 1985.

Comparison of ADCC and NK activities of peripheral blood mononuclear cells from patients at risk for acquired immune deficiency syndrome (AIDS), by J. Wisecarver, et al. AIDS RESEARCH 1(5):347-352, 1983-1984.

Inactivation by wet and dry heat of AIDS-associated retroviruses during factor VIII purification from plasma [letter], by J. A. Levy, et al. LANCET 1(8443):1456-1457, June 22, 1985.

Inactivation of the AIDS-causing retrovirus and other human viruses in antihemophilic plasma protein preparations by pasteurization, by J. Hilfenhaus, et al. VOX SANGUINIS 50(4):208-211, 1986.

Induction of antibody to asialo GM1 by spermatozoa and its occurrence in the sera of homosexual men with the acquired immune deficiency syndrome (AIDS), by S. S. Witkin, et al. CLINICAL AND EXPERIMENTAL IMMUNOLOGY 54(2): 346-350, November 1983.

Sera from patients with the acquired immunodeficiency syndrome inhibit production of interleukin-2 by normal lymphocytes, by J. P. Siegel, et al. JOURNAL OF CLINICAL INVESTIGATION 75(6):1957-1964, June 1985.

Serum angiotensin converting enzyme in the acquired immunodeficiency syndrome or related syndromes [letter], by D. Vittecoq, et al. PRESSE MEDICALE 15(16):758-759, April 19, 1986.

Serum beta 2-microglobulin and interferon in homosexual males: relationship to clinical findings and serologic status to the human T lymphotropic virus (HTLV-III), by L. H. Calabrese, et al. AIDS RESEARCH 1(6):423-438, 1984-1985.

Serum suppression of lymphocyte activation in vitro in acquired immunodeficiency disease, by S. Cunningham-Rundles, et al. JOURNAL OF CLINICAL IMMUNOLOGY 3(2):156-165, Apr8il 1983.

Startling AIDS-related discovery [modified hemoglobin blood substitute; work of C. Hsia], by M. McDonald. MACLEAN'S 98:42-43, July 15, 1985.

Tissue culture isolation of Toxoplasma from blood of a patient with AIDS, by J. M. Hofflin, et al. ARCHIVES OF INTERNAL MEDICINE 145(5):925-926, May 1985.

Vampire trade?, by D. Cottle. ARENA 75:38, 1986.

BLOOD—TESTING
Alternative sites for screening blood for antibodies to AIDS virus [letter]. NEW ENGLAND JOURNAL OF MEDICINE 313(318):1157-1158, October 31, 1985.

Screening blood donations for AIDS, by F. Peterson. FDA CONSUMER 19(4):5-11, May 1985.

Screening blood: public health and medical uncertainty, by C. Levine, et al. HASTINGS CENTER REPORT 15(4):8-11, August 1985.

Screening donated blood and plasma for HTLV-III antibody. Facing more than one crisis?, by M. T. Osterholm, et al. NEW ENGLAND JOURNAL OF MEDICINE 312(18):1185-1189, May 2, 1985.

BLOOD DONORS
Advances in the isolation of HTLV-III from patients with AIDS and AIDS-related complex and from donors at risk, by P. D. Markham, et al. CANCER RESEARCH 45(Suppl. 9):4588s-4591s, September 1985.

AIDS and blood donors [editorial], by A. I. Adams. MEDICAL JOURNAL OF AUSTRALIA 141(9):558, October 27, 1984.

AIDS: blood donor studies and screening programs, by H. S. Kaplan, et al. PROGRESS IN CLINICAL AND BIOLOGICAL RESEARCH 182:297-308, 1985.

AIDS blood screen approved, by J. Silberner. SCIENCE NEWS 127:148, March 9, 1985.

AIDS precautions for donors. SPARE RIB 161:45, December 1985.

DOD won't punish donors who have AIDS, by P. Smith. AIR FORCE TIMES 45:4, May 20, 1985.

HTLV-III and blood donors [editorial]. LANCET 1(8433):856, April 13, 1985.

HTLV-III antibodies in US Army blood donors in West Germany, by J. J. James. JAMA 254:1449, September 20, 1985.

HTLV-III testing of donor blood imminent; complex issues remain, by M. F. Goldsmith. JAMA 253:173-175+, January 11, 1985.

Human T-cell lymphotropic virus antibody screening: data survey on 33,603 German blood donors correlated to confirmatory tests,by P. Kühnl, et al. VOX SANGUINIS 49(5):327-330, 1985.

No lesbian blood, by S. Hyde. GAY COMMUNITY NEWS 12(27):1, January 26, 1985.

Red Cross new blood donation guidlines, by L. Goldsmith. GAY COMMUNITY NEWS 10(37):1, April 9, 1983.

Revised definition of persons who should refrain from donating blood and plasma. JAMA 254(14):1886, October 11, 1985.

Update: revised Public Health Service definition of persons who should refrain from donating blood and plasma—United States. MMWR 34(35):547-548, September 6, 1985.

Variables affecting T-lymphocyte subsets in a volunteer blood donor population by J. D. Lifson, et al. CLINICAL IMMUNOLOGY AND IMMUNOPATHOLOGY 36(2):151-160, August 1985.

AFRICA
Antibody to HTLV-III in blood donors in central Africa [letter], by P. Van de Perre, et al. LANCET 1(8424):336-337, February 9, 1985.

BRAZIL
AIDS and blood donors in Brazil [letter], by S. N. Wendel, et al. LANCET 2(8453):506, August 31, 1985.

FRANCE
AIDS: France to screen blood donors, by R. Walgate. NATURE 315:705, June 27, 1985.

BLOOD DONORS—FEMALE
Limiting factor VIII cryoprecipitate selection to female donors [letter], by A. Shore, et al. LANCET 1(8420):98-99, January 12, 1985.

BLOOD DONORS—TESTING
All blood donors must be tested for AIDS, by I. Lernevall. VARDFACKET 9(11): 24, June 13, 1985.

Asymptomatic blood donor with a false positive HTLV-III western blot, by M. S. Saag, et al. NEW ENGLAND JOURNAL OF MEDICINE 314:118, January 9, 1986.

Reasons behind blood donor screening, by R. W. Miller. FDA CONSUMER 19(9):31-34, November 1985.

Screening of all donors for preventing transmission of AIDS via blood, semen, tissues. LAKARTIDNINGEN 82(20):1881, May 15, 1985.

Screening tests for blood donors presumed to have transmitted the acquired immunodeficiency syndrome, by J. S. McDougal, et al. BLOOD 65(3):772-775, March 1985.

Testing donors for AIDS. AMERICAN FAMILY PHYSICIAN 32:251, August 1985.

—, by A. Finlayson. MACLEAN'S 98:49, May 27, 1985.

Testing of donor blood for AIDS agents, by A. Novick, et al. JAMA 253:3463-3465, June 21, 1985.

SPAIN
Screening for antibody to HTLV-III in blood donors of Liguria. BOLLETTINO DELL ISTITUTO SIEROTERAPICO MILANESE 64(5):363-366, 1985.

CARE
Aiding AIDS sufferers, by D. Miller. NEW ZEALAND NURSING JOURNAL 79(9):34, September 1986.

AIDS: allocating resources for research and patient care, by P. R. Lee. ISSUES IN SCIENCE AND TECHNOLOGY 2:66-73, Winter 1986.

AIDS and the caregiver, by J. Lieberman. CALIFORNIA NURSE 82(4):3, May 1986.

AIDS and the human services. Agencies face a whole range of problems, by J. J. O'Hara, et al. PUBLIC WELFARE 44(3):7-13, Summer 1986.

AIDS and succour, by N. Dickson. NURSING TIMES 80(41):18-19, October 9-15, 1985.

AIDS care in the community, by H. Schietinger. AUSTRALIAN NURSES JOURNAL 15(7):50-51, February 1986.

AIDS: 'isolate the disease, not the patient,' by P. Holmes. NURSING TIMES 81(6):15-16, February 6-12, 1985.

AIDS patient finds the best medicine in his struggle to survive—friends, family and faith, by S. Klein. PEOPLE WEEKLY 21:77-78+, January 30, 1984.

Alternative care helps firms reduce costs to treat AIDS, by S. Taravella. BUSINESS INSURANCE 19(39):1+, September 30, 1985.

Are AIDS caregivers homophobic?, by M. Helquist. ADVOCATE 425:30, July 23, 1985.

Are we abandoning the AIDS patient?, by W. J. Nelson, et al. RN 47(7):18-19, July 1984.

Care to AIDS patients: the cost impact on Medicare, by E. W. Smith. CARING 5(6):56-57, June 1986.

Companions for men with AIDS, by A. Cohen. GAY COMMUNITY NEWS 12(19):8, November 24, 1984.

Haven for AIDS outcasts. LIFE 7:78-82, January 1984.

Health care advocacy for AIDS patients, by R. L. Cecchi. QRB12(8):297-303, August 1986.

Health care and the politics of AIDS, by N. Freudenberg. HEALTH PAC BULLE-TIN 16(3):29, May 1985.

Holistic care of the AIDS victim, by A. Gillis. HEALTH CARE 26(3):34-35, April 1984.

How to care for an AIDS patient,by D. A. Coleman. RN 49(7):16-21, July 1986.

Justice, compassion needed in treating AIDS patients, by J. M. Cox. HEALTH PROGRESS 67(4):34-37, May 1986.

Life-sustaining care, by M. Helquist. ADVOCATE 443:21, April 1, 1986.

Love, growth and friendship: being an AIDS buddy, by G. Dale. ADVOCATE 448:8, June 10, 1986.

Management of suspected AIDS patients, by D. B. Stough, et al. JOURNAL OF THE ARKANSAS MEDICAL SOCIETY 80(4):169-172, September 1983.

Moving to meet needs of Haitians with AIDS, by A. Cohen. GAY COMMUNITY NEWS 13(15):1, October 26, 1985.

New York center helps homeless AIDS patients, by P. Freiberg. ADVOCATE 435:13, December 10, 1985.

Optimizing care for the AIDS patient, by A. S. Brodoff. PATIENT CARE 18(2):125-127+, January 30, 1984.

Transfer of AIDS patient—inhumane, by R. Oloughlin. ADVOCATE 3(82):10, December 8, 1983.

Where can an AIDS patient turn for care?, by S. A. DiTullio. AMERICAN JOURNAL OF HOSPICE CARE 3(2):4, March-April 1986.

SWITZERLAND
Memorandum from the Swiss Professional Commission for AIDS Problems on how to deal with AIDS patients and persons with antibodies to LAV/HTLV-III. KRANKEN- PFLEGE. SOINS INFIRMIERS 79(2):74-75, February 1986.

UNITED STATES
AIDS health care American style, by D. Altman. DEMOCRATIC LEFT 14(3):3, May 1986.

More effective and less costly AIDS health services, by D. Altman. CARING 5(6):52-55, June 1986.

CARE—HEALTH CARE WORKERS
Guidelines for the care of patients with AIDS [letter], by J. P. Paul. NEW ENGLAND JOURNAL OF MEDICINE 310(18):1194, May 3, 1984.

Learning to care for clients with AIDS—the practicum controversy by M. N. Bremner, et al. NURSING AND HEALTH CARE 7(5):250-253, May 1986.

Update on AIDS information for health care personnel. CANADIAN MEDICAL AS-SOCIATION JOURNAL 134(3):251, February 1, 1986.

CARE—HEALTH CARE WORKERS—INFECTION CONTROL
Precautions in care of patients with the acquired immunodeficiency syndrome [letter],by D. W. Blayney. ANNALS OF INTERNAL MEDICINE 101(2):275, August 1984.

CARE—HOME
Acquired immunodeficiency syndrome (AIDS) in home care: maximizing help-fulness and minimizing hysteria, by J. Lillard, et al. HOME HEALTHCARE NURSE 2(5):11-14+, November-December 1984.

AIDS and the home health care industry—Part II, by D. Borfitz. HOME HEALTH JOURNAL 4(12):27, December 1983.

AIDS beyond the hospital. 1. A home care plan for AIDS, by H. Schietinger. AMERICAN JOURNAL OF NURSING 86(9):1021-1028, September 1986.

AIDS: caring for your patient at home, by P. Jackson, et al. CANADIAN NURSE 82(3):18-22, March 1986.

AIDS epidemic: risk containment for home health care providers, by J. G. Turner, et al. FAMILY AND COMMUNITY HEALTH 8(3):25-37, November 1985.

AIDS home care and hospice program. A multidisciplinary approach to caring for persons with AIDS, by J. P. Martin. AMERICAN JOURNAL OF HOSPICE CARE 3(2):35-37, March-April 1986.

AIDS: the implications for home care, by M. G. Boland, et al. MCN 11(6):404-411, November-December 1986.

AIDS: a nurse's responsibility. Care plan for home care, by D. Dickinson. CALI-FORNIA NURSE 82(4):7, May 1986.

AIDS patients allowed to serve time at home. CORRECTIONS DIGEST 17(18): 10, August 27, 1986.

Caring for home patients . . . AIDS, by I. Goldstone. RNABC NEWS 17(6):21-22, November-December 1985.

Challenges in caring for the person with AIDS at home, by J. P. Martin. CARING 5(6):12-14+, June 1986.

Community. Home AIDS, by S. Robins. NURSING MIRROR 160(8):21-22, February 1985.

Guidelines for caring for the AIDS patient in the home setting, by E. C. Garvey. NITA 8(6):481-483, November-December 1985.

Home AIDS . . . district nurse's role in caring for the patient with acquired immune deficiency syndrome in his own home, by S. Robins. NURSING MIRROR 160(8):21-22, February 20, 1985.

Home care dealers help combat AIDS fears, by E. Beck. MEDICAL PRODUCTS SALES 16(12):21+, December 1985.

Home care for the AIDS patient: safety first, by K. Dhundale, et al. NURSING 16(9):34-36, September 1986.

Home care/hospice for the AIDS patient, by P. M. Gibbons. MASSACHUSETTS NURSE 54(7):5-6, July 1985.

Home care hospice program . . . AIDS, by J. Lieberman. CALIFORNIA NURSE 82(4):6-7, May 1986.

Home care of the client with AIDS, by J. K. Bryant. JOURNAL OF COMMUNITY HEALTH NURSING 3(2):69-74, 1986.

Home care plan for AIDS, by H. Schietinger. AMERICAN JOURNAL OF NURSING 86(9):1021-1028, September 1986.

No home means no home care for AIDS patients, by M. R. Traska. HOSPITALS 60(1):69-70, January 5, 1986.

Nursing care of AIDS victims . . . home care, by B. Stoller. JOURNAL OF PRACTICAL NURSING 35(4):26-30, December 1985.

Our first home care AIDS patient: Maria, by S. Brosnan. NURSING 16(9):37-39, September 1986.

CARE—HOME—INFECTION CONTROL
Precautions for the home care of patients with AIDS. CANADIAN MEDICAL ASSOCIATION JOURNAL 134(1):51+, January 1, 1986.

CARE—HOSPICE
AIDS home care and hospice program. A multidisciplinary approach to caring for persons with AIDS, by J. P. Martin. AMERICAN JOURNAL OF HOSPICE CARE 3(2):35-37, March-April 1986.

Community approach to AIDS through hospice. Louisiana program promotes high quality of life, by H. S. Kutzen. AMERICAN JOURNAL OF HOSPICE CARE 3(2):17-23, March-April 1986.

Ensuring quality hospice care for the person with AIDS, by J. P. Martin. QRB 12(10):353-358, October 1986.

Helping AIDS patients through unconditional love, by K. Mrgudic. AMERICAN JOURNAL OF HOSPICE CARE 3(2):5, March-April 1986.

Hospice, AIDS and the community . . . workshop on AIDS for the community, by C. J. Sheehan. CARING 5(6):34-37, June 1986.

Hospice care endorsed for AIDS patients. Michigan Hospice Organization. MICHIGAN HOSPITALS 22(8):25, August 1986.

Impact of the first gay AIDS patient on hospice staff, by S. Geis, et al. HOSPICE JOURNAL 1(3):17-36, Fall 1985.

Lodging of patients with AIDS as your guests: case studies are presented to discuss the role of nurses, by S. P. Hotzemer. AMERICAN JOURNAL OF HOSPICE CARE 3(2):28-31, March-April 1986.

Psychosocial aspects of hospice care for AIDS patients. Addressing these issues is a   key aspect of treatment, by K. Schoen. AMERICAN JOURNAL OF HOSPICE CARE 3(2):32-34, March-April 1986.

CANADA
Toronto to get hospice for AIDS patients. CANADIAN NURSE 82:15, March 1986.

CARE—HOSPITAL
Adequate precautions and extreme care: AIDS from inside the hospital, by R. Dobbins. VILLAGE VOICE 30:30-31, July 30, 1985.

Admitting AIDS patients, by L. Raffel. CONTEMPORARY LONGTERM CARE 8(12):54, December 1985.

AIDS and the accident and emergency department [letter], by W. G. Tennant, et al. ARCHIVES OF EMERGENCY MEDICINE 2(1):47-49, March 1985.

AIDS and the executive director. Perspectives in crisis management, by A. P. Brownstein. SCANDINAVIAN JOURNAL OF HAEMATOLOGY. SUPPLE-MENTUM 40:561-565, 1984.

AIDS and the hospital employer, by K. B. Stickler. HEALTH LAW VIGIL 8(26):1-4, December 27, 1985.

AIDS and hospital workers [letter], by M. B. McEvoy, et al. LANCET 1(8388): 1245, June 2, 1984.

AIDS awareness in the emergency department, by N. M. Holloway. CRITICAL CARE NURSE 6(2):90-93, March-April 1986.

AIDS cited as major administrative concern [interview], by V. Glesnes-Anderson. HOSPITALS 57(15):45-46, August 1, 1983.

AIDS: getting past the diagnosis and on to discharge planning, by P. H. Wolff, et al. CRITICAL CARE NURSE 6(4):76-81, July-August 1986.

AIDS: hospital guidelines, clinical clues. AHA panel hits exaggerated precautions, by D. Lefton. AMERICAN MEDICAL NEWS 26(48):1+, December 23-30, 1983.

AIDS in the emergency room, by V. Svesko. NEW YORK 18:36-37, September 23, 1985.

AIDS: a problem for intensive care, by R. A. Banks, et al. INTENSIVE CARE MEDICINE 11(4):169-171, 1985.

Boston City Hospital ousts man with AIDS, by C. Guilfoy. GAY COMMUNITY NEWS 12(20):1, December 1, 1984.

Boston hospital changes AIDS policy. GAY COMMUNITY NEWS 11(14):6, October 22, 1983.

Clinical care and research in AIDS, by P. Volberding, et al. HASTINGS CENTER REPORT 15(4):16-18, August 1985.

Clinical management of AIDS patients, by W. Melson. CALIFORNIA NURSE 82(4):10-12, May 1986.

First AIDS hospital set to open in July. MEDICAL WORLD NEWS 27(11):133-134, June 9, 1986.

Hospital report admits failings in AID case,by C. Guilfoy. GAY COMMUNITY NEWS 12(32):3, March 2, 1985.

HTLV-III exposure during cardiopulmonary resuscitation [letter], by S. M. Saviteer, et al. NEW ENGLAND JOURNAL OF MEDICINE 313(25):1606-1607, December 19, 1985.

Impact of AIDS-related cases on an inpatient therapeutic milieu, by H. J. Polan, et al. HOSPITAL AND COMMUNITY PSYCHIATRY 36(2):173-176, February 1985.

Interdisciplinary approach to dealing with the problems of AIDS patients at a tertiary medical center, by A. A. Cote, et al. HOSPITAL TOPICS 62(5):28-30, September-October 1984.

Is your facility an 'AIDS hospital,'? MODERN HEALTHCARE 15(22):5, October 25, 1985.

New infectious diseases impact hospital planning, by P. Hawrylyshyn. HEALTH CARE 28(3):34, April 1986.

New York hospital opens acute care AIDS unity, by T. L. Selby. AMERICAN NURSE 18(5):3+, May 1986.

Problems with Hepatitis B and HTLV III infections in hospital, by D. C. Shanson. JOURNAL OF STERILE SERVICE MANAGEMENT? 3(3):29-30, October 1985.

San Francisco General Hospital's AIDS/ARC care plan. CALIFORNIA NURSE 82(4):13, May 1986.

Small and rurals await impending AIDS crisis, by D. Burda. HOSPITALS 60(3): 71-73, February 5, 1986.

This century's catastrophe? (4). No isolation of AIDS patients in the hospital, by B. A. Ostby. SYKEPLEIEN 73(7A):28-30+, April 1986.

— (5). Fear of meeting AIDS patients, by T. Sorhus. SYKEPLEIEN 73(9):20-25,

CARE—NURSING

Acquired immune deficiency syndrome (AIDS) . . . critical care crossword, by A. L. Gilmour. CRITICAL CARE NURSE 4(5):134-135+, September-October 1984.

Acquired immune deficiency syndrome (AIDS): an update for nurses, by N. P. Guarda, et al. FLORIDA NURSE 34(10):1+, November 1985.

Acquired immune deficiency syndrome: a new challenge for nursing, by C. Carneiro. MASSACHUSETTS NURSE 52(6):1+, June 1983.

Administrative perspectives on care of patients with AIDS . . . the nurse administrator on the unit level, by D. Calliari. TOPICS IN CLINICAL NURSING 6(2):72-75, July 1984.

AIDS and the nurse. Part 1, by H. Goble, et al. AUSTRALIAN NURSES JOURNAL 15(7):37-41+, February 1986.

—. Part 2, by P. Kerr, et al. AUSTRALIAN NURSES JOURNAL 15(7):42+, February 1986.

—. Part 3, by M. Fine. AUSTRALIAN NURSES JOURNAL 15(7):43-44, February 1986.

AIDS: a challenge for contemporary nursing, Part 1, by J. G. Turner, et al. FOCUS ON CRITICAL CARE 13(3):53-61, June 1986. 1986.

—, Part 2, by J. G. Turner, et al. FOCUS ON CRITICAL CARE 13(4):41-50, August 1986.

AIDS—challenge nurses cannot fail to meet, by R. Wells. NURSING STANDARD 448:1, May 22, 1986.

AIDS: the challenge nurses have to face. NURSING JOURNAL OF INDIA 77(7): 177, July 1986.

AIDS—complex challenge of the 80s: nurses are in a good position to offer help, by C. Dunphy. WASHINGTON NURSE 15(2):1+, February 1985.

AIDS: guidelines for caring for AIDs patients, by C. Field. LAMP 42(1):21-21, February 1985.

AIDS: a neurological nursing challenge, by J. A. Sunder. TOPICS IN CLINICAL NURSING 6(2):67-71, July 1984.

AIDS: a new problem area for nursing personnel, by J. A. Lambregts. KRANKEN-PFLEGE 39(9):335-337, September 1985.

AIDS: a new task field for nurses, by J. A. Lambregts. TIJDSCHRIFT VOOR ZIEKENVERPLEGING 38(6):172-182, March 12, 1985.

AIDS: a nurse's responsibility. Care plan for home care, by D. Dickinson. CALIFORNIA NURSE 82(4):7, May 1986.

AIDS: a nurse's responsibility. Nursing's special challenge, by C. Morrisson. CALIFORNIA NURSE 82(4):1+, May 1986.

ANA reaffirms position on health care for AIDS patients. PENNSYLVANIA NURSE 41(2):7, February 1986.

ANA urges nurses to read CDC guidelines on AIDS. PENNSYLVANIA NURSE 41(2):6+, February 1986.

ANA urges use of CDC guidelines for care of AIDS patients. FLORIDA NURSE 34(10):3, November 1985.

As a nurse, I want to find out what the facts are on AIDS, by J. L. Phillips. CRITICAL CARE UPDATE 10(9):37-38, September 1983.

California VNAs train AIDS treatment corps. AMERICAN JOURNAL OF NURSING 84:1535, December 1984.

Caring for acquired immune deficiency syndrome patients . . . experiences of one AIDS nursing unit, by C. S. Viele, et al. ONCOLOGY NURSING FORUM 11(3):56-60, May-June 1984; also in NEW ZEALAND NURSING FORUM 13(1):7-11, February-March 1985.

Caring for the AIDS patient—fearlessly. NURSING (HORSHAM) 13(9):50-55, September 1983.

Caring for AIDS patients. NEW ZEALAND NURSING JOURNAL 77(4):5-6, April 1984.

Caring for AIDS patients in a compassionate way, by S. Butler. NURSING STANDARD 446:3, May 8, 1986.

Lodging of patients with AIDS as your guests: case studies are presented to discuss the role of nurses, by S. P. Hotzemer. AMERICAN JOURNAL OF HOSPICE CARE 3(2):28-31, March-April 1986.

My first AIDS patient, by L. Hadden. RN 49(3):51, March 1986.

Nursing care of patients suffering from acquired immunodeficiency syndrome, by C. P. Batten, et al. INFIRMIÈRE CANADIENNE 25(10):17-21, November 1983.

Nursing care plan for an AIDS patient. Nursing care must offer support and corrective measures in all areas—physical, psychological, social, by N. Bolash. PENNSYLVANIA NURSE 41(2):4-6, February 1986.

Nursing care plan for persons with AIDS. QRB12(10):361-365, October 1986.

Nursing diagnoses and care plans for ambulatory care patients with AIDS, by A. C. Howes. TOPICS IN CLINICAL NURSING 6(2):61-66, July 1984.

Nursing history of an AIDS patient, by E. Bages Mir, et al. REVISTA DE ENFERMERIA 8(88):20-25, November 1985.

Nursing the patient with AIDS, by C. Batten, et al. CANADIAN NURSE 79:19-22, November 1983.

Nursing the patient with AIDS calls for special care and knowledge, by P. M. Kenny. PENNSYLVANIA NURSE 38(4):6, April 1983.

Planning for the neurologically impaired AIDS patient, by E. Barker. JOURNAL OF NEUROSCIENCE NURSING 18(5):241, October 1986.

RN gives supportive care to patients dying of AIDS, by C. Donovan. AMERICAN NURSE 17(10):1+, November-December 1985.

San Francisco nurses provide AIDS care, by T. L. Selby. AMERICAN NURSE 18(2):1+, February 1986.

Strategic plan for the management of patients with AIDS, by S. Malik-Nitto, et al. NURSING MANAGEMENT 17(6):46+, June 1986.

VNA of Akron, Ohio. AIDS and the VNA, by P. Mahovich, et al. CARING 5(6):62-68, June 1986.

AFRICA
AIDS: Implications for South African nurses: I, by M. C. Heibst. CURA-TIONS 8(3):13-14+, September 1985.

—: II, by M. C. Heibst. CURATIONS 8(4):18-20, December 1985.

CARE—NURSING—PREGNANCY
Should pregnant women care for AIDS patients? [letter], by P. Solenberger. INFECTION CONTROL 6(5):180, May 1985.

CARE—NURSING HOME
Management of an AIDS patient in a nursing home, by H. J. Cools, et al. NEDER-LANDS TIJDSCHRIFT VOOR GENEESKUNDE 130(28):1285-1287, July 12, 1986.

Mobilizing to treat AIDS . . . nursing home staff, by R. C. Marlowe. PROVIDER 12(4):49-50, April 1986.

Should nursing homes take AIDS patients?, by R. B. Gebhardt. NURSING HOMES 35(2):13-15, March-April 1986.

CARE—PHYSICIANS
Caring for AIDS patients: the physician's risk and responsibility [editorial], by G. N. Burrow. CANADIAN MEDICAL ASSOCIATION JOURNAL 129(11):1181, December 1, 1983.

CARE—PREGNANCY
Caring for the infectious patient: risk factors during pregnancy, by I. Gurevich, et al. INFECTION CONTROL 5(10):482-488, October 1984.

CHILDREN
Acquired immune deficiency syndrome in childhood, by K. M. Shannon, et al. JOURNAL OF PEDIATRICS 106(2):332-342, February 1985.

Acquired immune deficiency syndrome in children, by J. M. Oleske, et al. PEDIATRIC INFECTIOUS DISEASE 2(2):85-86, March-April 1983.

Acquired immune deficiency syndrome in infants and children, by S. W. Thompson, et al. PEDIATRIC NURSING 11(4):278-280+, July-August 1985.

Acquired immunodeficiency syndrome in the child of a haemophiliac, by M. V. Ragni, et al. LANCET 1(8421):133-135, January 19, 1985.

Acquired immunodeficiency syndrome in children [editorial], by B. Garty, et al. HAREFUAH 107(9):262-263, November 1, 1984.

Acquired immunodeficiency syndrome in children, by F. Iwanczak, et al. POLSKI TYGODNIK LEKARSKI 40(9):245-248, March 4, 1985.

Acquired immunodeficiency syndrome in infants and children, by A. J. Ammann. ANNALS OF INTERNAL MEDICINE 103(5):734-737, November 1985.

—, by L. J. Bernstein, et al. PROGRESS IN ALLERGY 37:194-206, 1986.

Acquired immunodeficiency syndrome in older children, by P. Baudoux, et al. PEDIATRIE 40(3):213-218, April-May 1985.

Acquired immunodeficiency syndrome in a thalassemic child, by R. Paul, et al. PEDIATRIC INFECTIOUS DISEASE 5(2):274-276, March-April 1986.

Additional findings on the acquired deficiency syndrome, particularly in children, by J. Holy. CASOPIS LEKARU CESKYCH 122(45):1402, November 11, 1982.

AIDS babies: walls around children?, by L. Gentry. HUMAN DEVELOPMENT NEWS Fall 1985, p. 11-12.

AIDS in a child 5 1/2 years after a transfusion [letter], by M. J. Maloney, et al. NEW ENGLAND JOURNAL OF MEDICINE 312(19):1256, May 9, 1985.

AIDS in children, by G. Fontán. ANNALES ESPANOLES DE PEDIATRIA 23(3):157-162, September 1985.

AIDS in children: a review of the clinical, epidemiologic and public health aspects, by M. F. Rogers. PEDIATRIC INFECTIOUS DISEASE 4(3):230-236, May-June 1985.

AIDS in schoolchildren [letter], by P. M. Shah, et al. DEUTSCHE MEDIZINISCHE WOCHENSCHRIFT 110(42):1631, October 18, 1985.

AIDS: preschool and school issues, by J. L. Black. JOURNAL OF SCHOOL HEALTH 56(3):93-95, March 1986.

Altered distribution of T-lymphocyte subpopulations in children and adolescents with haemophilia, by N. L. Luban, et al. LANCET 1(8323):503-505, March 5, 1983.

Atypical presentation of childhood acquired immune deficiency syndrome mimicking Crohn's disease: nutritional considerations and management, by K. J. Benkov, et al. AMERICAN JOURNAL OF GASTROENTEROLOGY 80(4):260-265, April 1985.

Bacterial infection in the acquired immunodeficiency syndrome of children, by L. J. Bernstein, et al. PEDIATRIC INFECTIOUS DISEASE 4(5):472-475, September-October 1985.

Case study: a child with chronic pulmonary infiltrates. Part one, by B. Zeffren, et al. ANNALS OF ALLERGY 54(2):97-98+, February 1985.

Childhood acquired immune deficiency syndrome manifesting as acrodermatitis enteropathica, by T. K. Tong, et al. JOURNAL OF PEDIATRICS 108(3):426-428, March 1986.

Children and AIDS: implications for child welfare, by G. R. Anderson. CHILD WELFARE 63(1):62-73, January-February 1984.

Children with AIDS: part 2, by R. M. Klug. AMERICAN JOURNAL OF NURSING 86(10):1126-1132, October 1986.

Children with AIDS: a special dilemma, by M. W. Moon. MASSACHUSETTS NURSE 55(12):1+, December 1985.

Cytomegalovirus pyloric obstruction in a child with acquired immunodeficiency syndrome, by M. S. Victoria, et al. PEDIATRIC INFECTIOUS DISEASE 4(5): 550-552, September-October 1985.

Developmental abnormalities in infants and children with acquired immune deficiency syndrome (AIDS) and AIDS-related complex, by M. H. Ultmann, et al. DEVELOPMENTAL MEDICINE AND CHILD NEUROLOGY 27(5):563-571, October 1985.

Education and foster care of children infected with human T-lymphotropic virus type III/lymphadenopathy-associated virus. JAMA 254:1430+, September 20, 1985; also in MMWR 34(34):517-521, August 30, 1985.

Evidence against transmission of human T-lymphotropic virus/lymphadenopathy-associated virus (HTLV-III/LAV) in families of children with the acquired immunodeficiency syndrome, by J. E. Kaplan, et al. PEDIATRIC INFECTIOUS DISEASE 4(5):468-471, September-October 1985.

Expressions of HTLV-III infection in a pediatric population, by S. Pahwa, et al. ADVANCES IN EXPERIENTAL MEDICINE AND BIOLOGY 187:45-51, 1985.

Guidelines for enrolling children with AIDS set up in two states. PHI DELTA KAPPAN 66:448-449, February 1985.

Guidelines for people responsible for education and day care of children with HTLV-III/LAV infection, by G. F. Smith. CANADIAN MEDICAL ASSOCIATION JOURNAL 135(2):134-136, July 15, 1986.

Hepatitis in children with acquired immune deficiency syndrome. Histopathologic and immunocytologic features, by L. F. Duffy, et al. GASTROENTEROLOGY 90(1):173-181, January 1986.

HTLV-III infection in brains of children and adults with AIDS encephalopathy, by G. M. Shaw, et al. SCIENCE 227:177-181, January 11, 1985.

IgG subglass deficiencies in children with suspected AIDS [letter],by J. A. Church, et al. LANCET 1(8371):279, February 4, 1984.

Immune deficiency syndrome in children [letter], by F. Rosner, et al. JAMA 250(22):3046, December 9, 1983.

Immunodeficient and 'backward' child, by G. Kliman, et al. HOSPITAL PRACTICE 19(5):108-110, 112, 114, May 1984.

In New Jersey a pediatrician tends the littlest victims, by G. Breu. PEOPLE 23:46-47, June 17, 1985.

Infection with human T-lymphotropic virus type III/lymphadenopathy-associated virus: considerations for transmission in the child day care setting, by K. L. MacDonald, et al. REVIEWS OF INFECTIOUS DISEASES 8(4):606-612, July-August 1986.

Is there an acquired immune deficiency syndrome in infants and children?, by A. J. Ammann. PEDIATRICS 72(3):430-432, September 1983.

Laboratory investigation of pediatric acquired immunodeficiency syndrome, by A. J. Ammann, et al. CLINICAL IMMUNOLOGY AND IMMUNOPATHOLOGY 40(1):122-127, July 1986.

Life table analysis of children with acquired immunodeficiency syndrome, by R. Lampert, et al. PEDIATRIC INFECTIOUS DISEASE 5(3):374-375, May-June 1986.

Low circulating thymulin-like activity in children with AIDS and AIDS-related complex, by G. S. Incefy, et al. AIDS RESEARCH 2(2):109-116, Spring 1986.

Managing AIDS in children, by M. Boland, et al. MCN 9(6):384-389, November-December 1984.

Neurological complications in infants and children with acquired immune deficiency syndrome, by A. L. Belman, et al. ANNALS OF NEUROLOGY 18(5):560-566, November 1985.

New fears that children may catch AIDS, by O. Sattaur. NEW SCIENTIST 106:4, April 18, 1985.

New scarlet letter(s), pediatric AIDS, by J. A. Church, et al. PEDIATRICS 77(3): 423-427, March 1986.

Pediatric acquired immunodeficiency syndrome, by A. J. Ammann, et al. ANNALS OF THE NEW YORK ACADEMY OF SCIENCES 437:340-349, 1984.

Pediatric AIDS, by A. Rubinstein. CURRENT PROBLEMS IN PEDIATRICS 16(7): 361-409, July 1986.

Pediatric AIDS: a disease spectrum causally associated with HTLV-III infection, by W. P. Parks, et al. CANCER RESEARCH 45(Suppl. 9):4659s-4661s, September 1985.

Pre-AIDS in a child of a drug-addict. Clinical and laboratory description, by D. Pavesio, et al. MINERVA PEDATRICA 37(1-2):73-74, January 31, 1985.

Risk factors in pediatric AIDS [letter],by J. H. Joncas, et al. CANADIAN MEDICAL ASSOCIATION JOURNAL 132(6):614-615, March 15, 1985.

When should the acquired immunodeficiency syndrome be considered in children (AIDS)?, by A. Getlík. CESKOSLOVENSKA PEDIATRIE 89(8):485-4867, August 1984.

Young victims. TIME 120:79, December 27, 1982.

Youngest victims of AIDS, by M. Dobbin, et al. U.S. NEWS & WORLD REPORT 101(3): 71-72, July 7, 1986.

AFRICA
Unique pattern of HTLV-III (AIDS-related) antigen recognition by sera from African children in Uganda (1972), by C. Saxinger, et al. CANCER RESEARCH 45(Suppl. 9):4624s-4626s, September 1985.

ISRAEL
Impaired immune regulation in children and adolescents with hemophilia and thalassemia in Israel, by T. Umiel, et al. AMERICAN JOURNAL OF PEDIATRIC HEMATOLOGY/ONCOLOGY 6(4):371-378, Winter 1984.

SPAIN
Fourth case of AIDS in haemophiliac children in Seville [letter], by P. Noguerol, et al. LANCET 2(8409):986, October 27, 1984.

CHILDREN—CARE—NURSING
Nursing management of the pediatric AIDS patient, by L. Iazzetti. ISSUES IN COMPREHENSIVE PEDIATRIC NURSING 9(2):119-129, 1986.

CHILDREN—IMMUNOLOGY
Defective humoral immunity in pediatric acquired immune deficiency syndrome, by L. J. Bernstein, et al. JOURNAL OF PEDIATRICS 107(3):352-357, September 1985.

CHILDREN—OPHTHALMOLOGY
Perivasculitis of the retinal vessels as an important sign in children with AIDS-related complex, by P. Kestelyn, et al. AMERICAN JOURNAL OF OPHTHALMOLOGY 100(4):614-1615, October 15, 1985.

CHILDREN—PATHOLOGY
Pathogens in children with severe combined immune deficiency disease or AIDS, by D. Lauzon, et al. CANADIAN MEDICAL ASSOCIATION JOURNAL 135(1):33-38, July 1, 1986.

Pathologic appraisal of the thymus gland in acquired immunodeficiency syndrome in children. A study of four cases and a review of the literature, by V. V. Joshi, et al. ARCHIVES OF PATHOLOGY AND LABORATORY MEDICINE 109(2):142-146, February 1985.

Pathologic features of AIDS encephalopathy in children: evidence for LAV/HTLV-III infection of brain, by L. R. Sharer, et al. HUMAN PATHOLOGY 17(3):271-284, March 1986.

Pathologic pulmonary findings in children with the acquired immunodeficiency syndrome: a study of ten cases, by V. V. Joshi, et al. HUMAN PATHOLOGY 16(3):241-246, March 1985.

Progressive encephalopathy in children with acquired immune deficiency syndrome, by L. G. Epstein, et al. ANNALS OF NEUROLOGY 17(5):488-496, May 1985.

Spontaneous resolution of cryptosporidiosis in a child with acquired immunodeficiency syndrome [letter], by C. D. Berkowitz, et al. AMERICAN JOURNAL OF DISEASES OF CHILDREN 189(10):967, October 1985.

CHILDREN—TREATMENT
Serum lactate dehydrogenase levels in adults and children with acquired immune deficiency syndrome (AIDS) and AIDS-related complex: possible indicator of B cell lymphoproliferation and disease activity. Effect of intravenous gammaglobulin on enzyme levels, by B. A. Silverman, et al. AMERICAN JOURNAL OF MEDICINE 78(5):728-736, May 1985.

CIVIL RIGHTS
AFL/CIO supports gay rights—AIDS. GUARDIAN 36(4):4, October 26, 1983.

AIDS activists—confidentiality issue, by C. Guilfoy. GAY COMMUNITY NEWS 12(5):1, August 11, 1984.

AIDS and civil rights, by A. Press, et al. NEWSWEEK 106(21):86+, November 18, 1985.

AIDS and confidentiality [letter], by W. H. Foege. NATURE 306(5938):10, November 3-9, 1983.

AIDS and gay rights collide in closings, by Helquist, et al. IN THESE TIMES 8(41):1, October 31, 1984.

AIDS and the rights of the well, by B. Amiel. MACLEAN'S 98:11, September 30, 1985.

AIDS court case raises many serious right of privacy questions, by H. R. Halper. BUSINESS AND HEALTH 3(6):51-52, May 1986.

AIDS crisis/what the ACLU must do, by T. Stoddard. CIVIL LIBERTIES 355:1, Fall 1985.

AIDS: discrimination issues, by G. Tillet. LAMP 42(8):25+, October 1985.

AIDS, hepatitis B and the problems of confidentiality [letter], by R. C. Hitchcock. BRITISH DENTAL JOURNAL 159(8):243, October 19, 1985.

AIDS hunt: precaution or privacy violation? NEWSWEEK 106:27, September 2, 1985.

AIDS—issues in Rights Bill hearing, by L. Goldsmith. GAY COMMUNITY NEWS 11(36):1, March 31, 1984.

AIDS panic blamed in defeat of rights bill, by C. Guilfoy. GUARDIAN 38(3):5, October 16, 1985.

AIDS patients' confidentiality is medical records challenge, by C. A. Siegner. MODERN HEALTHCARE 15(24):86, November 22, 1985.

AIDS reportability—confiding in gov, by C. Guilfoy. GAY COMMUNITY NEWS 11(27):6, January 28, 1984.

AIDS researcher fights eviction, by B. Nelson. GAY COMMUNITY NEWS 11(14):6, October 22, 1983.

AIDS researcher wins eviction battle, by C. Smith. GAY COMMUNITY NEWS 12(17):3, November 10, 1984.

AIDS: victim's rights vs. the public's, by T. Philip, et al. ALBERTA REPORT 13: 32-33, September 1, 1986.

AIDS worker: confentiality prime concern, by B. Egerton. OUT 2(9):5, August 1984.

Cincinnatians nervous about confidentiality, by J. Zeh. GAY COMMUNITY NEWS 12(21):1, December 8, 1984.

Colorado to keep list of HTLV-3 positives, by M. Cocoves. GAY COMMUNITY NEWS 13(11):1, September 28, 1985.

Complaint filed for AIDS/bias, by P. Byron. GAY COMMUNITY NEWS 11(7):1, September 3, 1983.

Confidential matters, by S. Budiansky. NATURE 304:478, August 11, 1983.

Confidentiality, informed consent and untoward social consequences in research on a "new killer disease" (AIDS), by R. Purtilo, et al. CLINICAL RESEARCH 31(4):464-472, October 1983.

Constitutional rights of AIDS carriers. HARVARD LAW JOURNAL 99(6):1274-1292, April 1986.

Detaining patients with AIDS. BRITISH MEDICAL JOURNAL 291(6502):1102, October 19, 1985.

Dispute over AIDS patient priority, by T. Beardsley. NATURE 310:174, July 19, 1984.

Doctors' efforts to control AIDS spark battles over civil liberties, by M. Chase. WALL STREET JOURNAL 205:23+, February 8, 1985.

Drug test advances, civil rights abuses. BODY POLITIC 128:22, July 1986.

Fear about confidentiality jeopardizes study, by J. Cort. ADVOCATE 4(8):10, November 27, 1984.

Florida county fired AIDS victims illegally. CIVIL LIBERTIES 356:3, Winter 1986.

Florida fires workers who have AIDS, by C. Guilfoy GAY COMUNITY NEWS 12(29):1, February 9, 1985.

Florida man wins AIDS discrimination appeal, by D. Walter. ADVOCATE 438:17, January 21, 1986.

Keeping confidential, by P. H. Ridout, et al. POLICY OPTIONS/OPTIONS POLI-TIQUES 7:41-43, July-August 1986.

Man with ARC cites confidentiality breach, by C. Guilfoy. GAY COMMUNITY NEWS 13(8):3, August 31, 1985.

Massachusetts House crushes Gay Rights Bill, 88-65, by C. Gulfoy. GAY COM-MUNITY NEWS 13(12):1, October 5, 1985.

Massachusetts House passes Bill for HTLV-3 confidentiality, by S. Poggi. GAY COMMUNITY NEWS 13(44):1, May 31, 1986.

Massachusetts passes law to grant HTLV-3 confidentiality, by K. Westheimer. GAY COMMUNITY NEWS 14(2):1, July 20, 1986.

Research center urges privacy for AIDS subjects, by P. Frieberg. ADVOCATE 409:87, December 11, 1984.

Society's survival first, then victims' rights: AIDS plague, by Richard Restak. HUMAN EVENTS 45:18+, October 5, 1985.

CLASSIFICATION
Serological characterization of HTLV-III infection in AIDS and related disorders, by J. E. Groopman, et al. JOURNAL OF INFECTIOUS DISEASES 153(4):736-742, April 1986.

Serological characterization of human T-cell leukemia (lymphotropic) virus, type I (HTLV-I) small envelope protein, by M. J. Newman,e t al. VIROLOGY 150:106-116, April 15, 1986.

Serotypes of Cryptococcus neoformans in patients with AIDS [letter], by M. G. Rinaldi, et al. JOURNAL OF INFECTIOUS DISEASES 153(3):642, March 1986.

Walter Reed staging classification for HTLV-III/LAV infection, by R. R. Redfield, et al. NEW ENGLAND JOURNAL OF MEDICINE 314:131-132, January 9, 1986.

CLINICS
Acquired immune deficiency syndrome and the fertility clinic, by G. D. Ball. FERTILITY AND STERILITY 45(2):172-174, February 1986.

COLLEGES
AIDS on campus: what you should know, by R. P. Keeling. AGB REPORTS 28(2):24-28, March-April 1986.

AIDS on campuses: concern goes beyond health as officials prepare to handle flood of questions, by L. Biemiller. CHRONICLE OF HIGHER EDUCATION 31(5):40-41, October 2, 1985.

College fears for new AIDS measures. NURSING STANDARD 390:1, March 28, 1985.

College health group sees no reason to isolate AIDS victims. THE CHRONICLE OF HIGHER EDUCATION 31:33+, October 16, 1985.

Presence of AIDS victims poses no risk to others on campuses, committee says, by L. Biemiller. CHRONICLE OF HIGHER EDUCATION 31:25-26, December 11, 1985.

CONFERENCES

Acquired immune deficiency syndrome (AIDS)—a multidisciplinary enigma [clinical conference]. WESTERN JOURNAL OF MEDICINE 140(1):66-81, January 1984.

Acquired immune deficiency syndrome: A status report. The statement of a World Health Organization meeting. SERVIR 33(5):259-269, September-October 1985.

AIDS-associated syndromes. Proceedings of the International Conference on AIDS-Associated Syndromes. December 8-9, 1984, Irvine, California. ADVANCES IN EXPERIMENTAL MEDICINE AND BIOLOGY 187:1-181, 1985.

AIDS conference looks at the personal side, by C. Guilfoy. GAY COMMUNITY NEWS 12(37):3, April 6, 1985.

AIDS conference ponders the ethics of research, by C. Guilfoy. GAY COMMUNITY NEWS 12(42):1, May 11, 1985.

AIDS conference yields new warnings, by S. Burke. OUT 3(7):1, May 1985.

AIDS education need; conference highlight, by H. W. Jaffe. CORRECTIONS TODAY 48:49-50+, April 1986.

AIDS, ethics, and the blood supply. A report of a conference of the American Blood Commission and the Hastings Center, Institute of Society, Ethics and the Life Sciences, January 29 and 30, 1985, by W. V. Miller, et al. TRANSFUSION 25(2):174-175, March-April 1985.

AIDS: winter conference update, by R. A. Kiel. CORRECTIONS TODAY 48(3): 32+, May 1986.

Alternative health approaches to AIDS: conference, by Wolhandle. GAY COMMUNITY NEWS 13(34):8, March 15, 1986.

Atlanta AIDS conference begins, by N. Fain. ADVOCATE 420:24, May 14, 1985.

Cancer and AIDS. 19th annual San Francisco Cancer Symposium. San Francisco, Calif., March 2-4, 1984. FRONTIERS OF RADIATION THERAPY AND ONCOLOGY 19:1-184, 1985.

CDC to host AIDS risk reduction conferences, by N. Fain. ADVOCATE 415:24, March 5, 1985.

Conference takes stock of diversity and unity, by Larson, et al. GAY COMMUNITY NEWS 13(20):3, November 30, 1985.

Conference vigil lobbying in Washington, by D. France. GUARDIAN 36(3):4, October 19, 1983.

Epidemic of acquired immune deficiency syndrome (AIDS) and Kaposi's sarcoma. First workshop of the European Study Group on AIDS/KS, Naples, June 25, 1983. ANTIBIOTICS AND CHEMOTHERAPY 32:1-164, 1983.

Europe convenes 1st AIDS Conference, by N. Fain. ADVOCATE 3(89):20, March 6, 1984.

First International Conference on the Acquired Immunodeficiency Syndrome, by I. H. Frazer, et al. MEDICAL JOURNAL OF AUSTRALIA 143(1):31-3, July 8, 1985.

First National Canadian Conference on AIDS, by S. Poggi. GAY COMMUNITY NEWS 12(50):2, July 6, 1985.

From The National Institutes of Health. Summary of the National Institutes of Health Research Workshop on the Epidemiology of the Acquired Immuno-deficiency Syndrome (AIDS), by R. Edelman. JOURNAL OF INFECTIOUS DISEASES 150(2):295-303, August 1984.

Gloom in the Palais des Congres: an AIDS conference offers little hope for a cure, by J. Murphy, et al. TIME 128():51, July 7, 1986.

Health Conference aims for diversity, by C. Irvine. GAY COMMUNITY NEWS 12(1):3, July 14, 1984.

Initial European AIDS symposium, by S. Gesenhues. ZFA 60(2):82-83, January 20, 1984.

International Conference on Acquired Immunodeficiency Syndrome. 14-17 April 1985, Atlanta, Georgia. ANNALS OF INTERNAL MEDICINE 103(5):653-781, November 1985.

International issues at AAPHR Conference, by M Helquist. ADVOCATE 429:11, September 17, 1985.

Lesbian/Gay Health Conference, by J. Thomas, et al. OFF OUR BACKS 16(5):1, May 1986.

MAAFS-NEAFS combined meeting, Atlantic City, New Jersey, April 25-27, 1984. CRIME LABORATORY DIGEST 11(3):57, July 1984.

Manner of speaking—Quebec AIDS Conference, by Courte, et al. BODY POLITIC 128:19, July 1986.

New Hampshire AIDS Conference cites discrimination, by S. Janicki. GAY COM-MUNITY NEWS 13(31):3, February 22, 1986.

NIH Conference. Acquired immunodeficiency syndrome: epidemiologic, clinical, i immunologic, and therapeutic considerations, by A. S. Fauci, et al. ANNALS OF INTERNAL MEDICINE 100(1):92-106, January 1984.

—. The acquired immunodeficiency syndrome: an update, by A. S. Fauci, et al. ANNALS OF INTERNAL MEDICINE 102(6):800-813, June 1985.

NIH scientific workshops on acquired immune deficiency syndrome. PUBLIC HEALTH REPORTS 98(4):318-319, July-August 1983.

Pulmonary complications of the acquired immunodeficiency syndrome. Report of a National Heart, Lung, and Blood Institute workshop, by J. F. Murray, et al. NEW ENGLAND JOURNAL OF MEDICINE 310(25):1682-1688, June 21, 1984.

Radiologic-pathologic correlation conference: SUNY Upstate Medical Center. Progressive lung disease in a homosexual man, by E. G. Theros, et al. AJR 140(5):897-902, May 1983.

Report from the First International Congress on AIDS held at Atlanta: the American society threatened by sexually transmitted disease numbering more than 25, by C. Ikegami. KANGOGAKU ZASSHI 49(9):1074-1076, September 1985.

Report of a WHO meeting on AIDS. INTERNATIONAL NURSING REVIEW 32(3): 80-83, May-June 1985.

Seminar discusses 'AIDS: issues in the workplace,' by N. P. Guarda, et al. FLORIDA NURSE 35(2):5, February 1986.

Symposium on HTLV. Bethesda, Maryland, December 6 & 7, 1984. CANCER RESEARCH 45(Suppl. 9):4520s-4711s, September 1985.

Symposium on infections in the compromised host. The acquired immunodeficiency syndrome, by D. J. LaCamera, et al. NURSING CLINICS OF NORTH AMERICA 20(1):241-256, March 1985.

Tenth annual Eastern Claims Conference: AIDS—only the tip of the iceberg? by A. G. Clarke. BEST'S REVIEW 86:131-132, April 1986.

Thirteenth annual UCLA symposium. Abstracts: acquired immune deficiency syndrome. JOURNAL OF CELLULAR BIOCHEMISTRY 8A(Suppl):1-23, 1984.

Vocal gay presence at Atlanta Conference, by J. Beldekas. GAY COMMUNITY NEWS 12(43):3, May 18, 1985.

Women's Studies Conference: sex & culture, by B. Duren. GAY COMMUNITY NEWS 12(39):7, April 20, 1985.

World Health Organization workshop: conclusions and recommendations on acquired immunodeficiency syndrome. JAMA 253(23):3385-3386, June 21, 1985; also in MMWR 34(19):275-276, May 17, 1985.

COUNSELLING

Ban sought on gay counselors, by J. Zeh. GAY COMMUNITY NEWS 12(37):1, April 6, 1985.

Lovers of AIDS victims: psychosocial stresses and counseling needs, by S. B. Geis, et al. DEATH STUDIES 10(1):43-53, 1986.

Need for psychosocial research on AIDS and counseling laterrentions for AIDS victims, by R. T. Kinnier. JOURNAL OF COUNSELING AND DEVELOPMENT 64(7):472-473, March 1986.

Psychological support and counseling for patients with acquired immune deficiency syndrome (AIDS), by D. Miller, et al. GENITOURINARY MEDICINE
61(4):273-278, August 1985.

DENTISTRY
Acquired immune deficiency syndrome (AIDS)—complications in dental treat-
ment. Report of a case, by B. Hurlen, et al. INTERNATIONAL JOURNAL OF
ORAL SURGERY 13(2):148-150, April 1984.

Acquired immune deficiency syndrome: dental considerations, by B. E. Evans.
NEW YORK STATE DENTAL JOURNAL 49(9):649-652, November 1983.

AIDS—acquired immunodeficiency syndrome, its importance for the dentist, by
B. Maeglin. SCHWEIZERISCHE MONATSSCHRIFT FUR ZAHNMEDIZIN
95(8):697-699, August 1985.

AIDS and its significance to dentistry, by J. Hardie. CANADIAN DENTAL
ASSOCIATION JOURNAL 49(8):565-569, August 1983.

AIDS: information for dentists. New York State Department of Health. NEW
YORK JOURNAL OF DENTISTRY 54(6):256, September-October 1984.

AIDS: recent findings and their dental implications, by E. Bucci, et al. MINERVA
STOMATOLOGICA 35(4):247-252, April 1986.

Attention, prison dentists: CDC issues warning on AIDS. CORRECTIONS DI-
GEST 14(19):9-10, September 7, 1983.

Dental care for the AIDS patient: the dentist's perspective, by L. Brooks. TEXAS
HOSPITALS 40(6):9, November 1984.

Dental care for the AIDS patient: the infection control practitioner's perspective,
by C. Hardy. TEXAS HOSPITALS 40(5):9-10, October 1984.

Gay men challenge dentists on AIDS, Hep B, by C. Guilfoy. GAY COMMUNITY
NEWS 13(4):3, August 3, 1985.

Killer spit? Dentists worry about catching AIDS, by C. Milner, et al. ALBERTA RE-
PORT 12:21, September 2, 1985.

Significance of AIDS to dentists and dental practice, by D. R. Davis, et al. JOUR-
NAL OF PROSTHETIC DENTISTRY 52(5):736-738, November 1984.

Treatment of dental patients with acquired immune deficiency syndrome (AIDS),
by E. M. Moskowitz. NEW YORK JOURNAL OF DENTISTRY 54(3):119-120,
March 1984.

AUSTRALIA
AIDS and dentists in Australia [news], by C. H. Wall. BRITISH DENTAL
JOURNAL 158(10):380, May 25, 1985.

DIAGNOSIS
Abdominal CT in acquired immunodeficiency syndrome by R. B. Jeffrey, Jr., et al.
AJR 146(1):7-13, January 1986.

Acquired immune deficiency syndrome. Distinctive features of bone marrow biopsies, by S. A. Geller, et al. ARCHIVES OF PATHOLOGY AND LABORA-TORY MEDICINE 109(2):138-141, February 1985.

Acquired immunodeficiency syndrome (AIDS). Case reports and diagnosis, by O. Braun-Falco, et al. MUENCHENER MEDIZINISCHE WOCHENSCHRIFT 125(48):1135-1139, December 2, 1983.

Acquired immunodeficiency syndrome: cerebral computed tomographic manifestations, by M. A. Whelan, et al. RADIOLOGY 149(2):477-484, November 1983.

AIDS and its early-stage clinical signs, by S. L. Valle, et al. DUODECIM 102(7): 405-412, 1986.

AIDS blood test: qualified success [ELISA test], by J. Silberner. SCIENCE NEWS 128:84, August 10, 1985.

AIDS: blood test trials inconclusive, by S. Budiansky. NATURE 316:96, July 11, 1985.

AIDS: a clinical diagnosis, hence one with pitfalls, by S. A. Danner. NEDER-LANDS TIJDSCHRIFT VOOR GENEESKUNDE 129(11):481-483, Mach 16, 1985.

AIDS diagnosis uncertain, by S. Yanchinski. NEW SCIENTIST 105:24, February 7, 1985.

Aids to the laboratory diagnosis of AIDS [editorial], by R. Penny. PATHOLOGY 16(4):375-377, October 1984.

Analysis of serum samples positive for HTLV-III antibodies, by J. C. Petricciani, et al. NEW ENGLAND JOURNAL OF MEDICINE 313:47-48, July 4, 1985.

Bacterial expression of the acquired immunodeficiency syndrome retrovirus p24 gag protein and its use as a diagnostic reagent, by D. J. Dowbenko, et al. PROCEEDINGS OF THE NATIONAL ACADEMY OF SCIENCES 82(22): 7748-7752, November 1985.

Bone marrow biopsies in patients with the acquired immunodeficiency syndrome, by B. M. Osborne, et al. HUMAN PATHOLOGY 15(11):1048-1053, November 1984.

Bone marrow examination and culture in the diagnosis of acquired immunode-ficiency syndrome (AIDS) [letter], by J. Pasternak, et al. ARCHIVES OF INTERNAL MEDICINE 143(7):1495, July 1983.

Brain biopsies in patients with acquired immune deficiency syndrome, by L. B. Moskowitz, et al. ARCHIVES OF PATHOLOGY AND LABORATORY MEDI-CINE 108(5):368-371, May 1984.

Bronchoalveolar lavage in acquired immunodeficiency syndrome [letter],by A. Venet, et al. LANCET 2(8340):53, July 2, 1983.

—, by Y. M. Chung. MILITARY MEDICINE 149(9):518+, September 1984.

Cetus technique detects AIDS virus. CHEMICAL AND ENGINEERING NEWS 64:8, April 21, 1986.

Colonic biopsies have a high diagnostic yield in AIDS, by H. Rotterdam, et al. AMERICAN FAMILY PHYSICIAN 27:191, May 1983.

CT of acquired immunodeficiency syndrome , by E. M. Bursztyn, et al. AJNR 5(6):7110714, November-December 1984.

Demonstration of Isospora belli by acid-fast stain in a patient with acquired immune deficiency syndrome, by E. Ng, et al. JOURNAL OF CLINICAL MICROBIOLOGY 20(3):384-386, September 1984.

Diagnosis and management of acquired immune deficiency syndrome in intra-venous drug users, by D. Shine. ADVANCES IN ALCOHOL AND SUB-STANCE ABUSE 5(1-2):25-34, 1985-1986.

Diagnosis and management of mycobacterial infection and disease in persons with human T-lymphotropic virus type III/lymphadenopathy-associated virus infection. MMWR 35(28):448-452, July 18, 1986.

Diagnosis of HTLV-III infection by ultrastructural examination of germinal centers in lymph node—a case report, by T. F. Warner, et al. AIDS RESEARCH 2(1): 43-50, February 1986.

Differential diagnosis at the bedside. Mycoplasma pneumonia or AIDS?, by O. Karg, et al. MUENCHENER MEDIZINISCHE WOCHENSCHRIFT 125(35):72-73, September 2, 1983.

Difficulties in the diagnosis of acquired immune deficiency syndrome [letter], by E. G. Wilkins, et al. JOURNAL OF CLINICAL PATHOLOGY 37(11):1316-1317, November 1984.

Dual diagnosis: AIDS and addiction, by L. Caputo. SOCIAL WORK 30:360-364, July-August 1985.

Electron microscopy of the intestine and rectum in acquired immunodeficiency syndrome, by W. O. Dobbins, 3d, et al. GASTROENTEROLOGY 88(3):738-749, March 1985.

False-positive results in the detection of anti-LAV/HTLV-III antibodies by enzyme i immunoassay, by H. Näher, et al. HAUTARZT 37(6):338-340 June 1986.

First case of AIDS in Salzburg. Important diagnostic hint by determination of neopterin, by K. Wessely, et al. WIENER KLINISCHE WOCHENSCHRIFT 97(2):88-90, January 18, 1985.

Heated sera and laboratory tests [letter], by S. I. Vas, et al. ANNALS OF INTERNAL MEDICINE 103(2)308, August 1985.

HTLV-III in symptom-free seronegative persons, by S. Z. Salaguddin, et al. LANCET 2(8417-8418):1418-1420, December 22, 1984.

IASP (or IBA), not AIDS [letter],by J. F. Soothill. LANCET 1(8323):526, March 5, 1983.

Identification of C or D virus-type particles in the germinal centers of lymph nodes sampled at the lymphadenopathy stage of the acquired immunodeficiency syndrome [letter], by a. Le Tourneau, et al. PRESSE MEDICALE 15(3):121, January 25, 1986.

Immunologic laboratory tests in acquired immunodeficiency syndrome (AIDS) and suspected AIDS, by H. I. Joller-Jemelka, et al. SCHWEIZERISCHE MEDIZIN-ISCHE WOCHENSCHRIFT 115(4):125-132, January 26, 1985.

Indications for and diagnostic efficacy of open-lung biopsy in the patient with acquired immunodeficiency syndrome (AIDS),by H. I. Pass, et al. ANNALS OF THORACIC SURGERY 41(3):307-312, March 1986.

Is presence of interferon predictive for AIDS? [letter], by E. Buimovici-Klein, et al. LANCET 2(8345):344, August 6, 1983.

Leishmaniasis or AIDS? [letter], by A. de la Loma, et al. TRANSACTIONS OF THE ROYAL SOCIETY OF TROPICAL MEDICINE AND HYGIENE 79(3):421-422, 1985.

Limited usefulness of lymphocytopenia in screening for AIDS in hospital patients, by W. J. Boyko, et al. CANADIAN MEDICAL ASSOCIATION JOURNAL 133(4):293, August 15, 1985.

Lymph node biopsy in lymphadenopathy syndrome and AIDS [letter], by H. Müller, et al. DEUTCHE MEDIZINISCHE WOCHENSCHRIFT 110(36):1391, September 6, 1985.

Lymphocyte phenotyping by fluorescence microscopy and flow cytometry: results in homosexual men and heterosexual controls, by J. T. Newman,e t al. AIDS RESEARCH 1(2):127-134, 1983-1984.

Lymphoma versus AIDS [letter],by J. H. Mead, et al. AMERICAN JOURNAL OF CLINICAL PATHOLOGY 80(4):546-547, October 1983.

Lytic infection by British AIDS virus and development of rapid cell test for antiviral antibodies, by A. Karpas, et al. LANCET 2(8457):695-697, September 28, 1985.

Multivesicular rosettes, a possible marker of acquired immunodeficiency syndrome (AIDS) in the endothelial cells of the splenic sinusoids [letter], by E. Feliu, et al. MEDICINA CLINICA 83(3):129, June 16, 1984.

Mycobacterial culture in acquired immunodeficiency syndrome [letter], by J. A. Girón, et al. ANNALS OF INTERNAL MEDICINE 98(6):1028-1029, June 1983.

Mycobacteriosis in AIDS: easy to miss the correct diagnosis, by R. Grubb, et al. LAKARTIDNINGEN 82(25):2349-2351, June 19, 1985.

New biphasic culture system for isolation of mycobacteria from blood of patients with acquired immune deficiency syndrome, by O. G. Berlin, et al. JOURNAL OF CLINICAL MICROBIOLOGY 20(3):572-574, September 1984.

Nondiagnosis of acquired immunodeficiency syndrome [editorial], by G. T. Hensley, et al. ARCHIVES OF PATHOLOGY AND LABORATORY MEDICINE 110(4):307-308, April 1986.

Pointer to AIDS diagnosis found. CHEMICAL INDUSTRY 8:276, April 16, 1984.

Preclinical determination of AIDS disease by a series of tests [letter], by R. B. Bhalla, et al. CLINICAL CHEMISTRY 32(7):1426-1427, July 1986.

Presence of ultrastructural markers of AIDS in rectal biopsies at the early stage of the disease [letter], by C. Leport, et al. GASTROENTEROLOGIE CLINIQUE ET BIOLOGIQUE 8(12):983-984, December 1984.

Prognostic value of histopathology in persistent generalized lymphadenopathy in homosexual men [letter], by R. Fernandez, et al. NEW ENGLAND JOURNAL OF MEDICINE 309(3):185-186, July 21, 1983.

Pseudo-AIDS [letter],by D. A. Walker, et al. LANCET 2(8345):344, August 6, 1983.

Quantitative changes in T helper or T suppressor/cytotoxic lymphocyte subsets that distinguish acquired immune deficiency syndrome from other immune subset disorders, by J. L. Fahey, et al. AMERICAN JOURNAL OF MEDICINE 76(1):95-100, January 1984.

Radiographic findings in acquired immune deficiency syndrome, by W. T. Miller, et al. APPLIED RADIOLOGY 14(3):86-8, May-June 1985.

Radiographic immune deficiency syndrome (AIDS) and pre-AIDS, by A. E. Pitchenik, et al. AMERICAN REVIEW OF RESPIRATORY DISEASE 131(3): 393-396, March 1985.

Rapid detection of immunoreactive interferon-alpha in AIDS [letter], by S. R. Abbott, et al. LANCET 1(8376):564, March 10, 1984.

Recommendations: diagnosis of AIDS used by the Centers for Disease Control. EUROPEAN JOURNAL OF CANCER AND CLINICAL ONCOLOGY 20(2): 169-173, February 1984.

Renal ultrasound in acquired immune deficiency syndrome, by R. M. Schaffer, et al. RADIOLOGY 153(2):511-513, November 1984.

Safe method for identifying cryptosporidium cysts in the faeces of patients with suspected AIDS, or those infected with other serious concomitant pathogens [letter], by J. E. Williams, et al. JOURNAL OF CLINICAL PATHOLOGY 38(11):1313-1314, November 1985.

Serological analysis of a subgroup of human T-lymphotropic retroviruses (HTLV-III) associated with AIDS, by J. Schüpbach, et al. SCIENCE 224(4648):503-505, May 4, 1984.

Serum marker may identify potential AIDS victims. AMERICAN JOURNAL OF NURSING 84:177, February 1984.

Surgical biopsy for persistent generalized lymphadenopathy, by H. J. Rashleigh-Belcher, et al. BRITISH JOURNAL OF SURGERY 73(3):183-185, March 1986.

Surgical considerations in the diagnosis and management of AIDS, by M. T. Lotze. AIDS RESEARCH 2(2):141-148, Spring 1986.

Suspected AIDS: an approach that helps patients, whatever the diagnosis, by J. T. Wheeler. CONSULTANT 25(18):102-103+, December 1985.

Urinary excretion of modified nucleosides in patients with acquired immune deficiency syndrome (AIDS) and individuals at high risk of AIDS, by A. Fischbein, et al. CANCER DETECTION AND PREVENTION 8(1-2):271-277, 1985.

Urinary neopterin, a useful marker for AIDS?, [letter], by M. Perna, et al. LANCET 1(8436):1048, May 4, 1985.

Use of beta-2 microglobulin in the diagnosis of AIDS, suspected AIDS, and pre-clinical AIDS, by S. Zolla-Pazner, et al. ANNALS OF THE NEW YORK ACADEMY OF SCIENCES 437:526-529, 1984.

Value of digestive endoscopic examination in acquired immunodeficiency syndrome (45 cases), by J. Cosnes, et al. ANNALES DE GASTROENTER-OLOGIE ET D'HEPATOLOGIE 22(3):123-128, May-June 1986.

Value of electroencephalography in AIDS [letter], by W. Enzensberger, et al. LANCET 1(8436):1047-1048, May 4, 1985.

Value of haematological screening for AIDS in an at risk population, by J. N. Weber, et al. GENITOURINARY MEDICINE 61(5):325-329, October 1985.

Value of lymph node biopsy in unexplained lymphadenopathy in homosexual men, by R. K. Brynes, et al. JAMA 250(10):1313-1317, September 9, 1983.

Value of the cytological examination of the bronchoalveolar lavage fluid in patients with acquired immunodeficiency syndrome and related syndromes, by P. Fouret, et al. ANNALS OF PATHOLOGY 6(1):45-52, 1986.

Virological diagnosis of HTLV-III infections, by J. Suni, et al. DUODECIM 102(7): 423-428, 1986.

When is AIDS not AIDS? [letter], by R. D. Maw, et al. LANCET 2(8409):986, October 27, 1984.

Your role in the diagnosis and management of AIDS, by R. D. Smith. PATHOLO-GIST 37(9):609-611, September 1983.

HAITI
Malnutrition or AIDS in Haiti? [letter], by J. W. Mellors, et al. NEW ENGLAND JOURNAL OF MEDICINE 310(17):1119-1120, April 26, 1984.

UNITED STATES
AIDS: Ohio update and comments on diagnosis, by J. C. Neff. OHIO STATE MEDICAL JOURNAL 80(2):135-138, February 1984.

Beta 2-microglobulin as a prognostic marker for development of AIDS [letter], by R. B. Bhalla, et al. CLINICAL CHEMISTRY 31(8):1411-1412, August 1985.

Beta-2 microglobulin: a sensitive non-specific marker for acquired immune deficiency syndrome, by P. Francioloi, et al. EUROPEAN JOURNAL OF CLINICAL MICROBIOLOGY 3(1):68-69, February 1984.

DIAGNOSIS—SURGERY

Role of surgery in the prognosis of AIDS and related syndromes. Case reports, by F. Badellino, et al. MINERVA MEDICA 77(9-10):March 10, 1986.

DRUG ABUSE

Acquired immune deficiency syndrome. Review of the literature. Apropos of a pre-AIDS case in a heroin addict, by F. Valentini, et al. MINERVA MEDICA 77(1-2): 7-11, January 14, 1986.

Acquired immunodeficiency syndrome and infection with hepatitis viruses in i ndividuals abusing drugs by injection, by D. M. Novick, et al. BULLETIN ON NARCOTICS 38(1-2):15-25, January-June 1986.

Acquired immunodeficiency syndrome in a drug addict with Kaposi's sarcoma and chronic hepatitis B [letter], by A. García Díez, et al. MEDICINA CLINICA 83(12):518, October 20, 1984.

Acquired immunodeficiency syndrome: apropos of a case in an intravenous heroin user [letter], by A. Pintor Escobar, et al. MEDICINA CLINICA 82(1):42, January 14, 1984.

Acquired immunodeficiency syndrome in the prodromal phase in a drug addict [letter], by F. Cardellach, et al. MEDICINA CLINICA 81(14):645-646, November 5, 1983.

Additional recommendations to reduce sexual and drug abuse-related transmission of human T-lymphotropic virus type III/lymphadenopathy-associated virus. JAMA 255(14):1843-1844+, April 11, 1986; also in: MMWR 35(10): 152-155, March 14, 1986.

AIDS and drug use. An overview of the epidemiology, virus, symptoms, and the relationship with intravenous drug use, by J. H. Moerkerk, et al. TIJD-SCHRIFT VOOR ALCOHOL, DRUGS EN ANDERE PSYCHOTROPE STOFFEN 11(1):41+, 1985.

AIDS and the substance abuse treatment clinician [editorial], by J. Imhof, et al. JOURNAL OF SUBSTANCE ABUSE AND TREATMENT 2(3):137, 1985.

AIDS, drug abuse, and mental health [editorial], by H. A. Pincus. PUBLIC HEALTH REPORTS 99(2):106-108, March-April 1984.

AIDS-like immunologic alterations in clinically unaffected drug users, by G. Fiorini, et al. AMERICAN JOURNAL OF CLINICAL PATHOLOGY 84(3):354-357, September 1985.

AIDS studied among drug users. ADAMHA NEWS 11(11):1+, November 1985.

Central-nervous-system toxoplasmosis in homosexual men and parenteral drug abusers, by B. Wong, et al. ANNALS OF INTERNAL MEDICINE 100(1):36-42, January 1984.

Community-acquired opportunistic infections and defective cellular immunity in heterosexual drug abusers and homosexual men, by C. B. Small, et al. AMERICAN JOURNAL OF MEDICINE 74(3):433-441, March 1983.

Diagnosis and management of acquired immune deficiency syndrome in intra-venous drug users, by D. Shine. ADVANCES IN ALCOHOL AND SUB-STANCE ABUSE 5(1-2):25-34, 1985-1986.

Difference in the behavior of T-lymphocyte populations in heroin and methadone addicts, by M. A. Brugo, et al. BOLLETTINO DELL ISTITUTO SIEROTERAPI-CO MILANESE 62(6):517-523, 1983.

Drug abuse and AIDS: troubling connections, by G. De Stafano. ADVOCATE 449:47, June 24, 1986.

Drug abusers 'most likely' to spread AIDS virus by needles, by N. Casey. NURSING STANDARD 433:8, February 6, 1986.

Drug-linked AIDS cases up. CORRECTIONS DIGEST 17(10):10, May 7, 1986; also in NARCOTICS CONTROL DIGEST 16(9):2, April 30, 1986.

Dual diagnosis: AIDS and addiction, by L. Caputo. SOCIAL WORK 30:360-364, July-August 1985.

Epidemic of acquired immunodeficiency syndrome (AIDS) and suggestions for its control in drug abusers, by M. Marmor, et al. JOURNAL OF SUBSTANCE ABUSE AND TREATMENT 1(4):237-247, 1984.

Epidemic of AIDS related virus (HTLV-III/LAV) infection among intravenous drug abusers, by J. R. Robertson, et al. BRITISH MEDICAL JOURNAL 292(6519):527-529, Feburary 22, 1986.

Epidemic of AIDS related virus infection among intravenous drug abusers [letter],by R. P. Brettle. BRITISH MEDICAL JOURNAL 292(6336):1671, June 21, 1986.

Epidemiology of the Acquired Immunodeficiency Syndrome in intravenous drug abusers, by J. P. Koplan, et al. ADVANCES IN ALCOHOL AND SUB-STANCE ABUSE 5(1 & 2):13-23, Fall 1985-Winter 1986.

Fatal toxoplasmosis of the central nervous system in a heroin user with acquired i immunodeficiency disease, by S. K. Murthy, et al. NEW YORK STATE JOURNAL OF MEDICINE 84(9):464-466, September 1984.

Free needles for drug users weighed as anti-AIDS tactic. CRIMINAL JUSTICE NEWSLETTER 16(24):4-5, December 16, 1985.

"Free" needles for intravenous drug users at risk for AIDS: current developments in New York City, by D. C. Des Larlais, et al. NEW ENGLAND JOURNAL OF MEDICINE 313:1476, December 5, 1985.

House panel holds hearing on AIDS and IV drug abuse. NARCOTICS CONTROL DIGEST 15(25-26):5-6, December 11, 1985.

HTLV-III exposure among drug users, by H. M. Ginzburg, et al. CANCER RESEARCH 45(Suppl. 9):4605s-4608s, September 1985.

HTLV-III in persons with intravenous drug abuse. Correlation of antibodies against HTLV-III with neopterin and TH/TS, by P. Hengster, et al. DEUTSCHE MEDIZINISCHE WOCHENSCHRIFT 111(12):453-457, March 21, 1986.

Intravenous amphetamine abuse, primary cerebral mucormycosis, and acquired immunodeficiency, by M. S. Micozzi, et al. JOURNAL OF FORENSIC SCIENCES 30(2):504-510, April 1985.

Intravenous drug abusers and the acquired immunodeficiency syndrome (AIDS). Demographic, drug use, and needle-sharing patterns, by G. H. Friedland, et al. ARCHIVES OF INTERNAL MEDICINE 145(8):1413-1417, August 1985.

Intravenous drug users and the acquired immune deficiency syndrome, by H. M. Ginzburg. PUBLIC HEALTH REPORTS 99(2):206-212, March -April 1984.

Major medical problems and detoxification treatment of parenteral drug-abusing alcoholics, by D. M. Novick. ADVANCES IN ALCOHOL AND SUBSTANCE ABUSE 3(4):87-105, 1984.

Monocyte function in intravenous drug abusers with lymphadenopathy syndrome and in patients with acquired immunodeficiency syndrome: selective impairment of chemotaxis, by G. Po.i, et al. CLINICAL AND EXPERIMENTAL IMMUNOLOGY 62(1):136-142, October 1985.

Natural killer cells in intravenous drug abusers with lymphadenopathy syndrome, by G. Poli, et al. CLINICAL AND EXPERIMENTAL IMMUNOLOGY 62(1):128-135, October 1985.

New evidence could link drugs to AIDS. RN 46:20, June 1983.

New Jersey AIDS patients often drug abusers, by S. Hartnett. NEW JERSEY NURSE 16(2):13, March-April 1986.

Pre-AIDS in a child of a drug-addict. Clinical and laboratory description, by D. Pavesio, et al. MINERVA PEDATRICA 37(1-2):73-74, January 31, 1985.

Prevalence of HTLV-III infection among New Haven, Connecticut, parenteral drug abusers in 1982-1983, by R. D'Aquila, et al. NEW ENGLAND JOURNAL OF MEDICINE 314:117-118, January 9, 1986.

Prevalence of HTLV-III/LAV antibodies among intravenous drug users attending treatment programs in California: a preliminary report, by N. Levy, et al. NEW ENGLAND JOURNAL OF MEDICINE 314:446, February 13, 1986.

Prolonged incubation period of AIDS in intravenous drug abusers: epidemiological evidence in prison inmates, by J. P. Hanrahan, et al. JOURNAL OF INFECTIOUS DISEASES 150(2):263-266, August 1984.

Rapid spread of HTLV-III infection among drug addicts in Italy [letter], by G. Angarano, et al. LANCET 2(8467):1302, December 7, 1985.

Recreational drugs: relationship to AIDS, by J. J. Goedert. ANNALS OF THE NEW YORK ACADEMY OF SCIENCES 437:192-199, 1984.

Risk reduction for the acquired immunodeficiency syndrome among intravenous drug users, by D. C. Des Jarlais, et al. ANNALS OF INTERNAL MEDICINE 103(5):755-759, November 1985.

Sharing of needles among users of intravenous drugs, by J. L. Black, et al. NEW ENGLAND JOURNAL OF MEDICINE 314:446, February 13, 1986.

Spontaneous rupture of the spleen due to acquired immunodeficiency syndrome in an intravenous drug abuser, by H. G. Mirchandani, et al. ARCHIVES OF PATHOLOGY AND LABORATORY MEDICINE 109(12):1114-1116, December 1985.

State plans to trace sex, needle partners. OUT 4(5):1, April 1986.

GREAT BRITAIN
UK case of AIDS in an intravenous drug abuser [letter], by S. J. Winterton, et al. LANCET 1(8439):1223, May 25, 1985.

DRUG ADDICTS
See: DRUG ABUSE

ECONOMICS
Administration asks additional 45 million: AIDS, by D. Walter. ADVOCATE 428: 10, September 3, 1985.

AIDS aid, by S. Moorsom. NEW SOCIETY August 8, 1986, p. 12-13.

AIDS: allocating resources for research and patient care, by P. R. Lee. ISSUES IN SCIENCE AND TECHNOLOGY 2:66-73, Winter 1986.

AIDS amendment angers cancer institute [news] by B. J. Culiton. SCIENCE 226(4678):1056, November 30, 1984.

AIDS and Medicaid. The role of Medicaid in treating those with AIDS, by J. Luehrs, et al. PUBLIC WELFARE 44(3):20-28, Summer 1986.

AIDS budget doubled, by S. Hyde. GAY COMMUNITY NEWS 11(7):1, September 3, 1983.

AIDS costs: employers and insurers have reasons to fear expensive epidemic. WALL STREET JOURNAL 206:1+, October 18, 1985.

AIDS: financial implications for Michigan, by D. W. Benfer, et al. MICHIGAN HOSPITALS 22(8):13-16, August 1986.

AIDS funding decisions lack consensus opinion, by J. Firshei. HOSPITALS 60(1):35, January 5, 1986.

AIDS funding jeopardized by veto, by D. Nelson. GAY COMMUNITY NEWS 10(48):3, June 25, 1983.

AIDS funds approved. BODY POLITIC 91:19, March 1983.

AIDS grant. ADAMHA NEWS 9(20):1, November 18, 1983.

AIDS meets funding drought, by W. Doherty. SCIENCE FOR PEOPLE 15(3):5, May 1983.

AIDS: more for research and treatment [news], by T. Beardsley. NATURE 317(6037):466, October 10-16, 1985.

AIDS: more money promised, by S. Budiansky. NATURE 303:365, June 2, 1983.

AIDS patients' bills add up to trouble, by L. Punch. MODERN HEALTHCARE 14(7):49, May 15, 1984.

AIDS plan unveiled but funding in question by S. Hyde. GAY COMMUNITY NEWS 12(36):3, March 30, 1985.

AIDS research. Big enough spending? [news], by S. Budiansky. NATURE 304(5926):478, August 11-17, 1983.

AIDS research funding proposals more than double. AMERICAN FAMILY PHYSICIAN 32:18, October 1985.

AIDS research funding stalled; diagnostic test advances. AMERICAN FAMILY PHYSICIAN 30:18, August 1984.

AIDS rodeo benefit, by P. Byron. GAY COMMUNITY NEWS 11(13):3, October 15, 1983.

AIDS: US administration's parsimony criticized, by S. Budiansky. NATURE 313:725, February 28, 1985.

AIDS work funded. OUT 3(2):4, December 1984.

Alternative care helps firms reduce costs to treat AIDS, by S. Taravella. BUSI-NESS INSURANCE 19(39):1+, September 30, 1985.

Apuzzo blasts NYC/lack of money for AIDS service, by P. Freiberg. ADVOCATE 413:9, February 5, 1985.

Avalanche of new cash, by C. Norman. SCIENCE 230:1358, December 20, 1985.

Billions needed for AIDS research. BODY POLITIC 118:29, September 1985.

Boston AIDS Committee receives $150,000, by s. Hyde. GAY COMMUNITY NEWS 12(32):3, March 2, 1985.

Boston "walk for life" raises over $300,000, by K. Westheimer. GAY COMMUNITY NEWS 13(46):3, June 14, 1986.

Broadway benefit raises half a million for AIDS, by S. Greco. ADVOCATE 423:49, June 25, 1985.

Cases up, funding down. BODY POLITIC 125:23, April 1986.

Coalition forms for test-site funding. OUT 4(5):6, April 1986.

Congress close to doubling AIDS SPD, by L. Bush. ADVOCATE 3(71):8, July 7, 1983.

Congress likely to halt shrinkage in AIDS funds, by C. Norman. SCIENCE 231(4744):1364-1365, March 21, 1986.

Congress, NIH open coffers for AIDS, by G. Kolata. SCIENCE 221(4609):436+, July 29, 1983.

Congress readies AIDS funding transfusion, by C. Norman. SCIENCE 230(4724):418-419, October 25, 1985.

Congressional Committee/AIDS funding, by D. Walter. ADVOCATE 417:12, April 2, 1985.

Cost of AIDS, by R. Wingerter. IN THESE TIMES 10(26):22, May 28, 1986.

Cost of ignorance, by R. Davenport-Hines. TIMES LITERARY SUPPLEMENT July 18, 1986, p. 780.

Costly disease: the public bill for AIDS could be $5 billion by 1990, by G. Weiss. BARRON'S 65:32, April 22, 1985.

Curious way to fight AIDS: your tax dollars at work. HUMAN EVENTS 45:6, September 21, 1985.

Cuts in AIDS funding?, by D. Walter. ADVOCATE 440:10, February 18, 1986.

Doctor urges LA County to triple AIDS funding, by J. Cort. ADVOCATE 406:23, October 30, 1984.

Dubious test approved; funding cuts loom. BODY POLITIC 113:21, April 1985.

Dukakis announces $1.8 million AIDS grant, by S. Hyde. GAY COMMUNITY NEWS 13(7):3, August 24, 1985.

Economic impact of the first 10,000 cases of acquired immunodeficiency syndrome in the United States, by A. M. Hardy, et al. JAMA 255:209-211, January 10, 1986.

Economic implications: acquired immunodeficiency syndrome [editorial[, by C. H. Ramírez-Ronda. BOLETIN—ASOCIACION MEDICA DE PUERTO RICO 77(4):132-133, April 1985.

'Fast-buck' artists are making a killing on AIDS, by S. Ticer. BUSINESS WEEK December 2, 1985, p. 85-86.

Financial implications of AIDS, by S. D. Sedaka, et al. CARING 5(6):38-39+, June 1986.

Financing extinction in the tropics, by D. Coules. NOT MAN APART 15(4):14, May 1985.

Footing the bill, by B. Maschinot. IN THESE TIMES 9(37):4, October 2, 1985.

Forum: the costs of treatment, by J. Gildea. HEALTH COST MANAGEMENT 3(1):16-18, January-February 1986.

Funding improves for AIDS groups, by K. Popert. BODY POLITIC 1(6):11, September 1984.

Gala night for singing [opera stage benefit in East Hampton, N.Y.]. OPERA NEWS 50:32, November 1985.

Gala with a grim side [Hollywood fundraiser], by W. R. Doerner. TIME 126:30+, September 30, 1985.

Gay leaders ask Congress for more AIDS funding, by D. Walter. ADVOCATE 422:16, June 11, 1985.

GLC promises cash help to AIDS voluntary effort, by J. Meldrum. NEW STATES-MAN 108:8, December 21, 1984.

Good friends: raising funds for AIDS. ADVOCATE 3(74):25, August 18, 1983.

Governor compromises on vetoed AIDS funds, by M. Helquist. ADVOCATE 431:23, October 15, 1985.

Governor flipflops on AIDS funding, by B. Nelson. GAY COMMUNITY NEWS 10(50):3, July 9, 1983. 10(50):2, July 9, 1983.

Grants to study ADM aspects of AIDS. ADAMHA NEWS 12(1):1+, January 1986.

Higher AIDS budget proposed, by Bisticas-Cocoves. GAY COMMUNITY NEWS 13(5):1, August 10, 1985.

Hollywood bash to combat AIDS, by B. Barol. NEWSWEEK 106:80-81, September 30, 1985.

Hollywood Bowl AIDS benefit, by S. Anderson. ADVOCATE 3(78):13, October 13, 1983.

House Committee doubles '86 AIDS research money, by M. Cocoves. GAY COMMUNITY NEWS 13(11):3, September 28, 1985.

House OKs record AIDS funding, by Bush, et al. ADVOCATE 3(79):8, October 27, 1983.

Industry trade groups give money for AIDS education and research. THE NA-TIONAL UNDERWRITER (LIFE & HEALTH INSURANCE EDITION) 90:2, March 22, 1986.

Kennedy introduces $25M AIDS package, by K. Westheimer. GAY COMMUNITY NEWS 13(41):1, May 3, 1986.

Koch official defends city's AIDS spending, by P. Freiberg. ADVOCATE 416:12, March 19, 1985.

Koch raises NY AIDS funding, by P. Freiberg. ADVOCATE 419:16, April 30, 1985.

Making a buck off AIDS, by J. Irving. GAY COMMUNITY NEWS 13(28):2, February 1, 1986.

Making capital out of AIDS, by R. Butt. TIMES November 20, 1986, p. 20.

Massachusetts cuts AIDS funding, by C. Guilfoy. GAY COMMUNITY NEWS 12(48):1, June 22, 1985.

Money for AIDS; British spending too little, US research will need control. NATURE 304:671-672, August 25, 1983.

More AIDS money , by S. Budiansky. NATURE 304(5928):677, August 25-31, 1983

—, by T. Beardsley. NATURE 318(6044):306, November 28-December 4, 1985.

More federal AIDS research grants, by N. Fain. ADVOCATE 3(71):18, July 7, 1983.

More for AIDS in '85 budget request, by J. Ryan. GAY COMMUNITY NEWS 11(30):1, February 18, 1984.

More funding needed in rising AIDS crisis, by S. Martz. IN THESE TIMES 9(36):3, September 25, 1985.

More US funds for AIDS , by T. Beardsley. NATURE 316(6027):384, August 1-7, 1985.

Moynihan Bill requires PHS provide funds: AIDS, by D. Walter. ADVOCATE 427: 21, August 20, 1985.

Native Americans, PWA's protest health costs , by Bisticas-Cocoves. GAY COM- MUNITY NEWS 13(13):1, October 12, 1985.

New funds for AIDS drug centers , by D. M. Barnes. SCIENCE 233(4762):414, July 25, 1986.

New PHS grants awarded for research on AIDS. PUBLIC HEALTH REPORTS 98(3):228, May-June 1983.

NIAID to fund nine new AIDS studies. PUBLIC HEALTH REPORTS 99(3):324, May-June 1984.

NIDA AIDS grant, by K. Callen. ADAMHA NEWS 9(21):2, December 1983.

Non-partisan agency slams insufficient AIDS supp, by C. Guilfoy. GAY COM- MUNITY NEWS 12(35):7, March 23, 1985.

NW AIDS fund announced. NORTHWEST PASSAGE 23(13):7, August 1983.

Other AIDS crisis: who pays for the treatment? WASHINGTON MONTHLY 17:25-31, January 1986.

PHS steps up activities and increases grant support to combat acquired immune deficiency syndrome. PUBLIC HEALTH REPORTS 97:589, November-December 1982.

President's 1987 budget request. ADAMHA NEWS 12(3):1+, March 1986.

Price of AIDS, by S. Meyer. MIAMI /SOUTH FLORIDA MAGAZINE January 26, 1986.

Protection money , by L. Gubernick. FORBES 136:216, November 4, 1985.

Public funding increased to halt spread of AIDS, by E. F. Kuntz. CITY AND STATE HEALTH FINANCES 2(7):2+, September 1985.

Reagan doubles fiscal '84 AIDS funds, by L. Bush. ADVOCATE 3(78):20, October 13, 1983.

Reagan—1984 Health Emergency Bill, by B. Nelson. GAY COMMUNITY NEWS 11(2):1, July 23, 1983.

Reagan seeks $50M AIDS cut, by G. Gottlieb. GAY COMMUNITY NEWS 13(31): 1, February 15, 1986.

Senate approves $22m for AIDS, by Bisticas-Cocoves. GAY COMMUNITY NEWS 13(16):1, November 2, 1985.

600 rally/march for AIDS fund, by L. Goldsmith. GAY COMMUNITY NEWS 10(49):1, July 2, 1983.

SSI benefits approved AIDS patients, by P. Byron. GAY COMMUNITY NEWS 10(44):1, May 29, 1983.

Star-studded gala raises $1 mil. for AIDS research. JET 69:56, October 7, 1985.

State proposes $1.8M for AIDS, by C. Guilfoy. GAY COMMUNITY NEWS 12(42): 1, May 11, 1985.

Thousands demand AIDS funding. BODY POLITIC 95:19, July 1983.

Thousands demand more AIDS funding, by B. Nelson. GAY COMMUNITY NEWS 10(42):1, May 14, 1983.

Too little aid for AIDS, by J. Randal. TECHNOLOGY REVIEW 87(6):10-13+, August-September 1984.

Tough AIDS-funding fight predicted, by D. Walter. ADVOCATE 413:8, February 5, 1985.

$12 million cut in Reagan's AIDS budget, by D. Walter. ADVOCATE 416:16, March 19, 1985.

United States administration's parsimony criticized [news], by S. Budiansky. NATURE 313(6005):725, February 28-March 6, 1985.

United States funds AIDS education, by N. Fain. ADVOCATE 422:26, June 11, 1985.

Welcome but inadequate cash to fight AIDS, by M. Sargent. NURSING STANDARD 417:1, October 3, 1985.

Your money or your life—David Groat, by L. Goldsmith. GAY COMMUNITY NEWS 10(33):3, March 12, 1983.

GREAT BRITAIN
Acquired immune deficiency syndrome and epidemic of infection with human immunodeficiency virus: costs of care and prevention in an inner London district, by A. M. Johnson, et al. BRITISH MEDICAL JOURNAL 293(6545):489-492, August 23, 1986.

Money for AIDS; British spending too little, US research will need control. NATURE 304:671-672, August 25, 1983.

UK money for AIDS, by M. Clarke. NATURE 318(6045):401, December 5, 1985.

HAITI
AIDS funding and research hiked; Haitians' risk debated. AMERICAN FAMILY PHYSICIAN 28:17-18, September 1983.

EDUCATION
Aftercare instruction: AIDS brochure, by M. M. Hughes. JEN 9(6):340-342, November-December 1983.

AIDS and health education, by N. Freudenberg. HEALTH PAC BULLETIN 16(4):29, July 1985.

AIDS and hysterria a problem of health education, by N. J. Flumara. HEALTH VALUES 7(6):3, November-December 1983.

AIDS and the right to know, by J. Alter, et al. NEWSWEEK 108(7):46-47, August 18, 1986.

AIDS: be informed. WORLD HEALTH November 1985, p. 6.

AIDS brochure for distribution to patients, by M. M. Hughes. JEN 9(6):340-342, November-December 1983.

AIDS: California publishes booklet providing helpful info. CORRECTIONS DIGEST 14(16):4-6, July 27, 1983; also in CRIME CONTROL DIGEST 17(30): 4-6, July 29, 1983; NARCOTICS CONTROL DIGEST 13(16):3-5, August 3, 1983; TRAINING AIDS DIGEST 8(8):5-7, August 1983.

AIDS: a commentary . . . school health, by P. R. Nader. JOURNAL OF SCHOOL HEALTH 56(3):107-108, March 1986.

AIDS circular. NEW SCIENTIST 99:393, August 11, 1983.

AIDS data-sharing: help sought to combat bias, by C. Frank. AMERICAN BAR ASSOCIATION JOURNAL 76:22, January 1, 1986.

AIDS dilemma: recent court decisions place a burden of persuasion on public schools, by J. Beckham. NAASP BULLETIN 70(489):91-95, April 1986.

AIDS education: the city's closet case, by P. Byron. VILLAGE VOICE 30:33, May 28, 1985.

AIDS education for staff, by H. Schietinger. JOURNAL OF CONTINUING EDUCATION IN NURSING 17(1)3-4, January-February 1986.

AIDS education need; conference highlight, by H. W. Jaffe. CORRECTIONS TODAY 48:49-50+, April 1986.

AIDS epidemic creates educational, product demands, by E. Beck. MEDICAL PRODUCTS SALES 16(12):1+, December 1985.

AIDS fact book, by E. Mabrey. DELAWARE ALTERNATIVE PRESS 6(2):17, January 1984.

AIDS: getting the facts, by M. L. Stein. EDITOR AND PUBLISHER, THE FOURTH ESTATE 118:16-17, November 2, 1985.

AIDS guidelines urge common-sense care, by S. B. Young, et al. AIR FORCE TIMES 46:34, November 25, 1985.

AIDS—a health education challenge, by Z. Kurtz. HEALTH EDUCATION JOURNAL 44(4):169-171, 1985.

AIDS: an information perspective, by L. Kabbash, et al. BIBLIOTHECA MEDICA CANADIANA 8(2):71-78, 1986.

AIDS kids: the education of parents, by A. Mayo. VILLAGE VOICE 30:20, September 24, 1985.

AIDS lobby and education project proposed, by D. Slaw. GAY COMMUNITY NEWS 10(50):3, July 9, 1983.

AIDS newsletter available. CRIME CONTROL DIGEST 20(6):2, February 10, 1986.

AIDS: a risk for diabetes educators?, by C. A. Jenkins, et al. DIABETES EDUCATOR Suppl. 12:185-186, May 1986.

AIDS surveillance and health education: use of previously described risk factors to identify high-risk homosexuals, by R. O. Valdiserri, et al. AMERICAN JOURNAL OF PUBLIC HEALTH 74(3):259-260, March 1984.

AIDS—thorough information is never wasted, by E. Schmeltzer, et al. SYGEPLEJERSKEN 86(32):26-29, August 6, 1986.

AIDS to understanding [review article]. THE ECONOMIST 299:110, May 3, 1986.

Educating about AIDS, by J. Kosterlitz. NATIONAL JOURNAL 18:2044-2049, August 30, 1986.

Educating staff about AIDS eases hysteria. HOSPITALS 58(3):40+, February 1, 1984.

Education blitz necessary to reduce fear of AIDS, says infection control nurse, by J. Banning. CANADIAN NURSE 81(10):10, November 1985.

Education: a forum for attacking fear, by R. Wilkinson, et al. HOSPITALS 60(1): 60, January 1986.

Education For All Handicapped Children Act: coverage of children with acquired immune deficiency syndrome (AIDS), by N. L. Jones. JOURNAL OF LAW AND EDUCATION 15(2):195-206, Spring 1986.

Education still essential in fighting fear of AIDS. MEDICAL PRODUCTS SALES 16(11):77-78+, November 1985.

Explaining AIDS/Health Workers Forum, by L. Goldsmith. GAY COMMUNITY NEWS 10(27):3, January 29, 1983.

Fight against AIDS. First-level information and education. KRANKENPFLEGE. SOINS INFIRMIERS 78(10):49, October 1985.

Fighting AIDS with the facts and sound aseptic practice. OR MANAGER 1(9):1+, December 1985.

Free AIDS information materials available. PUBLIC HEALTH REPORTS 99:390, July-August 1984.

Frontlines: schools flunk on AIDS instruction, by Laura Fraser. MOTHER JONES 11:8, June 1986.

Grim ABC's of AIDS: a government report says children must be told about the disease, by B. Kantrowitz, et al. NEWSWEEK 108(18):66-67, November 3, 1986.

Health education and the politics of AIDS, by N. Freundenberg. HEALTH PAC BULLETIN 16(3):29-30, May-June 1985.

Health education: the advertising myth, by M. Pownall. NURSING TIMES 82(34): 19-20, August 20-26, 1986.

Learn more about AIDS, by M. Fearns. NURSING STANDARD 436:5, February 27, 1986.

Many groups offer AIDS information, support, by M. F. Goldsmith. JAMA 254: 2522-2523, November 8, 1985.

Mondale—need education—gay issues, by J. Ryan. GAY COMMUNITY NEWS 11(31):1, February 25, 1984.

New York AIDS Forum for black men/women, by C. Smith. GAY COMMUNITY NEWS 11(30):3, February 18, 1984.

NIJ offers a free manual on AIDS which every CJ Training Director needs. TRAIN-ING AIDS DIGEST 11(3):1-7, March 1986.

NIJ publishes huge manual on AIDS in prisons and jails. CORRECTIONS DIGEST 17(5):1-3, February 26, 1986; also in CRIME CONTROL DIGEST 20(8):3-5, February 24, 1986.

No need for panic about AIDS. Acquired immune deficiency disease, now frequent among male homosexuals in the United States, is not this century's black death. The most urgent need is to understand what is going on . NATURE 302(5911):749, April 28, 1983.

Public education on AIDS: not only the media's responsiblity, by W. Check. HASTINGS CENTER REPORT 15(4):27-31, August 1985.

Quandry of advice, by R. Bebout. BODY POLITIC 126:26, May 1986.

Questions and answers. CORPORATE SECURITY June 1986, p. 5.

Questions and answers about AIDS . . . patient education aid. PATIENT CARE 18(1):187-188, January 15, 1984.

Red Cross to educate public on AIDS: goal to dispel myths, by J. Cassell. PENNSYLVANIA NURSE 41(3):17, March 1986.

Red Cross to public: fight AIDS with facts, by L. Checco. PENNSYLVANIA NURSE 41(2):7-8, February 1986.

Request for proposals: NSA soliciting bids to produce three videotapes on AIDS. CRIME CONTROL DIGEST 20(43):10, October27, 1986.

Sound policies and expert advice are your best protection against AIDS, by K. McCormick. AMERICAN SCHOOL BOARD JOURNAL 173(5):36-37, May 1986.

Special challenge of AIDS: providing facts, calming fears. PUBLIC HEALTH REPORTS 99(1):99-100, January-February 1984.

Straight talk about AIDS. AMERICAN JOURNAL OF NURSING 83:1170, August 1983.

Test your knowledge of AIDS: a self-quiz, by F. R. Velazquez. MLO 18(8):40-42+, August 1986.

Time for honest talk on AIDS, by M. Adler. TIMES July 8, 1986, p. 10.

UC sets guide on AIDS. CALIFORNIA NURSE 79(2):1+, July-August 1983.

United States funds AIDS education, by N. Fain. ADVOCATE 422:26, June 11, 1985.

What (and why) you should know about . . . AIDS, by E. Copage. ESSENCE 14: 51, July 1983.

What you should know about AIDS, by K. McCoy. SEVENTEEN 44:24+, November 1985.

Your role as AIDS educator, by C. Hanks, et al. OHIO NURSES REVIEW 61(5): 12-13, May 1986.

GREAT BRITAIN
AIDS—a health education approach in West Glamorgan, by C. Griffiths, et al. HEALTH EDUCATION JOURNAL 44(4):172-173, 1985.

Students run Stanford AIDS education project, by G. Koskovich. ADVOCATE 455:17, September 16, 1985.

EDUCATION—POLITICS
What state officials should know about AIDS, by S. H. King. STATE GOVERN-MENT NEWS 28(9):8-10, September 1985.

EMPLOYMENT
AIDS and employment issues, by C. A. Klein. NURSE PRACTITIONER 11(5):87-88+, May 1986.

AIDS and SCBA: a threat to the fire service?, by W. D. Kipp. FIRE COMMAND 53:17, January 1986.

AIDS: the corporate response, by A. Halcrow. PERSONNEL JOURNAL 65(8): 123-127, August 1986.

AIDS costs: employers and insurers have reasons to fear expensive epidemic. WALL STREET JOURNAL 206:1+, October 18, 1985.

AIDS: an employer's dilemma, by R. S. Letchinger. PERSONNEL JOURNAL 63(2): 58-63, February 1986.

AIDS: here's how health experts and the legal community have viewed the disease: how some progressive businesses are working to enlighten their employees and peers; and what AIDS has meant to those living—and dying— with it. PERSONNEL JOURNAL 65:112-127, August 1986.

AIDS in the workplace. AAOHN JOURNAL 34(7):347-348, July 1986.

—. TRIAL 22(1):82-83, January 1986.

—, by A. Buzy. WASHINGTON NURSE 16(7):21, July-August 1986.

—, by A. Halcrow. PERSONNEL JOURNAL 64:10-11, October 1985.

—, by B. S. Murphy, et al. PERSONNEL JOURNAL 64:20+, December 1985.

—, by H. Z. Levine. PERSONNEL JOURNAL 63(3):56-64, March 1986.

—, by J. Aberth. MANAGEMENT REVIEW 74(12):49-51, December 1985.

—, by L. T. Duffie. CONTEMPORARY LONGTERM CARE 9(4):21-22, April 1986.

—, by M. Clark, et al. NEWSWEEK 108(1):62-63, July 7, 1986.

—, by P. G. Engel. INDUSTRY WEEK 228:28-30, February 3, 1986.

—, by W. L. Kandel. EMPLOYEE RELATIONS LAW JOURNAL 11(4):678-690, Spring 1986.

—: an epidemic fear. NATIONAL SAFETY AND HEALTH NEWS 133:34-39, January 1986.

AIDS in the workplace: facing the legal issues. CORPORATE SECURITY December 1985, pp. 2-3.

AIDS in the workplace. How to reach out to those among us, by C. Ryan. PUBLIC WELFARE 44(3):29-33, Summer 1986.

AIDS is no work environment risk with the correct protective measures, by I. Lernevall. VARDFACKET 9(7):22-23, April 4, 1985.

AIDS—meeting the challenge in the workplace. AAOHN JOURNAL 34(1):38-39+, January 1986 and 34(6)385-390, June 1986.

AIDS: minimising the occupational risks [editorial], by H. A. Waldron. BRITISH JOURNAL OF INDUSTRIAL MEDICINE 42(6):361-362, June 1985.

AIDS: no need for worry in the workplace [U.S. Public Health Service report]. NEWSWEEK 106:51, November 25, 1985.

AIDS on the job: bias appears hard to defend, by F. A. Silas. AMERICAN BAR ASSOCIATION JOURNAL 76:22, January 1, 1986.

AIDS poses employer dilemma, by S. Harris. AMERICAN HEALTH CARE ASSOCIATION JOURNAL 12(2):43-44, February 1986.

AIDS poses significant legal considerations for the work place, by C. D. Stromberg. BUSINESS AND HEALTH 3(3):50-51, January-February 1986.

AIDS: protecting members' rights and health, by C. Wcislo. LABOR NOTES 91:10, September 1986.

AIDS—risk and rights—response of the trade union movement, by D. Lowe. LAMP 42(6):26-28, August 1985.

AIDS tests workplace policies. MANAGEMENT WORLD 15:4, February 1986.

AIDS update: HTLV-III testing, immune globulins and employees with AIDS, by W. M. Valenti. INFECTION CONTROL 7(8):427-430, August 1986.

Black gay man battles United for job, by C. Smith. GAY COMMUNITY NEWS 12(23):3, December 22, 1984.

Corporate U.S. looks at workers with AIDS, by C. Harris. GAY COMMUNITY NEWS 13(32):3, March 1, 1986.

Decision backs phone employee, by K. Westheimer. GAY COMMUNITY NEWS 13(41):1, May 3, 1986.

Delta AIDS regulation takes quick nosedive, by D. Walter. ADVOCATE 416:14, March 19, 1985.

Delta backs down on AIDS policy, by C. Guilfoy. GAY COMMUNITY NEWS 12(31):1, February 23, 1985.

Delta bumps PWA from flight, later apologizes, by P. Freiberg. ADVOCATE 455:14, September 16, 1985.

DOJ opinion fuels AIDS firing debate, by D. Burda. HOSPITALS 60(15):30, August 5, 1986.

Employer seeks insurance money/man fired /AIDS, by S. Ager. ADVOCATE 417:17, April 2, 1985.

Fear and loathing in the workplace: what managers can do about AIDS, by I. Pave. BUSINESS WEEK November 25, 1985, p. 126.

Few companies have special policies for AIDS. COMPENSATION AND BENE-FITS REVIEW 18:6-7, March-April 1986.

Firing employees who have AIDS brings on new round of legal action, by C. R. Goerth. OCCUPATIONAL HEALTH AND SAFETY 54(10):28, October 1985.

Firing of AIDS victims in Florida touches off national policy debate. CRIME CONTROL DIGEST 19(5):10, February 4, 1985.

Flight attendants with AIDS fight friendly skies, by S. Kulieke. ADVOCATE 411:9, January 8, 1985.

Florida county fired AIDS victims illegally. CIVIL LIBERTIES 356:3, Winter 1986.

Florida fires workers who have AIDS, by C. Guilfoy GAY COMUNITY NEWS 12(29):1, February 9, 1985.

Frighten and be fired. THE ECONOMIST 299:29-30, June 28, 1986.

Infection control and employee health: update on AIDS, by W. M. Valenti. INFEC-TION CONTROL 6(2):85-86, February 1985.

Living with AIDS on the job, by S. Koepp, et al. TIME 128(8):48, August 25, 1986.

Phone Company fires Boston PWA, by J. Kiely. GAY COMMUNITY NEWS 14(4):1, August 3, 1986.

Recent developments: public health and employment issues generated by the AIDS crisis, by M. J. Lazzo, et al. WASHBURN LAW JOURNAL 25(3):505-535, 1986.

Stress management on the job, by C. Dunphy. WASHINGTON NURSE 15(2):9, February 1985.

Survey search: four studies of employers' responses to AIDS. HEALTH COST MANAGEMENT 3(1):7-15+, January-February 1986.

Twenty questions about AIDS in the workplace, by F. E. Kuzmits, et al. BUSI-NESS HORIZONS 29:36-42, July-August 1986.

United employee reinstated, by C. Guilfoy. GAY COMMUNITY NEWS 12(30):3, February 16, 1985.

United not friendly to workers with AIDS, by C. Guilfoy. GAY COMMUNITY NEWS 12(21):1, December 8, 1984.

What should employers do when AIDS strikes the work force?, by M. Braxton. RISK MANAGEMENT 33:64+, February 1986.

Workers and AIDS—Uncle Sam speaks [Public Health Service guidelines]. US NEWS & WORLD REPORT 99:14, November 25, 1985.

Workers who get AIDS: combating coworkers' fears, by B. McCormick. HOSPITALS 60(13):110, July 5, 1986.

EMPLOYMENT—ETHICS
AIDS in the workplace: the ethical ramifications, by R. Bayer, et al. BUSINESS AND HEALTH 3(3):30-34, January-February 1986.

EMPLOYMENT—TESTING
AIDS becoming an issue in pre-employment screening, other ways. SECURITY LETTER 16(16):1, August 15, 1986.

United takes AIDS testing stance. OUT 4(5):3, March 1986.

EPIDEMIOLOGY
Acquired immune deficiency syndrome. Epidemiologic update, by J. N. Kuritsky, et al. MINNESOTA MEDICINE 67(1):37-41, January 1984.

Acquired immune deficiency syndrome—epidemiology and etiology, by I. Ahmed. JOURNAL OF THE PAKISTAN MEDICAL ASSOCIATION 35(9): 269-271, September 1985.

Acquired immunodeficiency syndrome: epidemiology, virology, and immunology, by A. Weiss, et al. ANNUAL REVIEW OF MEDICINE 36:545-562, 1985.

Acquired immune deficiency syndrome: a new epidemic, by J. P. Griffin. CRITICAL CARE NURSE 3(2):21-24+, April-May 1983; also in HOME HEALTHCARE NURSE 1(1):17-18+, September-October 1983.

AIDS could plague the world, or not. NEW SCIENTIST 105:5, February 14, 1985.

AIDS: epidemiology update, by J. A. Bennett. AMERICAN JOURNAL OF NURSING 85(9):968-972, September 1984.

AIDS—etiology, pathogenesis and epidemiology, by A. Vaheri, et al. DUODECIM 102(7):396-403, 1986.

AIDS: a growing 'pandemic'?, by M. Clark. NEWSWEEK 105:71, April 29, 1985.

AIDS: homosexual plague, by M. Stanton Evans. HUMAN EVENTS 43:15, August 6, 1983.

AIDS—a new plague?, by I. Braveny. EUROPEAN JOURNAL OF CLINICAL MICROBIOLOGY 2(3):183-185, June 1983.

AIDS pandemic, by R. C. Gallo. DUODECIM 102(7):391-393, 1986.

AIDS: the plague that lays waste at noon, by J. E. Fortunato. WITNESS 68(9):6-9, September 1985.

379

AIDS: profile of an epidemic, by A. Cohen. GAY COMMUNITY NEWS 12(9):8, September 15, 1984.

AIDS—report of an epidemiological seminar, by J. M. Klopper. SOUTH AFRICAN MEDICAL JOURNAL 68(8):617-618, October 12, 1985.

AIDS: the twentieth century plague, by J. G. Bellows. COMPREHENSIVE THERAPY 11(11):3, November 1985.

Anatomy of an epidemic, by J. Lieberson. THE NEW YORK REVIEW OF BOOKS 30:17-22, August 18, 1983.

Another scourge plagues Africa, by J. Drury. LISTENER June 5, 1986, p. 10.

Battling a deadly new epidemic, by C. Wallis. TIME 121:53-55, March 28,1 983.

Containing the AIDS epidemic [letter]. JAMA 254(15):2059-2060.

Cries of plague for mysterious AIDS, by L. Wainwright. LIFE MAGAZINE 6:7, July 1983.

Current AIDS epidemiology and potential for nosocomial transmission, by D. K. Henderson. TOPICS IN CLINICAL NURSING 6(2):1-22, July 1984.

Description of an emerging epidemic: the acquired immunodeficiency syndrome (AIDS), by F. M. Muggia. GAN TO KAGAKU RYOHO 10(12):2429-2441, December 1983.

Despite increase in cases, AIDS not a public risk. WORLD HEALTH March 1984, p. 30-31.

Epidemic acquired immune deficiency syndrome: epidemiologic evidence for a transmissible agent, by D. P. Francis, et al. JOURNAL OF THE NATIONAL CANCER INSTITUTE 71(1):1-4, July 1983.

Epidemic of the acquired immunodeficiency syndrome: a need for economic and social planning, by J. E. Groopman, et al. ANNALS OF INTERNAL MEDICINE 99(2):259-261, August 1983.

Epidemic of acquired immunodeficiency syndrome triggering psychotic-psychogenic reactions, by M. Assel, et al. HAREFUAH 108(9):431-433, May 1, 1985.

Epidemic of the 80s: AIDS, by D. M. Price, et al. CANCER NURSING 7(4):283-290, August 1984.

Epidemic proportions, by J. Fishman. GAY COMMUNITY NEWS 11(7):5, September 3, 1983.

Epidemic spreads, by C. Doyle. OBSERVER May 1, 1983, p. 27.

Epidemiologic and clinical aspects of the acquired immune deficiency syndrome, by T. C. Quinn. DELAWARE MEDICAL JOURNAL 56(12):721-730, December 1984.

Epidemiologic and pathogenic aspects of AIDS, by G. Melino, et al. CLINICA TERAPEUTICA 112(6):537-546, March 31, 1985.

Epidemiologic aspects of acquired immunodeficiency syndrome (AIDS) in the United States: cases associated with transfusions, by J. W. Curran, et al. PROGRESS IN CLINICAL AND BIOLOGICAL RESEARCH 182:259-269, 1985.

Epidemiologic designs for the study of acquired immunodeficiency disease: options and obstacles, by A. S. Monto. REVIEWS OF INFECTIOUS DISEASES 6(5):720-725, September-October 1984.

Epidemiologic lessons from viral hepatitis B, by W. T. London. ANNALS OF THE NEW YORK ACADEMY OF SCIENCES 437:100-105, 1984.

Epidemiological and clinical aspects of acquired immunodeficiency syndrome, by N. Clumeck. REVUE MEDICALE DE BRUXELLES 7(4):271-274, April 1986.

Epidemiological investigation of AIDS, by K. H. Mayer. HASTINGS CENTER RE-PORT 15(Suppl. 12-15), August 1985.

Epidemiological trends of AIDS in the United States,by J. W. Curran, et al. CANCER RESEARCH 45(Suppl. 9):4602s-4604s, September 1985.

Epidemiology and prevention of the acquired immunodeficiency syndrome, by J. W. Curran. ANNALS OF INTERNAL MEDICINE 103(5):657-662, November 1985.

Epidemiology of acquired immune deficiency syndrome. FRONTIERS OF RADIATION THERAPY AND ONCOLOGY 2(2):67-72, 1984.

—, by H. W. Haverkos. ANTIBIOTIC CHEMOTHERAPY 32:18-26, 1983; also in DIAGNOSTIC IMMUNOLOGY 2(2)67-72, 1984.

—, by M. McEvoy. JOURNAL OF THE ROYAL SOCIETY OF HEALTH 105(3):88-90, June 1985.

—, by T. A. Peterman, et al. EPIDEMIOLOGIC REVIEWS 7:1-21, 1985.

—, by T. J. Spira, et al. PROGRESS IN ALLERGY 37:65-80, 1986.

Epidemiology of the Acquired Immunodeficiency Syndrome in intravenous drug abusers, by J. P. Koplan, et al. ADVANCES IN ALCOHOL AND SUB-STANCE ABUSE 5(1 & 2):13-23, Fall 1985-Winter 1986.

Epidemiology of the acquired immunodeficiency syndrome (AIDS) in the United States, by J. R. Allen. SEMINARS IN ONCOLOGY 11(1):4-11, March 1984.

Epidemiology of AIDS [letter], by G. Hunsmann, et al. KLINISCHE WOCHEN-SCHRIFT 63(13):616-617, July 1, 1985.

—, by J. L'age-Stehr. OFFENTLICHE GESUNDHEITSWESEN 47(8):343-348, August 1985.

—, by J. Seale. ZEITSCHRIFT FUR HAUTKRANKHEITEN 59(8):525-528, April 15, 1984.

—, by L. Pamnany. MEDICAL JOURNAL OF AUSTRALIA 140(8):506, April 14, 1984.

—, by W. R. Dowdle. PUBLIC HEALTH REPORTS 98(4):308-312, July-August 1983.

Epidemiology of AIDS: current status and future prospects, by J. W. Curran, et al. SCIENCE 229(4720):1352-1357, September 27, 1985.

Epidemiology of human lymphotrophic retroviruses: an overview, by W. A. Blattner, et al. CANCER RESEARCH 45(Suppl. 9):4598s-4601s, September 1985.

Epidemiology of human T-lymphotropic virus type III and the risk of the acquired immunodeficiency syndrome, by W. A. Blattner, et al. ANNALS OF INTERNAL MEDICINE 103(5):665-670, November 1985.

Grim projections for AIDS epidemic, by D. M. Barnes. SCIENCE 232:1589-1590, June 27, 1986.

Health: AIDS: epidemic of the '80s, by M. Horosko. DANCE MAGAZINE 60:76-78+, January 1986.

Is there an "AIDS plague"? HUMAN EVENTS 45:6+, May 18, 1985.

Journal of a plague year, by D. K. Mano. NATIONAL REVIEW 35:836-837, July 8, 1983.

Medical anthropology and the AIDS epidemic: a case study in San Francisco, by N. Spencer. URBAN ANTHROPOLOGY 12:141-159, Summer 1983.

Modern-day plague: the AIDS virus has found a niche in our society, and it acts as if it wants to stay, by J. Kaplan. NATURAL HISTORY 95:28+, February 1986.

Nasty new epidemic, by J. Seligmann. NEWSWEEK 105:72-73, February 4, 1985.

New epidemic: immune deficiency, opportunistic infections, and Kaposi's sarcoma, by J. Allen, et al. AMERICAN JOURNAL OF NURSING 82:1718-1722, November 1982.

Opportunistic infections in patients with AIDS: clues to the epidemiology of AIDS and the relative virulence of pathogens, by M. J. Blaser, et al. REVIEWS OF INFECTIOUS DISEASES 8(1):21-30, January-February 1986.

Outbreak of an acquired immunodeficiency syndrome associated with opportunistic infections and Kaposi's sarcoma in male homosexuals: an epidemic with forensic implications, by M. L. Taff, et al. AMERICAN JOURNAL OF FORENSIC MEDICINE AND PATHOLOGY 3(3):259-264, September 1982.

Plague and panic, by R. Porter. NEW SOCIETY December 12, 1986, p. 11-13.

Plague in the shadows, by F. Bentayou. CLEVELAND MAGAZINE 14:90+, November 1985.

Plague on all their homes? THE ECONOMIST 297:27-28+, November 2, 1985.

Plague years (I), by D. Black. ROLLING STONE March 28, 1985, p. 48-50+.

— (II), by D. Black. ROLLING STONE April 25, 1985, p. 35-36+.

Threat of AIDS widening to the general public [interview with J. Curran]. US NEWS & WORLD REPORT 99:66, August 5, 1985.

Trying to live with the AIDS plague, by P. Blauner. NEW YORK 18:51-52, June 17, 1985.

Widening scourge: lethal new ailment claims another group of victims, by J. E. Bishop. WALL STREET JOURNAL 200:1+, December 10, 1982.

—: part 2, epidemiology, by P. A. Selwyn. HOSPITAL PRACTICE 21(6):127-129+, June 15, 1986.

AFRICA
African form of the acquired immunodeficiency syndrome. Epidemiological reflections [letter], by D. Vittecoq, et al. PRESSE MEDICALE 13(42):2584, November 24, 1984.

EUROPE
Epidemiology of AIDS in Europe. EUROPEAN JOURNAL OF CANCER AND CLINICAL ONCOLOGY 20(2):157-164, February 1984.

FRANCE
Acquired immunodeficiency syndrome: epidemiological data in France and throughout the world, by J. B. Brunet, et al. BULLETIN DE L'ACADEMIE NATIONALE DE MEDECINE 168(1-2):278-281, January-February 1984.; also in REVUE FRANCAISE DE TRANSFUSION ET IMMUNO-HEMATOLOGIE 27(4):437-443, September 1984.

Epidemiological aspects of acquired immune deficiency syndrome in France, by J. B. Brunet, et al. ANNALS OF THE NEW YORK ACADEMY OF SCIENCES 437:334-339, 1984.

GREAT BRITAIN
Acquired immune deficiency syndrome and epidemic of infection with human immunodeficiency virus: costs of care and prevention in an inner London district, by A. M. Johnson, et al. BRITISH MEDICAL JOURNAL 293 (6545):489-492, August 23, 1986.

EPIDEMIOLOGY—ANIMALS
Epidemiologic aspects of an outbreak of acquired immunodeficiency in rhesus monkeys (Macaca mulatta), by N. W. Lerche, et al. LABORATORY ANIMAL SCIENCE 34(2):146-150, April 1984.

EPIDEMIOLOGY—ATTITUDES
Scism over the scourge, by C. Longley. TIMES December 23, 1986, p. 12.

Scourge spreads panic: as AIDS reaches around the globe, governments are galvanized into action, by M. S. Serrill, et al. TIME 126(17):50-52, October 28, 1985.

EPIDEMIOLOGY—CHILDREN
Epidemiology of pediatric acquired immunodeficiency syndrome, by A. Rubin-

stein, et al. CLINICAL IMMUNOLOGY AND IMMUNOPATHOLOGY 40(1):115-121, July 1986.

EPIDEMIOLOGY—HOMOSEXUALS

Plague on homosexuals? THE ECONOMIST 294:16-17, March 2, 1985.

ETHICS

Ethical dilemmas in caring for patients with the acquired immunodeficiency syndrome, by R. Steinbrook, et al. ANNALS OF INTERNAL MEDICINE 103(5):787-790, November 1985.

Ethical issues in AIDS research, by M. A. Grodin, et al. QRB12(10):347-352, October 1986.

Ethical issues in the care of patients with AIDS, by M. Cooke. QRB 12(10):343-346, October 1986.

Ethics and AIDS, by A. Jonsen. BULLETIN OF THE AMERICAN COLLEGE OF SURGEONS 70(6):16-18, June 1985.

Ethics of AIDS, by G. Allen. MACLEAN'S 98:44-48, November 18, 1985.

Ethics of AIDS research, by C. Patto. GAY COMMUNITY NEWS 12(33):8, March 9, 1985.

Ethics of a new disease, by G. Copello. ST LUKE'S JOURNAL OF THEOLOGY 29(2):91-95, March 1986.

How should we handle the ethical questions regarding information to donors and patients and the practical implications regarding deferral of donors and handling of donated blood in the event of introducing a screening test for HTLV-III as in order to prevent transmission of AIDS by blood transfusion?, by J. R. Bove, et al. VOX SANGUINIS 49(3):234-239, 1985.

'Looking' for the cause of AIDS [editorial], by D. Zucker-Franklin. NEW ENGLAND JOURNAL OF MEDICINE 308(14):837-838, April 7, 1983.

Moral, ethical, and legal aspects of infection control, by B. Parent. AMERICAN JOURNAL OF INFECTION CONTROL 13(6):278-280, December 1985.

ETIOLOGY

Acquired immune deficiency syndrome. Hypotheses on the etiology, by T. A. Kelly. MEDICAL HYPOTHESES 14(4):347-351, August 1984.

Acquired immune deficiency syndrome. A new disease of infectious origin? PRESSE MEDICALE 12(39):2453-2456, November 5, 1983.

Acquired immune deficiency syndrome: the causative agent and the evolving perspective, by P. J. Fischinger. CURRENT PROBLEMS IN CANCER 9(1):1-39, January 1985.

Acquired immune deficiency syndrome—epidemiology and etiology, by I. Ahmed. JOURNAL OF THE PAKISTAN MEDICAL ASSOCIATION 35(9): 269-271, September 1985.

Acquired immune deficiency syndrome (AIDS) HTLV-III/LAV; the causal agent and modes of transmission, by A. Smithies. HEALTH BULLETIN 44(4):234-238, July 1986.

Acquired immune deficiency syndrome (AIDS): speculations about its etiology and comparative immunology, by J. G. Sinkovics, et al. REVIEWS OF INFECTIOUS DISEASES 6(5):745-760, September-October 1984.

Acquired immune deficiency syndrome: viral infections and etiology, by D. Armstrong. PROGRESS IN MEDICAL VIROLOGY 30:1-13, 1984.

Acquired immunodeficiency syndrome: a discussion of etiologic hypotheses, by J. A. Sonnabend, et al. AIDS RESEARCH 1(2):107-120, 1983-1984.

AIDS and oncogenesis, by J. L. Ziegler. FRONTIERS OF RADIATION THERAPY AND ONCOLOGY 19:99-104, 1985.

AIDS breakthrough: cause of disease probably identified. CHEMICAL & ENGINEERING NEWS 62:6-7, April 30, 1984.

AIDS: the culprit found? DISCOVER 5:10-11, June 1984.

AIDS—etiology, pathogenesis and epidemiology, by A. Vaheri, et al. DUODECIM 102(7):396-403, 1986.

AIDS: is Retrovirus HTLV-III the causative agent?, by H. G. Thiele. IMMUNITAT UND INFEKTION 12(5):256-258, October 1984.

AIDS: research clues for etiology, by C. Lopez. SURVEY OF IMMUNOLOGIC RESEARCH 3(2-3):229-232, 1984.

AIDS—this century's catastrophe? 1. Origin and cause, by B. A. Ostby. SYKE-PLEIEN 73(5):12-17+, March 7, 1986.

Allogeneic leukocytes as a possible factor in induction of AIDS in homosexual men [letter], by G. M. Shearer. NEW ENGLAND JOURNAL OF MEDICINE 308(4):223-224, January 27, 1983.

Breakdown of P.G.E. 1 synthesis is responsible for the acquired immunodeficiency syndrome, by S. G. Marcus. MEDICAL HYPOTHESES 15(1):39-46, September 1984.

Can essential fatty acid deficiency predispose to AIDS? [letter], by U. N. Das. CANADIAN MEDICAL ASSOCIATION JOURNAL 132(8):900+, April 15, 1985.

Causation of AIDs revealed, by J. E. Groopman. NATURE 308:769, April 26, 1984.

Cause of acquired immune deficiency syndrome [letter]. JAMA 251(3):341-342, January 20, 1984.

Cause of acquired immunodeficiency syndrome—is it known?, by D. P. Francis, et al. PROGRESS IN CLINICAL AND BIOLOGICAL RESEARCH 182:277-283, 1985.

Cause of AIDS? [editorial]. LANCET 1(8385):1053-1054, May 12, 1984.

Concerning the genesis of AIDS, by J. Morgan. MEDICAL HYPOTHESES 13(1):29-30, January 1984 and 13(4):357-358, April 1984.

Considerations in searching for the cause of AIDS, by J. Teas. ANNALS OF THE NEW YORK ACADEMY OF SCIENCES 437:270-272, 1984.

Do human retroviruses cause multiple sclerosis? NEW SCIENTIST 108:30, December 5, 1985.

Dr. Robert Gallo, the medical sleuth who tracked the cause of AIDS, now tries to find the cure, by M. Brower. PEOPLE 22:49-50+, September 24, 1984.

Emergence of acquired immune deficiency syndrome, by K. R. McBride. QUEEN'S QUARTERLY 92(3):530-534, 1985.

Etiology of acquired immunodeficiency syndrome, by Kh. Odiseev. VUTRESHNI BOLESTI 24(2):7-9, 1985.

Etiology of AIDS [letter], by A. J. Ammann. JAMA 252(10):1281-1282, September 14, 1984.

Etiology of AIDS, by J. A. Sonnabend. AIDS RESEARCH 1(1):1-12, 1983-1984.

Etiology of AIDS: biological and biochemical characteristics of HTLV-III, by P. D. Markham, et al. ADVANCES IN EXPERIMENTAL MEDICINE AND BIOLOGY 187:13-34, 1985.

Family of human T-lymphotropic leukemia viruses: HTLV-I as the cause of adult T cell leukemia and HTLV-III as the cause of acquired immunodeficincy syndrome, by F. Wong-Staal, et al. BLOOD 65(2):253-263, February 1985.

Four theories about a mystery disease. ROLLING STONE p.20, February 3, 1983.

Fungal agent: microbiologist sites plant mould as possible cause of AIDS, by A. Lukits. EQUINOX 3:18, March-April 1984.

Gay plague, by M. VerMeulen. NEW YORK 15:52-54+, May 31, 1982.

Group-fantasy origins of AIDS, by C. G. Schmidt. JOURNAL OF PSYCHO-HISTORY 12(1):37-78, 1984.

Hot on the trail of the cause and cure of AIDS, by O. Timbs, et al. TIMES April 6, 1984, p. 11.

HTLV/III and the etiology of AIDS, by R. C. Gallo, et al. PROGRESS IN ALLERGY 37:1-45, 1986.

Human T-lymphotropic retrovirus (HTLV-III) as the cause of the acquired immuno-deficiency syndrome, by R. C. Gallo, et al. ANNALS OF INTERNAL MEDICINE 103(5):679-689, November 1985.

Immunologically oriented concept of the genesis of acquired immunodeficiency syndrome, by A. S. Mark, et al. MEDICAL HYPOTHESES 17(2):167-173, June 1985.

Is AIDS caused by a neurotropic virus? [letter], by W. Radding. JAMA 253(19): 2831, May 17, 1985.

Is human T-cell leukemia virus the cause of acquired immunodeficiency syndrome?, by Z. M. Rupniewska. ACTA HAEMATOLOGICA POLONICA 15(1-2):69-77, January-June 1984.

Isobutyl nitrite and AIDS. AMERICAN FAMILY PHYSICIAN 32:272, November 1985.

Lessening fears: contact does not spread AIDS, by C. Wallis, et al. TIME 127(7): 90, February 17, 1986.

Leukemia virus variant fingered as likely AIDS cause, by D. Franklin. SCIENCE NEWS 125:260, April 28, 1984.

Likely explanation of the etiology of AIDS, by S. Iwarson. NORDISK MEDICIN 99(8-9):200-201, 1984.

Multifactorial model for the development of AIDS in homosexual men, by J. A. Sonnabend, et al. ANNALS OF THE NEW YORK ACADEMY OF SCIENCES 437:177-183, 1984.

Origin of AIDS: a deadly visitor from our biological past, by M. Whitby. LISTENER March 27, 1986, p. 7-8.

Origin of the human AIDS virus [letter], by R. C. Desrosiers. NATURE 319(6056): 728, Feburary 27-March 5, 1986; 319:728, February 27, 1986.

Possible cause of acquired immune deficiency syndrome (AIDS) and other new diseases,by R. de Long. MEDICAL HYPOTHESES 13(4):395-397, April 1984.

Possible origin of human AIDS [letter], by P. K. Lewin. CANADIAN MEDICAL ASSOCIATION JOURNAL 132(10):1110, May 15, 1985.

—,by I. D. Mackie, et al. CANADIAN MEDICAL ASSOCIATION JOURNAL 133(6): 547-548, September 15, 1985.

Probable cause of AIDS identified. BIOSCIENCE 34:413, July-August 1984.

Prodromal syndromes in AIDS, by U. Mathur-Wagh, et al. ANNALS OF THE NEW YORK ACADEMY OF SCIENCES 437:184-191, 1984.

Recreational drugs: relationship to AIDS, by J. J. Goedert. ANNALS OF THE NEW YORK ACADEMY OF SCIENCES 437:192-199, 1984.

Scrofula followed by AIDS [letter], by A. Marchiando. EAR, NOSE, AND THROAT JOURNAL 63(3):197-198, March 1984.

387

Searching for the cause of the acquired immune deficiency syndrome, by R. D. Leavitt. EUROPEAN JOURNAL OF CLINICAL MICROBIOLOGY 3(1):79-84, February 1984.

Searching for the cause of AIDS: is HTLV the culprit?, by R. Bock. BIOSCIENCE 33:619-620, November 1983.

Seroepidemiological evidence for HTLV-III infection as the primary etiologic factor for acquired immunodeficiency syndrome, by M. G. Sarngadharan, et al. PROGRESS IN CLINICAL AND BIOLOGICAL RESEARCH 182:309-327, 1985.

Strong new candidate for AIDS agent [news], by J. L. Marx. SCIENCE 224(4648):475-477, May 4, 1984.

Tracing the origin of AIDS. NEW SCIENTIST 105:20, February 28, 1985.

—, by J. Seligmann. NEWSWEEK 103:101-102, May 7, 1984.

Transglutaminase: co-factor in aetiology of AIDS? [letter], by R. J. Ablin. LANCET 1(8432):813-814, April 6, 1985.

Viral etiologies of AIDS: facts and hypotheses, by F. Brun-Vézinet, et al. REVUE FRANÇAISE DE TRANSFUSION ET IMMUNO-HEMATOLOGIE 27(4):445-454, September 1984.

Virus identified as possible cause of simian AIDS, by R. Cowen. RESEARCH RE-SOURCES REPORTER 8(4):1-6, April 1984.

Why can't they find the agent causing AIDS? THE ECONOMIST 288:77, September 3, 1983.

AFRICA
Africa and the origin of AIDS [news], by C. Norman. SCIENCE 230(4730): 1141, December 6, 1985.

CANADA
Gay plague is invading Alberta, by J. Westaway. ALBERTA REPORT 10:33, February 21, 1983.

ETIOLOGY—HEMOPHILIACS
Coincidental appearance of LAV/HTLV-III antibodies in hemophiliacs and the on-set of the AIDS epidemic, by B. L. Evatt, et al. NEW ENGLAND JOURNAL OF MEDICINE 312(8):483-486, February 21, 1985.

ETIOLOGY—INFANTS—HAITI
Malnutrition and concomitant herpesvirus infection as a possible cause of immunodeficiency syndrome in Haitian infants [letter], by J. Goudsmit. NEW ENGLAND JOURNAL OF MEDICINE 309(9):554-555, September 1, 1983.

FAMILY
Acquired immunodeficiency syndrome in the wife of a hemophiliac, by A. E. Pitchenik, et al. ANNALS OF INTERNAL MEDICINE 100(1):62-65, January 1984.

AIDS in the family, by M. Blackwell. ESSENCE 16:54-56+, August 1985.

AIDS in the family [case of L. Nassaney], by S. Haller. PEOPLE 24:136-138+, November 18, 1985.

AIDS: the story of one family's pain, by J. McBride. US 3:38+, August 26, 1985.

AIDS: what it does to a family, by K. Barrett. LADIES' HOME JOURNAL 100:98+, November 1983.

Family gives refuge to a son who has AIDS, by J. Seligman,et al. NEWSWEEK 106:24, August 12, 1985.

Immunologic study of spouses and siblings of asymptomatic hemophiliacs, by M. V. Ragni, et al. SCANDINAVIAN JOURNAL OF HAEMATOLOGY. SUPPLE-MENTUM 40:373, 1984.

Iniquity of the fathers upon the children [editorial], by M. E. Alberts. JOURNAL OF THE IOWA MEDICAL SOCIETY 73(6):226, June 1983.

Living with AIDS: a mother's perspective, by B. Peabody. AMERICAN JOURNAL OF NURSING 86(1):45-46, January 1986.

Mothers of infants with the acquired immunodeficiency syndrome: evidence for both symptomatic and assymptomatic carriers, by G. B. Scott, et al. JAMA 253:363-366, January 18, 1985.

My husband has AIDS, by G. Blair. FAMILY CIRCLE 99:52+, February 11, 1986.

On Trojan horses and surrogate mothers [letter], by J. Kolins. NEW ENGLAND JOURNAL OF MEDICINE 311(1):53-54, July 5, 1984.

AFRICA
    Cluster of HTLV-III/LAV infection in an African family [letter], by T. Jonckheer, et al. LANCET 1(8425):400-401, February 16, 1985.

FAMILY—TRANSMISSION
    Postnatal transmission of AIDS-associated retrovirus from mother to infant, by J. B. Ziegler, et al. LANCET 1(8434):896-898, April 20, 1985.

FETUS
    Unborn babies and the AIDS virus, by W. Cooper. GUARDIAN February 4, 1986, p. 10.

GENETICS
    Aberrations in chromosomes of peripheral lymphocytes of male homosexuals predisposed to acquired immune deficiency syndrome, by G. Manolov, et al. AIDS RESEARCH 1(3):157-162, 1983-1984.

    Acquired immune deficiency syndrome . . . impact of heredity and East Indian sexual practices, by S. Khanna. NURSING JOURNAL OF INDIA 76(4):91-93, April 1985.

    Acquired immune deficiency syndrome: a study on impact of heredity, by S. Khanna. NURSING JOURNAL OF INDIA 76(4):91-93, April 1985.

    AIDS: does the control gene pX poison the lymphocytes?, by G. Miketta. FORT-SCHRITTE DER MEDIZIN 102(47-48):64-65, December 20, 1984.

Anti-genes attack AIDS virus, by J. Green. NEW SCIENTIST 111:23, August 28, 1986.

Association of the pX gene product of human T-cell leukemia virus type I with nucleus, by T. Kiyokawa, et al. VIROLOGY 147:462-465, December 1985.

Burkitt cell acute lymphoblastic leukemia with partial expression of T-cell markers and subclonal chromosome abnormalities in a man with acquired immunodeficiency syndrome, by M. Berman, et al. CANCER GENETICS AND CYTO-GENETICS 16(4):341-347, April 15, 1985.

Challenges and opportunities in biotechnology, by L. R. Overby. PROGRESS IN CLINICAL AND BIOLOGICAL RESEARCH 182:425-443, 1985.

Characterization of envelope and core structural gene products of HTLV-III with sera from AIDS patients, by W. G. Robey, et al. SCIENCE 228(4699):593-595, May 3, 1985.

Characterization of gp41 as the transmembrane protein coded by the HTLV-III/LAV envelope gene, by F. diM. Veronese, et al. SCIENCE 229:1402-1405, September 27, 1985.

Chromatin pattern and DNA content in acquired immune deficiency syndrome (AIDS): indicators of viral infection revealed by DNA image cytometry [letter], by W. Auffermann, et al. ANALYTICAL AND QUANTITATIVE CYTOLOGY 6(4):293-294, December 1984.

Chromosome aberrations in peripheral lymphocytes of male homosexuals, by G. Manolov, et al. CANCER GENETICS AND CYTOGENETICS 18(4):337-350, December 1985.

Cloning of AIDS genes brings vaccine near, by I. Anderson. NEW SCIENTIST 103:8, September 13, 1984.

Congenital rubella syndrome and diabetes: a review of epidemiologic, generic, and immunologic factors, by K. A. Shaver, et al. AMERICAN ANNALS OF THE DEAF 130:526-532, December 1985.

Deregulation of interleukin-2 receptor gene expression in HTLV-I-induced adult T-cell leukemia, by M. Krönke, et al. SCIENCE 228:1215-1217, June 7, 1985.

Determination of a splice acceptor site of pX gene in HTLV-I infected cells, by T. Okamoto, et al. VIROLOGY 143:636-639, June 1985.

Envelope gene-derived recombinant peptide in the serodiagnosis of human i immunodeficiency virus infection [letter], by T. F. Schulz, et al. LANCET 2(8498):111-112, July 12, 1986.

Expression in Escherichia coli of open reading frame gene segments of HTLV-III, by N. T. Chang, et al. SCIENCE 228:93-96, April 5, 1985.

Expression of the *pX* gene of HTLV-I: general splicing mechanism in the HTLV family, by M. Seiki, et al. SCIENCE 228:1532-1534, June 28, 1985.

Gene-cloners may have treatment for AIDS, by N. Heneson. NEW SCIENTIST 98:843, June 23, 1983.

Genes of AIDS-linked virus cloned, by D. Franklin. SCIENCE NEWS 126:164, September 15, 1984.

Genes of likely AIDS virus cloned. CHEMICAL AND ENGINEERING NEWS 62:7, September 17, 1984.

Genetic variation in HTLV-III/LAV over time in patients with AIDS or at risk for AIDS, by B. H. Hahn, et al. SCIENCE 232:1548-1553, June 20, 1986.

Genomic diversity of the acquired immune deficiency syndrome virus HTLV-III: different viruses exhibit greatest divergence in their envelope genes, by B. H. Hahn, et al. PROCEEDINGS OF THE NATIONAL ACADEMY OF SCI-ENCES USA 82(14):4813-4817, July 1985.

Genomic diversity of human T-lymphotropic virus type III (HTLV-III), by F. Wong-Staal, et al. SCIENCE 229:759-762, August 23, 1985.

Genomic heterogeneity of AIDS retroviral isolates from North America and Zaire, by S. Benn, et al. SCIENCE 230:949-951, November 22, 1985.

Homology of genome of AIDS-associated virus with genomes of human T-cell leukemia viruses, by S. K. Arya, et al. SCIENCE 225:927-930, August 31, 1984.

HTLV-III env gene products synthesized in E. coli are recognized by antibodies present in the sera of AIDS patients, by R. Crowl, et al. CELL 41(3):979-986, July 1985.

Identification of the gene responsible for human T-cell leukaemia virus transcrip-tional regulation, by A. J. Cann, et al. NATURE 318:571-574, December 12, 1985.

Infectious mutants of HTLV-III with changes in the 3' region and markedly reduced cytopathic effects, by A. G. Fisher, et al. SCIENCE 233(4764):655-659, August 8, 1986.

New HTLV-III/LAV protein encoded by a gene found in cytopathic retroviruses, by T. H. Lee, et al. SCIENCE 231:1546-1549, March 28, 1986.

Possible genetic susceptibility to the acquired immunodeficiency syndrome in hemophiliacs [letter], by L. Jacob, et al. ANNALS OF INTERNAL MEDICINE 104(1):130, January 1986.

Recombinant polypeptide from the endonuclease region of the acquired immune deficiency syndrome retrovirus polymerase (pol) gene detects serum anti-bodies in most infected individuals, by K. s. Steimer, et al JOURNALOF VIROLOGY 58(1):9-16, April 1986.

Replicative and cytopathic potential of HTLV-III/LAV with sor gene deletions, by J. Sodroski, et al. SCIENCE 231:1549-1553, March 28, 1986.

Researchers clone genes of AIDs-linked virus. BIOSCIENCE 34:685, December 1984.

Researchers discover new AIDS virus gene. CHEMICAL AND ENGINEERING NEWS 64:6, June 2, 1986.

Transfusion induced acquired immunodeficiency syndrome (AIDS) with Kaposi's sarcoma in a patient with congenital factor V deficiency, by E. Vélez-García, et al. AIDS RESEARCH 1(6):401-406, 1984-1985.

Vascular tumors produced by NIH/3T3 cells transfected with human AIDS Kaposi's sarcoma DNA, by S. C. Lo, et al. AMERICAN JOURNAL OF PATHOLOGY 118(1):7-13, January 1985.

x gene is essential for HTLV replication, by I. S. Y. Chen, et al. SCIENCE 229:54-58, July 5, 1985.

X-linked factor in acquired immunodeficiency syndrome? [letter], by M. F. Lyon, et al. LANCET 1(8327):768, Aprll 2, 1983.

AFRICA
Genetic variability of the AIDS virus: nucleotide sequence analysis of two isolates from African patients, by M. Alizon, et al. CELL 46(1):63-74, July 4, 1986.

INDIA
Acquired immune deficiency syndrome . . . impact of heredity and East Indian sexual practices, by S. Khanna. NURSING JOURNAL OF INDIA 76(4):91-93, April 1985.

HEALTH CARE WORKERS
See: HIGH RISK INDIVIDUALS—HEALTH CARE WORKERS

HETEROSEXUALS
Acquired immunodeficiency syndrome and female sexual partners of bisexual men [letter], by C. L. Soskolne. ANNALS OF INTERNAL MEDICINE 100(2): 312, February 1984.

Acquired immunodeficiency syndrome in a heterosexual population in Zaire, by P. Piot, et al. LANCET 2(8394):65-69, July 14, 1984.

AIDS goes hetero, by M. Castleman. MEDICAL SELF CARE 30:18, September 1985.

AIDS: the heterosexual connection. NEW SCIENTIST 100:644, December 1, 1983.

AIDS hits heterosexuals. SCIENCE NEWS 123:341, May 28, 1983.

AIDS: probing the heterosexual link. NEW SCIENTIST 107:15, September 19, 1985.

Anal intercourse as a possible factor in heterosexual transmission of HTLV-III to spouses of hemophiliacs [letter],by M. Melbye, et al. NEW ENGLAND JOURNAL OF MEDICINE 312(13):857, March 28, 1985.

Community-acquired opportunistic infections and defective cellular immunity in heterosexual drug abusers and homosexual men, by C. B. Small, et al. AMERICAN JOURNAL OF MEDICINE 74(3):433-441, March 1983.

Excessive concern about AIDS in two bisexual men, by G. P. Lippert. CANADIAN JOURNAL OF PSYCHIATRY 31(1):63-65, February 1986.

Female-to-male AIDS link found, by J. Silberner. SCIENCE NEWS 129:164-165, March 15, 1986.

Female-to-male transmission of AIDS [letter], by B. F. Polk. JAMA 254(22):3177-3178, December 13, 1985.

—, by H. W. Haverkos, et al. JAMA 254(8):1035-1036, August 23-30, 1985.

Female-to-male transmission of HTLV-III [letter]. JAMA 255(13):1703-1706, April 4, 1986.

Fever, cough, anal ulcer in a heterosexual man, by P. J. de Caprariis, et al. HOSPITAL PRACTICE 19(4):122+, April 1984.

Frequent transmission of HTLV-III among spouses of patients with AIDS-related complex and AIDS, by R. R. Redfield, et al. JAMA 253(11):1571-1573, March 15, 1985.

Heterosexual AIDS panic: a quear paradigm, by C. Patto. GAY COMMUNITY NEWS 12(29):3, February 9, 1985.

Heterosexual and homosexual patients with the acquired immunodeficiency syndrome. A comparison of surveillance, interview, and laboratory data, by M. E. Guinan, et al. ANNALS OF INTERNAL MEDICINE 100(2):213-218, February 1984.

Heterosexual partners: a large risk group for AIDS [letter], by D. C. Des Jarlais, et al. LANCET 2(8416):1346-1347, December 8, 1984.

Heterosexual promiscuity among African patients with AIDS [letter], by N. Clumck, et al. NEW ENGLAND JOURNAL OF MEDICINE 313(3):182, July 18, 1985.

Heterosexual transmission of AIDS [letter],by R. B. Pearce. JAMA 256(5):90-591, August 1, 1986.

Heterosexual transmission of the acquired immunodeficiency syndrome (AIDS), by M. Vogt, et al. DEUTSCHE MEDIZINISCHE WOCHENSCHRIFT 110(39): 1483-1487, September 27, 1985.

Heterosexual transmission of human T-lymphotropic virus type III/ lymphadenopathy-associated virus. JAMA 254:2051-2052, October 18, 1985; also in MMWR 34(37): 561-563, September 20, 1985.

Heterosexually acquired HTLV-III/LAV disease (AIDS-related complex and AIDS). Epidemiologic evidence for female-to-male transmission, by R. R. Redfield, et al. JAMA 254(15):2094-2096, October 18, 1985.

More heterosexual spread of HTLV-III virus seen , by M. F. Goldsmith. JAMA 253(23):3377-3379, June 21, 1985.

AFRICA
African AIDS points to heterosexual link, by O. Sattaur. NEW SCIENTIST 106:10-11, April 25, 1985.

AFRICA
AIDS in Africa: a heterosexuals' disease, by O. Sattaur. NEW SCIENTIST 104:9, October 18, 1984.

Female-to-male transmission of AIDS: a reexamination of the African sex ratio of cases [letter], by N. Padian, et al. JAMA 256(5):590, August 1, 1986.

HIGH RISK INDIVIDUALS
Acquired immunodeficiency syndrome in a patient with multiple risk factors, by S. B. Kalish, et al. ARCHIVES OF INTERNAL MEDICINE 143(12):2310-2311, December 1983.

Acquired immunodeficiency syndrome with Pneumocystis carinii pneumonia and Mycobacterium avium-intracellulare infection in a previously healthy patient with classic hemophilia. Clinical, immunologic, and virologic findings, by M. C. Poon, et al. ANNALS OF INTERNAL MEDICINE 98(3):287-290, March 1983.

AIDS and AIDS-related conditions: screening for populations at risk, by G. S. Carr, et al. NURSE PRACTITIONER 11(10):25-26+, October 1986.

AIDS and gay rights collide in closings, by Helquist, et al. IN THESE TIMES 8(41):1, October 31, 1984.

AIDS precautions for other high-risk groups? [letter], by R. S. Klein, et al. INFECTION CONTROL 5(10):466-467, October 1984.

AIDS risk category broadened. FDA CONSUMER 19(9):34, November 1985.

AIDS risk-group profiles in whites and members of minority groups [letter], by R. Bakeman, et al. NEW ENGLAND JOURNAL OF MEDICINE 315(3):191-192, July 17, 1986.

AIDS—risk groups, risk factors, measures. LAKARTIDNINGEN 82(11):958+, March 13, 1985.

Altered distribution of T-lymphocyte subpopulations in lymph nodes from patients with acquired immunodeficiency-like syndrome and hemophilia, by P. R. Meyer, et al. JOURNAL OF PEDIATRICS 103(3):407-410, September 1983.

CDC revises AIDS risk hierarchy, by Bisticas-Cocoves. GAY COMMUNITY NEWS 14(7):3, August 24, 1986.

Detection of two human T cell leukemia/lymphotropic viruses in cultured lymphocytes of a hemophiliac with acquired immunodeficiency syndrome, by E. L. Palmer, et al. JOURNAL OF INFECTIOUS DISEASES 151(3):559-563, March 1985.

Fourth case of AIDS in haemophiliac children in Seville [letter], by P. Noguerol, et al. LANCET 2(8409):986, October 27, 1984.

New AIDS risk groups identified. AMERICAN FAMILY PHYSICIAN 31:132, March 1985.

Patients at risk for AIDS-related opportunistic infection. Clinical manifestations and impaired gamma interferon production, by H. W. Murray, et al. NEW

ENGLAND JOURNAL OF MEDICINE 313(24):1504-1510, December 12, 1985.

Risk factor analysis among men referred for possible acquired immune deficiency syndrome, by G. R. Newell, et al. PREVENTIVE MEDICINE 14(1):81-91, January 1985.

Take no risks in AIDs care, by A. Fong, et al. RN 47:104, April 1984.

HAITI
Only homosexual Haitians, not all Haitians [letter], by R. Altema, et al. ANNALS OF INTERNAL MEDICINE 99(6):877-888, December 1983.

HIGH RISK INDIVIDUALS—DRUG ADDICTS
see: DRUG ABUSE

HIGH RISK INDIVIDUALS—HEALTH CARE WORKERS
Absence of antibodies to HTLV-III in health workers after hepatitis B vaccination, by J. L. Dienstag, et al. JAMA 254:1064-1066, August 23-30, 1985.

Acquired immune deficiency syndrome (AIDS): current status and implications for respiratory care practitioners, by T. J. Witek, Jr., et al. RESPIRATORY CARE 29(1):35-45, January 1984.

AIDS and health care in the laboratory, by N. Gilmore. CANADIAN JOURNAL OF MEDICAL TECHNOLOGY 47(4):267-268, December 1985.

AIDS and the health professions [editorial]. BRITISH MEDICAL JOURNAL 290 (6468):583-584, February 23, 1985.

—[letter]. BRITISH MEDICAL JOURNAL 290(6471):852-854, March 16, 1985.

AIDS and the home health care industry—Part II, by D. Borfitz. HOME HEALTH JOURNAL 4(12):27, December 1983.

AIDS and related conditions—infection control. Guidelines for health care workers involved in patient management and investigation, by R. Sher. SOUTH AFRICAN MEDICAL JOURNAL 68(12):843-848, December 7, 1985.

AIDS antibody in two health care workers. AMERICAN JOURNAL OF NURSING 85:1224-1225, November 1985.

AIDS: definition and guidelines for the health professional, by M. J. Healey, Jr. RADIOLOGIC TECHNOLOGY 57(3):233-235, January-February 1986.

AIDS . . . emergency care personnel, by M. F. Silverman. EMERGENCY: JOURNAL OF EMERGENCY SERVICES 18(5):44-46, May 1986.

AIDS exposure in health care workers, by R. D. Danielsen, et al. PHYSICIAN ASSISTANT 10(5):37-38+, May 1986.

AIDS: the impact on the health care worker, by G. I. Lusby. FRONTIERS OF RADIATION THERAPY AND ONCOLOGY 19:165-167, 1985.

AIDS, infectivity, and health care workers, by P. B. Kernoff. BRITISH JOURNAL OF HAEMATOLOGY 60(2):207-211, June 1985.

AIDS: an occupational hazard?, by R. L. Cooley, et al. JOURNAL OF THE AMERICAN DENTAL ASSOCIATION 107(1):28-31, July 1983.

AIDS: occupational implications for health care workers, by K. M. O'Laughlin, et al. OCCUPATIONAL HEALTH NURSING 32(3):134-136, March 1984.

AIDS precautions for clinical and laboratory staff. NEBRASKA NURSE 19(1):13, February 1986.

AIDS: precautions for health care employees, by S. Hecker. OREGON NURSE 49(1):34-35, February-March 1984.

AIDS: precautions for health care personnel, by D. LaCamera. TOPICS IN CLINICAL NURSING 6(2):45-52, July 1984.

AIDS: protecting the health care worker, by A. Beaufoy, et al. RNABC NEWS 17(6):18, November-December 1985.

AIDS references for health care providers, by S. Perdew. PENNSYLVANIA NURSE 41(3):16-17, March 1986.

AIDS risk found low for people with working with patients. CORRECTIONS DIGEST 16(10):6-7, May 8, 1985; also in CRIME CONTROL DIGEST 19(19):4, May 13, 1985.

AIDS toll on hospital workers, by M. Helquist. ADVOCATE 442:25, March 18, 1986.

Equipment handling risks from common and exotic pathogens, by J. Jeffries. JOURNAL OF STERILE SERVICE MANAGEMENT 3(6):4-8, April 1986.

Evaluation of the acquired immunodeficiency syndrome (AIDS) reported in health-care personnel—United States. MMWR 32(27):358-360, July 15, 1983.

Health care employees with AIDS—set policies before problems arise, by A. Dong. DIMENSIONS IN HEALTH SERVICE 63(6):43, September 1986.

Health care personnel and AIDS [letter], by L. Siegel. ARCHIVES OF INTERNAL MEDICINE 144(12):2431, December 1984.

Health care system under AIDS siege, by W. Curry. PHYSICIAN EXECUTIVE 12(2):4-6, March-April 1986.

Health care workers with AIDS [letter], by M. S. Cord. CANADIAN MEDICAL ASSOCIATION JOURNAL 134(6):573, March 15, 1986.

Health personnel may have gotten AIDS from patients. RN 48:6, December 1985.

Health worker's AIDS prompts investigation, by C. Guilfoy. GAY COMMUNITY NEWS 12(24):2, December 29, 1984.

Hospital workers with AIDS not in high-risk group. CORRECTIONS DIGEST 14(16):6-7, July 27, 1983.

Impact of AIDS on health care personnel, by K. H. Mayer. JOURNAL OF MEDICAL TECHNOLOGY 3(3):156-158+, March 1986.

Is it possible to contain the danger of AIDS to health care personnel?, by G. Melino, et al. NUOVI ANNALI D IGIENE E MICROBIOLOGIA 35(5):327-335, September-October 1984.

Is there a risk of AIDS for health care personnel?, by G. Melino, et al. NUOVI ANNALI D IGIENE E MICROBIOLOGIA 35(4):249-268, July-August 1984.

Is there risk to health care workers? AMERICAN JOURNAL OF NURSING 85:972, September 1985.

No special hazards caused by AIDS in the hospital. Information for hospital personnel, by A. Kümmel. KRANKENPFLEGE 39(9):312+, September 1985.

Precautions recommended in treating patients with AIDS [letter],by J. R. Masci, et al. NEW ENGLAND JOURNAL OF MEDICINE 308(3):156, January 20, 1983.

"Remember who you are" . . . working with people with AIDS, by C. Morrison. JEN 12(5):254-255, September-October 1986.

Risk of AIDS to health care workers [editorial], by A. M. Geddes. BRITISH MEDICAL JOURNAL 292(6522):711-722, March 15, 1986.

Risk of nosocomial infection with human T-cell lymphotropic virus type III/ lymphadenopathy-associated virus in a large cohort of intensively exposed health care workers,by D. K. Henderson, et al. ANNALS OF INTERNAL MEDICINE 104(5):644-647, May 1986.

Risk of seroconversion for acquired immunodeficiency syndrome (AIDS) in San Francisco health workers, by A. Moss, et al. JOURNAL OF OCCUPATIONAL MEDICINE 28(9):821-824, September 1986.

Survey of hospital personnel on the understanding of the acquired immunodeficiency syndrome, by W. M. Valenti, et al. AMERICAN JOURNAL OF INFECTION CONTROL 14(2):60-63, April 1986.

Update: evaluation of human T-lymphotropic virus type III/lymphadenopathy-associated virus infection in health-care personnel—United States. MMWR 34(38):575-578, September 27, 1985; also in CONNECTICUT MEDICINE 49(11):772, November 1985.

Update on acquired immune deficiency syndrome [letter], by L. Scarpinato. JOURNAL OF THE AMERICAN OSTEOPATHIC ASSOCIATION 82(7):452-454, March 1983.

Prospective evaluation of health-care workers exposed via parenteral or mucous-membrane routes to blood and body fluids of patients with acquired immuno-deficiency syndrome. JAMA 251(16):2071+, April 27, 1984; also in MMWR 33(13):181-182, April 6, 1984.

HIGH RISK INDIVIDUALS—HEALTH CARE WORKERS—INFECTION CONTROL
Protecting the health care worker . . . AIDS, by A. Beaufoy, et al. RNABC NEWS 17(6):18-19, November-December 1985.

HIGH RISK INDIVIDUALS—HEALTH CARE WORKERS—TRANSMISSION
Update: prospective evaluation of health-care workers exposed via the parenteral or mucous-membrane route to blood or body fluids from patients with acquired immunodeficiency syndrome—United States. MMWR 34(7):101-103, February 22, 1985.

HIGH RISK INDIVIDUALS—HEMOPHILIACS
Abnormalities of circulating lymphocyte subsets in haemophiliacs in an AIDS-free population, by R. Carr, et al. LANCET 1(8392):1431-1434, June 30, 1984.

Absence of Kaposi's sarcoma in hemophiliacs with the acquired immunode-ficiency syndrome [letter], by D. I. Cohn, et al. ANNALS OF INTERNAL MEDICINE 101(3): 401, September 1984.

Acid-labile alpha interferon. A possible immunodeficiency syndrome in hemo-philia, by M. E. Eyster, et al. NEW ENGLAND JOURNAL OF MEDICINE 309(10):583-586, September 8, 1983.

Acquired cellular immunodeficiency syndrome: 3 observations in hemophiliacs, by M. L. Miranda, et al. MEDICINA CLINICA 81(1):24-26, June 11, 1983.

Acquired immune deficiency syndrome (AIDS) in hemophiliacs: a hypothesis, by T. V. Shankey, et al. AIDS RESEARCH 1(1):83-90, 1983-1984.

Acquired immunodeficiency in haemophilia [editorial]. LANCET 1(8327):75, April 2, 1983.

Acquired-immunodeficiency-like syndrome in two haemophiliacs, by M. V. Ragni, et al. LANCET 1(8318):213-214, January 29, 1983.

Acquired immunodeficiency syndrome (AIDS) in hemophilia, by B. L. Evatt, et al. CLINICS IN LABORATORY MEDICINE 4(2):333-344, June 1984.

—, by J. M. Jason, et al. SCANDINAVIAN JOURNAL OF HAEMATOLOGY. SUPPLEMENTUM 40:349-356, 1984.

Acquired immunodeficiency syndrome (AIDS) in persons with hemophilia. JAMA 252:2679-2680, November 16, 1984.

Acquired immunodeficiency syndrome among patients with hemophilia. JAMA 250(24):3277-3278, December 23-30, 1983.

Acquired immunodeficiency syndrome and Mycobacterium avium-intracellulare bacteremia in a patient with hemophilia, by J. L. Elliott, et al. ANNALS OF INTERNAL MEDICINE 98(3):290-293, March 1983.

Acquired immunodeficiency syndrome and related syndromes in hemophiliacs: status throughout the world, by Y. Laurian, et al. REVUE FRANCAISE DE TRANSFUSION ET IMMUN0-HEMATOLOGIE 27(4):493-496, September 1984.

Acquired immunodeficiency syndrome and the treatment of hemophilia [letter], by V. Vicente, et al. MEDICINA CLINICA 81(5):231-232, July 16, 1983.

Acquired immunodeficiency syndrome, hepatitis, and haemophilia [editorial], by P. Jones. BRITISH MEDICAL JOURNAL 287(6407):1737-1738, December 10, 1983.

Acquired immunodeficiency syndrome in the child of a haemophiliac, by M. V. Ragni, et al. LANCET 1(8421):133-135, January 19, 1985.

Acquired immunodeficiency syndrome in a patient with hemophilia, by K. C. Davis, et al. ANNALS OF INTERNAL MEDICINE 98(3):284-286, March 1983.

Acquired immunodeficiency syndrome in patients with hemophilia, by B. L. Evatt, et al. ANNALS OF INTERNAL MEDICINE 100(4):499-504, April 1984.

Acquired immunodeficiency syndrome in persons with hemophilia, by P. H. Levine. ANNALS OF INTERNAL MEDICINE 103(5):723-726, November 1985.

Acquired immunodeficiency syndrome in the wife of a hemophiliac, by A. E. Pitchenik, et al. ANNALS OF INTERNAL MEDICINE 100(1):62-65, January 1984.

Aetiology of AIDS—antibodies to human T-cell leukaemia virus (type III) in haemophiliacs, by L. W. Kitchen, et al. NATURE 312(5992):367-369, November 22-28, 1984.

AIDS and haemophilia, by A. L. Bloom. BIOMEDICINE AND PHARMACO-THERAPY 39(7):355-365, 1985.

AIDS and hemophilia [letter], by R. J. Ablin, et al. AUSTRALIAN AND NEW ZEALAND JOURNAL OF MEDICINE 15(2):265-267, April 1985.

AIDS and haemophilia: morbidity and morality in a well defined population, by P. Jones, et al. BRITISH MEDICAL JOURNAL 291(6497):695-699, September 14, 1985.

AIDS and immunologic abnormalities in European and American hemophiliacs, by D. Green. SCANDINAVIAN JOURNAL OF HAEMATOLOGY. SUPPLE-MENTUM 40:367-369, 1984.

AIDS and preventive treatment in hemophilia [editorial], by J. F. Desforges. NEW ENGLAND JOURNAL OF MEDICINE 308(2):94-95, January 13, 1983.

AIDS' impact on hemophiliacs, by M. Helquist. ADVOCATE 451:23, July 22, 1986.

AIDS in a patient with hemophilia receiving mainly cryoprecipitate, by H. C. Gerstein, et al. CANADIAN MEDICAL ASSOCIATION JOURNAL 131(1):45-47, July 1, 1984.

AIDS surveillance in haemophilia, by H. M. Daly, et al. BRITISH JOURNAL OF HAEMATOLOGY 59(2):383-390, February 1985.

Anal intercourse as a possible factor in heterosexual transmission of HTLV-III to spouses of hemophiliacs [letter],by M. Melbye, et al. NEW ENGLAND JOURNAL OF MEDICINE 312(13):857, March 28, 1985.

Analysis of cytomegalovirus and Epstein-Barr virus antibody respOnses in treated hemophiliacs; implications for the study of acquired immune deficiency syndrome, by S. H. Cheeseman, et al. JAMA 252:83-85, July 6, 1984.

Blood transfusion, haemophilia, and AIDS [editorial]. LANCET 2(8417-8418): 1433-1435, December 22, 1984.

Changing patterns of acquired immunodeficiency syndrome in hemophilia patients—United States. MMWR 34(17):241-243, May 3, 1985; also in JAMA 253:2954-2955, May 24-31, 1985.

Development and early natural history of HTLV-III antibodies in persons with hemophilia, by M. E. Eyster, et al. JAMA 253:2219-2223, April 19, 1985.

Evidence for a 1980 HTLV-III infection in a currently asymptomatic B hemophiliac in Italy, by O. E. Vernier, et al. JAMA 254:1449-1450, September 20, 1985.

Haemophilia and AIDS [letter], by A. G. Bird, et al. LANCET 1(8421):162-163, January 19, 1985.

—, by A. L. Bloom. LANCET 1(8424):336, February 9, 1985.

Haemophilia, blood products and AIDS [letter], by D. G. Woodfield. NEW ZEALAND MEDICAL JOURNAL 97(748):51-52, January 25, 1984.

—, by E. W. Berry, et al. NEW ZEALAND MEDICAL JOURNAL 96(744):986, November 23, 1983.

Haemophilia, blood transfusion, and the AIDS virus [editorial], by J. S. Lilleyman. ARCHIVES OF DISEASE IN CHILDHOOD 61(2):105-107, February 1986.

Haemophiliac sues over AIDS. NEW SCIENTIST 102:5, May 17, 1984.

Hemophilia, AIDS and hepatitis. AMERICAN FAMILY PHYSICIAN 29:313-314, May 1984.

Hemophilia and acquired immune deficiency syndrome, by P. H. Levine, et al. PROGRESS IN CLINICAL AND BIOLOGICAL RESEARCH 182:287-296, 1985.

Hemophilia and the acquired immune deficiency syndrome (AIDS), by E. J. Sjamsoedin-Visser, et al. NEDERLANDS TIJDSCHRIFT VOOR GENEESKUNDE 127(23):1008-1009, June 4, 1983.

Hemophilia and the acquired immunodeficiency syndrome [letter], by O. D. Ratnoff, et al. ANNALS OF INTERNAL MEDICINE 102(3):412, March 1985.

Hemophilia and AIDS. AMERICAN FAMILY PHYSICIAN 31:318, January 1985.

Hemophilia and thrombocytopenia in a patient with impaired cellular immunity. A case report, by U. Zeithuber, et al. BLUT 48(6):392-395, June 1984.

Hemophilia, hepatitis, and the acquired immunodeficiency syndrome, by G. C. White, 2d, et al. ANNALS OF INTERNAL MEDICINE 98(3):403-404, March 1983.

Hemophilus influenzae bactermia in a patient with immunodeficiency caused by HTLV-III [letter], by D. L. Garbowit, et al. NEW ENGLAND JOURNAL OF MEDICINE 314(1):56, January 2, 1986.

HTLV-I antibody status in hemophilia patients treated with factor concentrates prepared from U.S. plasma sources and in hemophilia patients with AIDS, by T. L. Chorba, et al. THROMBOSIS AND HAEMOSTASIS 53(2):180-182, April 22, 1985.

HTLV-III antibodies and immunological alterations in hemophilia patients, by E. Seifried, et al. KLINISCHE WOCHENSCHRIFT 64(3):115-124, February 3, 1986.

HTLV-III antibody status and immunological abnormalities in haemophilic patients [letter], by E. H. Moffat, et al. LANCET 1(8434):935, April 20, 1985.

HTLV-III/LAV antibody and immune status of household contacts and sexual partners of persons with hemophilia, by J. M. Jason, et al. JAMA 255:212-215, January 10, 1986.

HTLV-III/LAV-seronegative, virus-negative sexual partners and household contacts of hemophiliacs [letter], by T. McFadden, et al. JAMA 255(13): 1702, April 4, 1986.

Human T-cell leukemia virus in lymphocytes of two hemophiliacs with the acquired immunodeficiency syndrome, by E. L. Palmer, et al. ANNALS OF INTERNAL MEDICINE 101(3):293-297, September 1984.

Human T cell leukemia virus type III antibody, lymphadenopathy, and acquired immune deficiency syndrome in hemophiliac subjects. Results of a prospective study, by J. K. Kreiss, et al. AMERICAN JOURNAL OF MEDICINE 80(3):345-350, March 1986.

Human T-lymphotropic retrovirus type III/lymphadenopathy-associated virus antibody: association with hemopiliacs' immune status and blood component usage, by J. Jason, et al. JAMA 253:3409-3415, June 21, 1985.

Human T-lymphotropic virus type III (HTLV-III) infection in seronegative haemophiliacs after transfusion of factor VIII, by C. A. Ludlam, et al. LANCET 2(8449):233-236, August 3, 1985.

Immunologic evaluation of hemophilia patients and their wives. Relationships to the acquired immunodeficiency syndrome, by R. D. deShazo, et al. ANNALS OF INTERNAL MEDICINE 99(2):159-164, August 1983.

Immunologic studies in asymptomatic hemophilia patients. Relationship to acquired immune deficiency syndrome (AIDS), by A. Landay, et al. JOURNAL OF CLINICAL INVESTIGATION 71(5):1500-1504, May 1983.

Immunologic study of spouses and siblings of asymptomatic hemophiliacs, by M. V. Ragni, et al. SCANDINAVIAN JOURNAL OF HAEMATOLOGY. SUPPLE-MENTUM 40:373, 1984.

Isolation of new lymphotropic retrovirus from two siblings with haemophilia B, one with AIDS, by E. Vilmer, et al. LANCET 1(8380):753-757, April 7, 1984.

Lymphoma presenting as a traumatic hematoma in HTLV-III antibody-positive hemophiliac, by M. V. Ragni, et al. NEW ENGLAND JOURNAL OF MEDICINE 313:640, September 5, 1985.

Preventive measures against HTLV-III/LAV infections among hemophiliacs and their relatives, by S. A. Evensen, et al. TIDSSKRIFT FOR DEN NORSKE LAEGEFORENING 106(1):19-21, January 10, 1986.

Pseudomembranous necrotizing bronchial aspergillosis. A variant of invasive aspergillosis in a patient with hemophilia and acquired immune deficiency syndrome, by N. K. Pervez, et al. AMERICAN REVIEW OF RESPIRATORY DISEASE 131(6):961-963, June 1985.

T-lymphocyte subpopulations in hemophiliacs and other groups at risk for the acquired immunodeficiency syndrome (AIDS), by T. Gallart. MEDICINA CLINICA 83(12):492-496, October 20, 1984.

Update: acquired immunodeficiency syndrome (AIDS) among patients with hemophilia—United States. MMWR 32(47):613-615, December 2, 1983.

Update: acquired immunodeficiency syndrome (AIDS) in persons with hemophilia. MMWR 33(42):589-591, October 26, 1984.

Update on acquired immune deficiency syndrome (AIDS) among patients with hemophilia A. CONNECTICUT MEDICINE 47(3):169-170, March 1983; also in MMWR 31(48):644-646+, December 10, 1982.

What is role of factor VIII therapy in inducing helper suppressor ratio reversals in hemophiliacs? [news], by T. Hager. JAMA 249(24):3277, June 24, 1983.

AUSTRALIA
Absence of AIDS in haemophiliacs in Australia treated from an entirely voluntary blood donor system [letter], by K. A. Rickard, et al. LANCET 2(8340): 50-51, July 2, 1983.

EUROPE
Acquired immunodeficiency syndrome and other possible immunological disorders in European haemophiliacs, by A. L. Bloom. LANCET 1(8392): 1452-1455, June 30, 1984.

FRANCE
AIDS, related syndromes and hemophilia: the situation in France and studies in progress, by J. P. Allain. REVUE FRANCAISE DE TRANSFUSION ET IMMUNOHEMATOLOGIE 27(4):459-461, September 1984.

Case of AIDS in a hemophilia B patient in France , by C. Gazengel, et al. REVUE FRANCAISE DE TRANSFUSION ET IMMUNOHEMATOLOGIE 27(4):479-486, September 1984.

402

FRANCE
LAV/HTLV-III seroconversion and disease in hemophiliacs treated in France, by D. Mathez, et al. NEW ENGLAND JOURNAL OF MEDICINE 314:118-119, January 9, 1986.

JAPAN
Distribution of the level of antibody to AIDS-assocated virus (LAV) in sera from AIDS or AIDS-related complex and Japanese hemophiliacs infected with AIDS-associated virus, by H. Tsuchie, et al. MICROBIOLOGYAND IMMUNOLOGY 29(11):1083-1087, 1985.

Occurence of AIDS in hemophiliacs in Japan, by T. Abe, et al. SEMINARS IN THROMBOSIS AND HEMOSTASIS 11(4):352-356, October 1985.

SPAIN
Acquired immunodeficiency syndrome (AIDS) in hemophiliacs. Clinical course and post-mortem examination of the first cases described in Spain by M. A. Díaz-Torres, et al. MEDICINA CLINICA 82(19):866-867, May 19, 1984.

AIDS in haemophilia patients in Spain [letter], by E. Lissen, et al. LANCET 1(8331):992-993, April 30, 1983.

AIDS in haemophiliacs in Spain [letter], by M. Leal, et al. LANCET 1(8423): 275, February 2, 1985.

UNITED STATES
Acquired immunodeficiency syndrome among patients attending hemophilia treatment centers and mortality experience of hemophiliacs in the United States, by R. E. Johson, et al. AMERICAN JOURNAL OF EPIDEMIOLO-GY 121(6):797-810, June 1985.

—, by O. Tello. LANCET 2(8417-8418):1472, December 22, 1985.

HIGH RISK INDIVIDUALS—HEMOPHILIACS—TREATMENT
Some complications of the therapy of classic hemophilia, by O. D. Ratnoff. JOURNAL OF LABORATORY AND CLINICAL MEDICINE 103(5):653-659, May 1984.

HIGH RISK INDIVIDUALS—HOMOSEXUALS
Aberrations in chromosomes of peripheral lymphocytes of male homosexuals redisposed to acquired immune deficiency syndrome, by G. Manolov, et al. AIDS RESEARCH 1(3):157-162, 1983-1984.

Abnormal lymphocyte response to exogenous interleukin-2 in homosexuals with acquired immune deficiency syndrome (AIDS) and AIDS related complex (ARC), by J. L. Murray, et al. CLINICAL AND EXPERIMENTAL IMMUNOLOGY 60(1):25-30, April 1985.

Acquired immunodeficiency in homosexual men, by H. H. Handsfield. AJR 139(4):832- 833, October 1982.

Acquired immunodeficiency syndrome (AIDS) in a homosexual male with tuberculosis and medullary hyperplasia [letter], by T. Martín Jiménez, et al. MEDICINA CLINICA 85(1):39-40, June 1, 1985.

403

Acquired immunodeficiency syndrome in a cohort of homosexual men. A six-year follow-up study, by H. W. Jaffe, et al. ANNALS OF INTERNAL MEDICINE 103(2):210-214, August 1985.

AIDS and the gay community: between the specter and the promise of medicine, by R. Bayer. SOCIAL RESEARCH 52:581-606, Fall 1985.

AIDS and the gay community: the doctor's role in counseling [editorial], by G. Leach, et al. BRITISH MEDICAL JOURNAL 290(6468):583, February 23, 1985.

AIDS and the gay man [letter], by N. R. Schram. NEW ENGLAND JOURNAL OF MEDICINE 310(19):1266-1267, May 10, 1984.

AIDS and homosexual panic [letter], by M. Rapaport, et al. AMERICAN JOURNAL OF PSYCHIATRY 142(12):1516, December 1985.

AIDS and a new gay generation, by D. Sadownick. ADVOCATE 432:8, October 29, 1985.

AIDS and sexual behavior reported by gay men in San Francisco, by L. McKusick, et al. AMERICAN JOURNAL OF PUBLIC HEALTH 75(5):493-496, May 1985.

AIDS behind anti-gay scare campaign, by F. Feldman. MILITANT 47(25):6, July 8, 1983.

AIDS: the gay epidemic, by F. Fisher. NEW SCIENTIST 96:713-715, December 16, 1982.

AIDS gay mens health crisis, by P. Byron. GAY COMMUNITY NEWS 11(3):8, July 30, 1983.

AIDS—its implications for South African homosexuals and the mediating role of the medical practitioner, by G. Isaacs, et al. SOUTH AFRICAN MEDICAL JOURNAL 68(5):327-330, August 31, 1985.

AIDS surveillance and health education: use of previously described risk factors to identify high-risk homosexuals, by R. O. Valdiserri, et al. AMERICAN JOURNAL OF PUBLIC HEALTH 74(3):259-260, March 1984.

Being gay is a health hazard, by B. Vinocur. THE SATURDAY EVENING POST 254:26+, October 1982.

Cryptosporidiosis in homosexual men, by R. Soave, et al. ANNALS OF INTERNAL MEDICINE 100(4):504-511, April 1984.

Gay business: the impact of AIDS, by P. Freiberg. ADVOCATE 437:10, January 7, 1986.

Gay cancer isn't gay anymore, by M. Horosko. DANCE MAGAZINE 57:72, February 1983.

Gay compromise syndrome, by J. McGlynn. NURSING MIRROR 156(12):20-22, March 23, 1983.

Gay crisis, crisis for all [editorial]. GUARDIAN 38(39):22, July 9, 1986.

Gay group sets 1984 for global actn, by D. France. GAY COMMUNITY NEWS 11(5):3, August 13, 1983.

Gay health organizations, by S. Kleinberg. ADVOCATE 3(98):24, July 10, 1984.

Gay perspective on AIDS, by R. Evans. NORTHWEST PASSAGE 23(11):10, June 1983.

Gay rights groups divided over HHS investigation, by D. Walter. ADVOCATE 449:17, June 24, 1986.

Gay rights victories . . . and setbacks. OFF OUR BACKS 17(8):10, August 1986.

Gay times and diseases, by Patrick J. Buchanan, et al. AMERICAN SPECTATOR 17:15+, August 1984.

Groups at high risk for AIDS [letter], by J. E. Ollé-Goig, et al. NEW ENGLAND JOURNAL OF MEDICINE 311(2):124, July 12, 1984.

Heckler finally meets with gay leaders, by D. Walter. ADVOCATE 411:11, January 8, 1985.

Heterosexual and homosexual patients with the acquired immunodeficiency syndrome. A comparison of surveillance, interview, and laboratory data, by M. E. Guinan, et al. ANNALS OF INTERNAL MEDICINE 100(2):213-218, February 1984.

Homosexual plague strikes new victims, by E. Keerdoja. NEWSWEEK 100:10, August 23, 1982.

Homosexuality: kick and kickback [editorial], by J. L. Fletcher. SOUTHERN MEDICAL JOURNAL 77(2):149-150, Febraury 1984.

Idiopathic thrombocytopenic purpura in homosexual men, by S. Karpatkin. ANNALS OF THE NEW YORK ACADEMY OF SCIENCES 237:58-64, 1984.

New gay renaissance: a change on the wind, by T. Hopkinson. RFD 47:29, Summer 1986.

Personal you: gay cancer isn't just gay anymore, by M. Horosko. DANCE MAGAZINE 57:72, February 1983.

Playing gay, by H. Johnson. US 3:55+, November 18, 1985.

Pursuing the 'gay plague,' by S. Riley. MACLEAN'S 95:20d, November 22, 1982.

Queer across the nation. GAY COMMUNITY NEWS 11(50):9, July 7, 1984.

Queers demand AIDS &, by S. Hyde. GAY COMMUNITY NEWS 12(33):6, March 9, 1985.

'Reasonable' discrimination against homosexuals [letter],by H. Warter. HOSPITAL PRACTICE 18(12):16+, December 1983.

Roy Cohn: a queer-baiter dies, by M. Bronski. GAY COMMUNITY NEWS 14(5):3, August 10, 1986.

Studies in homosexual patients with and without lymphadenopathy. Relationships to the acquired immune deficiency syndrome,by R. D. deShazo, et al. ARCHIVES OF INTERNAL MEDICINE 144(6):1153-1158, June 1984.

Understanding the gay reality, by J. S. Spong. CHRISTIAN CENTURY 103(3):62-63, January 22, 1986.

HIGH RISK INDIVIDUALS—HOMOSEXUALS—POLITICS
Queers go after Buckley, picket National Review, by B. Gelbert. GAY COMMUNITY NEWS 13(42):1, May 17, 1986.

HIGH RISK INDIVIDUALS—HOMOSEXUALS—WOMEN
Lesbians and AIDS, by J. Sky. LESBIAN INSIDER INSIGHTER INCITER 2(1):6, February 1986.

Lesbians/gays, by J. Hall. NORTHWEST PASSAGE 25(10):10, June 1985.

Lesbians take aim against AIDS, by K. Mcalister. LONGEST REVOLUTION 7:6, August 1983.

HIGH RISK INDIVIDUALS—LABORATORY WORKERS
AIDS and the laboratory worker [editorial], by A. Kellner. AMERICAN JOURNAL OF MEDICAL TECHNOLOGY 49(5):290, May 1983.

AIDS: are laboratorians at risk? MLO 17(4):9, April 1985.

AIDS—current concepts and implications for blood transfusion services and nursing staff, by C. J. Burrell, et al. AUSTRALIAN NURSES JOURNAL 14(7): 45-47, February 1985.

AIDS—a potential laboratory hazard?, by C. H. Collins. GAZETTE OF THE INSTITUTE OF MEDICAL LABORATORY SCIENCES 27(8):341-342, August 1983.

Guidelines for working with blood in Stockholm County. JORDEMODERN 99(6): 216-217, June 1986.

Impact of A.I.D.S. on laboratory medicine, by R. P. Rennie. CANADIAN JOURNAL OF MEDICAL TECHNOLOGY 47(4):266, December 1985.

Lab assistants at AIDS syposium, by I Lernevall. VARDFACKET 10(6):10, March 20, 1986.

Safe handling of laboratory samples from AIDS patients, by J. G. Roberts. IMLS GAZETTE 29(11):564-566, November 1985.

Safety in the forensic immunology laboratory, by W. W. Bond. CRIME LABORATORY DIGEST 13(1):15-24, January 1986.

What every laboratorian should know about AIDS part 1, by S. L. Haber. MLO 17(11):32-38, November 1985.

— part 2, by S. L. Haber. MLO 17(12):55-59, December 1985.

AIDS—current concepts and implications for blood transfusion services and nursing staff, by C. J. Burrell, et al. AUSTRALIAN NURSES JOURNAL 14(7): 45-47, February 1985.

AIDS epidemic: dilemmas facing nurse managers . . . how the University of California San Diego Medical Center has responded, by M. M. Jackson, et al. NURSING ECONOMICS 4(3):109-116, May-June 1986.

No cases of AIDS among nurses, by M. Allen. CANADIAN NURSE 81:13, May 1985.

Nurses and AIDS: do we know the facts?, by R. R. Caddace, et al. CALIFORNIA NURSE 82(4):4-5, May 1986.

Nurses most likely to have AIDS exposure, CDC data show. HOSPITAL EM-PLOYEE HEALTH 3(9):118-119, September 1984.

Nurses quit rather than treat AIDS patient. RN 46:11, August 1983.

Nursing the AIDS patient, by B. Bolding, et al. RNABC NEWS 17(6):15-17, November-December 1985.

Nursing AIDS: situations vacant, by J. Sherman. NURSING TIMES 81(49):19-20, December 4-10, 1985.

Nursing care. AIDS: real solution to keep AIDS away from sensationalism, by C. Nielsen, et al. SYGEPLEJERSKEN 85(43):18-21, October 23, 1985.

Nursing staff and AIDS: caution yes—fear no, by R. von Blarer. KRANKEN-PFLEGE. SOINS INFIRMIERS 79(1):23-26, January 1986.

Possible AIDS transmission is concern to nurses. AMERICAN FAMILY PHYSI-CIAN 28:17, July 1983.

Should nurses be told if a patient has AIDS? RN 48:10, November 1985.

To let nurses work in ignorance is despicable says College. Nurses not told patients had AIDS. NURSING STANDARD 380:1, January 17, 1985.

HIGH RISK INDIVIDUALS—NURSES—ATTITUDES
Nurses' attitudes regarding acquired immunodeficiency syndrome (AIDS), by P. Reed, et al. NURSING FORUM 21(4):153-156, 1984.

Nurses' fear of AIDS exceeds the risks. RN 47:13-14, January 1984.

HIGH RISK INDIVIDUALS—NURSES—SCHOOLS
Nurses urged to allay fears of AIDS in schools, by P. Cohen. NURSING STANDARD 418:1, October 10, 1984.

HIGH RISK INDIVIDUALS—TREATMENT
Thymosin in the early diagnosis and treatment of high risk homosexuals and hemophiliacs with AIDS-like immune dysfunction, by P. H. Naylor, et al. ANNALS OF THE NEW YORK ACADEMY OF SCIENCES 437:88-99, 1984.

Thymosin in the staging and treatment of HTLV-III positive homosexuals and hemophiliacs with AIDS-related immune dysfunction, by A. L. Goldstein, et al.

ADVANCES IN EXPERIMENTAL MEDICINE AND BIOLOGY 187:129-140, 1985.

HISTORY
Acquired immune deficiency syndrome: the past as prologue, by J. W. Curran, et al. ANNALS OF INTERNAL MEDICINE 98(3):401-403, March 1983.

AIDS in 1949? [letter], by G. Williams, et al. LANCET 2(8359):1136, November 12, 1983.

AIDS in 1968 [letter], by M. H. Witte, et al. JAMA 251(20):2657, May 25, 1984.

AIDS: what is now known: part 1, history and immunovirology, by P. A. Selwyn. HOSPITAL PRACTICE 21(5):67-76, May 15, 1986.

14th century black death type scenario, by P. Forbes. NEW STATESMAN November 7, 1986, p. 6-8.

History of an epidemic, by R. Bazell. THE NEW REPUBLIC 189:14-15+, August 1, 1983.

AFRICA
Evidence for exposure to HTLV-III in Uganda before 1973, by W. C. Saxinger, et al. SCIENCE 227:1036-1038, March 1, 1985.

EGYPT
AIDS: a disease of ancient Egypt? [letter], by R. J. Ablin, et al. NEW YORK STATE JOURNAL OF MEDICINE 85(5):200-201, May 1985.

HOMOSEXUALS
See: HIGH RISK INDIVIDUALS—HOMOSEXUALS

HOSPICE
See: CARE—HOSPICE

HOSPITALS
See: CARE—HOSPITAL, TRANSMISSION, TREATMENT

HOTLINES
See: AIDS—HOTLINES

IMMUNOLOGY
Abnormal lymphocyte response to exogenous interleukin-2 in homosexuals with acquired immune deficiency syndrome (AIDS) and AIDS related complex (ARC), by J. L. Murray, et al. CLINICAL AND EXPERIMENTAL IMMUNOLOGY 60(1):25-30, April 1985.

Abnormalities of B-cell activation and immunoregulation in patients with the acquired immunodeficiency syndrome, by H. C. Lane, et al. NEW ENGLAND JOURNAL OF MEDICINE 309(8):453-458, August 25, 1983.

Absence of antibodies against prostaglandins in sera of AIDS patients, by R. A. Knazek, et al. AIDS RESEARCH 2(2):73-76, Spring 1986.

Absence of antibodies to HTLV-III in health workers after hepatitis B vaccination, by J. L. Dienstag, et al. JAMA 254:1064-1066, August 23-30, 1985.

Absence of detectable IgM antibody during cytomegalovirus disease in patients with AIDS [letter], by J. Dylewski, et al. NEW ENGLAND JOURNAL OF MEDICINE 309(8):493, August 25, 1983.

Acquired immune deficiency syndrome: is disseminated aspergillosis predictive of underlying cellular immune deficiency?, by A. Schaffner. JOURNAL OF INFECTIOUS DISEASES 149(5):828-829, May 1984.

Acquired immune deficiency syndrome (AIDS): speculations about its etiology and comparative immunology, by J. G. Sinkovics, et al. REVIEWS OF INFECTIOUS DISEASES 6(5):745-760, September-October 1984.

Acquired immune dysfunction in homosexual men: immunologic profiles, by A. J. Ammann, et al. CLINICAL IMMUNOLOGY AND IMMUNOPATHOLOGY 27(3): 315-325, June 1983.

Acquired immunodeficiency syndrome and related syndromes. Critical analysis of biological tests of cell-mediated immunity, by J. C. Gluckman, et al. PRESSE MEDICALE 13(32):1937-1941, September 22, 1984.

Acquired immunodeficiency syndrome: epidemiology, virology, and immunology, by A. Weiss, et al. ANNUAL REVIEW OF MEDICINE 36:545-562, 1985.

Acquired immunodeficiency syndrome: state of immunological dysfunction in focus [editorial], by M. L. Santaella. BOLETIN-ASOCIACION MEDICA DE PUERTO RICO 75(9):391-392, September 1983.

Acquired neutrophil dysfunction in male homosexuals with the acquired immuno-deficiency syndrome [letter], by G. J. Ras, et al. SOUTH AFRICAN MEDICAL JOURNAL 65(22):873-874, June 2, 1984.

Activation of the AIDS retrovirus promoter by the cellular transcription factor, Sp1, by K. A. Jones, et al. SCIENCE 232:755-759, May 9, 1986.

Activation of monocyte-mediated tumoricidal activity in patients with acquired immunodeficiency syndrome, by E. S. Kleinerman, et al. JOURNAL OF CLINICAL ONCOLOGY 3(7):1005-1012, July 1985.

Activation of tissue macrophages from AIDS patients: in vitro response of AIDS alveolar macrophages to lymphokines and interferon-gamma, by H. W. Murray, et al. JOURNAL OF IMMUNOLOGY 135(4):2374-2377, October 1985.

Acute encephalopathy coincident with seroconversion for anti-HTLV-III, by C. A. Carne, et al. LANCET 2(8466):1206-1208, November 30, 1985.

AIDS and the current significance of serological studies for the presence of antibodies against LAV/HTLV III, by W. J. van Gestel. NEDERLANDS TIJDSCHRIFT VOOR GENEESKUNDE 129(5):233-234, February 2, 1985.

AIDS and organ transplantation [letter], by R. R. Bailey, et al. NEW ZEALAND MEDICAL JOURNAL 98(779):402-403, May 22, 1985.

AIDS: counting the bodies and the antibodies. NEW SCIENTIST 108:20, October 3, 1985.

AIDS: how the immune system works. CALIFORNIA NURSE 82(4):11, May 1986.

AIDS immunopathologic network a tangled web [news]. HOSPITAL PRACTICE 19(1):39-40+, January 1984.

AIDS-like immunologic alterations in clinically unaffected drug users, by G. Fiorini, et al. AMERICAN JOURNAL OF CLINICAL PATHOLOGY 84(3):354-357, September 1985.

AIDS—an immunologic reevaluation, by M. Seligmann, et al. NEW ENGLAND JOURNAL OF MEDICINE 311(20):1286-1292, November 15, 1984.

AIDS: the neurological connection, by J. Meer. PSYCHOLOGY TODAY 20:10, January 1986.

AIDS: a noncommunicable cofactor [letter], by R. J. Ablin. JAMA 253(23):3398-3399, June 21, 1985.

AIDS: some unanswered questions . . . human host's response to foreign organisms, by C. Carneiro. MASSACHUSETTS NURSE 54(3):1+, March 1985.

Analysis of T cell subsets in different clinical subgroups of patients with the acquired immune deficiency syndrome. Comparison with the 'classic' form of Kaposi's sarcoma, by A. Mittelman, et al. AMERICAN JOURNAL OF MEDICINE 78(6, Part 1):951-956, June 1985.

Antibodies against human T-cell leukemia virus (HTLV) in male homosexuals with acquired immunodeficiency syndrome, by R. Kurth, et al. MUENCHENER MEDIZINISCHE WOCHENSCHRIFT 125(48):1118-1123, December 2, 1983.

Antibodies against human T-cell leukemia virus type III in acquired immunodeficiency syndrome and persistent lymphadenopathy, by D. Wernicke, et al. DEUTSCHE MEDIZINISCHE WOCHENSCHRIFT 109(45):1709-1711, November 9, 1984.

Antibodies reactive with human T-lymphotropic retroviruses (HTLV-III) in the serum of patients with AIDS, by M. G. Sarngadharan,e t al. SCIENCE 224(4648):506-508, May 4, 1984.

Antibodies to the AIDS virus: methods of detection and clinical significance, by B. Hirschel. THERAPEUTISCHE UMSCHAU 43(2):128-132, February 1986.

Antibodies to cell membrane antigens associated with human T-cell leukemia virus in patients with AIDS, by M. Essex, et al. SCIENCE 220(4599):859-862, May 20, 1983.

Antibodies to the core protein of lymphadenopathy-associated virus (LAV) in patients with AIDS, by V. S. Kalyanaraman, et al. SCIENCE 225(4659):321-323, July 20, 1984.

Antibodies to HTLV-III and the lymphadenopathy syndrome in multitransfused betathalassemia patients, by M. DeMartino, et al. VOX SANGUINIS 49(3):230-233, 1985.

Antibodies to human T-lymphotropic virus type III and development of the acquired immunodeficiency syndrome in homosexual men presenting with immune throm- bocytopenia, by D. I. Abrams, et al. ANNALS OF INTERNAL MEDICINE 104(1):47-50, January 1986.

Antibodies to human T lymphotropic virus type III demonstrated by a dot immuno-binding assay, by G. Biberfeld, et al. SCANDINAVIAN JOURNAL OF IMMU-NOLOGY 21(3):289-292, March 1985.

Antibodies to human T-lymphotropic virus type III (HTLV-III) in saliva of acquired immunodeficiency syndrome (AIDS) patients and in persons at risk for AIDS, by D. W. Archibald, et al. BLOOD 67(3):831-834, March 1986.

Antibodies to a retrovirus etiologically associated with acquired immnodeficiency syndrome (AIDS) in populations with increased incidences of the syndrome. JAMA 252:608-609, August 3, 1984; also in MMWR 33(27):377-379, July 13, 1984.

Antibodies to simian T-lymphotropic retovirus type III in African green monkeys and recognition of STLV-III viral proteins by AIDS and related sera, by P. J. Kanki, et al. LANCET 1(8441):1330-1332, June 8, 1985.

Antibody finding may hasten AIDS vaccine. CHEMICAL ENGINEERING NEWS 64:5-6, May 26, 1986.

Antibody seronegative human T-lymphotropic virus type III (HTLV-III)-infected patients with acquired immunodeficiency syndrome or related disorders, by J. E. Groopman, et al. BLOOD 66(3):742-744, September 1985.

Antibody to HTLV-III in blood donors in central Africa [letter], by P. Van de Perre, et al. LANCET 1(8424):336-337, February 9, 1985.

Antibody to lymphadenopathy-associated virus in AIDS [letter], by D. D. Ho, et al. NEW ENGLAND JOURNAL OF MEDICINE 312(10):649-650, March 7, 1985.

Anti-HTLV-III antibody incidence [letter], by J. Goldbaum. MEDICAL JOURNAL OF AUSTRALIA 143(6):261-262, September 16, 1985.

Anti-lymphocyte antibodies in patients with the acquired immune deficiency syn-drome, by B. Dorsett, et al. AMERICAN JOURNAL OF MEDICINE 78(4):621-626, April 1985.

Autoantibodies to T cells in adult and pediatric AIDS, by A. Rubinstein, et al. ANNALS OF THE NEW YORK ACADEMY OF SCIENCES 437:508-512, 1984.

Autoimmunity and AIDS, by M. Helquist. ADVOCATE 438:22, January 21, 1986.

Autologous mixed lymphocyte reaction in man. XIV. Deficiency of the autologous mixed lymphocyte reaction in acquired immune deficiency syndrome (AIDS) and AIDS related complex (ARC). In vitro effect of purified interleukin-1 and i interleukin-2, by S. Gupta, et al. CLINICAL AND EXPERIMENTAL IMMU-NOLOGY 58(2):395-401, November 1984.

B-cell immunodeficiency in acquired immune deficiency syndrome, by A. J. Ammann, et al. JAMA 251(11):1447-1449, March 16, 1984.

411

Biological and biochemical characterization of a cloned Leu-3-cell surviving infection with the acquired immune deficiency syndrome retrovirus, by T. M. Folks, et al. JOURNAL OF EXPERIMENTAL MEDICINE 164(1):280-290, July 1, 1986.

Bronchoalveolar lavage cells and proteins in patients with the acquired immuno-deficiency syndrome. An immunologic analysis, by K. R. Young, Jr., et al. ANNALS OF INTERNAL MEDICINE 103(4):522-533, October 1985.

Cell-mediated immune responses in AIDS [letter],by E. Buimovici-Klein,et al. NEW ENGLAND JOURNAL OF MEDICINE 311(5):328-329, August 2, 1984.

Cell-mediated immunity to cytomegalovirus (CMV) and herpes simplex virus (HSV) antigens in the acquired immune deficiency syndrome: interleukin-1 and interleukin-2 modify in vitro responses, by J. F. Sheridan, et al. JOURNAL OF CLINICAL IMMUNOLOGY 4(4):304-311, July 1984.

Cell replication in an immunologically stimulated cell population in human bone marrow, by M. L. Greenberg, et al. ANNALS OF THE NEW YORK ACADEMY OF SCIENCES 459:67-72, 1985.

Cellular and T-lymphocyte subpopulation profiles in bronchoalveolar lavage fluid from patients with acquired immunodeficiency syndrome and pneumonitis, by J. M. Wallace, et al. AMERICAN REVIEW OF RESPIRATORY DISEASE 130(5):786-790, November 1984.

Cellular immune deficiency and polylymphadenopathy in the male sexual partners of a woman who died of acquired immunodeficiency (AIDS), by U. A. Baumann, et al. SCHWEIZERISCHE MEDIZINISCHE WOCHENSCHRIFT 114(12):415-418,   March 24, 1984.

Cellular immunity and the acquired immune deficiency syndrome: failure to secrete lymphokines and gamma interferon, by C. C. Hart, et al. SURVEY AND SYNTHETICS OF PATHOLOGY RESEARH 3(5):397-408, 1984.

Cellular targets of antilymphocyte antibodies in AIDS and LAS, by R. H. Tomar, et al. CLINICAL IMMUNOLOGY AND IMMUNOPATHOLOGY 37(1):37-47, October 1985.

Characterization of highly immunogenic p66/p51 as the reverse transcriptase of HTLV-III/LAV, by F. DiMarzo Veronese, et al. SCIENCE 231:1289-1291, March 14, 1986.

Circulating IgA immune complexes in AIDS, by M. M. Lightfoote, et al. IMMUNO-LOGICAL INVESTIGATIONS 14(4):341-345, August 1985.

Circulating immune complexes in AIDS [letter],by S. Gupta, et al. NEW ENGLAND JOURNAL OF MEDICINE 310(23):1530-1531, June 7, 1984.

Clinical and immunological findings in HTLV-III infection, by K. J. Krohn, et al. CANCER RESEARCH 45(Suppl. 9):4612s-4615s, September 1985.

Contribution of immunology to the positive and differential diagnosis of the acquired immunodeficiency syndrome. Immunologic mechanisms of the syndrome, by J. C. Gluckman, et al. BULLETIN DE L'ACADEMIE NA-TIONALE DE MEDECINE 168(1-2):282-287, January-February 1984.

Correlation between immunologic function and clinical subpopulations of patients with the acquired immune deficiency syndrome, by H. C. Lane, et al. AMERICAN JOURNAL OF MEDICINE 78(3):417-422, March 1985.

Cyclosporin immunosuppression as the possible cause of AIDS [letter],by K. W. Sell,et al. NEW ENGLAND JOURNAL OF MEDICINE 309(17):1065, October 27, 1983.

Cyclosporine-like substances not detected in patients with AIDS [letter],by H. F. Schran, et al. NEW ENGLAND JOURNAL OF MEDICINE 310(20):1324, May 17, 1984.

Cytomegalovirus-induced immunosuppression, by M. S. Hirsch, et al. ANNALS OF THE NEW YORK ACADEMY OF SCIENCES 478:8-15, 1984.

Cytotoxic effector mechanisms in AIDS, by S. Cunningham-Rundles, et al. ADVANCES IN EXPERIMENTAL MEDICINE AND BIOLOGY 187:97-110, 1985.

Decreased expression of human class II antigens on monocytes from patients with acquired immune deficiency syndrome. Increased expression with interferon-gamma, by W. Heagy, et al. JOURNAL OF CLINICAL INVESTIGATION 74(6):2089-2096, December 1984.

Decreased helper T lymphocytes in homosexual men. I. Sexual contact in high-i incidence areas for the acquired immunodeficiency syndrome, by J. J. Goedert, et al. AMERICAN JOURNAL OF EPIDEMIOLOGY 121(5):629-636, May 1985.

—. II. Sexual practices, by J. J. Goedert, et al. AMERICAN JOURNAL OF EPIDEMIOLOGY 121 (5):637-644, May 1985.

Decreased population of Leu-7+ natural killer cells in lymph nodes of homosexual men with AIDS-related persistent lymphadenopathy, by S. Jothy, et al. CANADIAN MEDICAL ASSOCIATION JOURNAL 132(2):141-144, January 15, 1985.

Defective B-lymphocyte function in homosexual men in relation to the acquired immunodeficiency syndrome, by S. G. Pahwa, et al. ANNALS OF INTERNAL MEDICINE 101(6):757-763, December 1984.

Defective in vitro T cell colony formation in the acquired immunodeficiency syndrome, by A. Winkelstein, et al. JOURNAL OF IMMUNOLOGY 134(1):151-156, January 1985.

Defective monocyte function in acquired immune deficiency syndrome (AIDS): evidence from a monocyte-dependent T-cell proliferative system, by H. E. Prince, et al. JOURNAL OF CLINICAL IMMUNOLOGY 5(1):21-25, January 1985.

Defective polymorphonuclear leukocyte migration in AIDS [letter], by G. J. Ras, et al. SOUTH AFRICAN MEDICAL JOURNAL 68(5):292-293, August 31, 1985.

Defective reticuloendothelial system Fc-receptor function in patients with acquired immunodeficiency syndrome, by B. S. Bender, et al. JOURNAL OF INFECTIOUS DISEASES 152(2):409-412, August 1985.

413

Defective T-cell response to PHA and mitogenic monoclonal antibodies in male homosexuals with acquired immunodeficiency syndrome and its in vitro correction by interleukin 2, by N. Ciobanu, et al. JOURNAL OF CLINICAL I IMMUNOLOGY 3(4):332-340, October 1983.

Deficiency of interferon-alpha generating capacity is associated with susceptibility to opportunistic infections in patients with AIDS, by C. Lopez, et al. ANNALS OF THE NEW YORK ACADEMY OF SCIENCES 437:39-48, 1984.

Deficient, HLA-restricted, cytomegalovirus-specific cytotoxic T cells and natural killer cells in patients with the acquired immunodeficiency syndrome, by A. H. Rook, et al. JOURNAL OF INFECTIOUS DISEASES 152(3):627-630, September 1985.

Deficient LAV I neutralising capacity of sera from patients with AIDS or related syndromes [letter], by F. Clavel, et al. LANCET 1(8433):879-880, April 3, 1985.

Deficient OKT4 epitope on helper T cells in a patient with SLE: confusion with AIDS, by W. Stohl. NEW ENGLAND JOURNAL OF MEDICINE 310:1531, June 7, 1984.

Demonstration of serum antibodies to cryptosporidium sp. in normal and immunodeficiency humans with confirmed infections, by P. N. Campbell,e t al. JOURNAL OF CLINICAL MICROBIOLOGY 18(1):165-169, July 1983.

Depressed interleukin 2 receptor expression in acquired immune deficiency and lymphadenopathy syndromes, by H. E. Prince, et al. JOURNAL OF IMMUNOLOGY 133(3):1313-1317, September 1984.

Detection of anti-HTLV-III antibodies in gammaglobulin preparations for intramuscular injection [letter], by N. Scheiermann, et al. DEUTSCHE MEDIZINISCHE WOCHENSCHRIFT 110(49):1912-1913, December 6, 1985.

Detection of IgG antibodies to lymphadenopathy-associated virus in patients with AIDS or lymphadenopathy syndrome,by F. Brun-Vezinet, et al. LANCET 1(8389):1253-1256, June 9, 1984.

Development and early natural history of HTLV-III antibodies in persons with hemophilia, by M. E. Eyster, et al. JAMA 253:2219-2223, April 19, 1985.

Diagnostic value of the determination of an interferon-induced enzyme activity: decreased 2',5'-oligoadenylate dependent binding protein activity in AIDS patient lymphocytes, by J. M. Wu, et al. AIDS RESEARCH 2(2):127-131, Spring 1986.

Differential antibody responses of individuals infected with AIDS-associated retroviruses surveyed using the viral core antigen p25 ga expressed in bacteria, by K. S. Steimer, et al. VIROLOGY 150(1):283-290, April 15, 1986.

Differential effects of interferon-alpha 2 and interleukin-2 on natural killer cell activity in patients with acquired immune deficiency syndrome, by M. M. Reddy, et al. JOURNAL OF BIOLOGICAL RESPONSE MODIFIERS 3(4): 379-386, August 1984.

Differential susceptibility to the acquired immunodeficiency syndrome retrovirus in cloned cells of human leukemic T-cell line Molt-4, by R. Kikukawa, et al. JOURNAL OF VIROLOGY 57(3):159-1162, March 1986.

Effects of alcohol on immune system, by T. Prugh. ADAMHA NEWS 12(1):3, January 1986.

Elevated adenosine deaminase and purine nucleoside phosphorylase activity in peripheral blood null lymphocytes from patients with acquired immune deficiency syndrome, by J. L. Murray, et al. BLOOD 65(6):1318-1324, June 1985.

Evaluation of serologic tests for Pneumocystis carinii antibody and antigenemia in patients with acquired immunodeficiency syndrome, by S. E. Maddison, et al. DIAGNOSTIC MICROBIOLOGY AND INFECTIOUS DISEASE 2(1):69-73, January 1984.

Evidence that immune deficiency after marrow transplantation is not caused by AIDS-associated retrovirus [letter], by K. Atkinson, et al. NEW ENGLAND JOURNAL OF MEDICINE 313(3):182-183, July 18, 1985.

Factor VIII products and disordered immune regulation [letter], by R. S. Gordon, Jr. LANCET 1(8331):991, April 30, 1983.

Functional integrity of T, B, and natural killer cells in homosexual subjects with prodromata and in patients with AIDS, by J. G. Bekesi, et al. ANNALS OF THE NEW YORK ACADEMY OF SCIENCES 437:28-38, 1984.

Functional T lymphocyte immune deficiency in a population of homosexual men who do not exhibit symptoms of acuqired immune deficiency syndrome, by G. M. Shearer, et al. JOURNAL OF CLINICAL INVESTIGATION 74(2):496-506, August 1984.

HLA-A,B,C and DR antigen frequencies in acquired immunodeficiency syndrome (AIDS) patients with opportunistic infections, by M. S. Pollack, et al. HUMAN IMMUNOLOGY 11(2):99-103, October 1984.

HTLV-I-specific antibody in AIDS patients and others at risk, by M. Robert-Guroff, et al. LANCET 2(8395):128-131, July 21, 1984.

HTLV-III antibodies in haematology staff [letter], by P. Jones, et al. LANCET 1(8422):217, January 26, 1985.

HTLV-III infection and epitope recognition by OKT4 monoclonal antibody [letter], by T. Hattori, et al. NEW ENGLAND JOURNAL OF MEDICINE 313(24):1543-1544, December 12, 1985.

HTLV-III-neutralizing antibodies in patients with AIDS and AIDS-related complex, by M. Robert-Guroff, et al. NATURE 316(6023):72-74, July 4-10, 1985.

HTLV-III peptide produced by recombinant DNA is immunoreactive with sera from patients with AIDS, by N. T. Chang, et al. NATURE 315(6015):151-154, May 9-15, 1985.

Human immunodeficiency virus and the adrenal medulla [letter]by C. D. Weiss. ANNALS OF INTERNAL MEDICINE 105(2):300, August 1986.

Human immunodeficiency virus infection in transplant recipients [letter], by C. Hiesse, et al. ANNALS OF INTERNAL MEDICINE 105(2):301, August 1986.

Human immunodeficiency viruses, by J. Coffin, et al. SCIENCE 232:697, May 9, 1986.

Human lymphocytopathic retroviruses (HLRV)? by J. W. Shields. NATURE 317:480, October 10, 1985.

Human recombinant interleukin-2 partly reconstitutes deficiency in-vitro immune responses of lyphocytes from patients with AIDS, by J. D. Lifson,e t al. LANCET 1(8379):698-702, March 1984.

Humoral and cellular immunity in uremia, by C. Irkec, et al. MIKROBIYOLOJI BULTENI 16(3):191-195, July 1982.

Humoral immune responses in healthy heterosexual, homosexual and vasec-tomized men and in homosexual men with the acquired immune deficiency syndrome, by S. S. Witkin, et al. AIDS RESEARCH 1(1):31-44, 1983-1984.

IgA deficiency and AIDS [letter], by M. Hepner, et al. JAMA 254(7):912, August 16,1985.

IgG-antibodies to HTLV-III in patients with AIDS, LAS, and persons at risk of AIDS in West Germany, by R. Hehlmann, et al. BLUT 50(1):13-18, January 1985.

IgM and IgG antibodies to HTLV-III in the lymphadenopathy syndrome and sub-jects at risk for AIDS [letter], by P. Pouletty, et al. BRITISH MEDICAL JOUR-NAL 291(6497):741, September 14, 1985.

IL-2 production and response in vitro by the leukocytes of patients with acquired immune deficiency syndrome, by J. M. Reuben, et al. LYMPHOKINE RE-SEARCH 4(2):103-116, Spring 1985.

Immune-cell augmentation (with altered T-subset ratio) is common in healthy homosexual men [letter], by J. L. Fahey, et al. NEW ENGLAND JOURNAL OF MEDICINE 308(14):842-843, April 7, 1983.

Immune complexes in the acquired immunodeficiency syndrome (AIDS): relation-ship to disease manifestation, risk group, and immunologic defect, by J. S. McDougal, et al. JOURNAL OF CLINICAL IMMUNOLOGY 5(2):130-138, March 1985.

Immune function and dysfunction in AIDS,by F. P. Siegal. SEMINARS IN ONCOLOGY 11(1):29-39, March 1984.

Immune system in AIDS, by J. Laurence. SCIENTIFIC AMERICAN 253(6):84-92, December 1985.

Immune thrombocytopenia in homosexual men [letter]. ANNALS OF INTERNAL MEDICINE 104(4):583-584, April 1986.

Immunity syndrome: new test, new ideas, by J. A. Miller. SCIENCE NEWS 123:197, March 26, 1983.

Immunocompromise syndrome in homosexual men. Prevalence of possible risk factors and screening for the prodrome using an accurate white cell count, by D. Goldmeier, et al. BRITISH JOURNAL OF VENEREAL DISEASES 59(2): 127-130, April 1983.

Immunoglobulin subclasses of antibodies to human T-cell leukemia/lymphoma virus I-associated antigens in acquired immune deficiency syndrome and lymphadenopathy syndrome, by J. Goudsmit, et al. JOURNAL OF VIROLOGY 53(1):287-291, January 1985.

Immunoglobulins in the acquired immunodeficiency syndrome [letter], by M. Fiorilli, et al. ANNALS OF INTERNAL MEDICINE 102(6):862-863, June 1985.

Immunohistochemical reactivity of anti-LAV p18 monoclonal antibody in lymph nodes from PGL and AIDS patients, by C. L. Parravicini, et al. BOLLETTINO DELL ISTITUTO SIEROTERAPICO MILANESE 64(5):422-424, 1985.

Immunohistological approach to persistent lymphadenopathy and its relevance to AIDS, by G. Janossy, et al. CLINICAL AND EXPERIMENTAL IMMUNOLOGY 59(2):257-266, February 1985.

Immunohistology of non-T cells in the acquired immunodeficiency syndrome, by G. S. Wood, et al. AMERICAN JOURNAL OF PATHOLOGY 120(3):371-379, September 1985.

Immunohistopathology of lymph nodes in HTLV-III infected homosexuals with persistent adenopathy or AIDS, by P. Biberfeld, et al. CANCER RESEARCH 45(Suppl. 9):4665s-4670s, September 1985.

Immunologic abnormalities among male homosexuals in New York City: changes over time, by M. Marmor, et al. ANNALS OF THE NEW YORK ACADEMY OF SCI-ENCES 437:312-319, 1984.

Immunologic abnormalities in the acquired immunodeficiency syndrome, by D. L. Bowen, et al. PROGRESS IN ALLERGY 37:207-223, 1986.

—, by H. C. Lane, et al. ANNUAL REVIEW OF IMMUNOLOGY 3:477-500, 1985.

Immunologic alterations in acquired immune deficiency syndrome, by M. S. Gottlieb, et al. ANTIOBIOTIC CHEMOTHERAPY 32:99-104, 1983.

Immunologic alterations in brochoalveolar lavage fluid in the acquired immunode-ficiency syndrome (AIDS), by J. A. Rankin, et al. AMERICAN REVIEW OF RESPIRATORY DISEASE 128(1):189-194, July 1983.

Immunologic aspects of AIDS, by M. S. Gottlieb. FRONTIERS OF RADIATION THERAPY AND ONCOLOGY 19:33-37, 1985.

—, by L. Hammerström, et al. LAKARTIDNINGEN 80(7):530+, February 16, 1983.

Immunologic characteristics of acquired immunodeficiency syndrome, by M. Velasco. REVISTA MEDICA DE CHILE 111(12):1299-1300, December 1983.

Immunologic findings in homosexual males with generalized lymphadenopathy. Prodromal state of acquired immunodeficiency syndrome?,by J. R. Kalden,e t al. KLINISCHE WOCHENSCHRIFT 61(21):1067-1073, November 2, 1983.

Immunologic profiles of adults with congenital bleeding disorders, by J. C. Goldsmith, et al. AIDS RESEARCH 1(3):163-179, 1983-1984.

Immunologic reconstitution in the acquired immunodeficiency syndrome, by H. C. Lane, et al. ANNALS OF INTERNAL MEDICINE 103(5):714-718, November 1985.

Immunologic studies of the acquired immune deficiency syndrome: relationship of immunodeficiency to extent of disease, by E. M. Hersh, et al. ANNALS OF THE NEW YORK ACADEMY OF SCIENCES 437:364-372, 1984.

Immunologic studies on the definition of impaired resistance in AIDS, by P. Kern, et al. OFFENTLICHE GESUNDHEITSWESEN 46(9):445-448, September 1984.

Immunologic study of spouses and siblings of asymptomatic hemophiliacs, by M. V. Ragni, et al. SCANDINAVIAN JOURNAL OF HAEMATOLOGY. SUPPLEMENTUM 40:373, 1984.

Immunological abnormalities in patients with the acquired immune deficiency syndrome (AIDS)—a review, by J. M. Dwyer, et al. CLINICAL IMMUNOLOGY REVIEWS 3(1):25-129, 1984.

Immunological and virological investigation in patients with lymphoadenopathy syndrome and in a population at risk for acquired immunodeficiency syndrome (AIDS), with particular focus on the detection of antibodies to human T-lymphotropic retroviruses (HTLV III), by M. C. Sirianni, et al. JOURNAL OF CLINICAL IMMUNOLOGY 5(4):261-268, July 1985.

Immunological changes in HTLV-III infections and AIDS, by K. Krohn, et al. DUODECIM 102(7):413-422, 1986.

Immunological characterizations of patients with acquired immune deficiency syndrome, acquired immune deficiency syndrome-related symptom complex, and a related life-style, by E. M. Hersh, et al. CANCER RESEARCH 44(12, Part 1):5894-5901, December 1984.

Immunological control of Epstein-Barr virus infection: possible lessons for AIDS, by M. A. Epstein. ANNALS OF THE NEW YORK ACADEMY OF SCIENCES 437:1-7, 1984.

Immunological findings associated with HTLV-III antibody positivity, by J. Antonen. ANNALS OF CLINICAL RESEARCH 17(2):81-85, 1985.

Immunological properties of the Gag protein p24 of the acquired immunodeficiency syndrome retrovirus (human T-cell leukemia virus type III, by M. G. Sarngadharan, et al. PROCEEDINGS OF THE NATIONAL ACADEMY OF SCIENCES USA 82(10):3481-3484, May 1985.

Immunological properties of HTLV-III antigens recognized by sera of patients with AIDS and AIDS-related complex and of asymptomatic carriers of HTLV-III

418

infection, by M. G. Sarngadharan, et al. CANCER RESEARCH 45(Suppl. 9):4574s-4577s, September 1985.

Immunological studies in acquired immunodeficiency syndrome. Functional studies of lymphocyte subpopulations, by B. Hofmann, et al. SCANDI-NAVIAN JOURNAL OF IMMUNOLOGY 21(3):235-243, March 1985.

Immunological studies in patients with acquired immune deficiency syndrome, by H. S. Panitch, et al. ANNALS OF THE NEW YORK ACADEMY OF SCIENCES 437:513-517, 1984.

Immunological studies of homosexual men with immunodeficiency and Kaposi's sarcoma, by R. W. Schroff, et al. CLINICAL IMMUNOLOGY AND IMMUNO-PATHOLOGY 27(3):300-314, June 1983.

Immunological studies of male homosexuals with the prodrome of the acquired immunodeficiency syndrome (AIDS),by E. M. Hershe t al. ADVANCES IN EXPERIMENTAL MEDICINE AND BIOLOGY 166:285-293, 1983.

Immunology of the acquired immunodeficiency syndrome, by P. W. McLaughlin, et al. HENRY FORD HOSPITAL MEDICAL JOURNAL 32(3):107-115, 1984.

Immunology of groups at risk for acquired immune deficiency syndrome, by W. Lang. FRONTIERS OF RADIATION THERAPY AND ONCOLOGY 19:43-51, 1985.

Immunopathogenesis of the acquired immunodeficiency syndrome, by D. L. Bowen, et al. ANNALS OF INTERNAL MEDICINE 103(5):704-709, November 1985.

Immunopathogenesis of AIDS, by A. J. Lewandowski. JOURNAL OF MEDICAL TECHNOLOGY 3(3):145-148+, March 1986.

Immunoperoxidase evaluation of lymph nodes from acquired immune deficiency patients, by M. Mangkornkanok-Mark, et al. CLINICAL AND EXPERIMENTAL IMMUNOLOGY 55(3):581-586, March 1984.

Immunopotentiation of impaired lymphocyte functions in vitro by isoprinosine in prodromal subjects and AIDS patients, by P. Tsang, et al. INTERNATIONAL JOURNAL OF IMMUNOPHARMACOLOGY 7(4):511-514, 1985.

Immunopurinogenic enzymatic activity in the acquired immunodeficiency syndrome, by E. Mejias, et al. ADVANCES IN EXPERIMENTAL MEDICINE AND BIOLOGY 295(Part A):275-280, 1986.

Immunoregulatory circuits in the acquired immune deficiency syndrome and related complex. Production of and response to interleukins 1 and 2, NK function and its enhancement by interleukin-2 and kinetics of the autologous mixed lymphocyte reaction, by J. Alcocer-Varela, et al. CLINICAL AND EXPERIMENTAL IMMUNOLOGY 60(1):31-38, April 1985.

Immunoregulatory lymphokines of T hybridomas from AIDS patients: constitutive and inducible suppressor factors, by J. Laurence, et al. SCIENCE 225(4657):66-69, July 6, 1984.

Immunoregulatory T cells in men with a new acquired immunodeficiency syndrome, by E. Benveniste, et al. JOURNAL OF CLINICAL IMMUNOLOGY 3(4):359-367, October 1983.

Immunosuppressants in patients with AIDS [letter], by A. Hausen, et al. NATURE 320(6058):114, March 13-19, 1986.

Impaired in vitro interferon, blastogenic, and natural killer cell responses to viral stimulation in acquired immune deficiency syndrome, by E. M. Hersh, et al. CANCER RESEARCH 45(1):406-410, January 1985.

Impaired mononuclear-cell proliferation in patients with the acquired immune deficiency syndrome results from abnormalities of both T lymphocytes and adherent mononuclear cells, by K. Shannon, et al. JOURNAL OF CLINICAL IMMUNOLOGY 5(4):239-245, July 1985.

Impaired production of lymphokines and immune (gamma) interferon in the acquired immunodeficiency syndrome, by H. W. Murray, et al. NEW ENGLAND JOURNAL OF MEDICINE 310(14):883-889, April 5, 1984.

In situ quantitation of lymph node helper, suppressor, and cytotoxic T cell subsets in AIDS, by G. S. Wood, et al. BLOOD 67(3):596-603, March 1986.

In vitro and in vivo studies with interleukin 2 (IL-2) and various immunostimulants in a patient with AIDS, by P. Vaith, et al. IMMUNITÄT UND INFEKTION 13(2):51-63, April 1985.

In vitro augmentation of interleukin-2 production and lymphocytes with the TAC antigen marker in patients with AIDS [letter],by K. Y. Tsang, et al. NEW ENGLAND JOURNAL OF MEDICINE 310(15):987, April 12, 1984.

Induction of cytolytic activity by anti-T3 monoclonal antibody. Activation of alloimmune memory cells and natural killer cells from normal and immunodeficiency individuals, by M. Suthanthiran, et al. JOURNAL OF CLINICAL INVESTIGATION 74(6):2263-2271, December 1984.

Infection and T lymphocyte subpopulations: changes associated with bacteremia and the acquired immunodeficiency syndrome, by J. A. Fishman, et al. DIAGNOSTIC IMMUNOLOGY 1(3):261-265, 1983.

Infection in the immunocompromised host, by J. Ô. Leyden. ARCHIVES OF DERMATOLOGY 121(7):855-857, July 1985.

Infection mechanism? by J. Palca. NATURE 319:170, January 16, 1986.

Inhibition of in vitro lymphocyte proliferation by serum from acquired immune deficiency syndrome patients depends on the ratio of cells to serum in culture, by A. K. Henning, et al. CLINICAL IMMUNOLOGY AND IMMUNOPATHOLOGY 33(2):258-267, November 1984.

Interleukin regulation of the immune system (IRIS) in male homosexuals with acquired immune deficiency disease syndrome, by M. A. Palladino, et al. ANNALS OF THE NEW YORK ACADEMY OF SCIENCES 437:535-539, 1984.

Interleukin 2 augmentation of natural killer cell activity in homosexual men with acquired immune deficiency syndrome, by M. M. Reddy, et al. INFECTION AND IMMUNITY 44(2):339-343, May 1984.

Interleukin-2 enhances the depressed natural killer and cytomegalovirus-specific cytotoxic activities of lymphocytes from patients with the acquired immune deficiency syndrome, by A. H. Rook, et al. JOURNAL OF CLINICAL INVESTIGATION 72(1):398-403, July 1983.

Interleukin 2 enhances the natural killer cell activity of acquired immunodeficiency syndrome patients through a gamma-interferon-independent mechanism, by A. H. Rook, et al. JOURNAL OF IMMUNOLOGY 134(3):1503-1507, March 1985.

Interleukin-2 production and response to exogenous interleukin-2 in a patient with the acquired immune deficiency syndrome (AIDS), by G. J. Hauser, et al. CLINICAL AND EXPERIMENTAL IMMUNOLOGY 56(1):14-17, April 1984.

Interleukin-2 production by persons with the generalized lymphadenopathy syndrome or the acquired immune deficiency syndrome, by C. H. Kirkpatrick, et al. JOURNAL OF CLINICAL IMMUNOLOGY 5(1):31-37, January 1985.

Lack of specific cell mediated immunity to cytomegalovirus in people at risk for AIDS, by M. C. Sirianni, et al. AIDS RESEARCH 1(2):99-105, 1983-1984.

Langerhans cell, as a representative of the accessory cell system, in health and disease, by G. J. Thorbecke, et al. IMMUNOBIOLOGY 168(3-5):313-324, December 1984.

Leukocyte subset analysis and related immunological findings in acquired immunodeficiency disease syndrome (AIDS) and malignancies, by E. M. Hersh, et al. DIAGNOSTIC IMMUNOLOGY 1(3):168-173, 1983.

Levamisole, immunostimulation, and the acquired immunodeficiency syndrome [letter], by N. Surapaneni, et al. ANNALS OF INTERNAL MEDICINE 102(2): 137, January 1985.

Locally synthesized antibodies in cerebrospinal fluid of patients with AIDS, by R. Ackermann, et al. JOURNAL OF NEUROLOGY 233(3):140-141, June 1986.

Lymphocyte-reactive antibodies in acquired imune deficiency syndrome, by R. C. Williams, Jr., et al. JOURNAL OF CLINICAL IMMUNOLOGY 4(2):118-123, March 1984.

Lymphocytotoxic antibodies against peripheral blood B and T lymphocytes in homosexuals with AIDS and ARC, by W. Pruzanski, et al. AIDS RESEARCH 1(3):211-220, 1983-1984.

Lymphocytotoxic antibodies to non-HLA antigens in the sera of patients with acquired immunodeficiency syndrome (AIDS), by M. S. Pollack, et al. PROGRESS IN CLINICAL AND BIOLOGICAL RESEARCH 133:209-213, 1983.

Lymphocytotoxic antibodies in the acquired immune deficiency syndrome (AIDS), by B. E. Kloster, et al. CLINICAL IMMUNOLOGY AND IMMUNOPATHOLOGY 30(2):330-335, February 1984.

421

Lymphotropic retroviruses (HTLV-I, -II, -III), by P. J. Fischinger, et el. CANCER RESEARCH 45(Suppl. 9):4694s-4699s, September 1985.

Major glycoprotein antigens that induce antibodies in AIDS patients are encoded by HLTV-III, by J. S. Allan, et al. SCIENCE 228:1091-1094, May 31, 1985.

Measuring antibodies may predict disease, by D. M. Barnes. SCIENCE 233:419, July 25, 1986.

Mechanism and modulation of immune dysfunction in AIDS associated syndromes, by J. G. Bekesi, et al. ADVANCES IN EXPERIMENTAL MEDICINE AND BIOLOGY 187:141-150, 1985.

Molecular level view gives immune system clues [news], by C. Marwick. JAMA 253(23):3371+, June 21, 1985.

Monoclonal antibody-defined beta 2-microglobulin-positive mononuclear cells in acquired immune deficiency syndrome, by S. Gupta. SCANDINAVIAN JOURNAL OF IMMUNOLOGY 22(4):357-361, October 1985.

Monoclonal immunoglobulins in HTLV-III-Positive sera [letter],by P. G. Sala, et al. CLINICAL CHEMISTRY 32(3):574, March 1986.

Monocyte function in the acquired immune deficiency syndrome. Defective chemotaxis, by P. D. Smith, et al. JOURNAL OF CLINICAL INVESTIGATION 74(6):2121-2128, December 1984.

Natural killer cell function and modulation by alpha IFN and IL2 in AIDS patients and prodromal subjects, by F. Lew, et al. JOURNAL OF CLINICAL AND LABORATORY IMMUNOLOGY 14(3):115-121, July 1984.

Naturally occurring antibodies reactive with sperm proteins: apparent deficiency in AIDS sera, by T. C. Rodman, et al. SCIENCE 228(4704):1211-1215, June 7, 1985.

Neutralization of the AIDS retrovirus by antibodies to a recombinant envelope glycoprotein, by L. A. Lasky, et al. SCIENCE 233(4760):209-212, July 11, 1986.

New immune booster: both legal and inexpensive, by M. Helquist. ADVOCATE 433:25, November 12, 1985.

New immunologic syndrome—AIDS, by W. Mazurkiewicz. PRZEGLAD DERMA-TOLOGICZNY 71(1):11-15, January-February 1984.

Noninfectious cofactors in susceptibility to AIDS: possible contributions of semen, HLA alloantigens and lack of natural resistance, by G. M. Shearer, et al. ANNALS OF THE NEW YORK ACADEMY OF SCIENCES 437:49-57, 1984.

Oligoclonal immunoglobulins in patients with the acquired immunodeficiency syndrome, by N. M. Papadopoulos, et al. CLINICAL IMMUNOLOGY AND IMMU-NOPATHOLOGY 35(1):43-36, April 1985.

Overview of clinical syndromes and immunology of AIDS, by A. S. Fauci, et al. TOPICS IN CLINICAL NURSING 6(2):12-18, July 1984.

Partial immune reconstitution in a patient with the acquired immunodeficiency syndrome, by H. C. Lane, et al. NEW ENGLAND JOURNAL OF MEDICINE 311(17):1099-1103, October 25, 1984.

Partial restoration of impaired interleukin-2 production and Tac antigen (putative interleukin-2 receptor) expression in patients with acquired immune deficiency syndrome by isoprinosine treatment in vitro, by K. Y. Tsang, et al. JOURNAL OF CLINICAL INVESTIGATION 75(5):1538-1544, May 1985.

Patients with acquired immunodeficiency syndrome (AIDS) have peripheral blood lymphocytes expressing plasma-cell differentiation antigens, by G. J. Ruiz-Argüelles, et al. REVISTA DE INVESTIGACION CLINICA 36(2):99-101, April-June 1984.

Precipitable immune complexes in healthy homosexual men, acquired immune deficiency syndrome and the related lymphadenopathy syndrome, by H. H. Euler, et al. CLINICAL AND EXPERIMENTAL IMMUNOLOGY 59(2):267-275, February 1985.

Presence of antibodies to the human T-cell leukemia virus HTLV I in German patients with symptoms of AIDS, by D. Wernicke, et al. HAMATOLOGIE UND BLUT-TRANSFUSION 29:338-341, 1985.

Presence of immunoglobulin D in endocrine disorders and diseases of immuno-regulation, including the acquired immunodeficiency syndrome, by N. M. Papadopoulos, et al. CLINICAL IMMUNOLOGY AND IMMUNOPATHOLOGY 32(2):248-252, August 1984.

Presence of viral antibodies to the human lymphoma-leukemia virus in patients with acquired immune deficiency syndrome, by M. Born, et al. EUROPEAN JOURNAL OF CLINICAL MICROBIOLOGY 3(1):77-78, February 1984.

Prevalence of antibodies to AIDS-associated retrovirus in single men in San Francisco [letter], by R. E. Anderson, et al. LANCET 1(8422):217, January 26, 1985.

Prevalence of antibody to LAV/HTLV-III among homosexual men in Seattle, by A. C. Collier, et al. AMERICAN JOURNAL OF PUBLIC HEALTH 76:564-565, May 1986.

Prospective observations of viral and immunologic abnormalities in homosexual males, by M. Lange, et al. ANNALS OF THE NEW YORK ACADEMY OF SCIENCES 437:350-363, 1984.

Qualitative analysis of immune function in patients with the acquired immunodeficiency syndrome. Evidence for a selective defect in soluble antigen recognition, by H. C. Lane, et al. NEW ENGLAND JOURNAL OF MEDICINE 313(2):79-84, July 11, 1985.

Quantitation of and neutralizing antibodies to AIDS-retroviruses; a novel system using HTLV-I carrying MT-4 cells, by S. Harada, et al. TANPAKUSHITSU KAKUSAN KOSO 30(13):1394-1407, December 1985.

Quantitation of beta 2-microglobulin and other immune characteristics in a prospective study of men at risk for acquired immune deficiency syndrome, by S. Zolla-Pazner, et al. JAMA 251(22):2951-2955, June 8, 1984.

Radioimmunoassay and enzyme-linked immunoassay of antibodies to the core protein (P24) of human T-lymphotropic virus (HTLVIII), by A. R. Neurath, et al. JOURNAL OF VIROLOGICAL METHODS 11(1):75-86, May 1985.

Red-cell alloantibody response in AIDS [letter],by G. Ramsey, et al. LANCET 2(8349):575, September 3, 1983.

Reduced ecto-5"-nucleotidase activity and enhanced OKT10 and HLA-DR expression on CD8 (T suppressor/cytotoxic) lymphocytes in the acquired immune deficiency syndrome: evidence of CD8 cell immaturity, by J. F. Salazar-Gonzalez, et al. JOURNAL OF IMMUNOLOGY 135(3):1778-1785, September 1985.

Selective defects in cytomegalovirus-and mitogen-induced lymphocyte proliferation and interferon release in patients with acquired immunodeficiency syndrome, by J. S. Epstein, et al. JOURNAL OF INFECTIOUS DISEASES 152(4):727-733, October 1985.

Serum immunoglobulin elevations in the acquired immunodeficiency syndrome (AIDS): IgG, IgA, IgM, and IgD, by Q. Chess, et al. DIAGNOSTIC IMMUNOLO-GY 2(3):148-153, 1984.

Severe acquired immune deficiency syndrome in male homosexuals: diminished capacity to make interferon-alpha in vitro associated with severe opportunistic infections, by C. Lopez, et al. JOURNAL OF INFECTIOUS DISEASES 148(6):962-966, December 1983.

Severe combined immunodeficiency associated with absent T4+ helper cells, by K. M. Edwards, et al. JOURNAL OF PEDIATRICS 105(1):70-72, July 1984.

Soluble factors inhibitory for T-cell-dependent immune responses in patients with the acquired immune deficiency syndrome and its prodromes, by J. Laurence, et al. ANNALS OF THE NEW YORK ACADEMY OF SCIENCES 437:518-525, 1984.

Soluble suppressor factors in patients with acquired immune deficiency syndrome and its prodrome. Elaboration in vitro by T lyphocyte-adherent cell interactions, by J. Laurence, et al. JOURNAL OF CLINICAL INVESTIGATION 72(6):2072-2081, December 1983.

Specific antibodies against human T cell leukemia virus found in AIDS patients,by K. Nagy, et al. ORVOSI HETILAP 125(26):1557-1560, June 24, 1984.

Specificity of lyphocytotoxic antibodies in AIDS and pre-AIDS patients, by V. Wicher, et al. AIDS RESEARCH 1(2):139-148, 1983-1984.

Spontaneous and interferon resistant natural killer cell energy in AIDS, by W. M. Mitchell, et al. AIDS RESEARCH 1(3):221-229, 1983-1984.

Suppressor function of T lymphocytes in the acquired immunodeficiency syndrome as assessed by allogeneic mixed lymphocyte culture, by R. Y. Lin, et al. JOURNAL OF CLINICAL AND LABORATORY IMMUNOLOGY 16(2):69-73, Feburary 1985.

Suppressor T cells and the immune response to tumors, by S. Schatten, et al. CRC CRITICAL REVIEWS IN IMMUNOLOGY 4(4):335-379, 1984.

Transient immunoglobulin and antibody production. Occurrence in two patients with common vairied immunodeficiency, by C. C. Zielinski, et al. ARCHIVES OF INTERNAL MEDICINE 143(10):1937-1940, October 1983.

Ultrastructural demonstration of retrovirus antigens with immuno-gold staining in prodromal acquired immune deficiency syndrome, by W. W. Feremans, et al. JOURNAL OF CLINICAL PATHOLOGY 37(12):399-1403, December 1984.

Unregulated production of virus and/or sperm specific anti-idiotypic antibodies as a cause of AIDS, by S. Hsia, et al. LANCET 1(8338):1212-1214, June 2, 1984.

Virologic, immunologic, and epidemiologic associations with AIDS among gay males in a low incidence area, by C. Rinaldo, et al. ANNALS OF THE NEW YORK ACADEMY OF SCIENCES 437:544-548, 1984.

Virus envelope protein of HTLV-III represents major target antigen for antibodies in AIDS patients, by F. Barin, et al. SCIENCE 228(4703):1094-1096, May 31, 1985.

AFRICA

Absence of immunosuppression in healthy subjects from eastern Zaire who are positive for HTLV-III antibody, by L. Kestens, et al. NEW ENGLAND JOURNAL OF MEDICINE 312:1517-1518, June 6, 1985.

Acquired immunodeficiency syndrome, chronic coccidiosis and Salmonella typhimurium septicemia in a couple from Zaire. Immunological functions and attempt at immunostimulation by thymopentin, by R. C. Martin-Du Pan, et al. SCHWEIZERISCHE MEDIZINISCHE WOCHENSCHRIFT 114(46):1645-1650, November 17, 1984.

HTLV-III antibody in East Africa [letter]. NEW ENGLAND JOURNAL OF MEDICINE 315(4):259-260, July 24, 1986.

Human T-cell leukemia virus (HTLV-I) antibodies in Africa, by W. Saxinger, et al. SCIENCE 225:1473-1476, September 28, 1984.

Immunologic findings in Texas homosexual men: relationship to the acquired immune deficiency syndrome, by J. T. Newman, et al. TEXAS MEDICINE 79(11):44-47, November 1983.

Immunological abnormalities in South African homosexual men, by R. Anderson, et al. SOUTH AFRICAN MEDICAL JOURNAL 64(4):119-122, July 23, 1983.

Immunological abnormalities in South African homosexuals—a non-infectious cofactor? [letter], by R. J. Ablin, et al. SOUTH AFRICAN MEDICAL JOUR-NAL 67(2):40-41, January 12, 1985.

Prevalence of antibodies to lymphadenopathy-associated retrovirus in African patients with AIDS, by F. Brun-Vézinet, et al. SCIENCE 226(4673):453-456, October 26, 1984.

Prevalence of HTLV-III antibodies in homosexual men in Johannesburg [letter], by R. Sher, et al. SOUTH AFRICAN MEDICAL JOURNAL 67(13):484, March 30, 1985.

AFRICA

Seroepidemiology of HTLV-III antibodies in a remote population of eastern Zaire, by R. J. Biggar, et al. BRITISH MEDICAL JOURNAL 290(6471): 808-810, March 16, 1985.

Sero-epidemiology of HTLV-III antibody in southern Africa, by S. F. Lyons, et al. SOUTH AFRICAN MEDICAL JOURNAL 67(24):961-962, June 15, 1985.

Seroepidemiological studies of HTLV-III antibody prevalence among selected groups of heterosexual Africans, by N. Clumeck, et al. JAMA 254:2599-2603, November 8, 1985.

AUSTRALIA

HTLV-III antibody in Sydney homosexual men [letter], by P. W. Robertson, et al. MEDICAL JOURNAL OF AUSTRALIA 143(6):261, September 16, 1985.

DENMARK

Occurrence of anti-HTLV-III antibodies in Danish high-risk homosexuals in 1982-83—seroconversion rate and risk of AIDS [letter], by B. Hoffmann, et al. AIDS RESEARCH 2(1):1-3, February 1986.

FRANCE

Antibodies to HTLV-III associated antigens in populations exposed to AIDS virus in France [letter], by D. Mathez, et al. LANCET a2(8400):460, August 25, 1984.

Immune status of AIDS patients in France: relationship with lymphadenopathy associated virus tropism, by D. Klatzmann, et al. ANNALS OF THE NEW YORK ACADEMY OF SCIENCES 437:228-237, 1984.

Immunological evaluation of acquired immune deficiency syndrome patients in France: preliminary results, by M. Cavaille-Coll, et al. ANTIOBIOTIC CHEMOTHERAPY 32:105-111, 1983.

GERMANY

Antibodies to adult T-cell leukemia virus (ATLV/HTLV-I) in AIDS patients and people at risk of AIDS in Germany, by G. Hunsmann, et al. MEDICAL MICROBIOLOGY AND IMMUNOLOGY 173(5):241-250, 1985.

Antibodies to HTLV-III in patients with acquired immunodeficiency or lympha-denopathy syndrome in West Germany [letter], by R. Hehlmann, et al. LANCET 2(8411):1094, November 10, 1984.

Presence of antibodies to human lymphoma-leukemia virus (HTLV-I) in Germans with symptoms of the acquired immunodeficiency syndrome (AIDS), by M. Born, et al. JOURNAL OF MEDICAL VIROLOGY 15(1):57-63, January 1985.

Prevalence of antibodies to HTLV-III in AIDS risk groups in West Germany, by V. Erfle, et al. CANCER RESEARCH 45(Suppl. 9):4627s-4629s, September 1985.

GERMANY
Seroepidemiology of HTLV-III (LAV) in the Federal Republic of Germany, by
G. Hunsmann, et al. KLINISCHE WOCHENSCHRIFT 63(5):233-235,
March 1, 1985.

GREAT BRITAIN
Longitudinal immunological studies on a cohort of initially symptom-free
homosexual men in London with respect to HTLV-III serology, by A. J.
Pinching, et al. ADVANCES IN EXPERIMENTAL MEDICINE AND
BIOLOGY 187:67-72, 1985.

Prevalence of antibody to human T-lymphotropic virus type III in AIDS and
AIDS-risk patients in Britain,by R. Cheingsong-Popov, et al. LANCET
2(8401):477-480, September 1, 1984.

Prevalence of HTLV-III infection in London. AMERICAN FAMILY PHYSICIAN
33:306, February 1986.

HAITI
Immunologic findings in healthy Haitians in Montreal, by A. Adrien, et al.
CANADIAN MEDICAL ASSOCIATION JOURNAL 133(5):401-406,
September 1, 1985.

ISRAEL
Immune derangements in asymptomatic male homosexuals in Israel: a pre-
AIDS condition?, by Z. T. Handzel, et al. ANNALS OF THE NEW YORK
ACADEMY OF SCIENCES 437:549-553, 1984.

Lack of antibodies to adult T-cell leukaemia virus and to AIDS virus in Israeli
Falashas [letter], by A. Karpas, et al. NATURE 319(6056):794, February
27-March 5, 1986.

ITALY
IgM and IgG antibodies to human T cell lymphotropic retrovirus (HTLV-III) in
lymphadenopathy syndrome and subjects at risk for AIDS in Italy, by F.
Aiuti, et al. BRITISH MEDICAL JOURNAL 291(6489):165-166, July 20,
1985.

Immunological and virological studies in a risk population for AIDS in Rome, by
F. Aiuti, et al. ANNALS OF THE NEW YORK ACADEMY OF SCIENCES
437:554-558, 1984.

JAPAN
Antibodies to HTLV I and III in sera from two Japanese patients, one with possible pre-AIDS [letter], by T. Aoki, et al. LANCET 2(8408):936-937, October 20, 1984.

Distribution of the level of antibody to AIDS-assocated virus (LAV) in sera
from AIDS or AIDS-related complex and Japanese hemophiliacs infected
with AIDS-associat- ed virus, by H. Tsuchie, et al. MICROBIOLOGYAND
IMMUNOLOGY 29(11):1083-1087, 1985.

SWITZERLAND
Antibodies to HTLV-III in Swiss patients with AIDS and pre-AIDS and in groups at risk for AIDS, by J. Schüpbach, et al. NEW ENGLAND JOURNAL OF MEDICINE 312(5):265-270, January 31, 1985.

Detection of anti-HTLV-III/LAV antibody by enzyme-linked immunosorbent assay in high-risk individuals in Switzerland 1974-1985, by J. Stroun, et al. EUROPEAN JOURNAL OF CLINICAL MICROBIOLOGY 4(6):583-586, December 1985.

Prevalence of antibodies against HTLV-III in various regions in Switzerland, by J. Schüpbach, et al. SCHWEIZERISCHE MEDIZINISCHE WOCHEN-SCHRIFT 115(30):1048-1054, July 27, 1985.

WEST INDIES
Seroepidemiology of human T-cell leukemia virus in the French West Indies: antibodies in blood donors and patients with lymphoproliferative diseases who do not have AIDS, by A. Calender, et al. ANNALS OF THE NEW YORK ACADEMY OF SCIENCES 437:175-176, 1984.

IMMUNOLOGY—BLOOD DONORS
Prevalence of HTLV-III antibody in American blood donors, by J. B. Schoor, et al. NEW ENGLAND JOURNAL OF MEDICINE 313:384, August 8, 1985.

IMMUNOLOGY—CHILDREN
Antibodies to AIDS-associated retrovirus distinguish between pediatric primary and acquired immunodeficiency diseases, by A. J. Ammann, et al. JAMA 253(21):3116-3118, June 7, 1985.

IMMUNOLOGY—FAMILY
Transient antibody to lymphadenopathy-associated virus/human T-lymphocyte virus type III and T-lymphocyte abnormalities in the wife of a man who developed the acquired immunodeficiency syndrome, by H. Burger, et al. ANNALS OF INTERNAL MEDICINE 103(4):545-547, October 1985.

IMMUNOLOGY—HEMOPHILIACS
Antibodies to human T-cell leukemia virus membrane antigens (HTLV-MA) in hemophiliacs, by M. Essex, et al. SCIENCE 221:1061-1064, September 9, 1983.

Antibody to human T-cell leukemia virus membrane antigens, beta 2-microglobulin levels, and thymosin alpha I levels in hemophiliacs and their spouses, by J. K. Kreiss, et al. ANNALS OF INTERNAL MEDICINE 100(2):178-182, February 1984.

Antibody to human T-lymphotropic virus type III in wives of hemophiliacs. Evidence for heterosexual transmission, by J. K. Kreiss, et al. ANNALS OF INTERNAL MEDICINE 102(5):623-626, May 1985.

Antibody to lymphadenopathy-associated virus in haemophiliacs with and without AIDS [letter],by R. B. Ramsey, et al. LANCET 2(8399):397-398, August 18, 1984.

IMMUNOLOGY—HEMOPHILIACS

Association of HTLV-III antibodies and cellular immune status of hemophiliacs, by C. Tsoukas, et al. NEW ENGLAND JOURNAL OF MEDICINE 311:1514-1515, December 6, 1984.

IMMUNOLOGY—HIGH RISK INDIVIDUALS
Antilymphocyte antibodies and seropositivity for retroviruses in groups at high risk for AIDS [letter], by D. D. Kiprov, et al. NEW ENGLAND JOURNAL OF MEDICINE 312(23):1517, June 6, 1985.

IMMUNOLOGY—TESTING
Simple method for determination of antibodies to AIDS associated virus (HTLV-II), by G. Biberfeld, et al. LAKARTIDNINGEN 81(39):3482-3483, September 26, 1984.

INFANTS
Acquired immune deficiency syndrome in infants and children, by S. W. Thompson, et al. PEDIATRIC NURSING 11(4):278-280+, July-August 1985.

Acquired immune deficiency syndrome in infants born of Haitian mothers [letter], by J. H. Joncas, et al. NEW ENGLAND JOURNAL OF MEDICINE 308(14): 842, April 7, 1983.

Acquired immunodeficiency in an infant: possible transmission by means of blood products, by A. J. Ammann, et al. LANCET 1(8331):956-958, April 30, 1983.

Acquired immunodeficiency syndrome in infants, by A. Rubinstein. AMERICAN JOURNAL OF DISEASES OF CHILDREN 137(9):825-827, September 1983.

—, by G. B. Scott, et al. NEW ENGLAND JOURNAL OF MEDICINE 310(2):76-81, January 12, 1984.

Acquired immunodeficiency syndrome in infants and children, by A. J. Ammann. ANNALS OF INTERNAL MEDICINE 103(5):734-737, November 1985.

—, by L. J. Bernstein, et al. PROGRESS IN ALLERGY 37:194-206, 1986.

AIDS baby in Miami, Fla. finally gets foster home. JET 65:5, January 16, 1984.

AIDS in the infant, by E. Vilmer, et al. REVUE FRANCAISE DE TRANSFUSION ET IMMUNO-HEMATOLOGIE 27(4):423-426, September 1984.

AIDS in infants, by S. Eliot. HEALTHSHARING 7(1):6, Winter 1985.

Babies born with AIDS, by J. Seligmann, et al. NEWSWEEK 108(12):70-71, September 22, 1986.

Developmental abnormalities in infants and children with acquired immune deficiency syndrome (AIDS) and AIDS-related complex, by M. H. Ultmann, et al. DEVELOPMENTAL MEDICINE AND CHILD NEUROLOGY 27(5):563-571, October 1985.

Immunologic dysfunction in infants infected through transfusion with HTLV-III, by R. F. Wykoff, et al. NEW ENGLAND JOURNAL OF MEDICINE 312(5):294-296, January 31, 1985.

429

Infection with two genotypes of Epstein-Barr virus in an infant with AIDS and lymphoma of the central nervous system, by B. Z. Katz, et al. JOURNAL OF INFECTIOUS DISEASES 153(3):601-604, March 1986.

Is there an acquired immune deficiency syndrome in infants and children?, by A. J. Ammann. PEDIATRICS 72(3):430-432, September 1983.

Mothers of infants with the acquired immunodeficiency syndrome: evidence for both symptomatic and assymptomatic carriers, by G. B. Scott, et al. JAMA 253:363-366, January 18, 1985.

Neurological complications in infants and children with acquired immune deficiency syndrome, by A. L. Belman, et al. ANNALS OF NEUROLOGY 18(5):560-566, November 1985.

Other factors to consider in infantile AIDS, by G. M. Shearer. NEW ENGLAND JOURNAL OF MEDICINE 311:189-191, July 19, 1984.

Perinatal AIDS. AMERICAN FAMILY PHYSICIAN 33:364+, February 1986.

Virus-like rods in a lymphoid line from an infant with AIDS [letter], by T. G. Burrage, et al. NEW ENGLAND JOURNAL OF MEDICINE 310(22):1461-1461, May 31, 1984.

AFRICA
Case of immune deficiency in a Zaire infant: AIDS?, by B. Massart, et al. REVUE MEDICALE DE LIEGE 40(10);433-438, May 15, 1985.

INFANTS—TRANSMISSION
Possible transmission of a human lymphotropic retrovirus (LAV) from mother to infant with AIDS [letter], by E. Vilmer, et al. LANCET 2(8396):229-230, July 28, 1984.

Postnatal transmission of AIDS-associated retrovirus from mother to infant, by J. B. Ziegler, et al. LANCET 1(8434):896-898, April 20, 1985.

INFANTS—TRANSMISSION—BLOOD TRANSFUSION
Transfusion-associated acquired immune deficiency syndrome in infants, by J. A. Church, et al. JOURNAL OF PEDIATRICS 105(5):731-737, November 1984.

Transfusion-associated acquired immunodeficiency syndrome in a twin infant, by F. Cox, et al. PEDIATRIC INFECTIOUS DISEASE 4(1):106-108, January-February 1985.

Transfusion-associated cytomegalovirus infection and acquired immune deficiency syndrome in an infant, by K. Shannon, et al. JOURNAL OF PEDIATRICS 103(6):859-863, December 1983.

Transfusion-induced AIDS in four premature babies [letter], by J. F. O'Duffy, et al. LANCET 2(8415):1346, December 8, 1984.

Transfusion-related acquired immunodeficiency syndrome and directed donations: would the national blood supply be safer with directed donations? by J. Umlas. HUMAN PATHOLOGY 17(2):108-110, February 1986.

Recommendations for assisting in the prevention of perinatal transmissions of HTLV-III/LAV and acquired immunodeficiency syndrome. JAMA 255:25-27+, January 3, 1986; also in MMWR 34(48):721-726+, December 6, 1985.

INFECTION CONTROL

Acquired immune deficiency syndrome. Infection control and public health law, by M. Mills, et al. NEW ENGLAND JOURNAL OF MEDICINE 314(14):931-936, April 3, 1986.

Acquired immune deficiency syndrome. Measures to be taken in blood transfusion establishments in order to protect the personnel], by J. Y. Muller. REVUE FRANCAISE DE TRANSFUSION ET IMMUNO-HEMATOLOGIE 27(4):567-570, September 1984.

Acquired immune deficiency syndrome. Recommendations to prevent transmission for hospitals and health care workers, by K. Crossley. MINNESOTA MEDICINE 69(4):211-213, April 1986.

Acquired immune deficiency syndrome (AIDS): precautions for clinical and laboratory staffs. EMERGENCY MEDICAL SERVICES 12(5):69, September-October 1983; also in MMWR 31(43):577-580, November 5, 1982.

Acquired immune deficiency syndrome (AIDS): precautions for clinical staff. CHART 83(5):7, May-June 1986.

Acquired immunodeficiency syndrome (AIDS): precautions for health-care workers and allied professionals. MMWR 32(34):450-451, September 2, 1983.

Acquired immunodeficiency syndrome: infection control guidelines for the G.I suite, by R. L. Messner. SGA JOURNAL 8(2):37-38, Fall 1985.

AIDS and infection control, by S. R. Perdew. CARING 5(6):22-26, June 1986.

AIDS and related conditions—infection control. Guidelines for health care workers involved in patient management and investigation, by R. Sher. SOUTH AFRICAN MEDICAL JOURNAL 68(12):843-848, December 7, 1985.

AIDS and the control of cell growth, by O. Sattaur. NEW SCIENTIST 102:20, May 10, 1984.

AIDS—aspects of infection control part 2, by E. A. Jenner. MIDWIFE, HEALTH VISITOR AND COMMUNITY NURSE 22(6):181-182+, June 1986.

AIDS infection control precautions, by M. A. Johnson. FRONTIERS OF RADIATION THERAPY AND ONCOLOGY 19:160-163, 1985.

Infection control and the hospitalized AIDS patient, by A. Adams, et al. INFECTION CONTROL 6(5):200-201, May 1985.

Infection control in the patient with AIDS, by P. J. Ungvarski. JOURNAL OF HOSPITAL INFECTION 5(Suppl. A):111-113, December 1984.

Infection control—a progress report, by R. P. Wenzel, et al. INFECTION CONTROL 6(1):9-10, January 1985.

Infection control update: AIDS, by P. Jemison-Smith, et al. CRITICAL CARE UPDATE 10(3):30-31, March 1983.

Royal Alexandra develops AIDS infection control protocol, by S. I. Hnatko. DIMENSIONS IN HEALTH SERVICE 62(8):25-28, September 1985.

Special report: infection-control guidelines for patients with the acquired immunodeficiency syndrome (AIDS), by J. E. Conte, Jr., et al. HOSPITAL TOPICS 62(2):44-48, March-April 1984.

Surveillance and control of infectious diseases: progress toward the 1990 objectives, by W. R. Dowdle. PUBLIC HEALTH REPORTS 98(3):210-218, May-June 1983.

Your role in the diagnosis and management of AIDS, by R. D. Smith. PATHOLOGIST 37(9):609-611, September 1983.

INFECTION CONTROL—HOSPITALS
Response of hospital infection control programs to the AIDS epidemic [editorial],by W. Schaffner. INFECTION 13(5):201-202, September-October 1985.

INFECTION CONTROL—LABORATORIES
AIDS and the lab: infection control guidelines, by W. M. Valenti. MLO 18(2):53-56, February 1986.

INFECTION CONTROL—LABORATORY WORKERS
Notes on handling the clinical specimens from patients with AIDS or similar conditions, by T. Kawai. RINSHO BYORI 31(12):1366-1368, December 1983.

INSURANCE
AIDS costs: employers and insurers have reasons to fear expensive epidemic. WALL STREET JOURNAL 206:1+, October 18, 1985.

AIDS, gay men and the insurance industry, by R. Mohr. GAY COMMUNITY NEWS 14(10):5, September 21, 1986.

AIDS insurance and health bills slated for votes, by K. Westheimer. GAY COMMUNITY NEWS 13(36):1, March 29, 1986.

AIDS-insurance investigation slated by NAIC, by J. Diamond. NATIONAL UNDERWRITER 89:8, December 27, 1985.

AIDS: the risks to insurers, the threat to equity, by G. M. Oppenheimer, et al. HASTINGS CENTER REPORT 16:18-22, October 1986.

AIDS victims can obtain health cover via state pooling arrangements, by L. Kocolowski. NATIONAL UNDERWRITER 89:3, October 4, 1985.

AIDS victims can obtain health cover via state shared-risk pools, by L. Kocolowski. NATIONAL UNDERWRITER 89:4+, September 28, 1985.

Ban on gay bias proposed by Insurance Council, by Bisticas-Cocoves. GAY COMMUNITY NEWS 13(47):1, June 21, 1986.

Benefits awarded to man caring for dying love,by R. Gillis. GAY COMMUNITY NEWS 13(17):1, November 9, 1985.

Care to AIDS patients: the cost impact on Medicare, by E. W. Smith. CARING 5(6):56-57, June 1986.

Council enacts tough insurance law, by D. Walter. ADVOCATE 449:12, June 24, 1986.

D.C. Insurance Law enacted, by D. Walter. ADVOCATE 454:22, September 2, 1986.

D.C. Insurance Law surviving, by J. McKnight. GAY COMMUNITY NEWS 14(7):1, August 24, 1986.

Employer seeks insurance money/man fired /AIDS, by S. Ager. ADVOCATE 417:17, April 2, 1985.

Group health insurers do not exclude AIDS cover. BUSINESS INSURANCE 19:61, September 30, 1985.

HTLV-III test sought as basis for insurance, by M. Cocoves. GAY COMMUNITY NEWS 13(10):1, September 21, 1985.

Insurance against AIDS?, by R. Blaun. NEW YORK 18:62-65, June 3, 1985.

Insurance industry must combat threat of AIDS to solvency, by L. s. Howard. NATIONAL UNDERWRITER 90:1+, March 22, 1986.

Insurers contend AIDS victims treated same as other policyholders, by M. J. Fisher. NATIONAL UNDERWRITER 89:1+, November 9, 1985.

Insurers gear up to examine impact of AIDS, by L. Kocolowski. NATIONAL UN-DERWRITER 89:4+, September 21, 1985.

Insurers: watchful but not worried, by T. Shahoda, et al. HOSPITALS 60(1):58, January 5, 1986.

Koch asks Cuomo to curb insurance discrimination, by P. Freiberg. ADVOCATE 438:17, January 21, 1986.

Life industry to plan fight against AIDS. NATIONAL UNDERWRITER 90:18, January 4, 1986.

Limiting right of insurers to use AIDS data called discrimination by ACLI, HIA. THE NATIONAL UNDERWRITER (LIFE & HEALTH INSURANCE EDITION) 90:2+, February 1, 1986.

Move to repeal DC AIDS insur. protect. rebuffed, by D. Walter. ADVOCATE 453:22, August 19, 1986.

San Francisco man files $5 million AIDS insurance suit, by M. Helquist. ADVO-CATE 442:23, March 18, 1986.

State regulators to probe impact of AIDS on insurance underwriting, by J. Diamond. THE NATIONAL UNDERWRITER 89:1+, December 28, 1985.

AIDS testing by insurers sparks acrimonious dabate. BEST'S REVIEW 86:100, February 1986.

Insurers need AIDS tests, doctor says. THE NATIONAL UNDERWRITER (LIFE & HEALTH INSURANCE EDITION) 89:4+, October 5, 1985.

Keep insurer AIDS tests: MD. THE NATIONAL UNDERWRITER (PROPERTY & CASUALTY INSURANCE EDITION) 89:3+, October 4, 1985.

Life firm using disputed AIDS test, by L. Kocolowski. NATIONAL UNDERWRITER 89:31, November 1, 1985.

Identification of HTLV-III/LAV or gene product and detection of antibodies in human sera, by N. C. Kan, et al. SCIENCE 231:1553-1555, March 28, 1986.

LAW ENFORCEMENT

AIDS and the police: a loaded gun?, by P. M. Wright. LAW AND ORDER 34(1): 38, January 1986.

AIDS concern grows in policing, by J. Nislow. LAW ENFORCEMENT NEWS 12(1):1+, January 6, 1986.

AIDS: a police hazard?, by H. V. Walker. THE POLICE CHIEF 51(7):21, July 1984.

Fresno police deputies adopt masks to guard against AIDS. CORRECTIONS DIGEST 16(22):6-7, October 23, 1985; also in CRIME CONTROL DIGEST 19(43):7, September 28, 1985.

Guild lawyers oppose San Francisco's sex police, by M. Burtle. GUILD NOTES 9(1):2, Winter 1985.

LAWS AND LEGISLATION

Acquired immune deficiency syndrome. Infection control and public health law, by M. Mills, et al. NEW ENGLAND JOURNAL OF MEDICINE 314(14):931-936, April 3, 1986.

Acquired immunodeficiency syndrome: legal issues in the department, by L. D. Moskowitz, et al. JEN 12(5):297-300, September-October 1986.

Addressing an epidemic: pending federal legislation on AIDS, by M. A. Kadzielski. REVIEW OF THE FEDERATION OF AMERICAN HEALTH SYSTEMS 19(3):48-49, May-June 1986.

AIDS also poses legal and political problems, by Phyllis Schlafly. HUMAN EVENTS 43:18, September 10, 1983.

AIDS and the AIDS virus (HIV): facts and implications for magistrates, by A. J. Pinching. MAGISTRATE 42(12):192-198, 1986.

AIDS bias ruling spurs debate, by D. B. Moskowitz, et al. ENGINEERING NEWS-RECORD 217:84, July 3, 1986.

AIDS bill denounced. REGISTER 62:2, October 5, 1986.

AIDS bills hit legislature, by J. A. Smith. CALIFORNIA NURSE 82(4):8, May 1986.

434

AIDS carrier arraigned on murder charges for spitting. CRIME CONTROL DIGEST 19(50):8-9, December 16, 1985.

AIDS case dismissed on legal technicality [news], by D. M. Barnes. SCIENCE 233(4762):414, July 25, 1986.

AIDS epidemic and gay bathhouses: a constitutional analysis, by J. A. Rabin. JOURNAL OF HEALTH POLITICS, POLICY AND LAW 10(4):729-747, Winter 1986.

AIDS in the workplace: facing the legal issues. CORPORATE SECURITY December 1985, pp. 2-3.

AIDS insurance and health bills slated for votes, by K. Westheimer. GAY COMMUNITY NEWS 13(36):1, March 29, 1986.

AIDS: the legal debate, by D. L. Wing. PERSONNEL JOURNAL 65(8):114-119, August 1986.

AIDS: a legal, medical, and social problem, by C. J. Postell. TRIAL 22(8):76-78, August 1986.

AIDS management: the federal role, by J. S. Oliver. JOURNAL OF MEDICAL TECHNOLOGY 3(3):159-166, March 1986.

AIDS: Pasteur plans to pursue patent: suit on virus [news], by R. Walgate, et al. NATURE 320(6058):96, March 13-19, 1986.

AIDS: Pasteur sues over patent, by T. Beardsley. NATURE 318:595, December 19-26, 1985.

AIDS patent negotiations break down, by C. Norman. SCIENCE 232:819, May 16, 1986.

AIDS patients: dealing with legal issues surrounding diagnosis and treatment, by E. K. Murphy. AORN JOURNAL 43(6):1208-1209+, June 1986.

AIDS poses significant legal considerations for the work place, by C. D. Stromberg. BUSINESS AND HEALTH 3(3):50-51, January-February 1986.

AIDS priority fight goes to court, by C. Norman. SCIENCE 231:11-12, January 3, 1986.

AIDS: public safety v. rights of victims, by N. N. Jurgens. ILLINOIS ISSUES 12:13-14, July 1986.

AIDS questions grow: lawsuits, voter initiatives, handicap laws surface, by P. Marcotte. AMERICAN BAR ASSOCIATION JOURNAL 72:28, November 1, 1986.

AIDS-related discrimination is illegal in NewYork, by P. Freiberg. ADVOCATE 453:16, August 19, 1986.

AIDS spreads to the courts, by A. Press. NEWSWEEK 106:61, July 1, 1985.

AIDS triggers painful legal battles, by T. Gest. US NEWS & WORLD REPORT 100(11):73-74, March 24, 1986.

AIDS: US and French institutes in patents struggle, by R. Walgate, et al. NATURE 317:373, October 3, 1985.

AIDS: US law delays drug testing, by T. Beardsley. NATURE 317:568, October 17, 1985.

AMA challenges Department of Justice ruling on employees with AIDS. CRIME CONTROL DIGEST 20(29):4-5, July 21, 1986; also in CORRECTIONS DI-GEST 17(15):8, July 16, 1986.

Antigay Congressman introduces AIDS bills, by D. Walter. ADVOCATE 435:20, December 10, 1985.

Are victims of AIDS 'handicapped' under federal law?, by T. J. Flygare. PHI DELTA KAPPAN 67:466-467, February 1986.

Atlanta battles gay bathhouse, by G. Cabrera. GAY COMMUNITY NEWS 12(38):1, April 13, 1985.

Bill for AIDS. NEW SCIENTIST 109:21, January 16, 1986.

California acts to protect blood, gays, by M. Lassell. ADVOCATE 419:14, April 30, 1985.

California Governor vetoes AIDS anti-discrimination. Bill, by M. Vandervelden. ADVOCATE 454:22, September 2, 1986.

California Senate fails to override AIDS funding veto, by M. Helquist. ADVOCATE 427:12, August 20, 1985.

Cincinnati Board okays measure protecting gays,by M. Tuhus. GUARDIAN 38(41):4, August 6, 1986.

Closing the baths: where will it end?, by S. Brookie. GAY COMMUNITY NEWS 12(22):3, December 15, 1984.

Congress and AIDS legislation, by D. Walter ADVOCATE 447:14, May 27, 1986.

Congress eyes proposals to curb AIDS. HUMAN EVENTS 45:5, December 7, 1985.

Controlling the baths and backroom bars, by M. Callen. VILLAGE VOICE 30:36, March 12, 1985.

Correspondence about handling evidence in cases of acquired immune defi-ciency syndrome (AIDS) [letter], by J. A. Kaye. AMERICAN JOURNAL OF FORENSIC MEDICINE AND PATHOLOGY 7(1):87-88, March 1986.

DC Council enacts tough insurance law, by D. Walter. ADVOCATE 449:12, June 24, 1986.

D.C. Insurance Law enacted, by D. Walter. ADVOCATE 454:22, September 2, 1986.

D.C. Insurance Law surviving, by J. McKnight. GAY COMMUNITY NEWS 14(7):1, August 24, 1986.

DC insurers barred from testing for AIDS, by J. Firshein. HOSPITALS 60(13): 50+, July 5, 1986.

DOJ opinion fuels AIDS firing debate, by D. Burda. HOSPITALS 60(15):30, August 5, 1986.

ERD rules AIDS ban discriminatory. OUT 4(8):3, June 1986.

Firing employees who have AIDS brings on new round of legal action, by C. R. Goerth. OCCUPATIONAL HEALTH AND SAFETY 54(10):28, October 1985.

Florida test case challenge of Justice Dept. ruling, by D. Walter. ADVOCATE 454:16, September 2, 1986.

"Good" and "bad" of California's 40 AIDS bills, by Bisticas-Cocoves. GAY COMMUNITY NEWS 13(44):3, May 31, 1986.

Health crisis: AIDS is now becoming a legal epidemic, too, by J. Hyatt. INC. 7:19-20, December 1985.

Hearing held in PWA case, by J. Kiely. GAY COMMUNITY NEWS 14(2):1, July 20, 1986.

Houston gay rights squashed in referendum, by S. Hyde. GAY COMMUNITY NEWS 12(28):1, February 2, 1985.

How the AIDS ruling affects us. DISABILITY 7(5):26, September 1986.

How will the law respond to AIDS?, by A. Affriol, et al.. JOURNAL OF PRACTICAL NURSING 35(4):31, December 1985.

Judge backs New York AIDS policy, by B. Norris. THE TIMES EDUCATIONAL SUPPLEMENT 3635:13, February 28, 1986.

Judge intervenes in bathhouse controversy, by S. Brooke. GAY COMMUNITY NEWS 12(15):1, October 27, 1984.

Justice Department: PWAs may be fired, by D. Walter. ADVOCATE 451:13, Juy 22, 1986.

LA Councilman proposes law banning AIDS bias,by Brooke, et al. ADVOCATE 425:21, July 23, 1985.

LA ordinance seeks to stop leper syndrome, by R. Hippler. GUARDIAN 37(45):5, Septemebr 18, 1985.

LA, West Hollywood ban AIDS discrimination, by Brooke, et al. ADVOCATE 429:13, September 17, 1985.

Law review offers articles on legal aspects of AIDS. CRIME CONTROL DIGEST 20(45):10, November 10, 1986.

Lawsuit on AIDS. NEWSWEEK 106:65, December 23, 1985.

Lawsuit over Rock's estate exposes scandal—and asserts a lover's right to know [case of M. Christian], by S. Haller. PEOPLE 24:52-54+, November 25, 1985.

Lawyers oppose most AIDS-related discrimination, by L. R. Reskin. AMERICAN BAR ASSOCIATION JOURNAL 72:34, June 1, 1986.

Legal: AIDS-related litigation looms over employers, by D. B. Thompson. INDUSTRY WEEK 227:26-28, December 9, 1985.

Legal aspects of AIDS part 1, by H. Creighton. NURSING MANAGEMENT 17(11):14+, November 1986.

Legal implications for health care providers, by M. a. Kadzielski. HEALTH PROG-RESS 67(4):48-52, May 1986.

Legal issues around the AIDS crisis, by P. Bucalo. CALIFORNIA NURSE 82(4): 14-15, May 1986.

Legal issues of AIDS, by A. D Hagerty. MICHIGAN HOSPITALS 22(8):22-24, August 1986.

Legislating AIDS away [editorial], by J. M. Dwyer. MEDICAL JOURNAL OF AUSTRALIA 143(7):276-277, September 30, 1985.

Legislation/confidentiality in AID research. ADVOCATE 416:109, March 19, 1985.

Legitimacy and paternity—HLA test—self-incrimination—AIDS. THE FAMILY LAW REPORTER: COURT OPINIONS 11(40):1515, August 20, 1985.

Los Angeles bans anti-AIDS discrimination, by M. Cocoves. GAY COMMUNITY NEWS 13(8):1, August 31, 1985.

Matlovich may push for D.C. ban on sex in baths, by D. Walter. ADVOCATE 420:10, May 14, 1985.

Medical experts challenge Justice Dept. memo, by D. Walter. ADVOCATE 454:14, September 2, 1986.

Moral, ethical, and legal aspects of infection control, by B. Parent. AMERICAN JOURNAL OF INFECTION CONTROL 13(6):278-280, December 1985.

Moynihan Bill requires PHS provide funds: AIDS, by D. Walter. ADVOCATE 427:21, August 20, 1985.

New twist in AIDS patent fight, by C. Norman. SCIENCE 232:308-309, April 18, 1986.

New York City grants Rights Bill to lesbians, gay men, by B. Gelbert. GAY COM-MUNITY NEWS 13(37):1, April 1, 1986.

New York locks up the "mineshaft", by Bisticas-Cocoves. GAY COMMUNITY NEWS 13(19):1, November 23, 1985.

New York officials reconsider closing baths, by P. Freiberg. ADVOCATE 433:14, November 12, 1985.

New York queers fight City Hall, by K. Westheimer. GAY COMMUNITY NEWS 13(20):1, November 30, 1985.

New York to introduce AIDS bill, by J. Aschkenasy. THE NATIONAL UNDER-WRITER (LIFE & HEALTH INSURANCE EDITION) 90:26, January 25, 1986.

NH bill would ban lesbian & gay blood,by C. Guilfoy. GAY COMMUNITY NEWS 12(30):1, February 16, 1985.

Patent battle of AIDS researchers, by D. Dickson. THE TIMES HIGHER EDUCA-TION SUPPLEMENT 673:12, September 27, 1985.

Potential liability for transfusion-associated AIDS, by P. J. Miller, et al. JAMA 253(23):3419-3424, June 21, 1985.

Power to shut bathhouses voted by House, by Bisticas-Cocoves. GAY COM-MUNITY NEWS 13(14):1, October 19, 1985.

Privacy provision signed into law. OUT 3(10):1, August 1985.

San Francisco Judge closes gay baths, sex clubs, by R. O'Loughlin. ADVOCATE 4(7):8, November 13, 1984.

San Francisco sex regulations tightened up, by C. Guilfoy. GAY COMMUNITY NEWS 12(25):1, January 12, 1985.

School law, by D. A. Splitt. EXECUTIVE EDUCATOR 8(3):12, March 1986.

Should the bathhouses be closed?, by P. Freiberg. ADVOCATE 41:8, March 5, 1985.

Will New York close the baths?, by L. Bush. VILLAGE VOICE 29:24+, December 18, 1984.

Winning smiles as the AIDS patent battle continues. NEW SCIENTIST 112:20, October 2, 1986.

FRANCE
AIDS: US and French institutes in patents struggle, by R. Walgate, et al. NATURE 317:373, October 3, 1985.

LAWS AND LEGISLATION—BLOOD TRANSFUSIONS
New Hampshire bill would ban lesbian and gay blood, by C. Guilfoy. GAY COM-MUNITY NEWS 12(30):1, February 16, 1985.

LAWS AND LEGISLATION—CIVIL RIGHTS
Massachusetts House crushes Gay Rights Bill, 88-65, by C. Gulfoy. GAY COM-MUNITY NEWS 13(12):1, October 5, 1985.

Massachusetts House passes Bill for HTLV-3 confidentiality, by S. Poggi. GAY COMMUNITY NEWS 13(44):1, May 31, 1986.

Massachusetts passes law to grant HTLV-3 confidentiality, by K. Westheimer. GAY COMMUNITY NEWS 14(2):1, July 20, 1986.

LAWS AND LEGISLATION—EMPLOYMENT
AIDS: a legal perspective on employer costs, by G. P. Cunningham. HEALTH COST MANAGEMENT 3(1):1-6, January-February 1986.

Employers can fire AIDS victims to keep the disease from spreading, DOJ rules. JUVENILE JUSTICE DIGEST 14(12):7-8, June 30, 1986; also in CRIME CONTROL DIGEST 20(26):8, June 30, 1986.

LAWS AND LEGISLATION—HEALTH CARE WORKERS
AIDS: responding to the crisis. Legal implications for health care providers, by M. A. Kadzielski. HEALTH PROGRESS 67(4):48-52, May 1986.

LAWS AND LEGISLATION—HOSPITALS
AIDS guidelines can reduce legal risks for hospitals, by D. L. Wing. HOSPITAL MANAGER 16(4):1-3, July-August 1986.

AIDS poses legal questions for hospital managers, by K. B. Stickler. HOSPITAL MANAGER 13(6):1-3, November-December 1983.

Hospitals face legal issues involving AIDS patients, employees, by J. D. Epstein, et al. TEXAS HOSPITALS 41(11):12-15, April 1986.

LAWS AND LEGISLATION—NURSES
Legislation affecting nursing practice. Legislation affecting occupational allied health groups. Legislation related to acquired immune deficiency syndrome, by C. La-Bar. STATE NURSING LEGISLATION QUARTERLY 4(2):1-23, Summer 1986.

LAWS AND LEGISLATION—TATTOOS
Tattoo trouble: fear of AIDS prompts a call for regulations, by B. Henker. ALBERTA REPORT 13:52-53, April 14, 1986.

LAWS AND LEGISLATION—TESTS
Patent dispute divides AIDS researchers [ELISA test], by C. Norman. SCIENCE 230:640-642, November 8, 1985.

LITERATURE
AIDS: a research and clinical bibliography. HEMATOLOGICAL ONCOLOGY 2(1):77-134, January-March 1984.

AIDS resource list. GAY COMMUNITY NEWS 11(32):4, March 3, 1984.

Computerized access to clinical nursing literature on AIDS, by S. M. Sparks. TOPICS IN CLINICAL NURSING 6(2):79-82, July 1984.

Computers, AIDS and literature, by R. Hall. ADVOCATE 3(76):34, September 15, 1983.

Gay dramatists pen new works/ "Age of AIDS", by M. Kearns. ADVOCATE 412:24, January 22, 1985.

Gay writers on disease & health, by Mitzel. GAY COMMUNITY NEWS 45:8, June 7, 1986.

New books examine the social and scientific issues surrounding AIDS. PUB-LISHERS WEEKLY 228:100+, September 13, 1985.

New books put human faces on—AIDS care. ADVOCATE 452:31, August 5, 1986.

New online AIDS library will be a central comprehensive source of information. COLLEAGUE ON CALL 3(5):8, October-November 1986.

Nursing literature on AIDS, by S. G. Fisher, et al. TOPICS IN CLINICAL NURSING 6(2):76-82, July 1984.

Quick-bibs: AIDS, by B. Ott. AMERICAN LIBRARIES 16:681, November 1985.

St. Martin's book to probe the AIDS mystery, by J. Davis. PUBLISHERS WEEKLY 223:30, April 29, 1983.

Summer reading on AIDS, by N. Fain. ADVOCATE 3(75):15, September 1, 1983.

MEDIA

Activists charge PBS AIDS show "unethical", by B. M. Gelbert. GAY COMMUNITY NEWS 13(36):2, March 29, 1986.

AIDS and the mythmakers, by B. Kochis. PROGRESSIVE 50(9):16, September 1986.

AIDS announcement raises questions, by J. Silberner. SCIENCE NEWS 128: 293, November 9, 1985.

AIDS awareness month, by D. Morris. GAY COMMUNITY NEWS 10(27):2, January 29, 1983.

AIDS, condoms and squeamish media, by R. Dorfman. QUILL 73:6-7, October 1985.

AIDS film honored, by C. Guilfoy. GAY COMMUNITY NEWS 13(3):12, July 27, 1985.

AIDS 1st leak cited on TV, by B. Gelbert. GAY COMMUNITY NEWS 13(39):1, April 19, 1986.

AIDS: journalism in a plague year, by David Nimmons. PLAYBOY 30:35+, October 1983.

AIDS material called "porno", by M. Helquist. ADVOCATE 430:22, October 1, 1985.

AIDS—organizing reporting, by C. Guilfoy. GAY COMMUNITY NEWS 11(18):3, November 19, 1983.

AIDS plagued by media, by M. Adams. HERIZONS 4(1):4, January 1986.

AIDS—putting the press together, by C. Patton. GAY COMMUNITY NEWS 11(23):3, December 24, 1983.

441

AIDS: what newspapers, radio and TV unfortunately grimly have to say . . . (various simple tools to fight against the spread of the virus), by L. Thiry. REVUE DE L'IN-FIRMIERE 36(6):30-32, March 1986.

All quiet on the tabloid front, by B. Morton. THE TIMES HIGHER EDUCATION SUPPLEMENT 658:13, June 14, 1985.

Anatomy of a media epidemic, by B. Odair. ALTERNATIVE MEDIA 14(3):10, Fall 1983.

Atypical AIDS cases draw world to town, by P. Thomas. MEDICAL WORLD NEWS 27(16):7+, August 25, 1986.

Beating the Mardi Gras media bash, by D. Grenville. BODY POLITIC 114:19, May 1985.

Chronicle: AIDS and the family paper, by Lisa Leff, et al. COLUMBIA JOURNAL-ISM REVIEW 24:11+, March-April 1986.

Early frost: the story behind NBC's AIDS dram, by A. Block. ADVOCATE 434:43, November 26, 1985.

Exploited for headlines. BODY POLITIC 126:22, May 1986.

Fighting for life [motion picture and television artists' views], by S. Haller. PEOPLE 24:28-33, September 23, 1985.

Filmmaker Arthur Bressa on AIDS, by M. Bronski. GAY COMMUNITY NEWS 13(17):10, November 9, 1985.

Gay papers bicker over AIDS coverage, by R. Oloughlin. MEDIAFILE 3(12):1, June 1983.

Hollywood love scenes: the scares, laughs, romance, by M. Murphy, et al. TV GUIDE 34:4+, February 8, 1986.

In the news: AIDS, by J. Richters. HEALTHRIGHT 2:4-7, August 1983.

Media hypes AIDS breakthrough/NIH, by N. Fain. ADVOCATE 3(75):14, September 1, 1983.

Media indicts woman—rumored AIDS, by C. Guilfoy. GAY COMMUNITY NEWS 11(35):7, March 24, 1984.

Media seething over bad blood, by E. Jackson. BODY POLITIC 92:11, April 1983.

NBC movie helped AIDS cause, gay leaders say, by B. Kenkelen. NATIONAL CATHOLIC REPORTER 22:6, November 22, 1985.

News analysis. Just another excuse to persecute?, by V. Scott. NURSING MIRROR 161(16):11, October 16, 1985.

PBS runs anti-black, anti-gay AIDS show, by B. Gelbert. GAY COMMUNITY NEWS 13(37):3, April 1, 1986.

Personal experience with AIDS. Courageous patient shares his ordeal through newspaper, by L. M. Keen. AMERICAN JOURNAL OF HOSPICE CARE 3(2):10-16, March-April 1986.

Public education on AIDS: not only the media's responsiblity, by W. Check. HASTINGS CENTER REPORT 15(4):27-31, August 1985.

Rating crisis coverage/AIDS/media, by N. Fain. ADVOCATE 3(77):24, September 29, 1983.

Royal College of Nursing. AIDS and the media. NURSING STANDARD 385:4, February 21, 1985.

—. Food for thought; facing reality. NURSING STANDARD 448:4, May 22, 1986.

—. Put to the test. NURSING STANDARD 379:4, January 10, 1985.

—. The real victims; rewarding cuts. NURSING STANDARD 418:4, October 10, 1984.

Signs of omission: press coverage of AIDS has left some things unsaid, by J. Alter. NEWSWEEK 106(13):25, Septemebr 23, 1985.

TV show hides main victims, by S. Garvey. IN THESE TIMES 8(32):21, August 22, 1984.

GREAT BRITAIN
Gonorrhoea in homosexual men and media coverage of the acquired immune deficiency syndrome in London 1982-3, by I. V. Weller, et al. BRITISH MEDICAL JOURNAL 289(6451):1041, October 20, 1984.

Tabloid terror from not-so-United Kingdom, by N. DeJongh. ADVOCATE 417:43, April 2, 1985.

MEDIA—ATTITUDES
TV news and Aids: how bad reporting scared America, by Edwin Diamond. TV GUIDE 31:4+, October 22, 1983.

MEDICAL ETHICS
AIDS and clinical ethics: honoring patients' dignity, by D. J. Roy, et al. DIMENSIONS IN HEALTH SERVICE 63(7):32-33, October 1986.

AIDS and ethics, by A. R. Jonsen, et al. ISSUES IN SCIENCE AND TECHNOLOGY 2:56-65, Winter 1986.

AIDS and the professional ethic, by C. Healy. AUSTRALIAN NURSES JOURNAL 14(7):10, February 1985.

AIDS: clarifying values to close in on ethical questions, by S. M. Steele. NURSING AND HEALTH CARE 7(5):246-248, May 1986.

AIDS: the emerging ethical dilemmas. HASTINGS CENTER REPORT 15(Suppl. 32):August 1985.

AIDS: an ethical challenge for our time, by C. Levine. QRB 12(8):273-277, August 1986.

443

AIDS, ethics, and the blood supply. A report of a conference of the American
Blood Commission and the Hastings Center, Institute of Society, Ethics and
the Life Sciences, January 29 and 30, 1985, by W. V. Miller, et al. TRANS-
FUSION 25(2):174-175, March-April 1985.

AIDS: evidence of the growing burden of ethical dilemmas in health care, by M. K.
Mitchell. NURSING AND HEALTH CARE 7(5):229, May 1986.

MEDICAL ETHICS—NURSING
AIDS: ethical duties of nurses, by S. J. Smith. CALIFORNIA NURSE 79(3):4,
September 1983.

MICROBIOLOGY
Acid-fast bacilli on buffy coat smears in the acquired immunodeficiency syn-
drome: a lesson from Hansen's bacillus, by B. S. Graham, et al.
SOUTHERN MEDICAL JOURNAL 77(2):246-248, February 1984.

MILITARY
AIDS incidence higher in older recruits, by P. Smith. AIR FORCE TIMES 46:3,
April 14, 1986.

AIDS-infected members limited to ConUS duty, by L. Famiglietti. AIR FORCE
TIMES 46:6, July 28, 1986.

AIDS panel recommends early medical discharge, by S. B. Young. AIR FORCE
TIMES 47:12+, October 20, 1986.

AIDS screening predicted for entire force, by P. J. Budahn. AIR FORCE TIMES
46:1+, October 21, 1985.

AIDS stretching VA's ability to treat veterans, by J. Firshein. HOSPITALS
60(4):33-34, February 20, 1986.

Army: spread of AIDS threatens readiness, by P. Smith. AIR FORCE TIMES
46:3+, August 26, 1985.

DOD: 40 with AIDS virus denied enlistment, by P. Smith. AIR FORCE TIMES
46:19, December 16, 1985.

DOD says two die from AIDS, over dozen afflicted, by P. Smith. AIR FORCE
TIMES 44:10, February 6, 1984.

DOD seeks suggestions on monitoring AIDS, by P. Smith. AIR FORCE TIMES
46:1+, August 12, 1985.

DOD won't punish donors who have AIDS, by P. Smith. AIR FORCE TIMES 45:4,
May 20, 1985.

First AIDS death in military gets cautious response, by K. Popert. BODY POLITIC
124:15, March 1986.

Gay man with AIDS wins discharge BT, by J. Ryan. GAY COMMUNITY NEWS
11(33):1, March 10, 1984.

Hill bars 'adverse action' against AIDS carriers, by P. J. Budahn. AIR FORCE
TIMES 47:10, November 3, 1986.

Retirement evaluation due AIDS-stricken sailor, by P. Smith. AIR FORCE TIMES 44:12, March 5, 1984.

Stevens: keep AIDS-positive civilians home,by A. Laurent. AIR FORCE TIMES 46:58, June 2, 1986.

United States troops and AIDS, by T. Beardsley. NATURE 316(6030):668, August 22-28, 1985.

GERMANY
HTLV-III/LAV-antibody-positive soldiers in Berlin [letter], by J. J. James, et al. NEW ENGLAND JOURNAL OF MEDICINE 314(1):55-56, January 2, 1986.

MILITARY—BLOOD DONORS
HTLV-III antibodies in US Army blood donors in West Germany, by J. J. James. JAMA 254:1449, September 20, 1985.

Pentagon delays policy on military blood donors, by Bisticas-Cocoves. GAY COMMUNITY NEWS 13(4):1, August 3, 1985.

MILITARY—CIVIL RIGHTS
Confidentiality in the military, by D. Walter. ADVOCATE 434:12, November 26, 1985.

MILITARY—STATISTICS
Services report 30 cases of AIDS, by P. Smith. AIR FORCE TIMES 44:26, May 14, 1984.

MILITARY—TESTING
AF gearing up for AIDS testing in March, by L. Famiglietti. AIR FORCE TIMES 46:7, November 25, 1985.

AIDS test ordered to screen recruits, by P. Smith. AIR FORCE TIMES 46:3, September 16, 1985.

AIDS testing for all troops to start September 1, by L. Famiglietti. AIR FORCE TIMES 46:1+, July 21, 1986.

AIDS testing opposed for civilians, dependents, by P. Smith. AIR FORCE TIMES 46:4, December 9, 1985.

AIDS: USAR testing starts in 1986, by B. Pratt. ARMY RESERVE MAGAZINE 32(2):15, Spring 1986.

AIDS: witchhunt aura surrounds Pentagon testing, by K. Gilberd. GUARDIAN 38(19):9, February 12, 1986.

Air Force plans to test 34,000 monthly for AIDS, by L. Famiglietti. AIR FORCE TIMES 46:3, May 26, 1986.

ANG joins in testing for AIDS, by P. Dalton. AIR FORCE TIMES 46:6, July 28, 1986.

ANG to begin screening members for AIDS, by P. Dalton. AIR FORCE TIMES 46:9, May 19, 1986.

Civilians exempted from AIDS testing, by P. Smith. AIR FORCE TIMES 46:28, February 10, 1986.

Deadline moved up for overseas AIDS tests, by L. Famiglietti. AIR FORCE TIMES 47:1+, September 22, 1986.

Early tests find fewer than 240 with AIDS, by P. Smith. AIR FORCE TIMES 46:3, May 26, 1986.

Military AIDS testing offers research bonus, by C. Norman. SCIENCE 232:818-820, May 16, 1986.

Military seeking test results, by M. Cocoves. GAY COMMUNITY NEWS 12(41):1, May 4, 1985.

Military test for viril antibodies: anti-gay, by T. Ensign. GUARDIAN 38(6):3, November 6, 1985.

Military to screen recruits for HTLV-III, by S. Poggi. GAY COMMUNITY NEWS 13(9):1, September 14, 1985.

Pentagon AIDS test that sparked furor. US NEWS & WORLD REPORT 99:12, September 9, 1985.

Pentagon orders mass HTLV-III screening, by Bisticas-Cocoves. GAY COMMUNITY NEWS 13(18):1, November 16, 1985.

Pentagon reviews policy on tests for AIDS virus, by S. B. Young. AIR FORCE TIMES 47:8, October 13, 1986.

Reserves to start AIDS tests Sept. 1, by P. Dalton. AIR FORCE TIMES 47:30, August 25, 1986.

SecDef decides to test active members for AIDS, by P. Smith. AIR FORCE TIMES 46:3, October 28, 1985.

SecDef issues guidelines for AIDS testing, by P. Smith. AIR FORCE TIMES 46:10, November 4, 1985.

Service groups say: "Don't take the test". BODY POLITIC 112:19, March 1985.

MILITARY—TRANSMISSION—BLOOD TRANSFUSION
AIDS virus in military blood donations drops. AIR FORCE TIMES 46:18, June 23, 1986.

MILITARY—TREATMENT
AF to begin use of AIDS drug when approved. AIR FORCE TIMES 47:6, October 6, 1986.

MINORITIES
People of color and AIDS: who's taking action, by Bisticas-Cocoves. GAY COMMUNITY NEWS 13(24):3, December 28, 1985.

MORTALITY
Acquired immunodeficiency syndrome among patients attending hemophilia treatment centers and mortality experience of hemophiliacs in the United

States, by R. E. Johson, et al. AMERICAN JOURNAL OF EPIDEMIOLOGY 121(6):797-810, June 1985.

AIDS and sudden death [letter], by C. H. Sherlock, et al. CANADIAN MEDICAL ASSOCIATION JOURNAL 129(10):1079, November 15, 1983.

AIDS: express train to death, by R. Wells. NURSING MIRROR 160(7):16-18, February 13, 1985.

AIDS: no threat from the dead: a doctor decried special care for victims' bodies, by S. Deaton. ALBERTA REPORT 13:32+, March 31, 1986.

AIDS patient who died too soon, by M. Turck. HOSPITAL PRACTICE 20(1):77+, January 15, 1985.

Autopsy pathology in the acquired immune deficiency syndrome, by C. M. Reichert, et al. AMERICAN JOURNAL OF PATHOLOGY 112(3):357-382, September 1983.

Bad blood: "gift of life" may be also an agent of death in some AIDS [acquired immuno deficiency syndrome] cases, by M. Chase. WALL STREET JOURNAL 203:1+, March 12, 1984.

Bobbi Campbell's brave fight against AIDS ends, by S. Kulieke. ADVOCATE 403:16, September 18, 1984.

Cela s'appelle la mort (LAV), by J. P. Richard. RELATIONS 45:244, October 1985.

Coffin as closet [editorial]. ADVOCATE 450:5, July 8, 1986.

Death and the erotic imagination, by M. Bronski. GAY COMMUNITY NEWS 14(8):8, September 7, 1986.

Death in the AIDS patient: role of cytomegalovirus [letter], by A. M. Macher, et al. NEW ENGLAND JOURNAL OF MEDICINE 309(23):1454, December 8, 1983.

Death in the family, by L. Van Gelder. ROLLING STONE February 3, 1983, p. 18-20+.

Deathly ill at centre stage, by A. Nelson. MACLEAN'S 98:58, June 24, 1985.

Disseminated Mycobacterium avium-intracellulare infection in homosexual men dying of acquired immunodeficiency, by P. Zakowski, et al. JAMA 248(22): 2980-2982, December 10, 1982.

DOD says two die from AIDS, over dozen afflicted, by P. Smith. AIR FORCE TIMES 44:10, February 6, 1984.

Dying to live/reflection on the Black Death, by G. Hannon. BODY POLITIC 117:27, August 1985.

Fatal cryptosporidiosis complicating Kaposi's sarcoma in an immunocompromised man, by M. Wittner, et al. AMERICAN JOURNAL OF THE MEDICAL SCIENCES 287(2):47-48, March-April 1984.

Fatal pulmonary pneumocystosis 2 years after multiple transfusions [letter], by G. Offenstadt, et al. PRESSE MEDICALE 13(39):2388-2389, November 3, 1984.

Fatal toxoplasmosis of the central nervous system in a heroin user with acquired immunodeficiency disease, by S. K. Murthy, et al. NEW YORK STATE JOURNAL OF MEDICINE 84(9):464-466, September 1984.

First AIDS death in military gets cautious response, by K. Popert. BODY POLITIC 124:15, March 1986.

Ginsberg meditates on death and eternity, by E. Shively. GAY COMMUNITY NEWS 13(34):7, March 15, 1986.

Immediate causes of death in acquired immunodeficiency syndrome, by L. Moskowitz, et al. ARCHIVES OF PATHOLOGY AND LABORATORY MEDICINE 109(8):735-738, August 1985.

In memoriam, by P. Wynne. ISSUES IN RADICAL THERAPY 11(3):8, 1984.

In memoriam: Bobbi Campbell 1952-1984. GAY COMMUNITY NEWS 12(8):11, September 8, 1984.

Looking death in the face, by B. Mahoney. AMERICAN PHOTOGRAPHER 16:98-102, April 1986.

Medical pathology conference. Respiratory failure in a 54-year-old man with hemophilia A, by J. H. Garcia, et al. ALABAMA JOURNAL OF MEDICAL SCIENCES 20(2):164-170, April 1983.

Mortality associated with mode of presentation in the acquired immune deficiency syndrome, by a. R. Moss, et al. JNCI 73(6):1281-1284, December 1984.

Mother tells how a blood donation, the gift of life, led to her young son's death from AIDS, by H. Kushnick. PEOPLE 21:62+, June 4, 1984.

Multiple infections and death in a homosexual man [clinical conference]. AMERICAN JOURNAL OF MEDICINE 75(5):855-867, November 1983.

Necropsy findings in acquired immunodeficiency syndrome: a comparison of pre-mortem diagnoses with postmortem findings, by A. N. Hui, et al. HUMAN PATHOLOGY 15(7):670-676, July 1984.

Necroscopic findings of variably acid-fast bacteria in a fatal case of acquired immunodeficiency syndrome and Kaposi's sarcoma,by A. R. Cantwell, Jr. GROWTH 47(2):129-134, Summer 1983.

New York jail cook dies from AIDS: not a high-risk group member. CORRECTIONS DIGEST 14(14):10, June 29, 1983.

Only months to live and no place to die, by J. Seligmann. NEWSWEEK 106:26, August 12, 1985.

Perhaps his death will help us to realize, by C. Jackson. GAY COMMUNITY NEWS 13(47):5, June 21, 1986.

Requiem for an AIDS victim, by D. K. Ciannella. WITNESS 68(9):10-11, September 1985.

Rock Hudson. PEOPLE WEEKLY 24:108+, December 23-30, 1985.

—, by G. Gottlieb. GAY COMMUNITY NEWS 14(7), August 24, 1986.

Rock Hudson AIDS case sends a message. U.S. NEWS & WORLD REPORT 99:12, August 5, 1985.

Rock Hudson and the war against AIDS, by J. Barber. MACLEAN'S 98:44, August 5, 1985.

Rock Hudson: the great gay hope, by S. Bronski. GAY COMMUNITY NEWS 13(7):7, August 24, 1985.

Rock Hudson has AIDS. ADVOCATE 427:22, August 20, 1985.

Rock Hudson: legacy of hope, by J. Adler. NEWSWEEK 106:36, October 14, 1985.

Rock Hudson: on camera and off, by J. Yarbrough. PEOPLE 24:34-41, August 12, 1985.

San Francisco's AIDS toll nears thousand, by I. Anderson. NEW SCIENTIST 102:8, April 12, 1984.

Suicide AIDS related. OUT 2(10):3, September 1984.

Texas attorney activist dies of AIDS, by H. Hod. ADVOCATE 3(86):11, January 24, 1984.

Texas attorney dies of AIDS. GAY COMMUNITY NEWS 11(25):3, January 14, 1984.

Wandering the woods in a season of death, by A. Troxier. RFD 45:39, Winter 1985.

Widows story: life after lover died of AIDS, by B. Hillard. ADVOCATE 421:5, May 28, 1985.

CANADA
Gay plague takes a life in Alberta, by F. Orr. ALBERTA REPORT 10:36, June 27, 1983.

GERMANY
AIDS fatalities in Hamburg (status: February 1985)—legal medicine aspects, by K. Püschel, et al. ZEITSCHRIFT FUR RECHTSMEDIZIN 95(2):113-121, 1985.

SWEDEN
First two fatal cases of AIDS in Sweden—diagnostic and therapeutic experiences, by E. Asbrink, et al. LAKARTIDNINGEN 81(15):1513-1516, April 11, 1984.

UNITED STATES
AIDS kills Virginia inmate. CORRECTIONS DIGEST 16(10):6, May 8, 1985.

Dumped AIDS patient dies in SF, by D. France. GAY COMMUNITY NEWS
11(16):3, November 5, 1983.

MORTALITY—HEMOPHILIACS
Fatal AIDS in a haemophiliac in the UK [letter], by H. M. Daly, et al. LANCET
2(8360):1190, November 19, 1983.

Fatal AIDS in a UK haemophiliac [letter], by H. M. Daly, et al. LANCET 1(8367):44,
January 1984.

ITALY
First case in Italy of fatal AIDS in a hemophiliac, by R. Kal Bo Zanon, et al.
ACTA HAEMATOLOGICA 75(1):34-37, 1986.

MORTALITY—PRISONS
First AIDS death reported in Maryland prison system. CORRECTIONS DIGEST
15(20):4-5, September 26, 1984.

MORTALITY—WOMEN
Listeriosis as a cause of maternal death: an obstetric complication of the acquired
immunodeficiency syndrome (AIDS), by C. V. Wetli, et al. AMERICAN JOUR-
NAL OF OBSTETRICS AND GYNECOLOGY 147(1):7-9, September 1, 1983.

NUTRITION
Deficiency in dietary gamma-linolenic and/or eicosapentaenoic acids may
determine individual susceptibility to AIDS, by M. E. Bégin, et al. MEDICAL
HYPOTHESES 20(1):1-8, May 1986.

Evaluation of body weight and nutritional status among AIDS patients, by P.
O'Sullivan, et al. AMERICAN DIETETIC ASSOCIATION JOURNAL 85:1483-
1484, November 1985.

Nutrition and the acquired immunodeficiency syndrome [letter], by R. S. Beach,
et al. ANNALS OF INTERNAL MEDICINE 99(4):565-566, October 1983.

Nutritional management of the AIDS patients, by R. R. Rago, et al. PHYSICIAN
ASSISTANT 10(10):89-90, October 1986.

Significance of altered nutritional status in acquired immune deficiency syndrome
(AIDS), by R. T. Chlebowski. NUTRITION AND CANCER 7(1-2):85-91, 1985.

OCCURRENCE
AIDS for all by the year 2000? [letter], by M. McEvoy, et al. BRITISH MEDICAL
JOURNAL 290(6466):463, February 9, 1985.

AIDS hits second tier cities, by M. Helquist. ADVOCATE 430:23, October 1,
1985.

AIDS in a bodybuilder using anabolic steroids [letter], by H. M. Sklarek, et al. NEW
ENGLAND JOURNAL OF MEDICINE 311(26):1701, December 27, 1984.

AIDS in Haitian-Americans: a reassessment, by E. Frank, et al. CANCER RE-
SEARCH 45(Supplement 9):4619s-4620s, September 1985.

AIDS incidence increases as experts continue investigations. AMERICAN FAMILY PHYSICIAN 33:328-329, March 1986.

AIDS likely to spread unless causes can be identified, by P. L. Polakoff. OCCU-PATIONAL HEALTH AND SAFETY February 1984, p. 44-45.

AIDS research and incidence on the rise. AMERICAN FAMILY PHYSICIAN 28:17, October 1983.

AIDS study finds virus is widespread. NEW SCIENTIST 106:3, April 25, 1985.

AIDS toll expected to soar, by M. Helquist. ADVOCATE 453:23, August 19, 1986.

AIDS toll rises. US NEWS & WORLD REPORT 97:80, November 26, 1984.

Incidence of AIDS [letter], by P. R. Gustafson. JAMA 254(6):751-752, August 9, 1985.

Incidence rate of acquired immunodeficiency syndrome in selected populations, by A. M. Hardy, et al. JAMA 253(2):215-220, January 11, 1985.

Increase in AIDS cases—anomaly or trend?, by Bill Kenkelen. NATIONAL CATHOLIC REPORTER 22:32, May 16, 1986.

Increase in high-grade lymphomas in young men, by C. C. Boring, et al. LANCET 1(8433):857-859, April 13, 1985.

International occurrence of the acquired immunodeficiency syndrome, by J. B. Brunet, et al. ANNALS OF INTERNAL MEDICINE 103(5):670-674, November 1985.

Notoriety of disease . . . famous people having diseases, by L. Klein. JOURNAL OF ENTEROSTOMAL THERAPY 12(6):191-192, November-December 1985.

Number of AIDS cases likely to escalate rapidly. CHEMICAL AND ENGINEERING NEWS 63:5, September 23, 1985.

PHS projects dramatic rise in AIDS cases, by D. Walter. ADVOCATE 451:22, July 22, 1986.

Report from the PHLS Communicable Disease Surveillance Centre. BRITISH MEDICAL JOURNAL 292(6533):1447-1448, May 31, 1986.

Searching for cases of AIDS in Britain, by S. Connor, et al. NEW SCIENTIST 98:361, May 12, 1983.

Three-year incidence of AIDS in five cohorts of HTLV-III infected risk group members, by J. J. Goedert, et al. SCIENCE 231:992-995, February 28, 1986.

Update: acquired immunodeficiency syndrome (AIDS)—United States. MMWR 32(30):389-391, August 5, 1983; also in subsequent issues.

World AIDS developments. BODY POLITIC 130:19, September 1986.

AFRICA

Acquired immune deficiency syndrome. A report of 2 South African cases, by G. J. Ras, et al. SOUTH AFRICAN MEDICAL JOURNAL 64(4):140-142, July 23, 1983.

Acquired immune deficiency syndrome in Belgium and its relation to Central Africa, by N. Clumeck, et al. ANNALS OF THE NEW YORK ACADEMY OF SCIENCES 437:264-269, 1984.

Acquired immune deficiency syndrome in Black Africans [letter], by N. Clumeck, et al. LANCET 1(8325):642, March 19, 1983.

Acquired immune deficiency syndrome in 3 patients from Zaire, by H. Taelman, et al. ANNALES DE LA SOCIETE BELGE DE MEDECINE TROPICALE 63(1):73-74, March 1983.

Acquired immunodeficiency syndrome in an African, by A. O. Obel, et al. EAST AFRICAN MEDICAL JOURNAL 61(9):724-726, September 1984.

Acquired immunodeficiency syndrome in African patients, by N. Clumeck, et al. NEW ENGLAND JOURNAL OF MEDICINE 310(8):492-497, February 23, 1984.

Acquired immunodeficiency syndrome (AIDS) in Africa. A review, by R. Cole-bunders, et al. TROPICAL DOCTOR 15(1):9-12, January 1985.

Acquired immunodeficiency syndrome (AIDS) in Africans, by C. Katlama, et al. ANNALES DE LA SOCIETE BELGE DE MEDECINE TROPICALE 64(4): 379-389, 1984.

Acquired immunodeficiency syndrome (AIDS) in Kinshasa, Zaire: clinical and epidemiological observations, by W. Odio, et al. ANNALES DE LA SOCIETE BELGE DE MEDECINE TROPICALE 65(4):357-361, 1985.

Acquired immunodeficiency syndrome in a couple from Zaire, by P. Le Bras, et al. REVISTA DE MEDICINA INTERNA 5(3):225-227, September 1984.

Acquired immunodeficiency syndrome in a heterosexual population in Zaire, by P. Piot, et al. LANCET 2(8394):65-69, July 14, 1984.

Acquired immunodeficiency syndrome in Rwanda, by P. Van de Pere, et al. LANCET 2(8394):62-65, July 14, 1984.

AIDS in Africa. NEW SCIENTIST 108:14, November 28, 1985.

AIDS in Johannesburg [letter], by R. Sher. SOUTH AFRICAN MEDICAL JOURNAL 68(3):137-138, August 3, 1985.

AIDS in tropical areas: Haitian and African foci, by H. Taelman et al. ANNALES DE LA SOCIETE BELGE DE MEDECINE TROPICALE 64(4):331-334, 1984.

AIDS in the USA and the RSA—an update [letter], by M. Malan. SOUTH AFRICAN MEDICAL JOURNAL 70(2):119, July 1986.

AFRICA
AIDS is running rampant through Africa. NEW SCIENTIST 110:26, June 26, 1986.

AIDS virus infection in Nairobi prostitutes: spread of the epidemic to East Africa, by J. K. Kreiss, et al. NEW ENGLAND JOURNAL OF MEDICINE 314:414-418, February 13, 1986.

Lack of evidence of HTLV-III endemicity in southern Africa, by S. F. Lyons, et al. NEW ENGLAND JOURNAL OF MEDICINE 312:1257-1258, May 9, 1985.

Prevalence of HTLV-III/LAV in household contacts of patients with confirmed AIDS and controls in Kinshasa, Zaire, by J. M. Mann, et al. JAMA 256(6): 721-724, August 8, 1986.

AUSTRALIA
Prodromal acquired immune deficiency syndrome in Australian homosexual men, by C. I. Smith, et al. MEDICAL JOURNAL OF AUSTRALIA 1(12): 561-563, June 11, 1983.

BELGIUM
Acquired immune deficiency syndrome in Belgium, by N. Clumeck. EURO-PEAN JOURNAL OF CLINICAL MICROBIOLOGY 3(1):59-60, February 1984.

Acquired immune deficiency syndrome in Belgium and its relation to Central Africa, by N. Clumeck, et al. ANNALS OF THE NEW YORK ACADEMY OF SCIENCES 437:264-269, 1984.

Acquired immunodeficiency syndrome (AIDS) in 2 homosexuals in Belgium, by J. Unger, et al. ACTA CLINICA BELGICA 38(6):401-405, 1983.

BRAZIL
Acquired immunodeficiency syndrome (AIDS): report of the 1st autochth-nous case in Brazil and immunological study, by V. Amato Neto, et al. REVISTA PAULISTA DE MEDICINA 101(4):165-168, July-August 1983.

CANADA
More AIDS appears in Alberta, by S. McCarthy, et al. ALBERTA REPORT 11:30, March 5, 1984.

CHILE
Acquired immunodeficiency syndrome: report of a case in Chile, by F. Figueroa, et al. REVISTA MEDICA DE CHILE 112(10):1057-1059, October 1984.

DENMARK
Acquired immunodeficiency syndrome (AIDS) in Denmark. A report from the Copenhagen study group of AIDS on the first 20 Danish patients, by J. Gerstoft, et al. ACTA MEDICA SCANDINAVICA 217(2):213-224, 1985.

AIDS and human T-cell leukemia/lymphoma virus III in Denmark, by G. Lange Wantzin. UGESKRIFT FOR LAEGER 147(5):389-391, January 28, 1985.

DENMARK
AIDS in Denmark and immunological parameters among homosexual Danish men with special reference to the prognosis of patients with low H/S rations. A report from the CAID, by J. Gerstoft, et al. ANTIBIOTIC CHEMOTHERAPY 32:127-137, 1983.

AIDS-induced decline of the incidence of syphilis in Denmark, by A. Poulsen, et al. ACTA DERMATO-VENEREOLOGICA 65(6):567-569, 1985.

EUROPE
Acquired immune deficiency syndrome (AIDS) in Europe. EUROPEAN JOURNAL OF CLINICAL MICROBIOLOGY 3(1):53-84, February 1984.

AIDS in Europe [letter], by J. Green, et al. BRITISH MEDICAL JOURNAL 287(6506):1715-1716, December 3, 1983.

AIDS in Europe, by P. Ebbesen, et al. BRITISH MEDICAL JOURNAL 287(6402):1324-1326, November 5, 1983.

AIDS reported in Eastern European countries, by P. Cummings. ADVOCATE 436:29, December 24, 1985.

European AIDS cases double annually, by P. Cumings. ADVOCATE 429:18, September 17, 1985.

First case of AIDS in the Tyrol, by I. Auhuber, et al. WIENER KLINISCHE WOCHENSCHRIFT 96(11):426-427, May 25, 1984.

Update: acquired immunodeficiency syndrome. CONNECTICUT MEDICINE 49(5):317-319, May 1985.

Update: acquired immunodeficiency syndrome—Europe. JAMA 253:1106+, February 2, 1985; also in subsequent issues; also in MMWR 33(43):607-609, November 2, 1984; also in subsequent issues.

FINLAND
Acquired immune deficiency syndrome. The first cases in Finland, by S. L. Valle, et al. ANNALS OF CLINICAL RESEARCH 15(5-6):203-205, 1983.

AIDS—the first cases in Finland, by H. Repo, et al. DUODECIM 100(11):656-657, 1984.

FRANCE
Acquired immune deficiency syndrome in France, by J. B. Brunet. EUROPEAN JOURNAL OF CLINICAL MICROBIOLOGY 3(1):66, February 1984.

Acquired immunodeficiency syndrome in France [letter], by J. B. Brunet, et al. LANCET 1(8326, Part 1):700-701, March 26, 1983.

AIDS in a Haitian couple in Paris [letter], by E. Dournon, et al. LANCET 1(8332):1040-1041, May 7, 1983.

GERMANY
Acquired immune deficiency syndrome in the Federal Republic of Germany, by J. L'age-Stehr. EUROPEAN JOURNAL OF CLINICAL MICROBI-OLOGY 3(1):61, February 1984.

Acquired immunodeficiency syndrome (AIDS) in male homosexuals in Frankfurt am Main, by E. B. Helm, et al. MUENCHENER MEDIZINISCHE WOCHENSCHRIFT 125(48):1129-1134, December 2, 1983.

AIDS and HTLV-III in West Germany: the status February 1985, by R. Hehlmann, et al. KLINISCHE WOCHENSCHRIFT 63(9):385-388, May 2, 1985.

AIDS in Germany: a failed challenge, by H. Fiedler. DEUTSCHE MEDIZI-NISCHE WOCHENSCHRIFT 110(47):1830-1831, November 22, 1985.

AIDS in West Germany [letter], by J. L'age-Stehr, et al. LANCET 2(8363): 1370-1371, December 10, 1983.

First case of AIDS in Salzburg. Important diagnostic hint by determination of neopterin, by K. Wessely, et al. WIENER KLINISCHE WOCHENSCHRIFT 97(2):88-90, January 18, 1985.

Incidence of AIDS cases in the Federal Republic of Germany and in Munich, by F. D. Goebel. KRANKENPFLEGE JOURNAL 24(7):32-33, July 1, 1986.

GREAT BRITAIN
Acquired immune deficiency syndrome in Britain, August 1983. BRITISH MEDICAL JOURNAL 287(6400):1205, October 22, 1983.

AIDS in a woman in England [letter],by C. L. Smith, et al. LANCET 2(8354): 846, October 8, 1983.

British AIDS; new cases cause alarm, by M. Clarke. NATURE 314(6006):5, March 7, 1985.

Estimating AIDS (UK) [letter], by M. McEvoy. LANCET 2(8466):1248, November 30, 1985.

Four more AIDS cases in Britain. NEW SCIENTIST 98:609, June 2, 1983.

Rising prevalence of human T-lymphotropic virus type III (HTLV-III) infection in homosexual men in London, by C. A. Carne, et al. LANCET 1(8440): 1261-1262, June 1, 1985.

HAITI
Acquired immune deficiency syndrome in infants born of Haitian mothers [letter], by J. H. Joncas, et al. NEW ENGLAND JOURNAL OF MEDICINE 308(14):842, April 7, 1983.

Acquired immunodeficiency syndrome in Haiti, by J. W. Pape, et al. ANNALS OF INTERNAL MEDICINE 103(5):674-678, November 1985.

AIDS in tropical areas: Haitian and African foci, by H. Taelman et al. ANNALES DE LA SOCIETE BELGE DE MEDECINE TROPICALE 64(4):331-334, 1984.

HONG KONG
First case of AIDS in Hong Kong [letter], by a. Y. Chan, et al. JAMA 254(6): 751, August 9, 1985.

INDIA
Nowhere to run, nowhere to hide . . . AIDS hits India, by K. M. Pierce, et al. TIME 128(9):36, September 1, 1986.

ISRAEL
First case of AIDS in a homosexual in Israel. Results of different therapeutic regimens, by R. Marilus, et al. ISRAEL JOURNAL OF MEDICAL SCIENCES 20(3):249-251, March 1984.

ITALY
AIDS in Italy [letter], by G. Rezza, et al. LANCET 2(8403):642, September 15, 1984.

JAMAICA
Acquired immune deficiency syndrome (AIDS) in a Jamaican, by C. Charles, et al. WEST INDIAN MEDICAL JOURNAL 33(2):130-133, June 1984.

JAPAN
AIDS in Japan. No screening of blood donors [news], by D. Swinbanks. NATURE 318(6044):306, November 28-December 4, 1985.

AIDS: undesirable import to Japan, by D. Swinbanks. NATURE 315:8, May 2, 1985.

Survey of the prevalence of AIDS-associated virus (LAV) infection in Japan, by H. Tsuchie, et al. JOURNAL OF INFECTION 10(3):272-276, May 1985.

MEXICO
Acquired immune deficiency syndrome. Clinical data and immunologic studies on 9 patients examined in Mexico, by C. Abud-Mendoza, et al. REVISTA DE INVESTIGACION CLINICA 36(4):311-319, October-December 1984.

Acquired immunodeficiency syndrome in Mexico [letter], by G. J. Ruiz-Argüelles, et al. REVISTA DE INVESTIGACION CLINICA 35(4):265-266, October-December 1983.

NEW ZEALAND
AIDS in New Zealand [letter], by S. D. Somerfield. NEW ZEALAND MEDICAL JOURNAL 98(774):160-161, March 13, 1985.

NORWAY
Acquired immunodeficiency syndrome (AIDS). Clinical, immunological, pathological, and microbiological studies of the first case diagnosed in Norway, by S. S. Froland, et al. SCANDINAVIAN JOURNAL OF GASTROENTEROLOGY 107:82-93, 1985.

PANAMA
Acquired immune deficiency syndrome. First confirmed case in Panamá, by M. M. de Ycaza, et al. REVISTA MEDICA DE PANAMA 10(1):66-73, January 1985.

PUERTO RICO
Acquired immunodeficiency syndrome (AIDS): experience in the Puerto Rico Medical Center, by C. Climent, et al. BOLETIN—ASOCIACION MEDICA DE PUERTO RICO 77(2):50-55, February 1985.

SAUDI ARABIA
Acquired immunodeficiency syndrome in Saudi Arabia. The American-Saudi connection, by H. A. Harfi, et al. JAMA 255:383-384, January 17, 1986.

SCANDINAVIA
Acquired immune deficiency syndrome in Scandinavia, by H. Repo, et al. EUROPEAN JOURNAL OF CLINICAL MICROBIOLOGY 3(1):65, February 1984.

SCOTLAND
Virus in Edinburgh, by M. Kohn. NEW SOCIETY May 2, 196, p. 11-13.

SPAIN
Acquired immunodeficiency syndrome (AIDS) in Spain [letter], by J. M. Arnau de Bolós, et al. MEDICINA CLINICA 82(18):827, May 12, 1984.

Acquired immunodeficiency syndrome in a male residing in Barcelona [letter], by R. Estruch, et al. MEDICINA CLINICA 81(14):645, November 5, 1983.

Iatrogenic AIDS? 2 possible cases in Barcelona [letter]. MEDICINA CLINICA 82(8):380-381, March 3, 1984.

SWEDEN
AIDS in homosexual men—the first cases in Sweden, by P. Pehrson, et al. LAKARTIDNINGEN 80(7):545-548, February 16, 1983.

SWITZERLAND
Acquired immune deficiency syndrome in Switzerland, by B. Somaini. EUROPEAN JOURNAL OF CLINICAL MICROBIOLOGY 3(1):67, February 1984.

AIDS in Switzerland, by B. Somaini. SCHWEIZERISCHE MEDIZINISCHE WOCHENSCHRIFT 114(16):538-544, April 21, 1984.

THAILAND
Acquired immune deficiency syndrome in Thailand, by H. Wilde, et al. ASIAN AND PACIFIC JOURNAL OF ALLERGY AND IMMUNOLOGY 3(1):104-107, June 1985.

Acquired immune deficiency syndrome in Thailand. A report of two cases, by A. Limsuwan, et al. JOURNAL OF THE MEDICAL ASSOCIATION OF THAILAND 69(3):164-169, March 1986.

THE NETHERLANDS
Acquired immune deficiency syndrome in The Netherlands, by C. M. Vandenbroucke-Grauls, et al. EUROPEAN JOURNAL OF CLINICAL MICROBIOLOGY 3(1):62, February 1984.

Acquired immunodeficiency syndrome in The Netherlands, by H. Bijkerk. NEDERLANDS TIJDSCHRIFT VOOR GENEESKUNDE 127(19):856, May 7, 1983.

Acquired immunodeficiency syndrome in The Netherlands and United States. NEDERLANDS TIJDSCHRIFT VOOR GENEESKUNDE 127(31):1414-1415, July 30, 1983.

AIDS in The Netherlands. Clinical and microbiological data on 36 cases, by S. A. Danner, et al. NETHERLAND JOURNAL OF MEDICINE 28(10):487-497, 1985.

Introduction of lymphotropic virus (LAV/HTLV-III) into the male homosexual community in Amsterdam, by R. A. Coutinho, et al. GENITOURINARY MEDICINE 62(1):38-43, February 1986.

TRINIDAD
Acquired immune deficiency syndrome in Trinidad. A report on two cases, by C. Bartholomew, et al. WEST INDIAN MEDICAL JOURNAL 32(3):177-180, September 1983.

AIDS on Trinidad [letter], by C. Bartholomew, et al. LANCET 1(8368):103, January 14, 1984.

UNITED KINGDOM
Acquired immune deficiency syndrome in the United Kingdom, by M. McEvoy. EUROPEAN JOURNAL OF CLINICAL MICROBIOLOGY 3(1): 63-64, February 1984.

UNITED STATES
Acquired immune deficiency syndrome in Kentucky, by J. M. Felser, et al. JOURNAL OF THE KENTUCKY MEDICAL ASSOCIATION 81(9):703-706, September 1983.

Acquired immune deficiency syndrome in West Virginia: an 'imported' disease, by J. M. Bernstein, et al. WEST VIRGINIA MEDICAL JOURNAL 80(8):153-156, August 1984.

Acquired immunodeficiency syndrome in Florida—a review, by C. L. MacLeod, et al. JOURNAL OF THE FLORIDA MEDICAL ASSOCIATION 71(9):712-717, September 1984.

Acquired immunodeficiency syndrome in New York City: evaluation of an active surveillance system, by M. E. Chamberland, et al. JAMA 254:383-387, July 19, 1985.

Acquired immunodeficiency syndrome in The Netherlands and United States. NEDERLANDS TIJDSCHRIFT VOOR GENEESKUNDE 127(31): 1414-1415, July 30, 1983.

UNITED STATES

Acquired immunodeficiency syndrome in the United States: an analysis of cases outside high-incidence groups, by M. E. Chamberland, et al. ANNALS OF INTERNAL MEDICINE 101(5):617-623, November 1984.

Acquired immunodeficiency syndrome in the United States: a selective review, by J. Layon, et al. CRITICAL CARE MEDICINE 14(9):819-827, September 1986.

AIDS cases low in U.S. heartland, by R. J. Donahue. NATIONAL UNDER-WRITER 90:4, March 29, 1986.

AIDS in Colorado: rumor and reality. COLORADO MEDICINE 30(11):314-317, November 1983.

AIDS in Houston, by P. I. Evans, et al. HOUSTON CITY MAGAZINE 9:56+, October 1985.

AIDS in Michigan. The public health approach, by R. Pope. MICHIGAN HOSPITALS 22(8):6-11, August 1986.

AIDS in New York City with particular reference to the psycho-social aspects, by N. Deuchar. BRITISH JOURNAL OF PSYCHIATRY 145:612-619, December 1984.

AIDS in Ohio. How the state is handling the problem, by K. S. Edwards. OHIO STATE MEDICAL JOURNAL 81(10):695-699+, October 1985.

AIDS in one city. An interview with Mervyn Silverman, Director of Health, San Francisco [interview by Stephen F. Morin], by M. Silverman. AMERICAN PSYCHOLOGIST 39(11):1294-1296, November 1984.

AIDS in South Carolina [editorial], by C. S. Bryan. JOURNAL OF THE SOUTH CAROLINA MEDICAL ASSOCIATION 79(8):452-453, August 1983.

AIDS in the USA and the RSA—an update [letter], by M. Malan. SOUTH AFRICAN MEDICAL JOURNAL 70(2):119, July 1986.

AIDS, a mysterious disease, plagues homosexual men from New York to California, by N. Faber, et al. PEOPLE WEEKLY 19:42-44, February 14, 1983.

AIDS on and off Broadway, by H. Popkin. LISTENER July 11, 1985, p. 15.

Case of AIDS in New Orleans, by S. R. Olive. JOURNAL OF THE LOUISIANA STATE MEDICAL SOCIETY 135(9):4-5+, September 1983.

Evaluation of the acquired immunodeficiency syndrome (AIDS) reported in healthcare personnel—United States. MMWR 32(27):358-360, July 15, 1983.

How common is HTLV-III infection in the United States? by S. L. Sivak, et al. NEW ENGLAND JOURNAL OF MEDICINE 313:1352, November 21, 1985.

UNITED STATES
Incidence of the acquired immunodeficiency syndrome in San Francisco, 1980-1983, by A. R. Moss, et al. JOURNAL OF INFECTIOUS DISEASES 152(1):152-161, July 1985.

—. FRONTIERS OF RADIATION THERAPY AND ONCOLOGY 19:14-20, 1985.

Update: acquired immunodeficiency syndrome in the San Francisco Cohort Study, 1978-1985. MMWR 34(38):573-575, September 27, 1985.

Update: acquired immunodeficiency syndrome—United States. JAMA 253:3386-3387+, June 21, 1985; also in MMWR 34(18):245-248, May 10, 1985.

USSR
AIDS reaches the Soviet Union, by B. Nahaylo. SPECTATOR October 4, 1986, p. 12-13.

Scientist allays fears about AIDS; claims fewer than 10 cases have been recorded in USSR. CURRENT DIGEST OF THE SOVIET PRESS 37:16+, December 25, 1985.

OCCURRENCE—ADOLESCENTS
More teens, women infected by AIDS virus, study shows, by P. Smith. AIR FORCE TIMES 46:6, July 28, 1986.

OCCURRENCE—BLACKS
AIDS in the black community, by D. Walter. ADVOCATE 454:10, September 2, 1986.

AIDS in a black Malian [letter], by D. Vittecoq, et al. LANCET 2(8357):1023, October 29, 1983.

OCCURRENCE—HAITIANS
Acquired immune deficiency in Haitians: opportunistic infections in previously healthy Haitian immigrants, by J. Vieira, et al. NEW ENGLAND JOURNAL OF MEDICINE 308(3):125-129, January 20, 1983.

Acquired immune deficiency syndrome in infants born of Haitian mothers [letter], by J. H. Joncas, et al. NEW ENGLAND JOURNAL OF MEDICINE 308(14): 842, April 7, 1983.

Acquired immunodeficiency in Haitians [letter], by M. Boncy, et al. NEW ENGLAND JOURNAL OF MEDICINE 308(23):1419-1420, June 9, 1983.

Acquired immunodeficiency syndrome among Haitians: an update, by M. A. Fischl, et al. ANNALS OF THE NEW YORK ACADEMY OF SCIENCES 437:325-333, 1984.

AIDS in Haitian immigrants [letter], by R. A. Fralick. CANADIAN MEDICAL ASSOCIATION JOURNAL 130(10):1266, May 15, 1984.

AIDS in Haitian immigrants and in a Caucasian woman closely associated with Haitians, by M. Laverdière, et al. CANADIAN MEDICAL ASSOCIATION JOURNAL 129(11):1209, 1212, December 1, 1983.

AIDS in a hospital worker [letter], by A. Belani, et al. LANCET 1(8378):676, March 24, 1984.

Perspectives on the future of AIDS, by T. C. Quinn. JAMA 253(2):247-249, January 1985.

OCCURRENCE—HEMOPHILIACS
AIDS in hemophilia, by M. W. Hilgartner, et al. ANNALS OF THE NEW YORK ACADEMY OF SCIENCES 437:466-471, 1984.

AIDS in hemophiliacs. AMERICAN FAMILY PHYSICIAN 32:222, July 1985.

OCCURRENCE—HETEROSEXUALS
AIDS in a heterosexual population. AMERICAN FAMILY PHYSICIAN 31:292, February 1985.

OCCURRENCE—HOMOSEXUALS
Acquired immunodeficiency syndrome (AIDS) in homosexual men—a new public health concern, by O. A. Strand. NIPH ANNALS 5(2):41-49, December 1982.

Acquired immunodeficiency syndrome in four homosexuals, by W. Rozenbaum, et al. PRESSE MEDICALE 12(18):1149-1154, April 23, 1983.

Acquired immunodeficiency syndrome in gay men, by H. W. Jaffe, et al. ANNALS OF INTERNAL MEDICINE 103(5):662-664, November 1985.

AIDS in the 'gay' areas of San Francisco [letter], by A. R. Moss, et al. LANCET 1(8330):923-924, Apri 23, 1983.

OCCURRENCE—PHYSICIANS
Patients of doctor with AIDS symptoms tested, by L. Famiglietti. AIR FORCE TIMES 46:3, January 20, 1986.

OCCURRENCE—WOMEN
Immunodeficiency among female sexual partners of males with acquired immune deficiency syndrome (AIDS)—New York. MMWR 31(52):697-698, January 7, 1983.

Immunodeficiency in female sexual partners of men with the acquired immunodeficiency syndrome, by C. Harris, et al. NEW ENGLAND JOURNAL OF MEDICINE 308(20):1181-1184, May 19, 1983. OCCURRENCE—GREAT BRITAIN HTLV-III infection and AIDS in a Zambian nurse resident in Britain [letter], by A. E. Raine, et al. LANCET 2(8409):985, October 27, 1984.

More teens, women infected by AIDS virus, study shows, by P. Smith. AIR FORCE TIMES 46:6, July 28, 1986.

OPHTHALMOLOGY
Acquired immune deficiency syndrome. Ophthalmic manifestations in ambulatory patients, by P. R. Rosenberg, et al. OPHTHALMOLOGY 90(8):874-878, August 1983.

Acquired immune deficiency syndrome. Pathogenic mechanisms of ocular disease, by J. S. Pepose, et al. OPHTHALMOLOGY 92(4):472-484, April 1985.

Acquired immunodeficiency syndrome (AIDS): the disease and its ocular manifestations, by J. A. Mines, et al. INTERNATIONAL OPHTHALMOLOGY CLINICS 26(2):73-115, Summer 1986.

Acquired immune deficiency syndrome retinpathy, pneumocystis, and cotton-wool spots [editorial], by W. R. Freeman, et al. AMERICAN JOURNAL OF OPHTHALMOLOGY 9892):235-237, August 15, 1984.

AIDS: a growing cause of blindness, by L. P. Wahl. JOURNAL OF VISUAL IMPAIRMENT AND BLINDNESS 80:544, January 1986.

Analysis of retinal cotton-wool spots and cytomegalovirus retinitis in the acquired immunodeficiency syndrome [letter], by J. S. Pepose, et al. AMERICAN JOURNAL OF OPHTHALMOLOGY 95(1):118-120, January 1983.

Assessing ophthalmic signs in patients with AIDS, by P. Stoer, et al. JOURNAL OF OPHTHALMIC NURSING AND TECHNOLOGY 4(6):6-10, November-December 1985.

Bilateral fungal corneal ulcers in a patient with AIDS-related complex, by C. Santos, et al. AMERICAN JOURNAL OF OPHTHALMOLOGY 102(1):118-119, July 15, 1986.

Caution. AIDS virus present: handle with care! . . . ophthalmic examination equipment, by N. Garber. JOURNAL OF OPHTHALMIC NURSING AND TECHNOLOGY 4(6):22-25, November-December 1985.

Clinical and histologic findings in opportunistic ocular infections. Part of a new syndrome of acquired immunodeficiency, by N. M. Newman, et al. ARCHIVES OF OPHTHALMOLOGY 101(3):396-401, March 1983.

Concurrent herpes simplex and cytomegalovirus retinitis and encephalitis in the acquired immune deficiency syndrome (AIDS), by J. S. Pepose, et al. OPHTHALMOLOGY 91(12):1669-1677, December 1984.

Culture-proven cytomegalovirus retinitis in a homosexual man with the acquired immunodeficiency syndrome, by D. M. Bachman, et al. OPHTHALMOLOGY 89(7):797-804, July 1982.

Cytomegalovirus retinitis in the acquired immunodeficiency syndrome (AIDS). Light-microscopical, ultrastructural and immunohistochemical examination of a case, by O. A. Jensen, et al. ACTA OPHTHALMOLOGICA 62(1):1-9, February 1984.

Cytomegalovirus retinitis in a young homosexual male with acquired immunodeficiency, by J. Neuwirth, et al. OPHTHALMOLOGY 89(7):805-808, July 1982.

Cytomegalovirus retinitis: a manifestation of the acquired immune deficiency syndrome (AIDS), by A. H. Friedman, et al. BRITISH JOURNAL OF OPHTHALMOLOGY 67(6):372-380, June 1983.

Diffuse toxoplasmic retinchoroiditis in a patient with AIDS, by D. W. Parke, 2d, et al. ARCHIVES OF OPHTHALMOLOGY 104(4):571-575, April 1986.

Disseminated bilateral chorioretinitis due to Histoplasma capsulatum in a patient withthe acquired immunodeficiency syndrome, by A. Macher, et al. OPHTHALMOLOGY 92(8):1159-1164, August 1985.

Eye disorders in 4 patients with acquired immunodeficiency syndrome, by M. F. Hoogesteger, et al. NEDERLANDS TIJDSCHRIFT VOOR GENEESKUNDE 129(1):24-25, January 5, 1985.

Histological study of retinal necrosis due to cytomeglovirus in AIDS , by P. Dhermy, et al. BULLETIN DES SOCIETES D'OPHTHALMOLOGIE DE FRANCE 84(4):381-384, April 1984.

Human T-cell leukemia/lymphotropic virus type III in the conjunctival epithelium of a patient with AIDS, by L. S. Fujikawa, et al. AMERICAN JOURNAL OF OPHTHALMOLOGY 100(4):507-509, October 15, 1985.

Impact of the AIDS epidemic on corneal transplantation [editorial], by J. S. Pepose, et al. AMERICAN JOURNAL OF OPHTHALMOLOGY 100(4):610-613, October 15, 1985.

Microvascular aspects of acquired immune deficiency syndrome retinopathy, by D. A. Newsome, et al. AMERICAN JOURNAL OF OPHTHALMOLOGY 98(5): 590-61, November 1984.

Ocular effects in acquired immune deficiency syndrome, by J. S. Schuman, et al. MOUNT SINAI JOURNAL OF MEDICINE 50(5):443-446, September-October 1983.

Ocular findings in the acquired immunodeficiency syndrome, by A. Gal, et al. BRITISH JOURNAL OF OPTHAMOLOGY 68(4):238-241, April 1984.

Ocular manifestations of the acquired immune deficiency syndrome, by G. N. Holland. INTERNATIONAL OPHTHALMOLOGY CLINICS 25(2):179-187, Summer 1985.

Ocular manifestations of AIDS, by S. J. Bass. JOURNAL OF THE AMERICAN OPTOMETRIC ASSOCIATION 55(10):765-769, October 1984.

Oculomotor cranial nerve palsey associated with acquired immunodeficiency syndrome, by M. K. Jack, et al. ANNALS OF OPHTHALMOLOGY 16(5):460-462, May 1984.

Ophthalmic involvement in acquired immunodeficiency syndrome, by A. G. Palestine, et al. OPHTHALMOLOGY 91(9):1092-1099, September 1984.

Ophthalmologic findings in acquired immune deficiency syndrome (AIDS), by M. Khadem, et al. ARCHIVES OF OPHTHALMOLOGY 102(2):201-206, February 1984.

Ophthalmoscopic manifestations observed in AIDS, by P. Le Hoang, et al. BULLETIN DES SOCIETES D'OPHTALMOLOGIE DE FRANCE 84(4):377-380, April 1984.

Perivasculitis of the retinal vessels as an important sign in children with AIDS-related complex, by P. Kestelyn, et al. AMERICAN JOURNAL OF OPHTHALMOLOGY 100(4):614-1615, October 15, 1985.

Prospective study of the ophthalmologic findings in the acquired immune deficiency syndrome, by W. R. Freeman, et al. AMERICAN JOURNAL OF OPHTHALMOLOGY 97(2):133-142, February 1984.

Retinal cotton-wool patches in acquired immunodeficiency syndrome [letter]. NEW ENGLAND JOURNAL OF MEDICINE 307(27):1704-1705, December 30, 1982.

Retinal lesions of the acquired immune deficiency syndrome, by A. H. Friedman. TRANSACTIONS OF THE AMERICAN OPHTHALMOLOGICAL SOCIETY 82: 447-491, 1984.

Retinal manifestations of acquired immunodeficiency syndrome (AIDS). Report of a case, by G. Buckman, et al. ANNALS OF OPHTHALMOLOGY 16(12): 1136-1138, December 1984.

Retinal manifestations of the acquired immune deficiency syndrome (AIDS): cytomegalovirus, candida albicans, cryptococcus, toxoplasmosis and Pneumocystis carinii, by J. S. Schuman, et al. TRANSACTIONS OF THE OPHTHALMOLOGICAL SOCIETIES OF THE UNITED KINGDOM 103(Part 2):177-190, 1983.

AFRICA
Prospective study of the ophthalmologic findings in the acquired immune deficiency syndrome in Africa, by P. Kestelyn, et al. AMERICAN JOURNAL OF OPHTHALMOLOGY 100(2):230-238, August 15, 1985.

OPHTHALMOLOGY—TESTING
Should corneal transplant donors be screened for human T-cell lymphotropic virus type III antibody? [editorial], by C. E. Margo. ARCHIVES OF OPHTHALMOLOGY 103(11):1643, November 1985.

OPHTHALMOLOGY—TREATMENT
Alpha-interferon administration in cytomegalovirus retinitis, by S. W. Chou, et al. ANTIMICROBIAL AGENTS AND CHEMOTHERAPY 25(1):25-28, January 1984.

Parenterally administered acyclovir for viral retinitis associated with AIDS [letter], by J. A. Schulman, et al. ARCHIVES OF OPHTHALMOLOGY 102(12):1750, December 1984.

ORGAN DONORS—TESTING
Testing donors of organs, tissues, and semen for antibody to human T-lymphotropic virus type III/lymphadenopathy-associated virus. JAMA 253:3391, June 21, 1985.

PATHOLOGY
Abnormal in vitro proliferation and differentiation of T colony forming cells in AIDS patients and clinically normal male homosexuals, by Y. Lunardi-Iskandar, et al. CLINICAL AND EXPERIMENTAL IMMUNOLOGY 60(2):285-293, May 1985.

Acquired immune deficiency syndrome. No evidence of the presence of cyclosporine, by H. F. Schran, et al. AMERICAN JOURNAL OF MEDICINE 77(5): 797-804, November 1984.

Acquired immune deficiency syndrome (AIDS) and generalized lymphadenopathy, by P. Francioli. REVUE MEDICALE DE LA SUISSE ROMANDE
103(12):1063-1068, December 1983.

Acquired immune deficiency syndrome (AIDS): disease characteristics and oral
manifestations, by D. T. Wofford, et al. JOURNAL OF THE AMERICAN
DENTAL ASSOCIATION 111(2):258-261, August 1985.

Acquired immune deficiency syndrome: laboratory findings, clinical features, and
leading hypotheses, by W. El-Sadr, et al. DIAGNOSTIC IMMUNOLOGY 2(2):
73-85, 1984.

Acquired immune deficiency syndrome—related lymphadenopathies presenting
in the salivary gland lymph nodes, by J. R. Ryan, et al. ARCHIVES OF OTO-
LARYNGOLOGY 111(8):554-556, August 1985.

Acquired immunodeficiency syndrome (AIDS)—a new pathology involving the
respiratory system, by F. Mihaltan. REVISTA DE IGIENA BACTERIOLOGIE,
VIRUSOLOGIE, PARAZITOLOGIE, EPIDEMIOLOGIE, PNEUMOFITIZI-
OLOGIE, PNEUMOFTIZIOLOGIA 34(4):313-317, October-December 1985.

Acquired immunodeficiency syndrome: anatomo-pathological report of 2
necropsy cases,by V. L. Delmonte, et al. REVISTA DO INSTITUTO DE
MEDICINA TROPICAL DE SAO PAULO 26(4):222-227, July-August 1984.

Acquired immunodeficiency syndrome in a patient with no known risk factors: a
pathological study, by A. D. Burt, et al. JOURNAL OF CLINICAL PATHOLO-
GY 37(4):471-474, April 1984.

Acquired immunodeficiency syndrome: an ultrastructural study, by G. S. Sidhu, et
al. HUMAN PATHOLOGY 16(4):377-386, April 1985.

Acquired immunodeficiency syndrome with progressive multifocal leukoencephalopathy and monoclonal B-cell proliferaion, by J. L. Ho, et al. ANNALS
OF INTERNAL MEDICINE 100(5):693-696, May 1984.

Adaptation of lymphadenopathy associated virus (LAV) to replication in EBV-
transformed B lymphoblastoid cell lines, by L. Montagnier, et al. SCIENCE
225:63-66, July 6, 1984.

AIDS and lymphadenopathy [editorial], by M. J. Godley. BRITISH JOURNAL OF
SURGERY 73(3):170-171, March 1986.

AIDS dementia complex: II. Neuropathology, by B. A. Navia, et al. ANNALS OF
NEUROLOGY 19(6):525-535, June 1986.

AIDS—etiology, pathogenesis and epidemiology, by A. Vaheri, et al. DUODECIM
102(7):396-403, 1986.

AIDS—general characteristics and new clues in the studies of etiopathogenesis
of the syndrome—the role of HTLV, by K. Jonderko. WIADOMOSCI
LEKARSKIE 38(15):1061-1066, August 1, 1985.

AIDS: histopathological aspects, by P. R. Millard. JOURNAL OF PATHOLOGY
143(4): 223-239, August 1984.

AIDS: a primary concern for the pathologist, by S. Jothy, et al. CANADIAN JOURNAL OF MEDICAL TECHNOLOGY 47(4):269-270, December 1985.

AIDS retrovirus induced cytopathology: giant cell formation and involvement of CD4 antigen, by J. D. Lifson, et al. SCIENCE 232:1123-1127, May 30, 1986.

Alterations of functional subsets of T helper and T suppressor cell populations in acquired immunodeficiency syndrome (AIDS) and chronic unexplained lymphadenopathy, by J. K. Nicholson, et al. JOURNAL OF CLINICAL IMMUNOLOGY 5(4):269-274, July 1985.

Asymptomatic lymphadenopathy and other early presentations of AIDS, by D. I. Abrams. FRONTIERS OF RADIATION THERAPY AND ONCOLOGY 19:59-65, 1985.

B-cell abnormalities in AIDS [letter]. NEW ENGLAND JOURNAL OF MEDICINE 310(4):258-259, January 26, 1984.

Burkitt lymphoma in acquired immune deficiency syndrome, by D. R. Radin, et al. JOURNAL OF COMPUTER ASSISTED TOMOGRAPHY 8(1)173-174, February 1984.

Burkitt's lymphoma in AIDS: cytogenetic study, by J. Whang-Peng, et al. BLOOD 63(4):818-822, April 1984.

Cerebral immunoblastic lymphoma and the acquired immunodeficiency syndrome, by P. F. Bidet, et al. ANNALES FRANCAISES D'ANESTHESIE ET DE REANIMATION 3(6):443-445, 1984.

Cerebral lymphoma, a complication of the acquired immunodeficiency syndrome [letter],by A. P. Blanc, et al. PRESSE MEDICALE 13(14):884, March 31, 1984.

Cervical adenopathies in relation to AIDS. Course of histological aspects. Diagnostic and prognostic value, by C. Marche, et al. ANNALES D'OTO-LARYNGOLOGIE ET DE CHIRURGIE CERVICO-FACIALE 102(5):299-303, 1985.

Changes in B-lymphocytes in AIDS [letter],by G. J. Ruiz-Argüelles. SANGRE 29(2):223-224, 1984.

Changing patterns of disease, by B. Lorber. TRANSACTIONS AND STUDIES OF THE COLLEGE OF PHYSICIANS OF PHILADELPHIA 7(2):117-130, June 1985.

Chemiluminescence measurement in AIDS, lymphadenopathy and hemophilia patients, by L. Stöhr, et al. ZEITSCHRIFT FUR HAUTKRANKHEITEN 60(15): 1214-1223, August 1, 1985.

Clinical and laboratory findings in ten Milwaukee patients with the acquired immunodeficiency syndrome or prodromal syndromes, by P. A. Turner, et al. WISCONSIN MEDICAL JOURNAL 84(4):19-22, April 1985.

Clinical and pathologic findings of the liver in the acquired immune deficiency syndrome (AIDS), by B. J. Glasgow, et al. AMERICAN JOURNAL OF CLINICAL PATHOLOGY 83(5):582-588, May 1985.

Clinical aspects of the acquired immune deficiency syndrome in the United Kingdom, by J. N. Weber, et al. BRITISH JOURNAL OF VENEREAL DISEASES 60(4);253-257, August 1984.

Clinical aspects of confirmed AIDS, by J. P. Coulaud, et al. BULLETIN DE L'ACADEMIE NATIONALE DE MEDECINE 168(1-2):267-270, January-February 1984.

Clinical microbiology of acquired immune deficiency syndrome (AIDS), by C. B. Inderlied, et al. JOURNAL OF MEDICAL TECHNOLOGY 2(3):167-173+, March 1985.

Clinical picture and etiopathogenesis of AIDS, by W. Mazurkiewicz. PRZEGLAD DERMATOLOGICZNY 72(2):185-191, March-April 1985.

Clinical spectrum of the acquired immunodeficiency syndrome: implications for comprehensive patient care, by P. A. Volberding. ANNALS OF INTERNAL MEDICINE 103(5):729-733, November 1985.

Clinical spectrum of HTLV-III in humans, by J. E. Groopman. CANCER RE-SEARCH 45(Suppl. 9):4649s-4651s, September 1985.

Clinical spectrum of human retroviral-induced diseases, by W. J. Urba, et al. CANCER RESEARCH 45(Suppl. 9):4637s-4643s, September 1985.

Clinical symptomatology of the acquired immunodeficiency syndrome (AIDS) and related disorders, by J. E. Groopman. PROGRESS IN ALLERGY 37:182-193, 1986.

Clonal analysis of T lymphocytes in the acquired immunodeficiency syndrome. Evidence for an abnormality affecting individual helper and suppressor T cells, by J. B. Margolick, et al. JOURNAL OF CLINICAL INVESTIGATION 76(2):709-715, August 1985.

Concentric effects of the acquired immune deficiency syndrome [editorial], by E. N. Brandt, Jr. PUBLIC HEALTH REPORTS 99(1):1-2, January-February 1984.

Consultation and collaborative studies on AIDS offered by New Center and Registry at the Armed Forces Institute of Pathology. PUBLIC HEALTH REPORTS 101:108, January-February 1986.

Critical analysis of T cell subset and function evaluation in patients with persistent generalized lymphadenopathy in groups at risk for AIDS,by M. Cavaille-Coll, et al. CLINICAL AND EXPERIMENTAL IMMUNOLOGY 57(3):511-519, September 1984.

Cytofluorographic analysis of lymph nodes from patients with the persistent generalized lymphadenopathy (PGL) syndrome, by N. Levy, et al. DIAG-NOSTIC IMMUNOLOGY 3(1):15-23, 1985.

Cytologic findings in homosexual males with acquired immunodeficiency, by S. W. Lobenthal, et al. ACTA CYTOLOGICA 27(6):597-604, November-December 1983.

Decreased 5' nucleotidase activity in lymphocytes from asymptomatic sexually active homosexual men and patients with the acquired immune deficiency syndrome, by J. L. Murray, et al. BLOOD 64(5):1016-1021, November 1984.

Dendritic reticulum cells in AIDS-related lymphadenopathy, by M. Alavaikko, et al. EXPERIENTIA 41(9):1173-1175, September 15, 1985.

Detection of coronavirus-like particles in homosexual men with acquired immunodeficiency and related lymphadenopathy syndrome, by P. Kern, et al. KLINISCHE WOCHENSCHRIFT 63(2):68-72, January 15, 1985.

Diagnostic pathology in the acquired immunodeficiency syndrome. Surgical pathology and cytology experience with 67 patients, by J. B. Amberson, et al. ARCHIVES OF PATHOLOGY AND LABORATORY MEDICINE 109(4):345-351, April 1985.

Diagnostic potential for human malignancies of bacterially produced HTLV-I envelope protein, by K. P. Samuel, et al. SCIENCE 226:1074-1097, November 30, 1984.

Direct polyclonal activation of human B lymphocytes by the acquired immune deficiency syndrome virus, by S. M. Schnittman, et al. SCIENCE 233:1084-1086, September 5, 1986.

Disproportionate expansion of a minor T cell subset in patients with lymphadenopathy syndrome and acquired immunodeficiency syndrome, by D. e. Lewis, et al. JOURNAL OF INFECTIOUS DISEASES 151(3):555-559, March 1985.

Distinct IgG recognition patterns during progression of subclinical and clinical infection with lymphadenopathy associated virus/human T lymphotropic virus, by J. M. Lange, et al. BRITISH MEDICAL JOURNAL 292(6515):228-230, January 25, 1986.

Distinctive follicular hyperplasia in the acquired immune deficiency syndrome (AIDS) and the AIDS related complex. A pre-lymphomatous state for B cell lymphomas, by P. R. Meyer, et al. HEMATOLOGICAL ONCOLOGY 2(4):319-347, October-December 1984.

Elevated levels of interferon-induced 2'-5' oligoadenylate synthetase in generalized persistent lymphadenopathy and the acquired immunodeficiency syndrome, by S. E. Read, et al. JOURNAL OF INFECTIOUS DISEASES 152(3):66-472, September 1985.

Epstein-Barr virus and chronic lymphadenomegaly in male homosexuals with acquired immunodeficiency syndrome (AIDS), by H. Lipscomb, et al. AIDS RESEARCH 1(1):59-82, 1983-1984.

Evaluation of natural killer cell activity in patients with persistent generalized lymphadenopathy and acquired immunodeficiency syndrome, by P. C. Creemers, et al. CLINICAL IMMUNOLOGY AND IMMUNOPATHOLOGY 36(2):141-150, August 1985.

Evidence for HTLV-III in T-cells from semen of AIDS patients: expression in primary cell culture, long-term mitogen-stimulated cell cultures, and cocultures with a permissive T-cell line, by D. Zagury, et al. CANCER RESEARCH 45(Suppl. 9):4595s-4597s, September 1985.

Exogenous interleukin-2 and mitogen responses in AIDS patients [letter], by M. Cavaille-Coll, et al. LANCET a1(8388):1245, June 2, 1984.

Expression of beta 2 microglobulin on the surface of mononuclear cells in patients with acquired immune deficiency syndrome (AIDS, and AIDS-related complex (ARC), by S. Gupta. ADVANCES IN EXPERIMENTAL MEDICINE AND BIOLOGY 187:111-115, 1985.

Follicular dendritic cells and virus-like particles in AIDS-related lymphadenopathy, by J. A. Armstrong, et al. LANCET 2(8399):370-372, August 18, 1984.

Follow-up at 41/2 years on homosexual men with generalized lymphadenopathy [letter], by U. Mathur-Wagh, et al. NEW ENGLAND JOURNAL OF MEDICINE 313(24):1542-1543, December 12, 1985.

Generalized lymphadenopathy syndrome related to AIDS. Histopatholgic aspects of the lymph nodes, by C. Marche, et al. BULLETIN DE L'ACADEMIE NATIONALE DE MEDECINE 168(1-2):271-277, January-February 1984.

Generalized tuberculosis in a patient with acquired immunodeficiency syndrome, by A. de la Loma, et al. JOURNAL OF INFECTION 10(1):57-59, January 1985.

Helper suppressor T cells—AIDS, by N. Fain. ADVOCATE 3(78):22, October 13, 1983.

High-grade non-Hodgkin's lymphoma in patients with AIDS, by J. L. Ziegler, et al. ANNALS OF THE NEW YORK ACADEMY OF SCIENCES 437:412-419, 1984.

Histopathological aspects of lymph nodes in the prodromal phase of the acquired immunodeficiency syndrome and related conditions, by J. Diebold, et al. ARCHIVES D'ANATOMIE ET DE CYTOLOGIE PATHOLOGIQUES 32(4):253-254, 1984.

Histopathological changes in the thymus gland in the acquired immune deficiency syndrome, by A. E. Davis, Jr. ANNALS OF THE NEW YORK ACADEMY OF SCIENCES 437:493-502, 1984.

Histopathological studies of lymphadenopathy in AIDS: tentative classification. Preliminary report, by C. Marche, et al. ANTIBIOTIC CHEMOTHERAPY 32:76-86, 1983.

Histopathological study of lymph nodes in patients with lymphadenopathy or acquired immune deficiency syndrome, by c. Marche, et al. EUROPEAN JOURNAL OF CLINICAL MICROBIOLOGY 3(1):75-76, February 1984.

Histopathology of the acquired immune deficiency syndrome, by C. Urmacher, et al. PATHOLOGY ANNUAL 20(Part 1):197-220, 1985.

HTLV-positive T-cell lymphoma/leukaemia in an AIDS patient [letter], by M. Kobayashi, et al. LANCET 1(8390):1361-1362, June 16, 1984.

HTLV-III viremia in homosexual men with generalized lymphadenopathy, by J. E. Kaplan, et al. NEW ENGLAND JOURNAL OF MEDICINE 312:1572-1573, June 13, 1985.

Human lymphoblastoid interferon treatment of Kaposi's sarcoma in the acquired immune deficiency syndrome. Clinical response and prognostic parameters, by E. P. Gelmann, et al. AMERICAN JOURNAL OF MEDICINE 78(5):737-741, May 1985.

Human lymphocyte subpopulations in lymphadenopathies in homosexual men, by P. Rácz, et al. ADVANCES IN EXPERIMENTAL MEDICINE AND BIOLOGY 186:1069-1076, 1985.

Human T-cell leukemia/lymphoma syndrome [serology positive for HTLV-I antibodies], by E. S. Christian, et al. AMERICAN FAMILY PHYSICIAN 32:155-1260, July 1985.

Human T-cell leukemia/lymphoma viruses: clinical and epidemiologic features, by W. A. Blattner, et al. CURRENT TOPICS IN MICROBIOLOGY AND IMMUNOLOGY 115:67-88, 1985.

Human T-lymphotropic retroviruses in adult T-cell leukemia-lymphoma and acquired immune deficiency syndrome, by P. S. Sarin, et al. JOURNAL OF CLINICAL IMMUNOLOGY 4(6):415-423, November 1984.

Hypothesis: the pathogenesis of AIDS. Activation of the T- and B-cell cascades, by A. S. Evans. YALE JOURNAL OF BIOLOGY AND MEDICINE 57(3):317-327, May-June 1984.

Immature sinus histiocytes in the lymphadenopathic stage of AIDS: relationship to polyclonal B-cell activation? [letter], by J. J. Van den Oord, et al. JOURNAL OF PATHOLOGY 145(1):63-64, January 1985.

Increased frequency of HLA-DR5 in lymphadenopathy stage of AIDS [letter],by R. W. Enlow, et al. LANCET 2(8340):51-52, July 2, 1983.

Inflammatory neuropathy in homosexual men with lymphadenopathy, by W. I. Lipkin, et al. NEUROLOGY 35(10):1479-1483, October 1985.

Interferon production in male homosexuals with the acquired immune deficiency syndrome (AIDS) or generalized lymphadenopathy, by J. Abb, et al. INFECTION 12(4):240-242, July-August 1984.

Interferon-related leukocyte inclusions in acquired immune deficiency syndrome: localization in T cells, by P. M. Grimley, et al. AMERICAN JOURNAL OF CLINICAL PATHOLOGY 81(2):147-155, February 1984.

Iron and iron binding proteins in persistent generalised lymphadenopathy and AIDS [letter],by B. S. Blumberg, et al. LANCET 1(8372):347, February 11, 1984.

Is there correlation of T cell proliferative functions and surface marker phenotypes in patients with acquired immune deficiency syndrome or lymphadenopathy syndrome?, by J. C. Gluckman, et al. CLINICAL AND EXPERIMENTAL IMMUNOLOGY 60(1):8-16, April 1985.

Long-term cultivation of T-cell subsets from patients with acquired immune deficiency syndrome, by J. A. Levy, et al. CLINICAL IMMUNOLOGY AND IMMUNOPATHOLOGY 35(3):328-336, June 1985.

Long-term cultures of HTLV-III-infected T cells: a model of cytopathology of T-cell depletion in AIDS, by D. Zagury, et al. SCIENCE 231:850-853, February 21, 1986.

Longitudinal assessment of persistent generalized lymphadenopathy (PGL) in homosexual men, by U. Mathur-Wagh, et al. ADVANCES IN EXPERI-MENTAL MEDICINE AND BIOLOGY 187:93-96, 1985.

Longitudinal study of a patient with acquired immunodeficiency syndrome using T cell subset analysis, by R. L. Siegel, et al. ADVANCES IN EXPERIMENTAL MEDICINE AND BIOLOGY 166:295-303, 1983.

Longitudinal study of persistent generalised lymphadenopathy in homosexual men: relation to acquired immunodeficiency syndrome, by U. Mathur-Wagh, et al. LANCET 1(8385):1033-1038, May 12, 1984.

Lymph node pathology of HTLV and HTLV-associated neoplasms, by E. S. Jaffe, et al. CANCER RESEARCH 45(Suppl. 9):4662s-4664s, September 1985.

Lymphadenopathies in homosexual men. Relationships with the acquired immune deficiency syndrome, by H. L. Ioachim, et al. JAMA 250(10):1316-1309, September 9, 1983.

Lymphadenopathy. AMERICAN FAMILY PHYSICIAN 29:257+, February 1984.

Lymphadenopathy and antibodies to HTLV-III in homosexual men. Clinical, laboratory and epidemiological features, by U. Bienzle, et al. KLINISCHE WOCHENSCHRIFT 63(13):597-602, July 1, 1985.

Lymphadenopathy-associated viral antibody in AIDS. Immune correlations and definition of a carrier state, by J. Laurence, et al. NEW ENGLAND JOURNAL OF MEDICINE 311(20):1269-1273, November 15, 1984.

Lymphadenopathy associated virus and its etiological role in AIDS, by L. Montagnier, et al. INTERNATIONAL SYMPOSIUM OF THE PRINCESS TAKAMATSU CANCER RESEARCH FUND 15:319-331, 1984.

Lymphadenopathy-associated virus: from molecular biology to pathogenicity, by L. Montagnier. ANNALS OF INTERNAL MEDICINE 103(5):689-693, November 1985.

Lymphadenopathy-associated-virus infection and acquired immunodeficiency syndrome, by J. C. Gluckman, et al. ANNUAL REVIEW OF IMMUNOLOGY 4:97-117, 1986.

Lymphadenopathy associated virus infection of a blood donor-recipient pair with acquired immunodeficiency syndrome, by P. M. Feorino, et al. SCIENCE 225:69-72, July 6, 1984.

Lymphadenopathy-associated virus isolated from bronchoalveolar lavage fluid in AIDS-related complex with lymphoid interstitial pneumonitis, by J. M. Ziza, et al. NEW ENGLAND JOURNAL OF MEDICINE 313:183, July 18, 1985.

Lymphadenopathy associated virus: its role in the pathogenesis of AIDS and related diseases, by L. Montagnier. PROGRESS IN ALLERGY 37:46-64, 1986.

471

Lymphadenopathy associated virus (L.A.V.): its association with AIDS or prodromes, by F. Barré-Sinoussi, et al. ADVANCES IN EXPERIMENTAL
MEDICINE AND BIOLOGY 187:35-43, 1985.

Lymphadenopathy: endpoint or prodrome? Update of a 24-month prospective
study, by D. I. Abrams, et al. ANNALS OF THE NEW YORK ACADEMY OF
SCIENCES 437:207-215, 1984.

—? Update of a 36-month prospective study, by D. I. Abrams, et al. ADVANCES
IN EXPERIMENTAL MEDICINE AND BIOLOGY 187:73-84, 1985.

Lymphadenopathy in a heterogenous population at risk for the acquired immunodeficiency syndrome (AIDS)—a morphologic study, by J. Domingo, et al.
AMERICAN JOURNAL OF CLINICAL PATHOLOGY 80(4):649-654, November 1983.

Lymphadenopathy in patients at risk for acquired immunodeficiency syndrome.
Histopathology and histochemistry, by M. Raphael, et al. ARCHIVES OF
PATHOLOGY AND LABORATORY MEDICINE 109(2):128-132, February
1985.

Lymphadenopathy syndrome in two thalassemic patients after LAV contamination by blood transfusion, by F. Boiteux, et al. NEW ENGLAND JOURNAL OF
MEDICINE 312:648-649, March 7, 1985.

Lymphocyte phenotypes in patients with highly reduced T inducer to T cytotoxic/
suppressor ratio, by f. Herrman. CLINICAL AND EXPERIMENTAL IM-
MUNOLOGY 56(2):476-478, May 1984.

Lymphocyte subsets in patients with acquired immunodeficiency syndrome
(AIDS), aids-related complex (ARC), and acute viral infections, by D. E. Lewis,
et al. TRANSACTIONS OF THE ASSOCIATION OF AMERICAN PHYSICIANS
97:197-204, 1984.

Lymphocytic subsets in the acquired immunodeficiency syndrome [letter], by S.
Gupta, et al. ANNALS OF INTERNAL MEDICINE 99(4):566-567, October
1983.

Mechanisms of T-cell functional deficiency in the acquired immunodeficiency syndrome, by G. V. Quinnan Jr, et al. ANNALS OF INTERNAL MEDICINE 103(5):
710-714, November 1985.

Monocytoid B lymphocytes: their relation to the patterns of the acquired immunodeficiency syndrome (AIDS) and AIDS-related lymphadenopathy, by C. C.
Sohn, et al. HUMAN PATHOLOGY 16(10):979-985, October 1985.

More on ultrastructure of AIDS lymph nodes [letter], by S. P. Hammar, et al. NEW
ENGLAND JOURNAL OF MEDICINE 310(14):924, April 5, 1984.

Morphological alterations in the lymphoreticular system in acquired immunodeficiency syndrome, by P. I. Liu, et al. ANNALS OF CLINICAL AND LABORA-
TORY SCIENCE 15(3):212-218, May-June 1985.

Morphological findings in the lymphadenopathy syndrome (LAS) and acquired
immunodeficiency syndrome (AIDS), by S. Falk et al. DEUTSCHE MEDIZI-
NISCHE WOCHENSCHRIFT 111(18):714-718, May 2, 1986.

New infectious diseases and new aspects of infectious diseases. VERHAND-LUNGEN DER DEUTSCHEN GESELLSCHAFT FUR INNERE MEDIZIN 20(Part 1):1-44, 1984.

Nonneoplastic AIDS syndromes, by M. S. Gottlieb. SEMINARS IN ONCOLOGY 11(1):40-46, March 1984.

Patho-anatomical studies in patients dying of AIDS, by S. Lauland, et al. ACTA PATHOLOGICA, MICROBIOLOGICA, ET IMMUNOLOGICA SCANDINAVICA 94(3):201-221, May 1986.

Pathogenesis of the acquired immune deficiency syndrome (AIDS), by M. C. Heng. CUTIS 32(3):255-257, September 1983.

Pathogenesis of AIDS [letter], by J. Melov. MEDICAL JOURNAL OF AUSTRALIA 140(3):177-178, February 4, 1984.

Pathogenesis of B cell lymphoma in a patient with AIDS, by J. E. Groopman, et al. BLOOD 67(3):612-615, March 1986.

Pathologic-anatomic findings in acquired immunologic deficiency syndrome (AIDS), by M. Krause, et al. VASA 13(2):99-106, 1984.

Pathologic features of the lung in the acquired immune deficiency syndrome (AIDS): an autopsy study of seventeen homosexual males, by G. Nash, et al. AMERICAN JOURNAL OF CLINICAL PATHOLOGY 81(1):6-12, January 1984.

Pathophysiologic aspects of lymphokines, by D. T. Boumpas, et al. CLINICAL IM-MUNOLOGY REVIEWS 4(2):201-240, 1985.

Pathophysiology and clinical aspects of acquired immunologic deficiency syn-drome (AIDS), by F. D. Goebel. OFFENTLICHE GESUNDHEITSWESEN 48(5):225-227, May 1986.

Persistent generalized lymphadenopathy: immunological and mycological investi-gations, by J. Torssander, et al. ACTA DERMATO-VENEREOLOGICA 65(6): 515-520, 1985.

Persistent lymphadenopathy in patients at risk of contracting acquired immune deficiency syndrome, by J. P. Clauvel, et al. EUROPEAN JOURNAL OF CLINICAL MICROBIOLOGY 3(1):72, February 1984.

Phagocytic and fungicidal activity of monocytes from patients with acquired immunodeficiency syndrome [letter], by R. G. Washburn, et al. JOURNAL OF INFECTIOUS DISEASES 151(3):565-566, March 1985.

Phenotypic and functional correlations in circulating lymphocytes of prodromal homosexuals and patients with AIDS, by P. H. Tsang, et al. JOURNAL OF CLINICAL AND LABORATORY IMMUNOLOGY 17(1):7-11, May 1985.

Plasmapheresis increases T4 lymphocytes in a patient with AIDS, by R. H. Tomar, et al. AMERICAN JOURNAL OF CLINICAL PATHOLOGY 81(4):518-521, April 1984. NURSES ANA surveys state nurses' associations on AIDS. PULSE OF THE MONTANA STATE NURSES ASSOCIATION 23(4):1, April 1986.

473

Podiatric implications of acquired immunodeficiency syndrome, by C. Abramson. JOURNAL OF THE AMERICAN PODIATRIC MEDICAL ASSOCIATION 76(3): 124-136, March 1986.

Prevalence, clinical manifestations, and immunology of herpesvirus infections in the acquired immunodeficiency syndrome, by G. V. Quinnan, Jr., et al. ANNALS OF THE NEW YORK ACADEMY OF SCIENCES 437:200-206, 1984.

Primary lymph node pathology in AIDS and AIDS-related lymphadenopathy, by E. P. Ewing, Jr., et al. ARCHIVES OF PATHOLOGY AND LABORATORY MEDICINE 109(11):977-981, November 1985.

Raised serum neopterin levels and imbalances of T-lymphocyte subsets in viral diseases, acquired immune deficiency and related lymphadenopathy syndromes, by P. Kern, et al. BIOMEDICINE AND PHARMACOTHERAPY 38(8):407-411, 1984.

Rectal epithelium in the acquired immunodeficiency syndrome [letter], by D. C. Snover. ANNALS OF INTERNAL MEDICINE 102(2):278-279, February 1985.

Reduced Ia-positive Langerhans' cells in AIDS [letter]. NEW ENGLAND JOURNAL OF MEDICINE 311(13):857-858, Septemebr 27, 1984.

Reduced Langerhans' cell Ia antigen and ATPase activity in patients with the acquired immunodeficiency syndrome, by D. V. Belsito, et al. NEW ENGLAND JOURNAL OF MEDICINE 310(20):1279-1282, May 17, 1984.

Researchers find that AIDS patients have defects in T and B cells, by P. Randall. NEWS & FEATURES FROM NIH November 1983, p. 8.

Revision of case definition of acquired immunodeficiency syndrome for national reporting—United States. ANNALS OF INTERNAL MEDICINE 103(3):402-403, September 1985; also in JAMA 254(5):599-600, August 2, 1985 and MMWR 34(25):373-375, June 28, 1985.

Selective tropism of lymphadenopathy associated virus (LAV) for helper-inducer T lymphocytes, by D. Klatzmann, et al. SCIENCE 225(4657):59-63, July 6, 1984.

Special pathologico-anatomical aspects of AIDS—acquired immune deficiency syndrome, By G. R. Krueger, et al. ZEITSCHRIFT FUR HAUTKRANKHEITEN 59(8):507-522, April 15, 1984.

Syndrome of unexplained generalized lymphadenopathy in young men in New York City. Is it related to the acquired immune deficiency syndrome?, by B. Miller, et al. JAMA 251(2):242-246, January 13, 1984.

T and B cell reactions in AIDS and AIDS risk groups, by J. Kekow, et al. IMMUNITÄT UND INFEKTION 13(1):26-28, February 1985.

T-cell imbalances in blood and lymph nodes from patients with acquired immune deficiency syndrome or AIDS-related complex, by C. E. Grossi, et al. ALABAMA JOURNAL OF MEDICAL SCIENCES 22(2):160-163, April 1985.

T cell malignancies and human T cell leukemia (lymphotropic) retroviruses (HTLV), by P. S. Sarin, et al. PROGRESS IN CLINICAL AND BIOLOGICAL RE-SEARCH 184:445-456, 1985.

T cell malignancies and human T cell leukemia virus, by R. C. Gallo, et al. SEMI-NARS IN ONCOLOGY 11(1):12-17, March 1984.

T cell proliferation and ablation. A biologic spectrum of abnormalities induced by the human T cell lymphotropic virus group, by S. Broder. PROGRESS IN ALLERGY 37:224-243, 1986.

T cell ratios in AIDS [letter], by A. J. Pinching. BRITISH MEDICAL JOURNAL 287(6406):1716-1717, December 3, 1983.

T-cells and sympathy, by R. Massa. VILLAGE VOICE 30:110, April 23, 1985.

T-lymphocyte subset phenotypes: a multisite evaluation of normal subjects and patients with AIDS, by M. F. La Via, et al. DIAGNOSTIC IMMUNOLOGY 3(2): 75-82, 1985.

T4 lymphocyte in AIDS [editorial], by R. S. Kalish, et al. NEW ENGLAND JOUR-NAL OF MEDICINE 313(2):112-113, July 11, 1985.

'Trojan Horse' leukocytes in AIDS [letter], by D. J. Anderson, et al. NEW ENGLAND JOURNAL OF MEDICINE 309(16):984-985, October 20, 1983.

Ultrastructural markers in acquired immune deficiency syndrome [letter], by J. M. Orenstein, et al. ARCHIVES OF PATHOLOGY AND LABORATORY MEDI-CINE 108(11):845-849, November 1984.

Ultrastructural markers in AIDS [letter]. LANCET 2(8344):284, July 30, 1983.

Ultrastructural markers in LAV-HTLV III virus infection: study of the rectal mucosa in 16 patients, by P. Bruneval, et al. GASTROENTEROLOGIE CLINIQUE ET BIOLOGIQUE 10(4):328-333, April 1986.

Ultrastructural markers of AIDS [letter], by G. S. Sidhu, et al. LANCET 1(8331): 990-991, April 30, 1983.

Ultrastructural markers of lymph nodes in patients with acquired immune defi-ciency syndrome and in homosexual males with unexplained persistent lymphadenopathy. A quantitative study, by R. M. Onerheim, et al. AMERI-CAN JOURNAL OF CLINICAL PATHOLOGY 82(3):380-388, September 1984.

Ultrastructure of AIDS lymph nodes [letter]. NEW ENGLAND JOURNAL OF MEDICINE 309(19):1188-1190, November 10, 1983.

Unexplained persistent lymphadenopathy in homosexual men and the acquired immune deficiency syndrome, by J. W. Gold, et al. MEDICINE 64(3):203-213, May 1985.

Unusual cytoplasmic body in lymphoid cells of homosexual men with unexplained lymphadenopathy. A preliminary report, by E. P. Ewing, Jr., et al. NEW ENG-LAND JOURNAL OF MEDICINE 308(14):819-822, April 7, 1983.

475

Viral type particles in the germinal centers during a lymphadenopathic syndrome related to AIDS, by A. Le Tourneau, et al. ANNALS OF PATHOLOGY 592): 137-142, 1985.

Virus-like particles in AIDS-related lymphadenopathy [letter], by J. H. Humphrey. LANCET 2(8403):643, September 15, 1984.

CANADA
Vancouver Lymphadenopathy-AIDS Study: 1. Persistent generalized lymphadenopathy, by M. T. Schechter, et al. CANADIAN MEDICAL ASSOCIATION JOURNAL 132(11):1273-1279, June 1, 1985.

—: 2. Seroepidemiology of HTLV-III antibody, by E. Jeffries, et al. CANADIAN MEDICAL ASSOCIATION JOURNAL 132(12):1373-1377, June 15, 1985.

—: 3. Relation of HTLV-III seropositivity, immune status and lymphadeno-pathy, by W. J. Boyko, et al. CANADIAN MEDICAL ASSOCIATION JOURNAL 133(1):28-32, July 1, 1985.

—: 4. Effects of exposure factors, cofactors and HTLV-III seropositivity on number of helper T cells, by M. T. Schechter, et al. CANADIAN MEDICAL ASSOCIATION JOURNAL 133(4):286-292, August 15, 1985.

EUROPE
Clinical features of AIDS in Europe. EUROPEAN JOURNAL OF CANCER AND CLINICAL ONCOLOGY 20(2):165-167, February 1984.

GERMANY
Lymphadenopathy and a lower T-helper/suppressor cell (Th/Ts) ration in homosexual men in West Germany. Studies of 147 patients to evaluate the individual risk of acquiring AIDS, by M. Heitmann, et al. HAUTARZT 36(2):90-95, February 1985.

GREAT BRITAIN
Clinical findings and serological evidence of HTLV-III infection in homosexual contacts of patients with AIDS and persistent generalised lymphadeno-pathy in London, by B. G. Gazzard, et al. LANCET 2(8401):480-483, September 1, 1984.

GREECE
Lymphadenopathy associated virus in AIDS, lymphadenopathy associated syndrome, and classic Kaposi patients in Greece [letter],by G. Papae-vangelou, et al. LANCET 2(8403):642, September 15, 1984.

ITALY
Persistent generalized lymphadenopathy: pre-AIDS. First description of a case observed in Italy, by G. B. Gabrielli, et al. MINERVA MEDICA 75(44):2653-2658, November 17, 1984.

PATHOLOGY—CHILDREN
Epstein-Barr virus infection in a child with acquired immunodeficiency syndrome, by J. C. Jackler, et al. AMERICAN JOURNAL OF DISEASES OF CHILDREN 139(10):1000-1004, October 1985.

T cell surface antigen expression on lymphocytes of patients with AIDS during in vitro mitogen stimulation, y C. G. Munn, et al. CANCER IMMUNOLOGY AND IMMUNOTHERAPY 18(3):141-148, 1984.

PHARMACEUTICAL INDUSTRY
Drug hike protestors claim they were sold out, by S. Poggi. GAY COMMUNITY NEWS 13(44):2, May 31, 1986.

PHARMACEUTICALS
AIDS business: drug firms anticipate big market in products for immune disorder, by M. Chase. WALL STREET JOURNAL 207:1+, June 26, 1986.

PHARMACISTS
Apothecary, by J. Stamps. RFD 36:20, Fall 1983.

Apothecary—cancer, by Stamps, et al. RFD 34:24, Spring 1983.

PHYSICIANS
Acquired immune deficiency syndrome. Implications for the practicing physician, by B. Varkey. POSTGRADUATE MEDICINE 73(5):138+, May 1983.

Acquired immune deficiency syndrome. A perspective for the medical practitioner, by R. J. Sherertz. MEDICAL CLINICS OF NORTH AMERICA 69(4): 637-655, July 1985.

Acquired immunodeficiency syndrome and the emergency physician, by W. F. Skeen. ANNALS OF EMERGENCY MEDICINE 14(3):267-273, March 1985.

AIDS and the gay community: the doctor's role in counseling [editorial], by G. Leach, et al. BRITISH MEDICAL JOURNAL 290(6468):583, February 23, 1985.

AIDS and the physician, by C. P. Erwin. WISCONSIN MEDICAL JOURNAL 82(10):5, October 1983.

AIDS and the physician's fear of contagion, by e. H. Loewy. CHEST 89(3):325-326, March 1986.

AIDS in a surgeon [letter], by J. J. Sacks. NEW ENGLAND JOURNAL OF MEDICINE 313(16):1017-1018, October 17, 1985.

AIDS—its implications for South African homosexuals and the mediating role of the medical practitioner, by G. Isaacs, et al. SOUTH AFRICAN MEDICAL JOURNAL 68(5):327-330, August 31, 1985.

Angry New York doctor turns south-of-the-border smuggler to treat patients in danger of AIDS, by S. Haller. PEOPLE 23(16):139-140+, October 14, 1985.

Dr. Cornwall was obsessed with AIDS . . . the most difficult person I've worked with, by L. Moran. NURSINGLIFE 5(1):30-31, January-February 1985.

Doctors' efforts to control AIDS spark battles over civil liberties, by M. Chase. WALL STREET JOURNAL 205:23+, February 8, 1985.

Doctors explode myths about AIDS. JET 68:24-27, August 19, 1985.

Duties, fears and physicians, by E. H. Loewy. SOCIAL SCIENCE & MEDICINE 22(12):1363-1366, 1986.

How does the medical profession protect itself? by W. Williams. JOURNAL OF THE LOUISIANA STATE MEDICAL SOCIETY 137(9):53-55, September 1985.

Impact of the acquired immunodeficiency syndrome on medical residency training, by R. M. Wachter. NEW ENGLAND JOURNAL OF MEDICINE 314:177-180, January 16, 1986.

Institute of Medicine launches assessment of AIDS programs, by C. Norman. SCIENCE 231:1500, March 28, 1986.

MD diagnosed with bias, by A. Lesk. BODY POLITIC 125:19, April 1986.

Michael Gottlieb, M.D.: challenge of AIDS research, by M. Helquist. ADVOCATE 451:32, July 22, 1986.

New York doctor granted new lease in AIDS eviction, by P. Freiberg. ADVOCATE 4(8):10, November 27, 1984.

Physician knowledge and concerns about AIDS, by E. Barrett-Connor. WESTERN JOURNAL OF MEDICINE 140(4):652-653, April 1984.

Physician surveillance and the AIDS crisis [editorial], by D. W. Fisher. HOSPITAL PRACTICE 20(9):8, September 15, 1985.

Physicians should report cases of acquired immune deficiency syndrome [editorial], by D. P. Drotman. ARCHIVES OF INTERNAL MEDICINE 143(12): 2247, December 1983.

Physicians urge mandatory AIDS testing, by V. Kimble. AIR FORCE TIMES 47:8+, November 24, 1986.

Practitioner and AIDS, by M. B. Gregg. JOURNAL OF THE MEDICAL ASSOCI-ATION OF GEORGIA 73(8):555-556, August 1984.

Professional demands, human frailties. Doctors respond to AIDS, by C. Wiebe. NEW PHYSICIAN 35(1):14-17+, January-February 1986.

What does the dermatologist need to know about the new disease AIDS?, by N. Sönnichsen, et al. DERMATOLOGISCHE MONATSSCHRIFT 170(3):153-159, 1984.

What every Ohio physician should know about AIDS, by S. Porter. OHIO STATE MEDICAL JOURNAL 81(10):704-705+, October 1985.

What should a doctor tell a patient? [hemophiliac boy and AIDS antibody test], by P. Klass. DISCOVER 6:20-21, October 1985.

PHYSICIANS—TESTING
What Delaware's physicians should know about HTLV-III antibody testing, by P. R. Silverman, et al. DELAWARE MEDICAL JOURNAL 57(5):331-332, May 1985.

Activist urges unified plan on AIDS test, by P. Freiberg. ADVOCATE 4(8):12, November 27, 1984.

Activists campaign to fight AIDS initiative, by P. Freiberg. ADVOCATE 456:14, September 30, 1986.

Activists, FDA clash over HTLV-III test, by B. Nelson. GAY COMMUNITY NEWS 12(34):1, March 16, 1985.

AIDS activism against all odds, by S. Ault. GUARDIAN 38(26):10, April 2, 1986.

AIDS activist gets state job, by C. Guilfoy. GAY COMMUNITY NEWS 13(3):3, July 27, 1985.

AIDS activists—confidentiality issue, by C. Guilfoy. GAY COMMUNITY NEWS 12(5):1, August 11, 1984.

AIDS activists demand legislative action, by S. Connor. GAY COMMUNITY NEWS13(17):1, November 9, 1985.

AIDS also poses legal and political problems, by Phyllis Schlafly. HUMAN EVENTS 43:18, September 10, 1983.

AIDS and the disabiliy rights movement, by M. Owen. DISABILITY 7(2):14, March 1986.

AIDS and politics, by J. Foster. CALIFORNIA NURSE 82(4):9, May 1986.

AIDS and politics of despair, by M. Pally. ADVOCATE 436:8, December 24, 1985.

AIDS and public policy. NATIONAL REVIEW 35:796, July 8, 1983.

AIDS forum: politics & science collide, by C. Guilfoy. GAY COMMUNITY NEWS 12(31):3, February 23, 1985.

AIDS—health—politics, by D. Feinberg. GAY COMMUNITY NEWS 11(19):8, November 26, 1983.

AIDS lobby and education project proposed, by D. Slaw. GAY COMMUNITY NEWS 10(50):3, July 9, 1983.

AIDS: Moral Majority intervenes [news], by P. David. NATURE 304(5923):201, July 21-27, 1983.

AIDS: the politicization of an epidemic, by D. Altman. SOCIALIST REVIEW 78:93, November 1984.

AIDS: US company rejects UK decision, by M. Clarke. NATURE 316:759, August 29, 1985.

Alarm on AIDS: government bias feared, by C. Frank. AMERICAN BAR ASSOCI-ATION JOURNAL 71:22, December 1985.

At risk: while the Reagan administration dozes and scientists vie for glory, the deadly AIDS [acquired immune deficiency syndrome] epidemic has put the

479

entire nation at risk, by D. Talbot, et al. MOTHER JONES 10:28-37, April 1985.

Axelrod warns of pressure to shut bathhouses, by P. Freiberg. ADVOCATE 418:10, April 16, 1985.

Banning the baths: AIDS and gay rights, by R. O'Loughlin. GUARDIAN 37(4):5, October 24, 1984.

Bay area bathowners balk at restrictions, by C. Guilfoy. GAY COMMUNITY NEWS 12(22):1, December 15, 1984.

Boston official roasted—AIDS joke, by L. Goldsmith. GAY COMMUNITY NEWS 11(35):1, March 24, 1984.

California questions LaRouche signatures, by Bisticas-Cocoves. GAY COMMUNITY NEWS 13(46):1, June 14, 1986.

CDC charged with sabotaging AIDS research, by Bisticas-Cocoves. GAY COMMUNITY NEWS 14(11):1, September 28, 1986.

CIA/CDC/AIDS political alliance, by C. Shively. GAY COMMUNITY NEWS 10(50): 5, July 9, 1983.

Cincinnati rebuts threat to gay AIDS counselors, by J. Zeh. GAY COMMUNITY NEWS 12(38):1, April 13, 1985.

City officials withdraw Cambridge AIDS policy, by K. Westheimer. GAY COMMUNITY NEWS 13(38):1, April 12, 1986.

Colorado to keep list of HTLV-3 positives, by M. Cocoves. GAY COMMUNITY NEWS 13(11):1, September 28, 1985.

Congressman AIDS, by T. Johnson. LOS ANGELES 124, January 1986.

Dukakis presence at AIDS event draws fire, by S. Poggi. GAY COMMUNITY NEWS 13(2):3, October 5, 1985.

Epidemics and the Government, by G. Wilson. THE GAO REVIEW 19(2):26-27+, Spring 1984.

Ex-Carter official hired by gay group, by L. Bush. ADVOCATE 3(75):8, September 1, 1983.

FDA responses to the challenges of AIDS, by H. M. Meyer, Jr. PUBLIC HEALTH REPORTS 98(4):320-323, July-August 1983.

Federal Government intensifies its efforts in the mental health aspects of AIDS, by B. Runck. HOSPITAL AND COMMUNITY PSYCHIATRY 37(3):219-221, March 1986.

Federal officials back use of consent forms, by C. Guilfoy. GAY COMMUNITY NEWS 12(10):1, September 22, 1984.

Federal response to the AIDS epidemic, by P. R. Lee, et al. HEALTH POLICY 6(3):259-267, 1986.

Feds AIDS action lacking, by L. Bush. ADVOCATE 3(76):8, September 15, 1983.

Florida AIDS victim deported, by D. France. GUARDIAN 36(6):4, November 9, 1983.

Gay body politics, by R. Kaye. IN THESE TIMES 7(39):12, October 29, 1983.

Gay representatives lobby for AIDS policy, by J. Ryan. GAY COMMUNITY NEWS 12(24):1, December 29, 1984.

GOP Senators hold briefing on AIDS, by D. Walter. ADVOCATE 428:18, September 3, 1985.

Government irresponsible on AIDS, says Fettner. OUT 3(12):3, October 1985.

Government's response to fears about acquired immunodeficiency syndrome, by R. Deitch. LANCET 1(8427):530-531, March 2, 1985.

Grassroots action/Gov. vagueness, by E. Jackson. BODY POLITIC 96:15, September 1983.

Grassroots petition demands AIDS response, by M. Cocoves. GAY COMMUNITY NEWS 12(47):3, June 15, 1985.

Hart disappointing on gay issues, by J. Ryan. GAY COMMUNITY NEWS 11(36):3, March 31, 1984.

Health Director closes Bay Area sex businesses, by C. Guilfoy. GAY COMMUNITY NEWS 12(14):1, October 20, 1984.

Health education and the politics of AIDS, by N. Freundenberg. HEALTH PAC BULLETIN 16(3):29-30, May-June 1985.

Health office set up/Koch pressured, by B. Nelson. GAY COMMUNITY NEWS 10(36):1, April 2, 1983.

Health officials close baths and sex clubs. BODY POLITIC 1(8):17, November 1984.

Injunct against NY march denied, by P. Byron. GAY COMMUNITY NEWS 10(49): 1, July 2, 1983.

Issues of morality dominate Houston's politics, by B. Sablatura. IN THESE TIMES 9(41):8, October 30, 1985.

KGB: Pentagon is responsible for AIDS, by Ralph de Toledano. HUMAN EVENTS 46:9, March 29, 1986.

Koch's postulates and the search for the AIDS agent, by R. M. Krause. PUBLIC HEALTH REPORTS 99(3):291-299, May-June 1984.

—, by R. M. Krause. REVIEWS OF INFECTIOUS DISEASES 6(2):270-279, March-April 1984.

LaRouche advocates "spread panic, not AIDS", by D. Walter. ADVOCATE 435: 21, December 10, 1985.

LaRouche AIDS initiative, by P. Freiberg. ADVOCATE 453:10, August 19, 1986.

LaRouche behind bigoted Calif. AIDS referendum. GUARDIAN 38(39):5, July 9, 1986.

LaRouche-supported initiative on AIDS policy in California spurs debate on handling disease, by J. R. Emshwiller. WALL STREET JOURNAL 208:38, August 11, 1986.

Latest great idea from Mayor Koch is a real winner! NARCOTICS CONTROL DIGEST 15(20):7, October 2, 1985.

Lyndon La Rouche initiative: AIDS quarantine, by P. Freiberg. ADVOCATE 446:12, May 13, 1986.

Medical caution/political judgment [editorial]. BODY POLITIC 93:8, May 1983.

Message from Secretary Heckler, by M. M. Heckler. FDA DRUG BULLETIN 15(3):26, October 1985.

Minnesota Board to seek sex partner notification, by Bisticas-Cocoves. GAY COMMUNITY NEWS 13(41):1, May 3, 1986.

New York activists fight eviction of PWA's survivor, by B. Gelbert. GAY COMMUNITY NEWS 13(38):1, April 12, 1986.

On AIDS jokes—public officials, by E. Rofes. GAY COMMUNITY NEWS 11(36):5, March 31, 1984.

OTA critical of AIDS initiative, by C. Holden. SCIENCE 227(4691):1182-1183, March 8, 1985.

Palm Spring Mayor protests AIDS hotel, by C. Love. ADVOCATE 4(7):12, November 13, 1984.

Parson cites AIDS/urges bar ban, by K. Orr. BODY POLITIC 97:11, October 1983.

Political consequences of AIDS, by Fowler, et al. SOCIALIST WORKER 76:5, August 1983.

Political medicine [editorial]. GUARDIAN 37(42):22, August 21, 1985.

Political posturing over AIDS, by L. Bush. ADVOCATE 3(74):20, August 18, 1983.

Politics of AIDS, by F. Barnes. THE NEW REPUBLIC 193:11-12+, November 4, 1985.

—, by L. Van Gelder. MS 11(11):103, May 1983.

—, by Payne, et al. SCIENCE FOR THE PEOPLE 16(5):17, September 1984.

Politics of AIDS—a tale of two states [Texas and Montana], by A. Trafford, et al. US NEWS & WORLD REPORT 99(21):70-71, November 18, 1985.

Politics of disease, by R. Kaye. ADVOCATE 441:52, March 4, 1986.

Politics of an epidemic, by K. Kelley. GUARDIAN 35(32):1, May 11, 1983.

Politics of a plague, by C. Krauthammer. THE NEW REPUBLIC 189:18-21, August 1, 1983.

Proposed government AIDS list draws fire, by S. Kulieke. ADVOCATE 404:14, October 2,1 984.

Seattle AIDS Action Committee, by G. Bakan. NORTHWEST PASSAGE 24(2):7, September 1983.

Stop the LaRouche panic!, by P. Drucker. AGAINST THE CURRENT 455:17, September 16, 1985.

Task Force to meet president aide, by S. Hyde. GAY COMMUNITY NEWS 10(47): 1, June 18, 1983.

United States new right linked to New Zealand homophobes, by S. Poggi. GAY COMMUNITY NEWS 13(10):1, September 21, 1985.

United States policy on AIDS hit, by Bisticas-Cocoves. GAY COMMUNITY NEWS 13(3):3, July 27, 1985.

Useless "plague politics". BODY POLITIC 124:26, March 1986.

CANADA
Ontario removes Haitians from list, by E. Jackson. BODY POLITIC 99:8, December 1983.

FRANCE
AIDS: politics of premature French claim of cure, by R. Walgate. NATURE 318:3, November 7, 1985.

GREAT BRITAIN
British AIDS Action Committee formed, by L. Taylor. ADVOCATE 3(81):15, November 24, 1983.

POLITICS—TESTS
Politics and test of AIDS, by S. Norman. RFD 44:53, Fall 1985.

PREGNANCY
Acquired immunodeficiency (AIDS) in pregnancy, by L. P. Jensene, et al. AMERICAN JOURNAL OF OBSTETRICS AND GYNECOLOGY 148(8):1145-1146, April 15, 1984.

AIDS in pregnancy, by A. Loveman, et al. JOGN NURSING15(2):91-93, March-April 1986.

AIDS in pregnancy, donors and tears. SCIENCE NEWS 128:187, September 21, 1985.

CDC reports caution obstetric personnel, patients about AIDS virus, by A. Ropp. NAACOG NEWSLETTER 13(6):1+, June 1986.

PREGNANCY—HEALTH CARE WORKERS
Infection control and the pregnant health care worker, by W. M. Valenti. AMERICAN JOURNAL OF INFECTION CONTROL 14(1):20-27, February 1986.

PREVENTION
Acquired immunodeficiency syndrome (AIDS)—clinical course and prevention, by E. Sandström, et al. LAKARTIDNINGEN 80(7):529-530, February 16, 1983.

AIDS and preventive treatment in hemophilia [editorial], by J. F. Desforges. NEW ENGLAND JOURNAL OF MEDICINE 308(2):94-95, January 13, 1983.

AIDS (and STD) prophylaxis: urgent need for an effective genital antiseptic [letter], by A. Comfort. JOURNAL OF THE ROYAL SOCIETY OF MEDICINE 79(5):311-312, May 1986.

AIDS epidemic: risk containment for home health care providers, by J. G. Turner, et al. FAMILY AND COMMUNITY HEALTH 8(3):25-37, November 1985.

AIDS in the workplace. How to prevent the transmission of the infection. INTERNATIONAL NURSES REVIEW 33(4/268):117-122+, July-August 1986.

AIDS investigators want input on prevention of disease. AMERICAN FAMILY PHYSICIAN 29:18, June 1984.

AIDS: it can be avoided, by J. H. Tanne. READER'S DIGEST 128:94-98, February 1986.

AIDS: a nurse's responsibility. Infection precautions in the community, by G. Lusby, et al. CALIFORNIA NURSE 82(4):16, May 1986.

AIDS prevention and treatment, by A. Ranki. DUODECIM 102(7):429-438, 1986.

AIDS: prevention strategies, by M. A. Conant. FRONTIERS OF RADIATION THERAPY AND ONCOLOGY 19:150-154, 1985.

AIDS: precautions, by B. Cox. ANNA JOURNAL 13(5):283, October 1986.

—, by C. B. Persons, et al. JOURNAL OF PRACTICAL NURSING 33(8):51-53, September-October 1983.

CDC: despite RN seroconversion, AIDS precautions adequate. HOSPITAL EMPLOYEE HEALTH 4(2):17-19, February 1985.

CDC guidelines for the prevention and control of nosocomial infections. Guideline for infection control in hospital personnel, by W. W. Williams. AMERICAN JOURNAL OF INFECTION CONTROL 12(1):34-63, February 1984.

CDC guidelines: recommendations for preventing transmission of AIDS. AORN JOURNAL 43(2):528+, February 1986.

CDC issues AIDS guidelines for health workers, by V. L. Bauknecht. AMERICAN NURSE 18(1):2+, January 1986.

CDC publishes AIDS precautions for health-care and allied professionals. EMER- GENCY DEPARTMENT NEWS 5(11):17, November 1983.

CDC recommendations for preventing transmission of AIDS during invasive pro- cedures. TEXAS NURSE 60(7):14, August 1986; also in OREGON NURSE 51(3):10, June 1986.

Comments on the CDC Guideline for Employees Health, by W. M. Valenti. IN- FECTION CONTROL 5(4):192-194, April 1984.

FDA issues guidelines to protect transfusion recipients from AIDS. HOSPITALS 57(12):59-60, June 16, 1983.

Hospitals stepping up effort to protect staff from AIDS. AMERICAN JOURNAL OF NURSING 83:1468+, October 1983.

Hospitalwide approach to AIDS. Recommendations of the Advisory Committee on Infections within Hospitals, by the American Hospital Association. INFEC- TION CONTROL 5(5):242-248, May 1984.

How to avoid catching AIDS, by A. Veitch, et al. GUARDIAN November 21, 1986, p. 21.

How to safeguard against AIDS, by C. Joyce. NEW SCIENTIST 102:8, May 31, 1984.

Infection control. EMS reacts—and overreacts—to the AIDS panic, by B. Smith. JOURNAL OF EMERGENCY MEDICAL SERVICE 8(8):24-29, August 1983.

Infection control and employee health: update on AIDS, by W. M. Valenti. INFEC- TION CONTROL 6(2):85-86, February 1985.

Infection control at home, by G. Lusby, et al. AMERICAN JOURNAL OF HOS- PITAL CARE 3(2):24-27, March-April 1986.

Infection control: gays and medicine age of AIDS, by E. Collins. BORDERLINES 4:4, Winter 1985.

Infection-control guidelines for patients with the acquired immunodeficiency syn- drome (AIDS), by J. E. Conte, Jr., et al. NEW ENGLAND JOURNAL OF MEDI- CINE 309(12):740-744, September 22, 1983.

Infection precautions in the community . . . at home, by G. Lusby, et al. CALI- FORNIA NURSE 82(4):16, May 1986.

Last word on avoiding AIDS, by J. H. Tanne. NEW YORK 18:28-34, October 7, 1985.

Laundry workers need AIDS guidelines. LAUNDRY NEWS 11(10):24, October 1985.

Minimizing the risk of contracting AIDS, by J. L. Marx. SCIENCE 219:1301, March 18, 1983.

New developments in the acquired immunodeficiency syndrome: are treatment, prevention, and control possible?, by J. M. Luce. RESPIRATORY CARE 31(2):113-116, February 1986.

New measures to contain AIDS. NURSING STANDARD 386:1, February 28, 1985.

New strategies for AIDS therapy and prophylaxis [letter], by E. C. M. Mariman, et al. NATURE 318(6045):414, December 5-11, 1985.

Precautions against acquired immunodeficiency syndrome [editorial]. LANCET 1(8317):164, January 22, 1983.

Precautions against transmittable disease, By K. S. Kawala. ILLINOIS MEDICAL JOURNAL 166(6):387, December 1984.

Precautions prevent transmission of HTLV-III virus, by J. Prescott. TEXAS HOS-PITALS 41(11):16-17, April 1986.

Preventing the acquired immunodeficiency syndrome [letter],by L. A. Hassell. NEW ENGLAND JOURNAL OF MEDICINE 309(22):1395, December 1, 1983.

Preventing the spread of AIDS [letter], by R. F. Wykoff. JAMA 255(13):1706-1707, April 4, 1986.

Prevention of acquired immune deficiency syndrome (AIDS): report of inter-agency recommendations. CONNECTICUT MEDICINE 47(6):361-362, June 1983; also in JAMA 249 (12)1544-1555, March 25, 1983 and MMWR 32(8): 101-103, March 4, 1983.

Prevention of acquired immunodeficiency syndrome [letter], by A. E. Pitchenick, et al. ANNALS OF INTERNAL MEDICINE 98(4):558-559, April 1983.

Prevention of AIDS [letter]. LANCET 2(8468):1362-1363, December 14, 1985.

Prevention of HTLV-III infection [letter],by P. R. Gustafson. JAMA 256(3):346-347, July 18, 1986.

Protect yourself against AIDS, CDC urges. RN 46:11, February 1983.

Protecting against A.I.D.S. NURSING 14:22, December 1984.

Protecting ourselves against AIDS, by R. Rodale. PREVENTION 37:17-18+, December 1985.

Recommendations for preventing transmission of infection with human T-lymphotropic virus type III/lymphadenopathy-associated virus during invasive procedures. ANNALS OF INTERNAL MEDICINE 104(6):824-825, June 1986; also in PENNSYLVANIA NURSE 41(7):3, July 1986.

Recommendations on preventing AIDS transmissions released. TEXAS HOS-PITALS 42(1):20-21, June 1986.

Society's survival first, then victims' rights: AIDS plague, by Richard Restak. HUMAN EVENTS 45:18+, October 5, 1985.

Stopping the AIDS epidemic, by P. Kawata. PUBLIC WELFARE 44(3):35, Summer 1986.

Struggling to save the next generation, by T. Prentice. TIMES October 28, 1986, p. 14.

Study proves condoms block AIDS virus, by M. Helquist. ADVOCATE 438:20, January 21, 1986.

Summary: recommendations for preventing transmission of infection with HTLV-III/LAV in the workplace. JAMA 254:3023-3024+, December 6, 1985.

Trying to head off AIDS, by S. Deaton. ALBERTA REPORT 12:32-33, September 16, 1985.

Trying to lock out AIDS, by J. Adler, et al. NEWSWEEK 106(12):65, September 16, 1985.

What can I do to avoid getting AIDS, doctor?, by A. S. Brodoff. PATIENT CARE 18(2):153-154+, January 30, 1984.

When will prevention of HTLV-III infection be possible?, by R. Tedder, et al. VACCINE 2(3):171-172, September 1984.

Who decides what AIDS protection is enough? RN 48:10, October, 1985.

CANADA
AIDS prevention underway in B.C., by K. Scholl. RNABC NEWS15(8):9-10, November-December 1983.

POLAND
AIDS: Poland's minister for prophylaxis, by V. Rich. NATURE 317:100, September 12, 1985.

PREVENTION—BLOOD DONORS—TESTING
Preventing AIDS transmission: should blood donors be screened? , by W. A. Check. JAMA 249(5):567-570, February 4, 1983.

PREVENTION—BLOOD TRANSFUSIONS
Avoiding AIDS with autologous transfusions [letter], by S. E. James. BRITISH MEDICAL JOURNAL 290(6471):854, March 16, 1985.

PREVENTION—EMPLOYMENT
Reducing the risk of job related disease, by R. Zack. LAW AND ORDER 33(2):59-60, February 1985.

Statement on the development of guidelines for the prevention of AIDS transmission in the workplace, by J. O. Mason. PUBLIC HEALTH REPORTS 101(1):6-8, January-Febraury 1986.

PREVENTION—HEALTH CARE WORKERS
AIDS—safety practices for clinical and research laboratories, by J. V. Federico, et al. INFECTION CONTROL 5(4):185-187, April 1984.

Entirely new hygienic guidelines for care of AIDS patients, by M. Meyer. SYGEPLEJERSKEN 85(45):20-22, November 6, 1985.

New safety rules for AIDS workers. NEW SCIENTIST 103:5, August 23, 1984.

PREVENTION—HOMOSEXUALS
New strategy to prevent the spread of AIDS among heterosexuals [editorial], by D. F. Echenberg. JAMA 254(15):2129-2130, October 18, 1985.

PREVENTION—HOSPITALS
AIDS: what precautions do you take in the hospital? by J. Bennett. AMERICAN JOURNAL OF NURSING 86(8):952-953, August 1986.

Coast hospital laundry manager calls yellow alert on AIDS linen. LAUNDRY NEWS 9(8):1+, August 1983.

Hospital guidelines on AIDS developed at UCSF. INFECTION CONTROL DI-GEST 4(8):3-4, August 1983.

Hospital hygiene. AIDS: preventing contamination in the hospital, by G. Ducel. KRANKENPFLEGE. SOINS INFIRMIERS 79(5):67-70, May 1986.

—. Notice of the Expert Federal Commission for AIDS on procedures to adopt in regard to patients with AIDS and to persons carrying anti-LAV/HTLV-III anti-bodies. KRANKENPFLEGE. SOINS INFIRMIERS 79(5):74-75, May 1986.

Prevention of in-hospital transmission of the acquired immune deficiency syndrome virus (HTLV III): current USA policy, by F. S. Rhame. JOURNAL OF HOSPITAL INFECTION 6(Suppl. C):53-66, December 1985.

PREVENTION—NURSES
Doubts over AIDs precautions spur RN resignation. AMERICAN JOURNAL OF NURSING 83:1258+, September 1983.

Guidelines to protect nurses from AIDS. NURSING STANDARD 379:1, January 10, 1985.

PREVENTION—PUBLIC HEALTH SERVICE
Public Health Service plan for the prevention and control of acquired immune deficiency syndrome (AIDS), by J. O. Mason. PUBLIC HEALTH REPORT 100:453-455, September-October 1985.

PREVENTION—SEX
Prevention of AIDS by modifying sexual behavior, by D. C. William. ANNALS OF THE NEW YORK ACADEMY OF SCIENCES 437:283-285, 1984.

Reducing the risk of acquiring AIDS . . . the condom, by M. S. Tillis. AAOHN JOURNAL 34(9):432-434, September 1986.

PRISONS
Acquired immunodeficiency syndrome in correctional facilities: a report of the National Institute of Justice and the American Correctional Association. MMWR 35(12):195-199, March 28, 1986.

Acquired immunodeficiency syndrome in male prisoners. New insights into an emerging syndrome, by G. P. Wormser, et al. ANNALS OF INTERNAL MEDICINE 98(3):297-303 March 1983.

AIDS behind bars: lies and manipulation, by T. Schrieber. GAY COMMUNITY NEWS 13(35):3, March 22, 1986.

AIDS cases found concentrated in few prisons, study finds. CRIMINAL JUSTICE NEWSLETTER 17(5):4-5, March 3, 1986.

AIDS in the prison system: some suggestions on how to prevent new outbreaks, by T. Bassinger. CORRECTIONS DIGEST 14(16):3-4, July 27, 1983.

AIDS patient isolated in prison, by D. Van Straten. OUT 4(5):5, March 1986.

AIDS-stricken inmate bites deputy; charged with attempted murder. CORRECTIONS DIGEST 17(12):3, June 4, 1986; also in CRIME CONTROL DIGEST 20(22):9-10, June 2, 1986.

Attention, prison dentists: CDC issues warning on AIDS. CORRECTIONS DIGEST 14(19):9-10, September 7, 1983.

Correctional officials may be closing their eyes to AIDS threat. LAW ENFORCEMENT NEWS 12(1):1+, January 6, 1986.

Corrections. CRIMINAL JUSTICE NEWSLETTER 15(20):7, October 15, 1984.

In prison with AIDS, by J. Jones. GUARDIAN 38(10):1, December 4, 1985.

Inmates dying from AIDS disease. CORRECTIONS DIGEST 14(13):7, June 15, 1983.

Interview: Michael Hennessey—Sheriff of San Francisco County, Calif., and authority on AIDS behind bars, by J. Nislow. LAW ENFORCEMENT NEWS 12(1):9-11+, January 6, 1986.

Look at AIDS inside: coming soon to a prison, by E. Mead. NORTHWEST PASSAGE 26(4):5, December 1985.

New AIDS risk: a term in jail. NEWSWEEK 106:98, October 28, 1985.

New Jersey prisoners file AIDS suit. GAY COMMUNITY NEWS 13(4):2, August 3, 1985.

NIC update, by N. Sabanosh. CORRECTIONS TODAY 48(4):22+, June 1986.

NIJ publishes huge manual on AIDS in prisons and jails. CORRECTIONS DIGEST 17(5):1-3, February 26, 1986; also in CRIME CONTROL DIGEST 20(8):3-5, February 24, 1986.

Officers suspended for refusing to transport inmate with AIDS. CRIME CONTROL DIGEST 17(42):3, October 24, 1983; also in CORRECTIONS DIGEST 14(22):8-9, October 19, 1983.

Police, court officials arraign AIDS victim in Rhode Island jail cell. CORRECTIONS DIGEST 16(26):5, December 18, 1985; also in CRIME CONTROL DIGEST 20(1):3-4, January 6, 1986.

Politics of AIDS in prison, by E. Mead. GAY COMMUNITY NEWS 13(25):5, January 11, 1986.

Prevalence of infection caused by AIDS and hepatitis B viruses in jailed people, by P. Crovari, et al. BOLLETTINO DELL ISTITUTO SIEROTERAPICO MILANESE 64(5):367-370, 1985.

Prisoner with AIDS: double isolation, by E. Bubbenmayer. GAY COMMUNITY NEWS 13(25):5, January 11, 1986.

Prolonged incubation period of AIDS in intravenous drug abusers: epidemiological evidence in prison inmates, by J. P. Hanrahan, et al. JOURNAL OF INFECTIOUS DISEASES 150(2):263-266, August 1984.

Responding to AIDS in prisons: the team approach, by J. J. Maffucci. CORRECTIONS TODAY 45:68+, December 1983.

Tough new problems for institutions: inmates with AIDS. CRIMINAL JUSTICE NEWSLETTER 16(17):1-2, September 3, 1985.

FRANCE
AIDS in French prisons, by I. Porras. CORRECTIONS TODAY 48:128, August 1986.

PRISONS—SEX
Condoms for prisoners: would fighting AIDS promote homosexual acts?, by L. Cohen, et al. ALBERTA REPORT 12:12-13, October 7, 1985.

PSYCHOLOGY AND PSYCHIATRY
Acquired immune deficiency syndrome (AIDS) and consultation-liaison psychiatry, by D. L. Wolcott, et al. GENERAL HOSPITAL PSYCHIATRY 7(4):280-293, October 1985.

Act of God—AIDS—fear of death, by J. Rule. BODY POLITIC 95:39, July 1983.

AIDS and community supportive services. Understanding and management of psychological needs, by T. Goulden, et al. MEDICAL JOURNAL OF AUSTRALIA 141(9):582-586, October 27, 1984.

AIDS and the gay community: the doctor's role in counseling [editorial], by G. Leach, et al. BRITISH MEDICAL JOURNAL 290(6468):583, February 23, 1985.

AIDS and the mind, by N. Fain. ADVOCATE 3(79):22, October 27, 1983.

AIDS and the new morality, by M. Godwin. GAY COMMUNITY NEWS 11(5):6, August 13, 1983.

AIDS dementia complex: I. Clinical features, by B. A. Navia, et al. ANNALS OF NEUROLOGY 19(6):517-524, June 1986.

AIDS: dilemmas for the psychiatric patient [letter], by D. Summerfield. LANCET 2(8498):112, July 12, 1986.

AIDS: dilemmas for the psychiatrist [letter], by A. J. Pinching. LANCET 1(8479):496-497, March 1, 1986.

AIDS impairs mental function. ADAMHA NEWS 11(8):1, August 1985.

AIDS in New York City with particular reference to the psycho-social aspects, by N. Deuchar. BRITISH JOURNAL OF PSYCHIATRY 145:612-619, December 1984.

AIDS: a living nightmare: psychosocial intervention by the GIA, by S. Lewis, et al. SGA JOURNAL 7(4):16-21, Spring 1985.

AIDS may force re-examination of values, by Ray Kerrison. HUMAN EVENTS 45:9, August 17, 1985.

AIDS: one psychosocial response, by J. P. Doherty. QRB12(8):295-297, August 1986.

AIDS-panic: AIDS-induced psychogenic states [letter], by G. O'Brien, et al. BRITISH JOURNAL OF PSYCHIATRY 147:91, July 1985.

AIDS-prompted behavior changes reported, by D. E. Riesenberg. JAMA 255: 171+, January 10, 1986.

AIDS: a public health disaster, by N. Heneson. NEW SCIENTIST 108:75-76, November 14, 1985.

AIDS: a threat to physical and psychological integrity, by L. J. Ryan. TOPICS IN CLINICAL NURSING 6(2):19-25, July 1984.

AIDS: what is now known: part 4, psychosocial aspects, treatment prospects, by P. A. Selwyn. HOSPITAL PRACTICE 21(10):125-128+, October 15, 1986.

Behavioral and psychosocial factors in AIDS. Methodological and substantive issues, by J. L. Martin, et al. AMERICAN PSYCHOLOGIST 39(11):1303-1308, November 1984.

Behind the mental symptoms of AIDS, by M. Norman. PSYCHOLOGY TODAY 18:12, December 1984.

Case study: "If I have AIDS, then let me die now," by S. Vinogradov, et al. HASTINGS CENTER REPORT 14:24-26, February 1984.

Celebrating life honoring courage, by W. K. Hale. GAY COMMUNITY NEWS 11(16):15, November 5, 1983.

Considering the psychosocial aspects of AIDS, by L. J. Redouty, et al. MICHIGAN HOSPITALS 22(8):17-21, August 1986.

Contracting AIDS as a means of committing suicide [letter], by R. J. Frances, et al. AMERICAN JOURNAL OF PSYCHIATRY 142(5):656, May 1985.

Counseling. Advice and sympathy for AIDS sufferers, by J. Sherman. HEALTH AND SOCIAL SERVICE JOURNAL 95(4976):1506-1507, November 28, 1985.

Countertransference issues in working with persons with AIDS, by J. Dunkel, et al. SOCIAL WORK 31(2):114-117, March-April 1986.

Dementia and AIDS. AMERICAN FAMILY PHYSICIAN 32:239+, August 1985.

Disabling fear of AIDS responsive to imipramine, by M. A. Jenike, et al. PSYCHO-SOMATICS 27(2):143-144, February 1986.

Findings in psychiatric consultations with patients with acquired immune deficiency syndrome, by J. W. Dilley, et al. AMERICAN JOURNAL OF PSYCHIATRY 142(1):82-86, January 1985.

Homophobia among physicians and nurses: an empirical study, by C. J. Douglas, et al. HOSPITAL AND COMMUNITY PSYCHIATRY 36(12):1309-1311, December 1985.

HTLV-III and psychiatric disturbance [letter], by c. S. Thomas, et al. LANCET 2(8451):395-396, August 17, 1985.

"If I have AIDS, then let me die now!" [case study], by S. Vinogradov, et al. HASTINGS CENTER REPORT 14:24-26, February 1984.

—. Commentary, by A. J. Levinson. HASTINGS CENTER REPORT 14(1):26, February 1984.

Neuropsychiatric aspects of acquired immune deficiency syndrome, by R. J. Loewenstein, et al. INTERNATIONAL JOURNAL OF PSYCHIATRY IN MEDICINE 13(4):255-260, 1983-1984.

Neuropsychiatric complications of AIDS, by R. S. Hoffman. PSYCHOSOMATICS 25(5):393-395+, May 1984.

Neuropsychiatric complications of AIDS: a literature review, by W. M. Detmer, et al. INTERNATIONAL JOURNAL OF PSYCHIATRY IN MEDICINE 16(1):21-29, 1986-1987.

New emphasis on psychosocial issues: AIDS studies, by N. Fain. ADVOCATE 421:24, May 28, 1985.

New psychopathologic findings in AIDS: case report, by E. J. Ermani, et al. JOURNAL OF CLINICAL PSYCHIATRY 46(6):240-241, June 1985.

Pinning down the psychosocial dimensions of AIDS, by S. Feinblum. NURSING AND HEALTH CARE 7(5):254-256, May 1986.

Pseudo-AIDS syndrome following from fear of AIDS, by D. Miller, et al. BRITISH JOURNAL OF PSYCHIATRY 146:550-551, May 1985.

Psychiatric aspects of AIDS, by R. Zumbrunnen, et al. SCHWEIZERISCHE RUNDSCHAU FUER MEDIZIN PRAXIS 73(43):1311-1312, October 23, 1984.

—, by S. E. Nichols, Jr. PSYCHOSOMATICS 24(12):1083-1089, December 1983.

Psychiatric problems of AIDS inpatients at the New York Hospital: preliminary report, by S. W. Perry, et al. PUBLIC HEALTH REPORTS 99(2):200-205, 1984.

Psychiatric staff response to acquired immune deficiency syndrome, by M. A. Cummings, et al. AMERICAN JOURNAL OF PSYCHIATRY 143:682, May 1986.

Psychic channel on AIDS, by J Ferguson. RFD 45:48, Winter 1985.

Psychological factors associated with AIDS under study. PUBLIC HEALTH RE-PORTS 100(3):345, May-June 1985.

Psychological impact of AIDS on gay men, by S. F. Morin, et al. AMERICAN PSY-CHOLOGIST 39(11):1288-1293, November 1984.

Psychological impact of AIDS on primary care physicians [letter],by L. McKusick, et al. WESTERN JOURNAL OF MEDICINE 144(6):751-752, June 1986.

Psychological themes in patients with acquired immune deficiency syndrome [letter], by L. R. Hays, et al. AMERICAN JOURNAL OF PSYCHIATRY 143(4): 551, April 1986.

Psychopathology complicating acquired immune deficiency syndrome (AIDS), by H. G. Nurnberg, et al. AMERICAN JOURNAL OF PSYCHIATRY 141(1):95-96, January 1984.

Psychosocial and ethical issues of AIDS health care programs, by D. G. Ostrow, et al. QRB 12(8):284-294, August 1986.

Psychosocial impact of acquired immune deficiency syndrome [letter], by H. Holtz, et al. JAMA 250(2):167, July 8, 1983.

Psychosocial impact of the acquired immunodeficiency syndrome, by M. Forstein. SEMINARS IN ONCOLOGY 11(1):77-82, March 1984.

Psychosocial impact of AIDS, by D. R. Rubinow. TOPICS IN CLINICAL NURSING 6(2):26-30, July 1984.

Psychosocial issues for people with AIDS, by d. W. Smith, et al. JOURNAL OF THE MEDICAL ASSOCIATION OF GEORGIA 73(8):535-536, August 1984.

Psychosocial reactions of persons with the acquired immunodeficiency syn-drome, by S. E. Nichols. ANNALS OF INTERNAL MEDICINE 103(5):765-767, November 1, 1985.

Psychosocial research is essential to understanding and treating AIDS, by T. J. Coates, et al. AMERICAN PSYCHOLOGIST 39(11):1309-1314, November 1984.

Reducing psychological complications for the critically ill AIDS patient, by J. D. Durham, et al. DIMENSIONS OF CRITICAL CARE NURSING 3(5):300-306, September-October 1984.

Responding to the psychological crisis of AIDS, by S. F. Morin, et al. PUBLIC HEALTH REPORTS 99(1):4-9, January-February 1984.

Three cases of AIDS-related psychiatric disorders, by J. R. Rundell, et al. AMERI-CAN JOURNAL OF PSYCHIATRY 143:777-778, June 1986.

UCLA psychological study of AIDS, by D. K. Wellisch. FRONTIERS OF RADIA-
TION THERAPY AND ONCOLOGY 19:155-158, 1985.

Venereophobia [letter]. BRITISH JOURNAL OF HOSPITAL MEDICINE 32(3):
155, September 1984.

Victimizing the victim. WOMANEWS 6(9):14, October 1985.

PSYCHOLOGY AND PSYCHIATRY—HEALTH CARE WORKERS
AIDS: psychosocial needs of the health care worker, by S. Simmons-Alling.
TOPICS IN CLINICAL NURSING 6(2):31-37, July 1984.

PSYCHOLOGY AND PSYCHAITRY—NURSES
Psycho nursing care of AIDS victims, by M. Fiske. CHART 83(5):+, May-June
1986.

PSYCHOLOGY AND PSYCHAITRY—TREATMENT
Treating victims of AIDS poses challenge to psychiatrists. Part 1, by K. Hausman.
PSYCHIATRIC NEWS 18(15):1+, August 5, 1983.

PUBLIC HEALTH
AIDS and community health issues, by S. Cowell. JOURNAL OF AMERICAN
COLLEGE HEALTH 33(6):253-258, June 1985.

AIDS and the threat to public health, by M. F. Silverman, et al. HASTINGS
CENTER REPORT 15(Suppl. 19-22), August 1985.

AIDS: a challenge for the public health, by E. D. Acheson. LANCET 1(8482):
662-666, March 22, 1986.

AIDS: Footdragging on public health, by M. Stanton Evans. HUMAN EVENTS
45:7, September 21, 1985.

AIDS guidelines too stringent [letter], by A. J. Pinching, et al. BRITISH MEDICAL
JOURNAL 290(6469):709-710, March 2, 1985.

—, by S. McKechnie. BRITISH MEDICAL JOURNAL 290(6473):1006, March 30,
1985.

AIDS is top priority for U.S. Public Health Service. FLORIDA NURSE 31(10):7+,
November 1983.

AIDS: once dismissd as the "gay plague," the disease has become the No. 1
public health menace, by M. Clark, et al. NEWSWEEK 106(7):20-24, August
12, 1985.

AIDS project inSeattle, Washington, by S. D. Helgerson. AMERICAN JOURNAL
OF PUBLIC HEALTH 74:1419, December 1984.

AIDS: public enemy no. 1. NEWSWEEK 101:95, June 6, 1983.

AIDS: a public health and psychological emergency, by W. F. Batchelor. AMERI-
CAN PSYCHOLOGIST 39(11):1279-1284, November 1984.

AIDS, public policy and biomedical research, by S. Panem. CHEST 85(3):416-
422, March 1984.

AIDS: responding to the crisis. A public policy agenda, by S. W. Gamble. HEALTH PROGRESS 67(4):30-33, May 1986.

Apuzzo assesses task force & community, by S. Hyde. GAY COMMUNITY NEWS 12(33):3, March 9, 1985.

Boston hires city AIDS coordinator, by C. Guilfoy. GAY COMMUNITY NEWS 11(32):1, March 3, 1984.

Call to battle: a national panel urges a campaign to alert an AIDS "catastrophe", by G. J. Church, et al. TIME 128(19):18-20, November 10, 1986.

CDC advises HTLV-3 test for all "at risk", by Bisticas-Cocoves. GAY COMMUNITY NEWS 13(37):1, April 1, 1986.

CDC bans "explicit sex" from AIDS education, by K. Westheimer. GAY COMMUNITY NEWS 13(26):1, January 18, 1986.

CDC charged with sabotaging AIDS research, by Bisticas-Cocoves. GAY COMMUNITY NEWS 14(11):1, September 28, 1986.

CDC: despite RN seroconversion, AIDS precautions adequate. HOSPITAL EMPLOYEE HEALTH 4(2):17-19, February 1985.

CDC guidelines for the prevention and control of nosocomial infections. Guideline for infection control in hospital personnel, by W. W. Williams. AMERICAN JOURNAL OF INFECTION CONTROL 12(1):34-63, February 1984.

CDC guidelines: recommendations for preventing transmission of AIDS. AORN JOURNAL 43(2):528+, February 1986.

CDC: "Hands off safe sex," by J. Irving. GAY COMMUNITY NEWS 13(31):2, February 15, 1986.

CDC issues AIDS guidelines for health workers, by V. L. Bauknecht. AMERICAN NURSE 18(1):2+, January 1986.

CDC issues HTLV-III screening guidelines, by C. Guilfoy. GAY COMMUNITY NEWS 12(27):1, January 26, 1985.

CDC publishes AIDS precautions for health-care and allied professionals. EMERGENCY DEPARTMENT NEWS 5(11):17, November 1983.

CDC recommendations for preventing transmission of AIDS during invasive procedures. TEXAS NURSE 60(7):14, August 1986; also in OREGON NURSE 51(3):10, June 1986.

CDC reports AIDS cases in U.S. top 15,000, by Bisticas-Cocoves. GAY COMMUNITY NEWS 13(22):3, December 14, 1985.

CDC reports first AIDS transmission from child to parent. AMERICAN FAMILY PHYSICIAN 33:17-18, March 1986.

CDC reports 10,000 diagnosed with AIDS, by M. Cocoves. GAY COMMUNITY NEWS 12(45):1, June 1, 1985.

CDC revises AIDS risk hierarchy, by Bisticas-Cocoves. GAY COMMUNITY NEWS 14(7):3, August 24, 1986.

CDC sees no need to test health workers for AIDS; two SNA's launch campaigns "to reduce anxiety." AMERICAN JOURNAL OF NURSING 86:200-202, February 1986.

CDC to host AIDS risk reduction conferences, by N. Fain. ADVOCATE 415:24, March 5, 1985.

CDC updates trends in AIDS epidemic. AMERICAN FAMILY PHYSICIAN 26: 290+, November 1982.

Commentary on 'Recommendations on the prevention and control of AIDS by the Public Health Service' [letter], by N. Schmacke, et al. OFFENTLICHE GESUNDHEITSWESEN 46(8):395-396, August 1984.

Consensus conference. The impact of routine HTLV-III antibody testing of blood and plasma donors on public health. JAMA 256(13):1778-1783, October 3, 1986.

Coolfont Report: a PHS plan for prevention and control of AIDS and the AIDS virus, by D. I. Macdonald. PUBLIC HEALTH REPORTS 101(4):341-348, July-August 1986.

Crisis in public health [San Francisco], by K. Leishman. THE ATLANTIC 256:18+, October 1985.

Health Director resigns, by J. Ryan. GAY COMMUNITY NEWS 12(15):1, October 27, 1984.

Health officials recommend contact tracing/HTLV3, by D. Walter. ADVOCATE 449:15, June 24, 1986.

Health officials seek ways to halt AIDS, by J. L. Marx. SCIENCE 219:271-272, January 21, 1983.

HHS announces new contract award, research initiatives in fight against AIDS. PUBLIC HEALTH REPORTS 98(6):622-623, November-December 1983.

HHS investigations centered on AIDS, by E. N. Brandt, Jr. US MEDICINE 20(2): 67-69, January 15, 1984.

HHS official resigns over AIDS policy, by C. Linebarger. ADVOCATE 443:14, April 1, 1986.

HHS rejects proposed ban on HTLV-3 test, by Bisticas-Cocoves. GAY COM-MUNITY NEWS 12(44):1, May 25, 1985.

HHS to screen new immigrants for HTLV-III, by Bisticas-Cocoves. GAY COM-MUNITY NEWS 13(31):1, February 22, 1986.

How a virus that is very hard to catch crossed the world; AIDS and public health, by J. Meldrum. NEW STATESMAN 110:14-15, September 27, 1985.

Implications of the acquired immunodeficiency syndrome for health policy, by E. N. Brandt, Jr. ANNALS OF INTERNAL MEDICINE 103(5):771-773, November 1985.

Interim advice from the Public Health Council concerning patients with acquired immunodeficiency syndrome, by S. A. Danner. NEDERLANDS TIJD-SCHRIFT VOOR GENEESKUNDE 128(42):2001-2002, October 20, 1984.

National Institutes of Health and Research into the acquired immune deficiency syndrome, by F. P. Witti, et al. PUBLIC HEALTH REPORTS 98(4):312-319, July-August 1983.

National Social Welfare Board's directions and general recommendations concerning AIDS. JORDEMODERN 98(7-8):246-251, July-August 1985.

Persistence of public health problems: SF, STD, and AIDS, by A. Yankauer. AMERICAN JOURNAL OF PUBLIC HEALTH 76:494-495, May 1986.

Proposals for the prevention and control of AIDS by the Public Health Department, by G. Jantzen. OFFENTLICHE GESUNDHEITSWESEN 45(10):544-545, October 1983.

Protecting New Yorkers' health: an interview with NY Health Commissioner Dr. David Axelrod. EMPIRE STATE REPORT 11:9-10+, August 1985.

Provisional Public Health Service inter-agency recommendations for screening donated blood and plasma for antibody to the virus causing acquired immunodeficiency syndrome. MMWR 34(1):1-5, January 11, 1985.

Public health and AIDS, by J. Foster, et al. CARING 5(6):4-11+, June 1986.

Public health implications of HIV infection, by A. B. Williams. NURSE PRACTITIONER 11(10):8-10+, October 1986.

Public response and public health: scientific, social and political interdigitations. Special session, by R. Enlow. ANNALS OF THE NEW YORK ACADEMY OF SCIENCES 437:290-311, 1984.

Recent developments: public health and employment issues generated by the AIDS crisis, by M. J. Lazzo, et al. WASHBURN LAW JOURNAL 25(3):505-535, 1986.

Uses of epidemiology in the development of health policy, by W. H. Foege. PUBLIC HEALTH REPORTS 99(3):233-236, May-June 1984.

What impact has the public health scare of A.I.D.S. had on your housekeeping department and how have you addressed it? EXECUTIVE HOUSEKEEPING TODAY 7(3):12-13, March 1986.

PUBLIC HEALTH SERVICE
Public Health Service sets new AIDS guidelines, by D. Walter. ADVOCATE 436:24, December 24, 1985.

Public Health Service's number one priority [editorial],by E. N. Brandt, Jr. PUBLIC HEALTH REPORTS 98(4):306-307, July-August 1983.

Public Health Service; program announcement; alternate testing sites to perform HTLV-III antibody testing. FEDERAL REGISTER 50(48):9909-9910, March 12, 1985.

QUARANTINE

AIDS: the impending quarantine, by R. Cohen. HEALTH PAC BULLETIN 16(4):9, July 1985.

AIDS quarantine measure for California ballot, by Bisticas-Cocoves. GAY COMMUNITY NEWS 13(44):1, May 31, 1986.

AIDS quarantines—government and us, by S. Hyde. GAY COMMUNITY NEWS 11(35):3, March 24, 1984.

Boston AIDS Conference discusses quarantine issue, by C. Guilfoy. GAY COMMUNITY NEWS 12(41):1, May 4, 1985.

Boston quarantine proposal withdrawn, by K. Westheimer. GAY COMMUNITY NEWS 13(2):1, December 28, 1985.

California to vote on AIDS quarantine, by J. Kiely. GAY COMMUNITY NEWS 13(50):3, July 6, 1986.

Call for quarantine, by C. Bowland. ADVOCATE 443:42, April 1, 1986.

College health group sees no reason to isolate AIDS victims. THE CHRONICLE OF HIGHER EDUCATION 31:33+, October 16, 1985.

LaRouche quarantine on November ballot. BODY POLITIC 129:19, August 1986.

Lyndon La Rouche initiative: AIDS quarantine, by P. Freiberg. ADVOCATE 446:12, May 13, 1986.

Quarantine and AIDS, by A. Novick. CONNECTICUT MEDICINE 49(2):81-83, February 1985.

Quarantine corner. PROCESSED WORLD 15:10, Winter 1985.

Quarantine is no way to fight AIDS, by C. Guilfoy. GAY COMMUNITY NEWS 13(21):8, Decemebr 7, 1985.

Quarantine of prostitutes with AIDS rumored, by K. Westheimer. GAY COMMUNITY NEWS 13(21):1, Decemebr 7, 1985.

Should AIDS victims be isolated? [interviews with R. Restak and C. Levine]. US NEWS & WORLD REPORT 99:50, September 30, 1985.

Texas backs off from "incorrigibles" quarantine, by Bisticas-Cocoves. GAY COMMUNITY NEWS 13(28):1, February 1, 1986.

Texas health official drops AIDS quarantine sup., by D. Walter. ADVOCATE 440:15, February 18, 1986.

Texas health officials seek quarantine, by S. Conn. GAY COMMUNITY NEWS 13(26):1, January 18, 1986.

Texas set to approve AIDS quarantine rule, by D. Walter. ADVOCATE 438:15, January 21, 1986.

Times poll: public support for quarantine tattoo, by M. Daniels. ADVOCATE 438:15, January 21, 1986.

United States mayors are told "don't quarantine," by D. Walter. ADVOCATE 441:22, March 4, 1986.

GREAT BRITAIN
British hospital attempts AIDS quarantine, by P. Cummings. ADVOCATE 432:22, October 29, 1985.

RELIGION
AIDS and ARC: a theological reflection on the Church's ministry, by J. Hanvey. MONTH 19:326-331, December 1986.

AIDS and the church, by E. E. Shelp, et al. CHRISTIAN CENTURY 102(27):797-800, September 11-18,1985.

AIDS and the churches: belated, growing response, by B. J. Stiles. CHRIS-TIANITY AND CRISIS 45(22):534-536, January 13, 1986.

AIDS and the common cup, by F. C. Senn. DIALOG 25(1):4-5, Winter 1986.

AIDS and communion. CHRISTIAN CENTURY 102:888, October 9, 1985.

AIDS and moral issues, by T. Johson. ADVOCATE 3(79):24, October 27, 1983.

AIDS: a Christian response. AMERICA 153:77, August 17-24, 1985.

AIDS epidemic and the communion cup, by Orville N. Griese. LINACRE QUARTERLY 53:15-25, May 1986.

AIDS hysteria and the common cup: take and drink, by R. W. Hovda. WORSHIP 60(1):67-73, January 1986.

AIDS ministers should urge that God is not punishing. REGISTER 62:2, December 7, 1986.

AIDS: ministry issues for chaplains, by J. Bohne. PASTORAL PSYCHOLOGY 34(3):173-192, Spring 1986.

AIDS: responding to the crisis. Pastoral care: helping patients on an inward journey, by L. J. Tibesar. HEALTH PROGRESS 67(4):41-47, May 1986.

AIDS scare prompts concern about communion, by V. F. A. Golphin. NATIONAL CATHOLIC REPORTER 22:6, November 1, 1985.

AIDS: a task for the churces, by E. Norman. TIMES October 13, 1986, p. 14.

Amen corner: AIDS hysteria and the common cup: take a drink, by R. W. Horda. WORSHIP 60:67-73, January 1986.

Belated, growing response; AIDS and the churches, by B. J. Stiles. CHRIS-TIANITY AND CRISIS 45:534-536, Jnuary 13, 1986.

Case study in pastoral counseling, by M. E. Johson. HEALTH PROGRESS 67(4):38-40, May 1986.

Catholics who fear AIDS don't have to drink from communion chalice. JET 69:28-29, December 9, 1985.

Christian view of AIDS, by S. S. Macauley. JOURNAL OF CHRISTIAN NURSING 3(2):32, Spring 1986.

Church as sanctuary: 1985's top story. CHRISTIAN CENTURY 102:1163-1165, December 18-25, 1985.

Church in the midst of the AIDS epidemic, by L. Ranck. ESA14(2):2-46, February 1986.

Churches and AIDS: responsibilities in mission, by L. Howell. CHRISTIANITY AND CRISIS 45:483-484, December 9, 1985.

Church's response to AIDS: is compassion waning in light of a so-called gay disease. CHRISTIANITY TODAY 29(17):50-51, November 22, 1985.

Common cup supported. CHRISTIAN CENTURY 103(6):169, February 19, 1986.

Compassion marks church service for AIDS victims. NATIONAL CATHOLIC REPORTER 21:6, January 18, 1985.

Congregation confronts AIDS, by M. Rankin. SHMATE 13:3, Fall 1985.

Dioceses' ministries gear up for AIDS epidemic, by Bill Kenkelen. NATIONAL CATHOLIC REPORTER 23:1+, December 12, 1986.

Excommunicated. CHRISTIAN CENTURY 103(5):112, February 5-12, 1986.

Falwell launches (another) anti-gay campaign, by M. Godwin. GAY COMMUNITY NEWS 13(3):2, July 27, 1985.

Falwell on antigay AIDS crusade, by M. Henson. GUARDIAN 35(40):5, July 27, 1983.

Falwell speaks—Cincinnati responds, by S. Hyde. GAY COMMUNITY NEWS 11(2):3, July 23, 1983.

Falwell's claim of God's judgement, by J. Real. ADVOCATE 3(73):10, August 4, 1983.

Forum advocates AIDS ministry, by K. Smith. NATIONAL CATHOLIC RE-PORTER 21:19, March 8, 1985.

Gay Catholic activist makes life, AIDS death educational opportunity for Baltimore church, by F. A. Vincent. NATIONAL CHURCH REPORTER 21:6-7, September 27, 1985.

God and the AIDS victim: Anglicans offer sympathy and debate morality, by W. Harbeck, et al. ALBERTA REPORT 13:40-41, March 24, 1986.

God as judge, God as savior, by H. S. Shoemaker. CHRISTIAN MINISTRY 17(1): 24-26, January 1986.

Health concerns and the common cup; Bishops liturgy committee. ORIGINS 15:475-477, January 2, 1986.

Justification of Rock Hudson: AIDS has a dual message for Christians, by C. Plantinga, Jr. CHRISTIANITY TODAY 15:16-17, October 18, 1985.

Keep common cup. CHRISTIAN CENTURY 103(1):9, January 1-8, 1986.

Ministerial ethics and AIDS, by G. T. Miller. CHRISTIAN MINISTRY 17(3):22-24, May 1986.

Ministers back AIDS education. NEW SCIENTIST 108:21, October 3, 1985.

Ministry to AIDS victims, by Francis A. Quinn. ORIGINS 16:224-226, September 4, 1986.

Pardon my morality, by T. Stafford. CHRISTIANITY TODAY 30(9):17, June 13, 1986.

Pastoral care and persons with AIDS. A means to alleviate physical, emotional, social, and spiritual suffering, by P. Murphy. AMERICAN JOURNAL OF HOSPICE CARE 3(2):38-40, March-April 1986.

Preaching to the infected, by M. Jones. SUNDAY TIMES December 14, 1986, p. 25.

Priest urges bishops: support work of Christ, by Peter Hebblethwaite. NATIONAL CATHOLIC REPORTER 23:7, November 14, 1986.

Priests AIDS deaths: shame, fear, compassion. NATIONAL CATHOLIC REPORTER 23:23-26, December 12, 1986.

Puzzling case of the nun with AIDS. RN 47:19, January 1984.

Religion—moralizing and AIDS, by K. Gordon. GAY COMMUNITY NEWS 11(22):6, December 17, 1983.

Religious leaders declare AIDS not God's punishment, by P. Freiberg. ADVOCATE 417:18, April 2, 1985.

Responding to, learning from AIDS: for starters: principles and theologies, by J. B. Nelson. CHRISTIANITY AND CRISIS 46:176-181, May 19, 1986.

Rev. Jerry Falwell/AIDS God's judgment, by Zeh, et al. ADVOCATE 3(74):15, August 18, 1983.

Such were some of you: a Christian response to homosexuals, by M. Braun. F FUNDAMENTALIST JOURNAL 4(3):22-24, March 1985.

CANADA
Great Calgary AIDS debate: wrath of God or mystery disease: Christians divide, by M. McKinley. ALBERTA REPORT 10:30, September 5, 1983.

How should Catholic hospitals respond to the AIDS problem? HOSPITAL PRO-GRESS 65:49-50, May 1984.

RELIGION—TESTING

Ministers delayed launch of AIDS test. NEW SCIENTIST107:16, August 8, 1985.

RESEARCH

Advances in research on AIDS, by C. H. Gu. CHUNG-HUA NEI KO TSA CHIH 24(10):627-629, October 1985.

AIDS: allocating resources for research and patient care, by P. R. Lee. ISSUES IN SCIENCE AND TECHNOLOGY 2:66-73, Winter 1986.

AIDS—clinical research criteria [letter], by G. Yales. HOSPITAL PRACTICE 20(8): 17, August 15, 1985.

AIDS discovery may unlock cancer secrets. NEW SCIENTIST 102:4, May 10, 1984.

AIDS: disease, research efforts advance, by J. Silberner. SCIENCE NEWS 127: 260-261, April 27, 1985.

AIDS figures mount as researchers seek answers to the puzzle. AMERICAN FAMILY PHYSICIAN 28:331+, September 1983.

AIDS group doubts study, by K. Popert. BODY POLITIC 124:15, March 1986.

AIDS: looking for the cure, by E. Dobson. FUNDAMENTALIST JOURNAL 4(9): 14, October 1985.

AIDS: new centres for clinical trials [news], by J. Palca. NATURE 322(6075):100, July 10-16, 1986.

AIDS protein made, by K. Wright. NATURE 319:525, February 13, 1986.

AIDS, public policy and biomedical research, by S. Panem. CHEST 85(3):416-422, March 1984.

AIDS: quest for a cure. CANADA AND THE WORLD 51:8-9, October 1985.

—, by J. Langone. DISCOVER 6:75+, January 1985.

AIDS research. Big enough spending? [news], by S. Budiansky. NATURE 304(5926):478, August 11-17, 1983.

AIDS research. Is there really a virus? [news], by G. Linnebank. NATURE 305(5932):264, September 22-28, 1983.

AIDS: a research and clinical bibliography. HEMATOLOGICAL ONCOLOGY 2(1):77-134, January-March 1984.

AIDS research and incidence on the rise. AMERICAN FAMILY PHYSICIAN 28:17, October 1983.

AIDS research and 'the window of opportunity,' by W. J. Curran. NEW ENGLAND JOURNAL OF MEDICINE 312(14):903-904, April 4, 1985.

AIDS research centers sought. ADAMHA NEWS 12(3):3, March 1986.

AIDS research: charting new directions, by E. N. Brandt, Jr. PUBLIC HEALTH REPORTS 99(5):433-435, September-October 1984.

AIDS research in new phase [news], by D. M. Barnes. SCIENCE 233(4761):282-283, July 18, 1986.

AIDS research, to review or not to review: by S. Budiansky. NATURE 305:349, September 29, 1983.

AIDS researchers track an elusive foe, by R. M. Baum. CHEMICAL AND ENGINEERING NEWS 62:15-16+, January 23, 1984.

AIDS: too hot to study: gays protest as the U of A drops research, by T. Philip. ALBERTA REPORT 11:26, June 4, 1984.

AIDS update: search for Agent X, by P. Taulbee. SCIENCE NEWS 123:245, April 16, 1983.

AMI hopes to convert Houston hospital into AIDS research and treatment center. REVIEW OF THE FEDERATION OF AMERICAN HEALTH SYSTEMS 19(2): 108-109, March-April 1986.

Anti-AIDS agents show varying early results in vitro and in vivo, by D. E. Riesenberg, et al. JAMA 254:2521+, November 8, 1985.

Attempts at the development of vaccines against adult T-cell leukemia, by M. Hayami. KANGO GIJUTSU 31(16):2214-2215, December 1985.

Blow to research, by W. Michaud. GAY COMMUNITY NEWS 13(34):5, March 15, 1986.

Chasing an AIDS cure, by R. Wood. GAY COMMUNITY NEWS 13(41):8, May 3, 1986.

Clinical care and research in AIDS, by P. Volberding, et al. HASTINGS CENTER REPORT 15(4):16-18, August 1985.

Consent form for AIDS research urged by Brandt, by S. Kulieke. ADVOCATE 405:8, October 16, 1984.

Coordination and managment of information on AIDS, by L. S. Garden. SYGEPLEJERSKEN 86(24):32-33+, June 1986.

Different kind of AIDS fight: scientists engage in a heated transatlantic duel, by C. Wallis, et al. TIME 127(19):86, May 12, 1986.

Doing research in an epidemic: confidentiality, by K. Mayer. GAY COMMUNITY NEWS 12(36):5, March 30, 1985.

Effects of a novel compound (AL 721) on HTLV-III infectivity in vitro, by P. S. Sarin, et al. NEW ENGLAND JOURNAL OF MEDICINE 313:1289-1290, November 14, 1985.

Fighting AIDS: the search for a cure, by J. Wilkinson. LISTENER October 17, 1985, p. 7-8.

Gay recruits needed for AIDS research, by K. Popert. BODY POLITIC 109:9, December 1984.

Giving researchers a hand, by M. Helquist. ADVOCATE 434:20, November 26, 1985.

Government awards $100 million to study AIDS drug, by D. Walter. ADVOCATE 453:14, August 19, 1986.

Hastings Center initiates AIDS study, by M. F. Goldsmith. JAMA 254:2527, November 8, 1985.

How Gallo got credit for AIDS discovery, by O. Sattaur. NEW SCIENTIST 105:3-4, February 7, 1985.

In search of the best drugs against AIDS, by D. M. Barnes. SCIENCE 233(4762): 419, July 25, 1986.

Investigation begins into spread of new AIDS virus. NEW SCIENTIST 110:25, April 10, 1986.

Investigators combine work to find key to AIDS. AMERICAN FAMILY PHYSICIAN 29:17, May 1984.

Investigators study AIDs epidemiology and drug treatment. AMERICAN FAMILY PHYSICIAN 32:206, December 1985.

Laboratory evaluation of AIDS, by D. A. Bergeron. JOURNAL OF MEDICAL TECHNOLOGY 3(3):152-155+, March 1986.

Law-medicine notes—AIDS research and 'the window of opportunity' [letter]. NEW ENGLAND JOURNAL OF MEDICINE 313(8):515-517, August 22, 1985.

Man who found the AIDS virus [Robert Gallo], by S. Schiefelbein. SCIENCE DIGEST 92:62-65+, July 1984.

Medical research: band-aids. THE ECONOMIST 288:22+, August 13, 1983.

Modulation in vitro of immune parameters in homosexual males with the preclinical complex of symptoms related to acquired immune deficiency syndrome by azimexon, by Y. Z. Patt, et al. JOURNAL OF BIOLOGICAL RESPONSE MODIFIERS 5(3):263-269, June 1986.

Molecular clone of HTLV-III with biological activity, by A. G. Fisher, et al. NATURE 316:262-265, July 18, 1985.

Molecular cloning and characterization of the HTLV-III virus associated with AIDS, by B. H. Hahn, et al. NATURE 312(5990):166-169, November 8-14, 1984.

Molecular cloning of AIDS-associated retrovirus, by P. A. Luciw, et al. NATURE 312(5996):760-763, December 20, 1984-January 2, 1985.

Molecular cloning of lymphadenopathy-associated virus, by M. Alizon, et al. NATURE 312(5996):757-760, December 20, 1984-January 2, 1985.

National AIDS Research Foundation formed, by M. Daniels. ADVOCATE 432:11, October 29, 1985.

New AIDS research guidelines released, by C. Guilfoy. GAY COMMUNITY NEWS 12(19):1, November 24, 1984.

New findings in race for AIDS cure, by K. McAuliffe. U.S. NEWS AND WORLD REPORT 100(16):71-72, April 28, 1986.

New York-Cornell becomes center for AIDS study. AMERICAN JOURNAL OF PUBLIC HEALTH 73:1193, October 1983.

New PHS grants awarded for research on AIDS. PUBLIC HEALTH REPORTS 98(3):228, May-June 1983.

Not there yet, but 'on our way' in AIDs research, scientists say, by M. F. Goldsmith. JAMA 253(23):3369-3371+, by June 21, 1985.

On the AIDS trail: work continues on test, cure, vaccine, by J. Silberner. SCIENCE NEWS 127:100, February 16, 1985.

Picking plays in AIDS research, by S. J. Smiurda. VENTURE 7:20, August 1985.

Planning more research on AIDS, by J. Maddox. NATURE 303(5916):377, June 2, 1983.

Protection of T cells against infectivity and cytopathic effect of GTLV-III in vitro, by H. Mitsuya, et al. INTERNATIONAL SYMPOSIUM OF THE PRINCESS TAKAMATSU CANCER RESEARCH FUND 15:277-288, 1984.

Pursuit of a cure (AIDS), by P. Ohlendorf. MACLEAN'S 98:36-37, August 12, 1985.

Recent progress in research on AIDS (acquired immune deficiency syndrome), by A. Pana, et al. RECENTI PROGRESSI IN MEDICINA 74(8):879-887, August 1983.

Research developments in AIDS [editorial], by J. A. Armstrong. MEDICAL JOURNAL OF AUSTRALIA 141(9):556-557, October 27, 1984.

Research on AIDS. FDA DRUG BULLETIN 12(3):21-23, December 1982.

Research reported at press seminar. ADAMHA NEWS 11(8):1, August 1985.

Researcher: tools exist to battle AIDS' spread, by G. Willis. AIR FORCE TIMES 47:8+, November 24, 1986.

Researchers tackle AIDS. HIGH TECHNOLOGY 5:8, May 1985.

Rx for AIDS: a grim race against the clock, by J. Carey. U.S. NEWS & WORLD REPORT 99(14):48-49, September 30, 1985.

505

Science base underlying research on acquired immune deficiency syndrome, by S. Taube, et al. PUBLIC HEALTH REPORTS 98(6):559-565, November-December 1983.

Scientific speculation continues in Atlanta, by Bistecas-Cocoves. GAY COMMUNITY NEWS 12(43):3, May 18, 1985.

Scientists honored for achievements in cancer research, by S. D. Levine. NEWS & FEATURES FROM NIH August 1984, p. 12-13.

Searching for AZT (azidothymidine): monthly search hint, by R. L. Stander. NLM TECH BULLETIN 210:15-17, October 1986.

Several NIH Institutes involved in tracking down cause of AIDS, by J. McCarthy. NEWS & FEATURES FROM NIH April 1983, p 12-13.

Support for DNCB research, by M. Helquist. ADVOCATE 446:21, May 13, 1986.

Synthesis of kappa light chains by cell lines containing an 8;22 chromosomal translocation derived from a male homosexual with Burkitt's lymphoma, by I. Magrath, et al. SCIENCE 222:1094-1098, December 9, 1983.

Top AIDS researcher testify, by M. Helquist. ADVOCATE 429:18, September 17, 1985.

Two steps closer to stopping AIDS. SCIENCE DIGEST 93:19, April 1985.

Ultrastructural and immunoelectron microscopic studies of cells with abnormal cytoplasmic inclusions in patients with AIDS, by M. Kostianovsky, et al. AIDS RESEARCH 1(3):181-196, 1983-1984.

Ultrastructural aspects of a cutaneous biopsy in acquired immune deficiency syndrome (AIDS), by P. Bruneval, et al. ANNALS OF PATHOLOGY 4(4):305-307, September-November 1984.

Ultrastructural comparison of the retroviruses associated with human and simian acquired immunodeficiency syndromes, by R. J. Munn, et al. LABORATORY INVESTIGATION 53(2):194-199, August 1985.

Unusual virus produced by cultured cells from a patient with AIDS, by A. Karpas. MOLECULAR BIOLOGY AND MEDICINE 1(4):457-459, November 1983.

Virus as a Rosetta stone: AIDS cases increase, but new research shows some signs of hope, by C. Wallis. TIME 124(19):91, November 5, 1984.

Vital clue to AIDS, by B. D. Johnson. MACLEAN'S 96:54, May 23, 1983.

Volunteers needed for AIDS study. OUT 3(6):1, April 1985.

AFRICA
Trailing AIDS in Central Africa, by P. Newmark. NATURE 315(6017):273, May 23-29, 1985.

FRANCE
AIDS research in France: different culture, same virus? by V. Elliott. SCIENCE NEWS 125:285-286, May 5, 1984.

GREAT BRITAIN
AIDS research in Britain, by D. Morris. GAY COMMUNITY NEWS 10(27):2, January 29, 1983.

ICELAND
Icelandic research. Slow virus infections and AIDS, by G. Pétursson, et al. NORDISK MEDICIN 101(5):160-161+, 1986.

RESEARCH—AUTOPSY
Acquired immune deficiency syndrome. Clinicopathologic study of 56 autopsies, by G. W. Niedt, et al. ARCHIVES OF PATHOLOGY AND LABORATORY MEDICINE 109(8):727-734, August 1985.

Acquired immune deficiency syndrome: postmortem findings, by L. A. Guarda, et al. AMERICAN JOURNAL OF CLINICAL PATHOLOGY 81(5):549-557, May 1984.

AIDS autopsy precautions, by A. E. Mass. PATHOLOGIST 39(11):20-21, November 1985.

Autopsy findings in the acquired immune deficiency syndrome, by K. Mobley, et al. PATHOLOGY ANNUAL 20(Part 1):45-65, 1985.

—, by H L. Schmidts, et al. PATOLOGE 7(1):8-21, January 1986.

—, by K. Welch, et al. JAMA 252(9):1152-1159, September 7, 1984.

RESEARCH—BLOOD
Reactivity of E. coli-derived trans-activating protein of human T lymphotropic virus type III with sera from patients with acquired immune deficiency syndrome, by A. D. Barone, et al. JOURNAL OF IMMUNOLOGY 137(2):669-673, July 1, 1986.

RESEARCH—ECONOMICS
United States Government AIDS research, by C. Shively. DELAWARE ALTERNATIVE PRESS 6(1):9, 1983.

United States mayors increase research funds, by L. Bush. ADVOCATE 3(72): 11, July 21, 1983.

SCHOOLS
AIDS in the schools: a special report, by S. Reed. PHI DELTA KAPPAN 67:494-498, March 1986.

AIDS issue hits the schools, by E. McGrath. TIME 126:61, September 9, 1985.

AIDS: majority would permit children to attend school with AIDS victim. GALLUP REPORT pp. 19-22, April 1986.

AIDS: preschool and school issues, by J. L. Black. JOURNAL OF SCHOOL HEALTH 56(3):93-95, March 1986.

AIDS, the schools, and policy issues, by J. H. Price. JOURNAL OF SCHOOL HEALTH 56(4):137-140, April 1986.

As AIDS spooks the schoolroom. US NEWS & WORLD REPORT 99(13):7, September 23, 1985.

Boys and girls come out to play? . . . shadow of AIDS has spread to the school playground, by C. Clementson. NURSING TIMES 82(7):19-20, February 12-18, 1986.

Boys with AIDS barred from classrooms, by L. Sherman. GAY COMMUNITY NEWS 13(7):2, August 24, 1985.

Cambridge, Boston schools revise AIDS policy, by K. Westheimer. GAY COMMUNITY NEWS 13(49):3, June 29, 1986.

Fear rules as officials slap classroom ban on AIDS boy [United States], by B. Norris. THE TIMES EDUCATIONAL SUPPLEMENT 3606:11, August 9, 1985.

Foster mom may sue to get AIDS kid in school. JET 68:23, April 15, 1985.

Frontlines: schools flunk on AIDS instruction, by Laura Fraser. MOTHER JONES 11:8, June 1986.

High school students' perceptions and misperceptions of AIDS, by J. H. Price, et al. JOURNAL OF SCHOOL HEALTH 55(3):107-109, March 1985.

HTLV-III in saliva of people with AIDS-related complex and healthy homosexual men at risk for AIDS, by J. E. Groopman, et al. SCIENCE 226(4673):447-449, October 26, 1984.

Is school for all? AIDS victims spark dilemma, by F. A. Silas. AMERICAN BAR ASSOCIATION JOURNAL 71:18-19, November 1985.

Mother with AIDS prompts school policy, by M. Schwartz. GAY COMMUNITY NEWS 12(46):2, June 8, 1985.

NEA sets guidelines to handle AIDS in schools. JET 69:37, October 28, 1985.

New AIDS policy set for Boston's school workers, by C. Guilfoy. GAY COMMUNITY NEWS 13(11):1, September 28, 1985.

New federal guidelines say children with AIDS can attend school. PHI DELTA KAPPAN 67:242+, November 1985.

Recommended guidelines for dealing with AIDS in the schools from the National Education Association. JOURNAL OF SCHOOL HEALTH 56(4):129-130, April 1986.

School attendance of children and adolescents with human T lyphotropic virus III/ lymphadenopathy-associated virus infection, by the American Academy of Pediatrics. Committee on School Health, Committee on Infectious Diseases. PEDIATRICS 77(3):430-432, March 1986.

School Boards ignore medical advice on AIDS. OUT 4(3):1, January 1986.

Schools await decision. BODY POLITIC 120:29, November 1985.

Schools try to abate fears about AIDS kids. JET 69:6, September 30, 1985.

GREAT BRITAIN
AIDS fear affects first UK school [Hampshire, England], by S. Bayliss. THE TIMES EDUCATIONAL SUPPLEMENT 3612:3, September 20, 1985.

UNITED STATES
Massachusetts AIDS policy defuses school furor, by C. Guilfoy. GAY COMMUNITY NEWS 13(10):3, September 21, 1985.

SCHOOLS—EDUCATION
Schools flunk on AIDS instruction, by L. Fraser. MOTHER JONES 11(4):8, June 1986.

SCHOOLS—LAWS AND LEGISLATION
School ordered to admit New Jersey girl with AIDS. JET 69:26, November 25, 1985.

SECONDARY CONDITIONS
Acquired ichthyosis in the acquired immunodeficiency syndrome [letter], by C. Bories, et al. PRESSE MEDICALE 13(25):1573, June 16, 1984.

Acquired immune deficiency syndrome and multiple tract degeneration in a homosexual man, by D. S. Horoupian, et al. ANNALS OF NEUROLOGY 15(5);502-505, May 1984.

Adrenal insufficiency as a complication of the acquired immunodeficiency syndrome, by L. W. Greene, et al. ANNALS OF INTERNAL MEDICINE 101(4):497-498, October 1984.

Adrenal necrosis in the acquired immunodeficiency syndrome, by M. L. Tapper, et al. ANNALS OF INTERNAL MEDICINE 100(2):239-241, February 1984.

Adrenocortical function in the acquired immunodeficiency syndrome [letter], by R. S. Klein, et al. ANNALS OF INTERNAL MEDICINE 99(4):566, October 1983.

AIDS and zinc deficiency [letter], by R. G. Weiner. JAMA 252(11):1409-1410, September 21, 1984.

AIDS dementia complex: I. Clinical features, by B. A. Navia, et al. ANNALS OF NEUROLOGY 19(6):517-524, June 1986.

AIDS exacerbates psoriasis, by T. M. Johnson, et al. NEW ENGLAND JOURNAL OF MEDICINE 313:1415, November 28, 1985.

AIDS linked to gamma interferon deficiency. CHEMICAL AND ENGINEERING NEWS 62:7, April 9, 1984.

Atypical neurologic symptoms in the course of acquired immunodeficiency syndrome (AIDS), by J. Kesselring, et al. DEUTSCHE MEDIZINISCHE WOCHENSCHRIFT 111(27):1058-1060, July 4, 1986.

Biliary tract obstruction in the acquired imunodeficiency syndrome, by S. J. Margulis, et al. ANNALS OF INTERNAL MEDICINE 105(2):207-210, August 1986.

Bone marrow abnormalities in the acquired immunodeficiency syndrome [letter], by C. M. Franco, et al. ANNALS OF INTERNAL MEDICINE 101(2):275-276, August 1984.

Bone marrow in the acquired immunodeficiency syndrome [letter], by R. A. Hromas, et al. ANNALS OF INTERNAL MEDICINE 101(6):877, December 1984.

Bone marrow in AIDS. A histologic, hematologic, and microbiologic study, by A. Castella, et al. AMERICAN JOURNAL OF CLINICAL PATHOLOGY 84(4):425-432, October 1985.

Case 32-1983. Acquired immunodeficiency syndrome and cranial-nerve abnormalities. NEW ENGLAND JOURNAL OF MEDICINE 309(6):359-369, August 11, 1983.

Digestive manifestations of the acquired immunodeficiency syndrome (AIDS): study in 26 patients, by E. René , et al. GASTROENTEROLOGIE CLINIQUE ET BIOLOGIQUE 9(4):327-335, April 1985.

Elevated beta 2-microglobulin and lysozyme levels in patients with acquired immune deficiency syndrome,by M. H. Grieco, et al. CLINICAL IMMUNOLO-GY AND IMMUNOPATHOLOGY 32(2):174-184, August 1984.

Elevated erythrocyte adenosine deaminase activity in patients with acquired immunodeficiency syndrome, by M. J. Cowan, et al. PROCEEDINGS OF THE NATIONAL ACADEMY OF SCIENCES USA 83(4):1089-1091, February 1986.

Elevated levels of interferon-induced 2'-5' oligoadenylate synthetase in generalized persistent lymphadenopathy and the acquired immunodeficiency syndrome, by S. E. Read, et al. JOURNAL OF INFECTIOUS DISEASES 152(3):66-472, September 1985.

Elevated urinary neopterin levels in patients with the acquired immunodeficiency syndrome (AIDS). A priliminary report, by H. Wachter, et al. HOPPE-SEYLER'S ZEITSCHRIFT FUER PHYSIOLOGISCHE CHEMIE 364(9):1345-1346, September 1983.

Encephalopathy in patients with LAV-HTLV-III infections, by J. Goudsmit, et al. NEDERLANDS TIJDSCHRIFT VOOR GENEESKUNDE 130(22):998-999, May 31, 1986.

Enteropathy associated with the acquired immunodeficiency syndrome,by D. P. Kotler, et al. ANNALS OF INTERNAL MEDICINE 101(4):421-428, October 1984.

Erythroblastopenia in acquired immunodeficiency syndrome (AIDS) [letter], by Y. N. Berner, et al. ACTA HAEMATOLOGICA 70(4):273, 1983.

Evaluation of abdominal pain in the AIDS patient, by D. A. Potter, et al. ANNALS OF SURGERY 199(3):332-339, March 1984.

Gastrointestinal involvement in acquired immunologic deficiency syndrome (AIDS), by R. Münch, et al. ZEITSCHRIFT FUR GASTROENTEROLOGIE 24(5):235-244, May 1986.

Gastrointestinal manifestations of the acquired immunodeficiency syndrome: a review of 22 cases, by B. Dworkin, et al. AMERICAN JOURNAL OF GASTRO-ENTEROLOGY 80(10):774-778, October 1985.

Gastrointestinal manifestations of AIDS, by E. René, et al. ANNALES DE GASTROENTEROLOGIE ET D'HEPATOLOGIE 21(6):389-391, December 1985.

Granulomatous involvement of the liver in patients with AIDS, by M. S. Orenstein, et al. GUT 26(11):1220-1225, November 1985.

Head and neck presentations of acquired immunodeficiency syndrome,by R. A. Rosenberg, et al. LARYNGOSCOPE 94(5, Part 1):642-646, May 1984.

Head lice linked with AIDS, by H. Wilce. THE TIMES EDUCATIONAL SUPPLE-MENT 3636:7, March 7, 1986.

Hematologic abnormalities in the acquired immune deficiency syndrome by J. L. Spivak, et al. AMERICAN JOURNAL OF MEDICINE 77(2):224-228, August 1984.

Hemolytic-uremic syndrome with the acquired immunodeficiency syndrome [letter], by R. V. Boccia, et al. ANNALS OF INTERNAL MEDICINE 101(5): 716-717, November 1984.

Hepatic involvement in the acquired immunodeficiency syndrome. Study of 20 cases, by J. F. Devars du Mayne, et al. PRESSE MEDICALE 14(21):1177-1180, May 25, 1985.

Highly abnormal B-cell function found in AIDS. HOSPITAL PRACTICE 18(10): 32+, October 1983.

Hypoalbuminemia, diarrhea, and the acquired immunodeficiency syndrome [letter], by R. R. Brinson. ANNALS OF INTERNAL MEDICINE 102(3):413, March 1985.

Low serum thymic hormone levels in patients with acquired immunodeficiency syndrome [letter], by M. Dardenne, et al. NEW ENGLAND JOURNAL OF MEDICINE 309(1):48-49, July 7, 1983.

Of AIDS and abdominal pain. EMERGENCY MEDICINE 16(14):107-108+, August 15, 1984.

Severe diarrhea in a patient with AIDS [letter], by J. M. Guerin, et al. JAMA 256(5): 591, August 1, 1986.

Surgical abdomen in the acquired immunodeficiency syndrome. Apropos of 4 cases, by A. Olivier, et al. CHIRURGIE 111(1):69-75, 1985.

Unidentified virus-like particles in the intestine of patients with the acquired immunodeficiency syndrome, by F. W. Chandler, et al. ANNALS OF INTERNAL MEDICINE 100(6):851-853, June 1984.

Urinary neopterin and biopterin levels in patients with AIDS and AIDS-related complex [letter], by J. P. Abita, et al. LANCET 2(8445):51-52, July 6, 1985.

AFRICA
  Severe digestive complications of AIDS in a group of patients from Zaire, by
    C. Jonas, et al. ACTA GASTROENTEROLOGICA BELGICA 47(4):396-
    402, July-August 1984.

SECONDARY CONDITIONS—PSYCHOLOGY AND PSYCHIATRY
  Psychosocial and neuropsychiatric sequelae of the acquired immunodeficiency
    syndrome and related disorders, by J. C. Holland, et al. ANNALS OF IN-
    TERNAL MEDICINE 103(5):760-764, November 1985.

  Psychosocial aspects of AIDS and AIDS-related complex: a pilot study, by J. N.
    Donlou, et al. JOURNAL OF PSYCHOSOCIAL ONCOLOGY 3(2):39-55,
    Summer 1985.

SECONDARY LESIONS
  Abdominal CT findings of disseminated Mycobacterium avium-intracellulare in
    AIDS, by D. A. Nyberg, et al. AJR 145(2):297-299, August 1985.

  Acalculous cholecystitis and cytomegalovirus infection in the acquired immuno-
    deficiency syndrome, by H. Kavin, et al. ANNALS OF INTERNAL MEDICINE
    104(1):53-54, January 1986.

  Acquired immune deficiency syndrome and the management of associated
    opportunistic infections, by N. Dozier, et al. DRUG INTELLIGENCE AND
    CLINICAL PHARMACY 17(11):798-807, November 1983.

  Acquired immune deficiency syndrome and pancytopenia, by J. L. Spivak, et al.
    JAMA 250(22):3084-3087, December 9, 1983.

  Acquired immune deficiency syndrome in a patient with prior sarcoidosis: case
    report with monocyte function studies, by S. Kalter, et al. TEXAS MEDICINE
    81(9):44-46, September 1985.

  Acquired immune deficiency syndrome presenting as recalcitrant Candida, by A.
    Babajews, et al. BRITISH DENTAL JOURNAL 159(4):106-108, August 24,
    1985.

  Acquired immunodeficiency syndrome (AIDS) in a homosexual male with tubercu-
    losis and medullary hyperplasia [letter], by T. Martín Jiménez, et al. MEDICINA
    CLINICA 85(1):39-40, June 1, 1985.

  Acquired immunodeficiency syndrome and lupus anticoagulant [letter], by W. D.
    Haire. ANNALS OF INTERNAL MEDICINE 105(2):301-302, August 1986.

  Acquired immunodeficiency syndrome and nonmenstrual toxic shock syndrome
    [letter], by J. Sparano, et al. ANNALS OF INTERNAL MEDICINE 105(2):300-
    301, August 1986.

  Acquired immunodeficiency syndrome and opportunistic infections [editorial], by
    R. de J. Pedro. REVISTA PAULISTA DE MEDICINA 101(4):123, July-August
    1983.

  Acquired immunodeficiency syndrome associated with Acanthamoeba infection
    and other opportunistic organisms, by M. M. Gonzalez, et al. ARCHIVES OF
    PATHOLOGY AND LABORATORY MEDICINE 110(8):749-751, August
    1986.

Acquired immunodeficiency syndrome: highlights on the diagnosis and management of opportunistic infections, by C. E. Lopez. JOURNAL OF THE MEDICAL ASSOCIATION OF GEORGIA 73(8):525-533, August 1984.

Acquired immunodeficiency syndrome: impact and implication for neurological system, by M. M. Beckham, et al. JOURNAL OF NEUROSCIENCE NURSING 18(1):5-10, February 1986.

Acquired immunodeficiency syndrome manifested as disseminated cryptococcosis, by G. Pittard, et al. JOURNAL OF EMERGENCY MEDICINE 3(4):275-279, 1985.

Acquired immunodeficiency syndrome, opportunistic infections, and malignancies in male homosexuals. A hypothesis of etiologic factors in pathogenesis, by J. Sonnabend, et al. JAMA 249(17):2370-2374, May 6, 1983.

Acquired immunosuppression syndrome associated with severe anguilluliasis [letter], by G. Pialoux, et al. PRESSE MEDICALE 13(32):1960, September 22, 1984.

Actinomycetales infection in the acquired immunodeficiency syndrome, by H. A. Holtz, et al. ANNALS OF INTERNAL MEDICINE 102(2):203-205, February 1985.

Acute Cryptosporidium enteritis without immunologic weakness [letter], by U. Laukamm-Josten, et al. DEUTSCHE MEDIZINISCHE WOCHENSCHRIFT. 110(25):1014-1015, June 21, 1985.

Acute illnesses associated with HTLV-III seroconversion [letter], by C. Farthing, et al. LANCET 1(8434):935-936, April 20, 1985.

Acute myelofibrosis and infection with the lymphadenopathy-associated virus/human T-lymphotropic virus type III [letter], by C. Darne, et al. ANNALS OF INTERNAL MEDICINE 104(1):130-131, January 1986.

Add coccidioidomycosis to AIDS. EMERGENCY MEDICINE 16(16):43+, September 30, 1984.

Adenosquamous carcinoma of the lung and the acquired immunodeficiency syndrome [letter], by L. E. Irwin, et al. ANNALS OF INTERNAL MEDICINE 100(1):158, January 1984.

AIDS and AIDS-related diseases—clinical manifestations and therapy, by A. Sönnerborg, et al. LAKARTIDNINGEN 82(20):1877-1880, May 15, 1985.

AIDS and associated syndromes: clinical manifestations, by C. Mayaud, et al. REVUE FRANCAISE DE TRANSFUSION ET IMMUNOHEMATOLOGIE 27(4):411-421, September 1984.

AIDS and fungal infections, by K. Holmberg, et al. LAKARTIDNINGEN 83(19): 1753-1759, May 7, 1986.

AIDS and gastroenterology, by A. Gelb, et al. AMERICAN JOURNAL OF GASTROENTEROLOGY 81(8):619-622, August 1986.

513

AIDS and hepatitis B [letter], by K. S. Froebel, et al. LANCET 1(8377):632, March 17, 1984.

AIDS and hepatitis B cannot be venereal diseases [letter], by J. R. Seale. CANADIAN MEDICAL ASSOCIATION JOURNAL 130(9):1109-1110, May 1, 1984.

AIDS and Hodgkin's disease, by S. L. Schoeppel, et al. FRONTIERS OF RADIA-TION THERAPY AND ONCOLOGY 19:66-73, 1985.

AIDS and parasitic infections, including Pneumocystis carinii and cryptosporidi-osis, by C. D. Berkowitz. PEDIATRIC CLINICS OF NORTH AMERICA 32(4): 933-952, August 1985.

AIDS and parasitism [letter], by R. B. Pearce, et al. LANCET 1(8391):1411, June 23, 1984.

AIDS and related conditions—infection control. Guidelines for health care workers involved in patient management and investigation, by R. Sher. SOUTH AFRICAN MEDICAL JOURNAL 68(12):843-848, December 7, 1985.

AIDS and the gut, by I. V. Weller. SCANDINAVIAN JOURNAL OF GASTRO-ENTEROLOGY 114:77-89, 1985.

AIDS as a handicapping condition. MENTAL DISABILITY LAW REPORTER 9(6): 402-406, November-December 1985.

AIDS-associated ultrastructural changes [letter], by Z. Schaff, et al. LANCET 1(8337):1336, June 11, 1983.

AIDS encephalopathy, by R. W. Price, et al. NEUROLOGIC CLINICS 4(1):285-301, February 1986.

AIDS enters the brain, by M. Small. SCIENCE DIGEST 94:18, April 1986.

AIDS in association with malignant melanoma and Hodgkin's disease [letter], by G. E. Moore, et al. JOURNAL OF CLINICAL ONCOLOGY 3(10):1437, October 1985.

AIDS in the human brain, by C. H. Fox, et al. NATURE 319:8, January 2, 1986.

AIDS in a patient with Crohn's disease, by J. M. Dhar, et al. BRITISH MEDICAL JOURNAL 288(6433):1802-1803, June 16, 1984.

AIDS may lead to a tuberculosis epidemic. DISCOVER 7:9, March 1986.

AIDS-related brain damage unexplained, by D. M. Barnes. SCIENCE 232:1091-1093, May 30, 1986.

AIDS related complex—conumdrum, by N. Fain. ADVOCATE 3(89):20, March 6, 1984.

AIDS-related complex with lymphoid intersitial pneumonitis [letter], by J. M. Ziza, et al. NEW ENGLAND JOURNAL OF MEDICINE 313(3):183, July 18, 1985.

AIDS-related lymphomas: evaluation by abdominal CT, by D. A. Nyberg, et al. RADIOLOGY 159(1):59-63, April 1986.

AIDS with central nervous system toxoplasmosis [letter], by D. Moskopp. JOURNAL OF NEUROSURGERY 62(3):459-460, March 1985.

AIDS with Mycobacterium avium-intracellulare lesions resembling those of Whipple's disease [letter]. NEW ENGLAND JOURNAL OF MEDICINE 309(21):1323-1325, November 24, 1983.

Alimentary tract biopsy lesions in the acquired immune deficiency syndrome, by H. Rotterdam, et al. PATHOLOGY 17(2):181-192, April 1985.

Altered distribution of T-lymphocyte subpopulations in lymph nodes from patients with acquired immunodeficiency-like syndrome and hemophilia, by P. R. Meyer, et al. JOURNAL OF PEDIATRICS 103(3):407-410, September 1983.

Angioimmunoblastic lymphadenopathy with dysproteinemia in homosexual men with acquired immune deficiency syndrome, by W. Blumenfeld, et al. ARCHIVES OF PATHOLOGY AND LABORATORY MEDICINE 107(11):567-569, November 1983.

Another cause of diarrhea in AIDS [letter], by H. Edelstein, et al. WESTERN JOURNAL OF MEDICINE 142(2);262, February 1985.

Assessment of therapy for pneumocystis carinii pneumonia. PCP Therapy Project Group, by H. W. Haverkos. AMERICAN JOURNAL OF MEDICINE 76(3):501-508, March 1984.

Associated focal and segmental glomerulosclerosis in the acquired immunodeficiency syndrome, by T. K. Rao, et al. NEW ENGLAND JOURNAL OF MEDICINE 310(11):6569-673, March 15, 1984.

Association between HTLV-III/LAV infection and and tuberculosis in Zaire [letter],by J. Mann, et al. JAMA 256(3):346, July 18, 1986.

Asymptomatic carriage of crptosporidium in the stool of a patient with acquired immunodeficiency syndrome [letter], by F. Zar, et al. JOURNAL OF INFECTIOUS DISEASES 151(1):195, January 1985.

Atypical Hodgkin's disease and the acquired immunodeficiency syndrome [letter], by R. G. Scheib, et al. ANNALS OF INTERNAL MEDICINE 102(4): 5544, April 1985.

Atypical myobacterial and cytomegalovirus infection of the duodenum in a patient with acquired immunodeficiency syndrome: endoscopic and histopathologic appearance, by J. G. Caya, et al. WISCONSIN MEDICAL JOURNAL 83(11): 33-36, November 1984.

Atypical subcutaneous infection associated with acquired immune deficiency syndrome, by M. H. Stoler, et al. AMERICAN JOURNAL OF CLINICAL PATHOLOGY 80(5):714-718, November 1983.

515

Bacteremia and fungemia in patients with the acquired immunodeficiency syndrome, by E. Whimbey, et al. ANNALS OF INTERNAL MEDICINE 104(4): 511-514, April 1986.

Bacteremia due to Mycobacterium avium-intracellulare in the acquired immunodeficiency syndrome, by A. M. Macher, et al. ANNALS OF INTERNAL MEDICINE 99(6):782-785, December 1983.

Bacterial bronchopneumopathies in patients with the acquired immunodeficiency syndrome [letter], by C. Mayaud, et al. PRESSE MEDICALE 15(16):760-761, April 19, 1986.

Bacterial pneumonia in patients with the acquired immunodeficiency syndrome, by B. Polsky, et al. ANNALS OF INTERNAL MEDICINE 104(1):38-41, January 1986.

Basal cell carcinoma in a man with acquired immunodeficiency syndrome [letter], by L. Slazinski, et al. JOURNAL OF THE AMERICAN ACADEMY OF DERMATOLOGY 11(1):140-141, July 1984.

Biologic health hazards: AIDS and hepatitis B, by B. Burgel. CALIFORNIA NURSE 81(6):4, July-August 1985.

Brain endothelial cells infected by AIDS virus , by D. M. Barnes. SCIENCE 233(4762):418-419, July 25, 1986.

Campylobacter fetus ssp fetus cholecystitis and relapsing bacteremia in a patient with acquired immunodeficiency syndrome, by E. E. Coster, et al. SOUTHERN MEDICAL JOURNAL 77(7):927-928, July 1984.

Cancer trends in a population at risk of acquired immunodeficiency syndrome, by R. J. Biggar, et al. JNCI 74(4):793-797, April 1985.

Capsule-deficiency Cryptococcus neoformans in AIDS patients [letter], by D. W. Mackenzie, et al. LANCET 1(8429):642, March 16, 1985.

Capsule-deficient cryptococci in AIDS [letter], by E. J. Bottone, et al. LANCET 2(8454):553, September 7, 1985.

Capsule-deficient Cryptococcus neoformans in AIDS patients [letter]. LANCET 1(8435):988-997, April 27, 1985.

—, by E. J. Bottone, et al. LANCET 1(8425):400, February 16, 1985.

Cardiac abnormalities in acquired immune deficiency syndrome, by L. Fink, et al. AMERICAN JOURNAL OF CARDIOLOGY 54(8):1161-1163, November 1, 1984.

Cardiac aspergillosis in acquired immune deficiency syndrome, by S. Henochowicz, et al. AMERICAN JOURNAL OF CARDIOLOGY 55(9):1239-1240, April 15, 1985.

Cardiac lesions in acquired immune deficiency syndrome (AIDS), by C. Cammarosano, et al. JOURNAL OF THE AMERICAN COLLEGE OF CARDIOLOGY 55(3):703-706, March 1985.

Central nervous system disease in acquired immunodeficiency syndrome: prospective correlation using CT, MR imaging, and pathologic studies, by M. J. Post, et al. RADIOLOGY 158(1):141-148, January 1986.

Central nervous system infections in the immunocompromised host, by D. Armstrong. INFECTION 12(Suppl. 1):S58-S64, 1984.

Central nervous system infections in patients with the acquired immune deficiency syndrome (AIDS), by A. A. Harris, et al. CLINICAL NEUROPHARMACOLOGY 8(3):201-210, 1985.

Central nervous system involvement in patients with acquired immune deficiency syndrome (AIDS), by B. S. Koppel, et al. ACTA NEUROLOGICA SCANDINAVICA 71(5):337-353, May 1985.

Central nervous system mass lesions in the acquired immunodeficiency syndrome (AIDS), by R. M. Levy, et al. JOURNAL OF NEUROSURGERY 61(1):9-16, July 1984.

Central-nervous-system toxoplasmosis in homosexual men and parenteral drug abusers, by B. Wong, et al. ANNALS OF INTERNAL MEDICINE 100(1):36-42, January 1984.

Central nervous system tuberculosis with the acquired immunodeficiency syndrome and its related complex, by E. Bishburg, et al. ANNALS OF INTERNAL MEDICINE 105(2):210-213, August 1986.

Cerebral toxoplasmosis [letter], by J. H. Sher. LANCET 1(8335):1225, May 28, 1983.

Cerebral toxoplasmosis in acquired immune deficiency syndrome, by R. Alonso, et al. ARCHIVES OF NEUROLOGY 41(3):321-323, March 1984.

Cerebral toxoplasmosis in acquired immuno deficiency syndeome. A comparative assisted tomographic and neuropathological study of a case, by A. Gaston, et al. NEURORADIOLOGY 27(1):83-86, 1985.

Cerebral toxoplasmosis in AIDS,by F. Christ, et al. ROFO: FORTSCHRITTE AUF DEM GEBIETE DER RONTGENSTRAHLEN UND DER NUKLEARMEDIZIN 144(2):230-231, February 1986.

Cerebral toxoplasmosis in AIDS: a simple laboratory technique for diagnosis, by A. Datry, et al. TRANSACTIONS OF THE ROYAL SOCIETY OF TROPICAL MEDICINE AND HYGIENE 78(5):679-680, 1984.

Cerebral toxoplasmosis in a patient with acquired imunodeficiency syndrome, by A. Danziger, et al. SURGICAL NEUROLOGY 20(4):332-334, October 1983.

Cerebral toxoplasmosis in two adults without known immunodeficiency [letter], by P. Hericord, et al. PRESSE MEDICALE 12(16):1017-1018, April 9, 1983.

Chronic adenopathies in persons exposed to the risk of acquired immunodeficiency syndrome [letter], by J. P. Clauvel, et al. PRESSE MEDICALE 13(23): 1456, June 2, 1984.

Chronic lymphocytic leukemia: an AIDS like disease? [letter], by N. E. Kay, et al. BRITISH JOURNAL OF HAEMATOLOGY 63(2):389-391, June 1986.

Clinical features of Pneumocystis pneumonia in the acquired immune deficiency syndrome, by L. A. Engelberg, et al. AMERICAN REVIEW OF RESPIRATORY DISEASE 180(4):689-694, October 1984.

Clinical manifestations and therapy of Isospora belli infection in patients with the acquired immunodeficiency syndrome, by J. A. DeHovitz, et al. NEW ENGLAND JOURNAL OF MEDICINE 315(2):87-90, July 10, 1986.

Clinical spectrum of infections in patients with HTLV-III-associated diseases, by J. W. Gold. CANCER RESEARCH 45(Suppl. 9):4652s-4654s, September 1985.

Clues to the early diagnois of Mycobacterium avium-intracellulare infection in patients with acquired immunodeficiency syndrome, by M. A. Polis, et al. ARCHIVES OF PATHOLOGY AND LABORATORY MEDICINE 109(5):465-466, May 1985.

CNS toxoplasmosis in acquired immunodeficiency syndrome, by S. L. Horowitz, et al. ARCHIVES OF NEUROLOGY 40(10):649-652, October 1983.

Coccidioidomycosis in acquired immune deficiency syndrome. Depressed humoral as well as cellular immunity, by C. J. Roberts. AMERICAN JOURNAL OF MEDICINE 76(4):734-736, April 1984.

Comparison of biopsy-proven Pneumocystis carinii pneumonia in acquired immune deficiency syndrome patients and renal allograft recipients, by R. P. Sterling, et al. ANNALS OF THORACIC SURGERY 38(5):494-499, November 1984.

Concurrent herpes simplex and cytomegalovirus retinitis and encephalitis in the acquired immune deficiency syndrome (AIDS), by J. S. Pepose, et al. OPHTHALMOLOGY 91(12):1669-1677, December 1984.

Continuous high-grade mycobacterium avium-intracellulare bacteremia in patients with the acquired immune deficiency syndrome, by B. Wong, et alf. AMERICAN JOURNAL OF MEDICINE 78(1):35-40, January 1985.

Correlation between gallium lung scans and fiberoptic bronchoscopy in patients with suspected Pneumocystis carinii pneumonia and the acquired immune deficiency syndrome, by D. L. Coleman, et al. AMERICAN REVIEW OF RESPIRATORY DISEASE 130(6):1166-1169, December 1984.

Correlation between serial pulmonary function tests and fiberoptic bronchoscopy in patients with Pneumocystis carinii pneumonia and the acquired immune deficiency syndrome, by D. L. Coleman, et al. AMERICAN REVIEW OF RESPIRATORY DISEASE 129(3):491-493, March 1984.

Cranial CT in acquired immunodeficiency syndrome: spectrum of diseases and optimal contrast enhancement technique, by M. J. Post, et al. AJR 145(5): 929-940, November 1985.

Cryptococcal arthritis in a patient with acquired immune deficiency syndrome. Case report and review of the literature, by D. D. Ricciardi, et al. JOURNAL OF RHEUMATOLOGY 13(2):455-458, April 1986.

Cryptococcal infections in patients with acquired immune deficiency syndrome, by R. H. Eng, et al. AMERICAN JOURNAL OF MEDICINE 81(1):19-21, July 1986.

Cryptococcal meningitis, herpes genitalis and oral candidiasis in a homosexual man with acquired immunodeficiency syndrome [letter], by J. Bras,e t al. NEDERLANDS TIJDSCHRIFT VOOR GENEESKUNDE 127(34):1553-1554, August 20, 1983.

Cryptococcal meningitis, herpes genitalis and oral immunodeficiency, by L. Zegerius, et al. NEDERLANDS TIJDSCHRIFT VOOR GENEESKUNDE 127(19):817-820, May 7, 1983.

Cryptococcal myocarditis in acquired immune deficiency syndrome, by W. Lewis, et al. AMERICAN JOURNAL OF CARDIOLOGY 55(9):1240, April 15, 1985.

Cryptococcosis and torulopsidosis of the skin and lung and epidermodysplasia verruciformis in AIDS (acquired immune deficiency syndrome), by I. Grimm. HAUTARZT 35(12):653-655, December 1984.

Cryptococcosis in the acquired immunodeficiency syndrome, by J. A. Kovacs, et al. ANNALS OF INTERNAL MEDICINE 103(4):533-538, October 1985.

Cryptosporidial enteritis in a homosexual male with an acquired immunodeficiency syndrome, by R. E. Petras, et al. CLEVELAND CLINIC QUARTERLY 50(1): 41-45, Spring 1983.

Cryptosporidiosis and AIDS, by D. L. Volker. ONCOLOGY NURSING FORUM 11(3):86, May-June 1984.

Cryptosporidiosis in the acquired immune deficiency syndrome, by D. A. Cooper, et al. PATHOLOGY 16(4):455-457, October 1984.

Cryptosporidiosis in homosexual men, by R. Soave, et al. ANNALS OF IN-TERNAL MEDICINE 100(4):504-511, April 1984.

Cryptosporidiosis of the stomach and small intestine in patients with AIDS, by R. N. Berk, et al. AJR 143(3):549-554, September 1984.

Cryptosporidium and the enteropathy of immune deficiency, by P. Ma. JOUR-NAL OF PEDIATRIC GASTROENTEROLOGY AND NUTRITION 3(4):488-490, September 1984.

Cryptosporidium causing severe enteritis in a Belgian immunocompetent patient, by J. Vandepitte, et al. ACTA CLINICA BELGICA 40(1):43-47, 1985.

Cryptosporidium enterocolitis in homosexual men with AIDS, by J. Gerstoft, et al. SCANDINAVIAN JOURNAL OF INFECTIOUS DISEASES 16(4):385-388, 1984.

Cryptosporidium in acquired immunodeficiency syndrome, by J. D. Cohen, et al. DIGESTIVE DISEASES AND SCIENCES 29(8):773-777, August 1984.

Cryptosporidium in patient with acquired immunodeficiency syndrome [letter], by C. Jonas, et al. LANCET 2(8356):964, October 22, 1983.

Cutaneous cryptococcosis resembling molluscum contagiosum in a patient with AIDS, by M. J. Rico, et al. ARCHIVES OF DERMATOLOGY 121(7):901-902, July 1985.

Cutaneous manifestations of AIDS, by G. E. Pierard, et al. REVUE MEDICALE DE LIEGE 41(6):189-198, March 15, 1986.

Cytomegalovirus and herpes simplex virus ascending myelitis in a patient with acquired immune deficiency syndrome, by T. Tucker, et al. ANNALS OF NEUROLOGY 18(1):74-79, July 1985.

Cytomegalovirus colitis. Report of the clinical, endoscopic, and pathologic findings in two patients with the acquired immune deficiency syndrome, by M. S. Meiselman, et al. GASTROENTEROLOGY 88(1, Part 1):171-175, January 1985.

Cytomegalovirus colitis in acquired immunodeficiency syndrome—a chronic disease with varying manifestations, by W. Levinson, et al. AMERICAN JOURNAL OF GASTROENTEROLOGY 80(6):445-447, June 1985.

Cytomegalovirus colitis in AIDS: radiographic findings in 11 patients, by E. J. Balthazar, et al. RADIOLOGY 155(3):585-589, June 1985.

Cytomegalovirus encephalitis in acquired immunodeficiency syndrome, by D. A. Hawley, et al. AMERICAN JOURNAL OF CLINICAL PATHOLOGY 80(6):874-877, December 1983.

Cytomegalovirus encephalitis in a patient with acquired immunodeficiency syndrome [letter], by C. Vital, et al. ARCHIVES OF PATHOLOGY AND LABORATORY MEDICINE 109(2):105-106, February 1985.

Cytomegalovirus esophagitis and gastritis in AIDS, by E. J. Balthazar, et al. AJR 144(6):1201-1204, June 1985.

Cytomegalovirus esophagogastritis in a patient with acquired immunodeficiency syndrome, by P. G. Freedman, et al. AMERICAN JOURNAL OF GASTROENTEROLOGY 80(6):434-437, June 1985.

Cytomegalovirus-induced demyelination associated with acquired immune deficiency syndrome, by L. B. Moskowitz, et al. ARCHIVES OF PATHOLOGY AND LABORATORY MEDICINE 108(11):873-877, November 1984.

Cytomegalovirus infection, ascending myelitis, and pulmonary embolus [letter], by P. H. Bagley, et al. ANNALS OF INTERNAL MEDICINE 104(4):587, April 1986.

Cytomegalovirus infection in homosexual men—relationship to AIDS, by W. L. Drew. FRONTIERS OF RADIATION THERAPY AND ONCOLOGY 19:38-42, 1985.

Cytomegalovirus infections in AIDS [letter], by H. L. Schmidts, et al. DEUTSCHE MEDIZINISCHE WOCHENSCHRIFT 110(20):818, May 17, 1985.

Decreased incidence of syphilis among homosexual men as a consequence of AIDS?, by L. Hellström, et al. LAKARTIDNINGEN 82(28-29):2529-2530, July 10, 1985.

Defective regulation of Epstein-Barr virus infection in patients with acquired immunodeficiency syndrome (AIDS) or AIDS-related disorders,by D. L. Birx, et al. NEW ENGLAND JOURNAL OF MEDICINE 314(14):874-879, April 3, 1986.

Dementia and AIDS. AMERICAN FAMILY PHYSICIAN 32:239+, August 1985.

Diarrhea and the acquired immunodeficiency syndrome, by C. Bories, et al. GASTROENTEROLOGIE CLINIQUE ET BIOLOGIQUE 9(4):354-360, April 1985.

Diarrhea and malabsorption associated with the acquired immunodeficiency syndrome (AIDS). NUTRITION REVIEWS 43:235-237, August 1985.

Diarrhea and malabsorption in acquired immune deficiency syndrome: a study of four cases with special emphasis on opportunistic protozoan infestations, by R. Modigliani, et al. GUT 26(2):179-187, February 1985.

Diarrhea caused by 'nonpathogenic amoebae' in patients with AIDS [letter], by K. V. Rolston, et al. NEW ENGLAND JOURNAL OF MEDICINE 315(3):192, July 17, 1986.

Diffuse alveolar damage and interstitial fibrosis in acquired immunodeficiency syndrome patients without concurrent pulmonary infection, by G. Ramaswamy , et al. ARCHIVES OF PATHOLOGY AND LABORATORY MEDICINE 109(5): 408-412, May 1985.

Diffuse immunoblastic sarcoma from benign lymphoid proliferation [letter], by J. L. Wade, 3d, et al. ANNALS OF INTERNAL MEDICINE 10094):765, May 1984.

Diffuse pulmonary gallium accumulation with a normal chest radiogram in a homosexual man with Pneumocystis carinii pneumonia. A case report, by S. C. Moses, et al. CLINICAL NUCLEAR MEDICINE 8(12):608-609, December 1983.

Disease in many guises, by C. Norman. SCIENCE 230:1019, November 29, 1985.

Disseminated CMV infection [letter], by D. P. Kotler, et al. JAMA 253(21):3093-3094, June 7, 1985.

Disseminated coccidioidomycosis in AIDS [letter], by D. I. Abrams, et al. NEW ENGLAND JOURNAL OF MEDICINE 310(15):986-987, April 12, 1984.

Disseminated coccidioidomycosis in a patient with acquired immune deficiency syndrome, by A. Kovacs, et al. WESTERN JOURNAL OF MEDICINE 140(3): 447-449, March 1984.

Disseminated cryptococcal infection, AIDS, Kaposi's sarcoma, chronic diarrhea, hepatitis B carrier, and cytomegalovirus, by M. Vongxaiburana. WEST VIRGINIA MEDICAL JOURNAL 81(11):248-251, November 1985.

Disseminated cryptococcosis in two AIDS patients. A contribution to cryptococcosis diagnosis in AIDS, by F. Staib, et al. DEUTSCHE MEDIZINISCHE WOCHENSCHRIFT 111(27):1061-1065, July 4, 1986.

Disseminated cryptococcosis presenting as herpetiform lesions in a homosexual man with acquired immunodeficiency syndrome, by L. K. Borton, et al. JOURNAL OF THE AMERICAN ACADEMY OF DERMATOLOGY 10(2 Pt 2): 387-390, February 1984.

Disseminated histoplasmosis associated with the acquired imune deficiency syndrome,by M. N. Taylor, et al. AMERICAN JOURNAL OF MEDICINE 77(3): 579-580, September 1984.

Disseminated histoplasmosis in the acquired immune deficiency syndrome, by L. J. Wheat, et al. ARCHIVES OF INTERNAL MEDICINE144(11):2147-2149, November 1984.

Disseminated histoplasmosis in patients with the acquired immune deficiency syndrome, by J. R. Bonner, et al. ARCHIVES OF INTERNAL MEDICINE 144(11):2178-2181, Novembr 1984.

Disseminated histoplasmosis, invasive pulmonary aspergillosis, and other opportunistic infections in a homosexual patient with acquired immune deficiency syndrome, by P. G. Jones, et al. SEXUALLY TRANSMITTED DISEASES 10(4):202-204, October-December 1983.

Disseminated infection due to mycobacterium avium-intreacellulare complex [letter], by B. C. West, et al. CHEST 85(5):710-711, May 1984.

Disseminated Mycobacterium avium-intracellulare infection in acquired immunodeficiency syndrome mimicking Whipple's disease,by J. S. Gillin, et al. GASTROENTEROLOGY 85(5):1187-1191, November 1983.

Disseminated Mycobacterium avium-intracellulare infection in homosexual men with acquired cell-mediated immunodeficiency: a histologic and immunologic study oftwo cases, by C. C. Sohn, et al. AMERICAN JOURNAL OF CLINICAL PATHOLOGY 79(2):247-252, February 1983.

Disseminated talc granulomatosis. An unusual finding in a patient with acquired immunodeficiency syndrome and fatal cytomegalovirus infection, by J. H. Lewis, et al. ARCHIVES OF PATHOLOGY AND LABORATORY MEDICINE 109(2);147-150, February 1985.

Disseminated tuberculosis and the acquired immunodeficiency syndrome [letter] by A. E. Pitchenik, et al. ANNALS OF INTERNAL MEDICINE 98(1):112, January 1983.

Disseminated tubuloreticular inclusions in acquired immunodeficiency syndrome (AIDS), by M. Kostianovsky, et al. ULTRASTRUCTURAL PATHOLOGY 4(4): 331-336, June 1983.

Emerging importance of infections due to the Mycobacterium avium-intracellulare complex [editorial], by D. Y. Rosenzweig. NEW YORK STATE JOURNAL OF MEDICINE 84(6):290, June 1984.

Enteric coccidiosis among patients with the acquired immunodeficiency syndrome, by M. E. Whiteside, et al. AMERICAN JOURNAL OF TROPICAL MEDICINE AND HYGIENE 33(6):1065-1072, November 1984.

Eosinophilic pustular folliculitis in patients with acquired immunodeficiency syndrome. Report of three cases, by F. F. Soeprono, et al. JOURNAL OF THE AMERICAN ACADEMY OF DERMATOLOGY 14(6):1020-1022, June 1986.

Evaluation of cerebral mass lesions in acquired immunodeficiency syndrome [letter], by A. E. Pitchenik, et al. NEW ENGLAND JOURNAL OF MEDICINE 308(18):1099, May 5, 1983.

Fever, cough, anal ulcer in a heterosexual man, by P. J. de Caprariis, et al. HOSPITAL PRACTICE 19(4):122+, April 1984.

Fitz-Hugh and Curtis syndrome in a homosexual man with impaired cell mediated immunity, by W. P. Winkler, et al. GASTROINTESTINAL ENDOSCOPY 31(1): 28-30, February 1985.

Fungal infections in patients with AIDS and AIDS-related complex, by K. Holmberg, et al. SCANDINAVIAN JOURNAL OF INFECTIOUS DISEASES. 18(3): 179-192, 1986.

Fungal stains in the acquired immunodeficiency syndrome [letter], by R. E. Stahl, et al. ANNALS OF INTERNAL MEDICINE 102(3):413, March 1985.

Ga-67 studies in a patient with acquired immunodeficiency syndrome and disseminated mycobacterial infection, by C. M. Malhotra, et al. CLINICAL NUCLEAR MEDICINE 10(2):96-98, February 1985.

Gastrointestinal cryptosporidiosis and sytomegalovirus enterocolitis, by d. F. Altman. FRONTIERS OF RADIATION THERAPY AND ONCOLOGY 19:88-90, 1985.

Gastrointestinal histoplasmosis in suspected acquired immunodeficiency syndrome, by C. M. Haggerty, et al. WESTERN JOURNAL OF MEDICINE 143(2):244-246, August 1985.

Gastrointestinal infections during AIDS [letter], by E. René, et al. LANCET 1(8382): 915, April 2, 1984.

Gastrointestinal sytomegalovirus infection in a homosexual man with severe acquired immunodeficiency syndrome, by S. L. Gertler, et al. GASTRO-ENTEROLOGY 85(6):1403-1406, December 1983.

Generalized lymphadenopathy in homosexual men: an update of the New York experience, by C. E. Metroka, et al. ANNALS OF THE NEW YORK ACADEMY OF SCIENCES 437:400-411, 1984.

Glomerular lesions in the acquired immunodeficiency syndrome, by V. Pardo,e t al. ANNALS OF INTERNAL MEDICINE 101(4):429-434, October 1984.

Hepatic lesions in AIDS, by C. Marche, et al. ARCHIVES D'ANATOMIE ET DE CYTOLOGIE PATHOLOGIQUES 32(2):120-121, 1984.

Hepatic vascular lesions in AIDS [letter], by J. F. Devars du Mayne. JAMA 254(1): 53-54, July 5, 1985.

Histoplasmosis diagnosed on peripheral blood smear from a patient with AIDS, by S. Henochowicz, et al. JAMA 253(21):3148, June 7, 1985.

Histoplasmosis in the acquired immune deficiency syndrome, by L. J. Wheat, et al. AMERICAN JOURNAL OF MEDICINE 78(2):203-210, February 1985.

Histoplasmosis in acquired immunodeficiency syndrome (AIDS): diagnosis by bone marrow examination [letter], by J. Pasternak, et al. ARCHIVES OF INTERNAL MEDICINE 143(10):2024, October 1983.

Histoplasmosis presenting with unusual skin lesions in acquired immunodeficiency syndrome (AIDS), by J. A. Hazelhurst, et al. BRITISH JOURNAL OF DERMATOLOGY 113·3):345-348, September 1985.

Hodgkin's disease and the acquired immunodeficiency syndrome [letter], by H. L. Ioachim, et al. ANNALS OF INTERNAL MEDICINE 101(6):876-877, December 1984.

—, by N. J. Robert, et al. ANNALS OF INTERNAL MEDICINE 101(1):142-143, July 1984.

Hodgkin's disease in AIDS complex patients. Report of four cases and tissue immunologic marker studies, by P. D. Unger, et al. CANCER 58(4):821-825, August 15, 1986.

Human cryptosporidiosis in the acquired immune deficiency syndrome, by L. A. Guarda, et al. ARCHIVES OF PATHOLOGY AND LABORATORY MEDICINE 107(11):562-566, November 1983.

Human cryptosporidiosis: spectrum of disease. Report of six cases and review of the literature, by S. D. Pitlik, et al. ARCHIVES OF INTERNAL MEDICINE 143(12):2269-2275, December 1983.

Human T-cell lymphotropic virus type III associated disorders. The spectrum in the heterosexual population, by P. S. Gill, et al. ARCHIVES OF INTERNAL MEDICINE 146(8):1501-1504, Augus 1986.

Humoral response to disseminated infection by Mycobacterium avium-Mycobacterium intracellulare in acquired immunodeficiency syndrome and hairy cell leukemia, by S. M. Winter, et al. JOURNAL OF INFECTIOUS DISEASES 151(3):523-527, March 1985.

Hyperalgesic pseudothrombophlebitis. New syndrome in male homosexual, by S. B. Abramson, et al. AMERICAN JOURNAL OF MEDICINE 78(2):317-320, February 1985.

Hypercalcemia and disseminated cytomegalovirus infection in the acquired immunodeficiency syndrome, by G. P. Zaloga, et al. ANNALS OF INTERNAL MEDICINE 102(3);331-333, March 1985.

Hypothesis: fungal toxins are involved in aspergillosis and AIDS, by R. D. Eichner, et al. AUSTRALIAN JOURNAL OF EXPERIMENTAL BIOLOGY AND MEDICAL SCIENCE 62(Part 4):479-484, August 1984.

Identification of Cryptosporidium in patients with the acquired immunologic syndrome [letter],by P. Payne, et al. NEW ENGLAND JOURNAL OF MEDICINE 309(10):613-614, September 8, 1983.

Identification of multiple cytomegalovirus strains in homosexual men with acquired immunodeficiency syndrome, by S. A. Spector, et al. JOURNAL OF INFECTIOUS DISEASES 150(6):953-956, December 1984.

Immune deficiency presenting as disseminated sporotrichosis,by S. E. Matter, et al. JOURNAL OF THE OKLAHOMA STATE MEDICAL ASSOCIATION 77(4): 114-117, April 1984.

Infection with Rhodococcus equi in AIDS [letter], by D. C. Sane, et al. NEW ENGLAND JOURNAL OF MEDICINE 314(1):56-57, January 2, 1986.

Infections due to Pneumocystis carinii and Mycobacterium avium-intracellulare in patients with acquired immune deficiency syndrome, by J. H. Shelhamer, et al. ANNALS OF THE NEW YORK ACADEMY OF SCIENCES 437:394-399, 1984.

Infections in AIDS patients, by J. Dryjanski, et al. CLINICAL HAEMATOLOGY 13(3):709-726, October 1984.

Infections in homosexual men, by S. Iwarson, et al. LAKARTIDNINGEN 80(7): 548-552, February 16, 1983.

Infectious complications of the acquired immune deficiency syndrome, by J. W. Gold, et al. ANNALS OF THE NEW YORK ACADEMY OF SCIENCES 437: 383-393, 1984.

Inoculation of cryptococcosis without transmission of the acquired immunodeficiency syndrome [letter], by J. B. Glaser, et al. NEW ENGLAND JOURNAL OF MEDICINE 313(4):266, July 25, 1985.

Intestinal infection with Mycobacterium avium in acquired immune deficiency syndrome (AIDS). Histological and clinical comparison with Whipple's disease, by R. I. Roth, et al. DIGESTIVE DISEASES AND SCIENCES 30(5):497-504, May 1985.

Intestinal perforation associated with cytomegalovirus infection in patients with acquired immune deficiency syndrome,by D. Frank, et al. AMERICAN JOURNAL OF GASTROENTEROLOGY 79(3):201-205, March 1984.

Intestinal protozoal infections in AIDS [letter],by R. B. Pearce. LANCET 2(8340): 51, July 2, 1983.

Intra-blood-brain-barrier synthesis of HTLV-III-specific IgG in patients with neurologic symptoms associated with AIDS or AIDS-related complex, by L. Resnick, et al. NEW ENGLAND JOURNAL OF MEDICINE 313:1498-1504, December 12, 1985.

Intracerebral-mass lesions in the acquired immunodeficiency syndrome (AIDS) [letter], by R. M. Levy, et al. NEW ENGLAND JOURNAL OF MEDICINE 309(23):1454-1455, December 8, 1983.

Intracerebral toxoplasmosis in patients with acquired immune deficiency syndrome, by M. Handler, et al. JOURNAL OF NEUROSURGERY 59(6):994-1001, December 1983.

Intracranial lesions in the acquired imunodeficiency syndrome. Radiological (computed tomographic) features, by C. M. Elkin, et al. JAMA 253(3):393-396, January 18, 1985.

Intracranial lesions in AIDS. AMERICAN FAMILY PHYSICIAN 32:206+, September 1985.

Intracranial space-occupying lesions in acquired immune deficiency syndrome patients, by R. B. Snow, et al. NEUROSURGERY 165(2):148-153, February 1985.

Intrathoracic adenopathy: differential feature of AIDS and diffuse lymphadenopathy syndrome by R. G. Ster,e t al. AJR 142(4):689-692, April 1984.

Isospora belli in a patient with acquired immunodeficiency syndrome, by R. Shein, et al. JOURNAL OF CLINICAL GASTROENTEROLOGY 6(6):525-528, December 1984.

Legionellosis in the acquired immunodeficiency syndrome [letter], by O. Guenot, et al. PRESSE MÉDICALE 13(35):2150-2151, October 6, 1984.

Lesions of the digestive mucosa in AIDS, by c. Marche, et al. ARCHIVES D'ANATOMIE ET DE CYTOLOGIE PATHOLOGIQUES 32(2):122-123, 1984.

Lesser AIDS and tuberculosis [letter], by J. J. Goedert, et al. LANCET 2(8445): 52, July 6, 1985.

Leukopenia, trimethoprim-sulfamethoxazole, and folinic acid [letter], by H. Hollander. ANNALS OF INTERNAL MEDICINE 102(1):138, January 1985.

Listeria monocytogenes bacteremia in the acquired immunodeficiency syndrome [letter], by f. X. Real, et al. ANNALS OF INTERNAL MEDICINE 101(6):883, December 1984.

Listeria monocytogenes meningitis in AIDS, by K. Koziol, et al. CANADIAN MEDICAL ASSOCIATION JOURNAL 135(1):43-44, July 1, 1986.

Listeria monocytogenes sepsis and small cell carcinoma of the rectum: an unusual presentation of the acquired immunodeficiency syndrome, by E. J. read, et al. AMERICAN JOURNAL OF CLINICAL PATHOLOGY 83(3):385-389, March 1985.

Listeria sepsis in AIDS [letter],by M. Thiel, et al. DEUTSCHE MEDIZINISCHE WOCHENSCHRIFT 111(8):316-317, Feburary 21, 1986.

Listeriosis and AIDS: an unfounded assumption [letter],by M. Boucher, et al. AMERICAN JOURNAL OF OBSTETRICS AND GYNECOLOGY 149(7):804-806, August 1, 1984.

Liver in the acquired immunodeficiency syndrome: a clinical and histologic study, by E. Lebovics, et al. HEPATOLOGY 5(2):293-298, March-April 1985.

526

Localization of cytomegalovirus proteins and genome during fulminant central nervous system infection in an AIDS patient, by C. A. Wiley, et al. JOURNAL OF NEUROPATHOLOGY AND EXPERIMENTAL NEUROLOGY 45(2):127-139, March 1986.

Lung complications in AIDS, by R. Weiske, et al. RADIOLOGE 26(1):3-9, January 1986.

Lupus anticoagulant in the acquired immunodeficiency syndrome, by E. J. Bloom, et al. JAMA 256(4):491-493, July 25, 1986.

Lymph node involvement in AIDS [letter]. UGESKRIFT FOR LAEGER 146(9): 672-673, February 27, 1984.

Lymphoid lesions associated with the acquired immunodeficiency syndrome, by H. L. Iochim, et al. AMERICAN JOURNAL OF SURGICAL PATHOLOGY 7(6): 543-553, September 1983.

Lymphoreticular malignancies in the setting of acquired immunodeficiency syndrome (AIDS). A potential model for evolution of hyman lymphid neoplasma, by A. Khojasteh, et al. MISSOURI MEDICINE 82(9):599-602, September 1985.

Maculopapular rash in a patient with acquired immunodeficiency syndrome. Disseminated histoplasmosis in acquired immunodeficiency syndrome (AIDS), by D. C. Kalter, et al. ARCHIVES OF DERMATOLOGY 121(11):1455-1456+, November 1985.

Malabsorption and mucosal abnormalities of the small intestine in the acquired Immunodeficiency syndrome, by J. S. Gillin, et al. ANNALS OF INTERNAL MEDICINE 102(5):619-622, May 1985.

Malignancies in the AIDS patient: natural history, treatment strategies, and preliminary results, by D. L. Longo, et al. ANNALS OF THE NEW YORK ACADEMY OF SCIENCES 237:421-430, 1984.

Malignant catarrhal fever parallel with AIDS. THE VETERINARY RECORD 117: 351-352, October 5, 1985.

Malignant lymphoreticular lesions in patients with immune disorders resembling acquired immunodeficiency syndrome (AIDS): review of 80 cases, by A. Khojasteh, et al. SOUTHERN MEDICAL JOURNAL 79(9):1070-1075, September 1986.

Management of infectious complications in acquired immunodeficiency syndrome, by I. H. Grant, et al. AMERICAN JOURNAL OF MEDICINE 81(1A):59-72, July 28, 1986.

Maxillofacial manifestations of acquired immunodeficiency syndrome, by P. Goudot, et al. REVUE DE STOMATOLOGIE ET DE CHIRURGIE MAXILLO-FACIALE 86(1):3-8, 1985.

Metastatic small-cell carcinoma of the lung in a patient with AIDS [letter], by N. J. Nusbaum. NEW ENGLAND JOURNAL OF MEDICINE 312(26):1706, June 27, 1985.

527

Microsporidiosis myositis in a patient with the acquired immunodeficiency syndrome, by D. K. Ledford, et al. ANNALS OF INTERNAL MEDICINE 102(5): 628-630, May 1985.

Molluscum contagiosum and the acquired immunodeficiency syndrome [letter], by M. Katzman, et al. ANNALS OF INTERNAL MEDICINE 102(3);413-414, March 1985.

—, by P. C. Lombardo, et al. ARCHIVES OF DEROMATOLOGY 121(7):834-835, July 1985.

Monilial enteritis in acquired immunodeficiency syndrome,by D. R. Radin, et al. AMERICAN JOURNAL OF ROENTGENOLOGY 141(6):1289-1290, December 1983.

Mononuclear and polymorphonuclear leucocyte dysfunction in male homosexuals with the acquired immunodeficiency syndrome (AIDS), by G. J. Ras, et al. SOUTH AFRICAN MEDICAL JOURNAL 66(21):806-809, November 24, 1984.

More evidence for brain disease in AIDS, by O. Sattaur. NEW SCIENTIST 108: 26, October 10, 1985.

Multifocal abnormalities of the gatrointestinal tract in AIDS, by S. D. Wall, et al. AMERICAN JOURNAL OF ROENTGENOLOGY 146(1):1-5, January 1986.

Multinucleated giant cells and HTLV-III in AIDS encephalopathy, by L. R. Sharer, et al. HUMAN PATHOLOGY 16(8):760, August 1985.

Multiple myeloma in a homosexual man with chronic lymphadenopathy, by L. A. Vandermolen, et al. ARCHIVES OF INTERNAL MEDICINE 145(4):745-746, April 1985.

Multiple opportunistic infections and neoplasms in the acquired immunodeficiency syndrome [editorial], by G. P. Wormser. JAMA 253(23)3441-3442, June 21, 1985.

Multiple sclerosis and human T-cell lymphotropic retroviruses, by H. Koprowski, et al. NATURE 318:154-160, November 14, 1985.

Multiple sclerosis and viruses, by P. Newmark. NATURE 318:101, November 14, 1985.

Mycobacteriosis and AIDS in hospitals, by G. E. Noel. CANADIAN MEDICAL ASSOCIATION JOURNAL 135(2):136, July 15, 1986.

Mycobacterium avium-complex infections and development of the acquired immunodeficiency syndrome: casual opportunist or causal cofactor?, by F. M. Collins. INTERNATIONAL JOURNAL OF LEPROSY AND OTHER MYCO-BACTERIAL DISEASES 54(3):458-474, September 1986.

Mycobacterium avium complex infections in patients with the acquired immunodeficiency syndrome, by C. C. Hawkins, et al. ANNALS OF INTERNAL MEDICINE 105(2):184-188, August 1986.

Mycobacterium avium-intracellulare: another scourge for individuals with the acquired immunodeficiency syndrome [editorial], by H. Masur. JAMA 248(22):3013, December 10, 1982.

Mycobacterium avium-intracellulare-associated colitis in a patient with the acquired immunodeficiency syndrome, by A. Wolke, et al. JOURNAL OF CLINICAL GASTROENTEROLOGY 6(3):225-229, June 1984.

Mycobacterium avium-intracellulare complex enteritis: pseudo-Whipple disease in AIDS, by M. E. Vincent, et al. AJR 144(5):921-922, May 1985.

Mycobacterium avium-intracellulare infection and possibly venereal transmission [letter], by P. J. de Caprariis, et al. ANNALS OF INTERNAL MEDICINE 101(5):721, November 1984.

Mycobacterium avium-Mycobacterium intracellulare from the intestinal tracts of patients with the acquired immunodeficiency syndrome: concepts regarding acquisition and pathogenesis, by B. Damsker, et al. JOURNAL OF INFECTIOUS DISEASES 151(1):179-181, January 1985.

Mycobacterium avium: a pathogen of patients with acquired immunodeficiency syndrome, by O. G. Berlin, et al. DIAGNOSTIC MICROBIOLOGY AND INFECTIOUS DISEASE 2(3):213-218, June 1984.

Mycobacterium gordonae in the acquired immunodeficiency syndrome [letter],by J. Chan, et al. ANNALS OF INTERNAL MEDICINE 101(3):400, September 1984.

Mycobacterium tuberculosis bacteremia in the acquired immunodeficiency syndrome, by B. R. Saltzman,e t al. JAMA 256(3):390-391, July 18, 1986.

Mycobacterium xenopi and the acquired immunodeficiency syndrome [letter], by F. T. Tecson-Tumang, et al. ANNALS OF INTERNAL MEDICINE 100(3):461-462, March 1984.

Mycobacterium xenopi infection in a patient with acquired imunodeficiency syndrome, by R. H. Eng, et al. CHEST 86(1):145-147, July 1984.

Myelodysplasia in the acquired immune deficiency syndrome, by D. R. Schneider, et al. AMERICAN JOURNAL OF CLINICAL PATHOLOGY 84(2): 144-152, August 1985.

Neurologic complications in acquired immunodeficiency syndrome (AIDS), by C. B. Britton, et al. NEUROLOGICAL CLINIC 2(2):315-339, May 1984.

Neurologic complications in acquired immunodeficiency syndrome (AIDS). A clinical, computer tomographic and neuropathologic case presentation with a review of the literature, by S. M. Pulst. NERVENARZT 55(8):407-412, August 1984.

Neurologic manifestations in acquired immunodeficiency syndrome (AIDS), by J. Kesselring. DEUTSCHE MEDIZINISCHE WOCHENSCHRIFT 111(27):1068-1073, July 4, 1986.

Neurologic manifestations of the acquired immunodeficiency syndrome, by G. Fenelon, et al. REVUE NEUROLOGIQUE 142(2):97-106, 1986.

Neurological complications appear often in AIDS, by C. Marwick. JAMA 253: 3379+, June 21, 1985.

Neurological complications now characterizing many AIDS victims [news], by P. Gapen. JAMA 248(22):2941-2942, December 10, 1982.

Neurological complications of acquired immune deficiency syndrome: analysis of 50 patients, by W. D. Snider, et al. ANNALS OF NEUROLOGY 14(4);403-418, October 1983.

Neurological disorders and AIDS. ADVOCATE 454:23, Septemebr 2, 1986.

Neurological manifestations of acquired immunodeficiency syndrome,by J. H. McArthur, et al. JOURNAL OF NEUROSCIENCE NURSING 18(5):242-249, October 1986.

Neurological manifestations of the acquired immunodeficiency syndrome (AIDS): experience at UCSF and review of the literature, by R. M. Levy, et al. JOURNAL OF NEUROSURGERY 62(4):475-495, April 1985.

Neurological syndromes complicating AIDS, by B. D. Jordan, et al. FRONTIERS OF RADIATION THERAPY AND ONCOLOGY 19:82-87, 1985.

Neuropathologic findings in the acquired immunodeficiency syndrome (AIDS), by K. Anders, et al. CLINICAL NEUROPATHOLOGY 5(1):1-20, January-February 1986.

Neuropathologic observations in acquired immunodeficiency syndrome (AIDS), by L. R. Sharer, et al. ACTA NEUROPATHOLOGICA 66(3):188-198, 1985.

Neuropathology of acquired immune deficiency syndrome, by L. B. Moskowitz, et al. ARCHIVES OF PATHOLOGY AND LABORATORY MEDICINE 108(11): 867-872, November 1984.

Neuropathology of AIDS, by A. Hirano, et al. NO TO SHINKEI 36(11):1136-1137, November 1984.

New complication of AIDS: thoracic myelitis caused by herpes simplex virus, by C. B. Britton, et al. NEUROLOGY 35(7):1071-1074, July 1985.

Non-Hodgkin's lymphoma in 90 homosexual men: relation to generalized lymphadenopathy and the acquired immunodeficiency syndrome, by J. L. Ziegler, et al. NEW ENGLAND JOURNAL OF MEDICINE 311(9):565-570, August 30, 1984.

Nontyphoidal Salmonella bacteremia as an early infection in acquired immunodeficiency syndrome, by E. J. Bottone, et al. DIAGNOSTIC MICROBIOLOGY AND INFECTIOUS DISEASE 2(3):247-250, June 1984.

Oat-cell carcinoma in transfusion-associated acquired immunodeficiency syndrome [letter], by R. J.\ Moser, 3d, et al. ANNALS OF INTERNAL MEDICINE 103(3):478, September 1985.

Occult infections with M. intracellulare in bone-marrow biopsy specimens from patients with AIDS [letter], by R. J. Cohen, et al. NEW ENGLAND JOURNAL OF MEDICINE 308(24):1476, June 16, 1983.

Occurrence of a new microsporidan: Enterocytozoon bieneusi n.g., n. sp., in the enterocytes of a human patient with AIDS, by I. Desportes, et al. JOURNAL OF PROTOZOOLOGY 32(2):250-254, May 1985.

Oral candidiasis and the acquired immunodeficiency syndrome [letter], by B. Romanowski, et al. ANNALS OF INTERNAL MEDICINE 101(3):400-401, September 1984.

Oral candidiasis and AIDS [letter], by M. Joy. NEW ENGLAND JOURNAL OF MEDICINE 311(21):1378-1379, November 22, 1984.

Oral candidiasis as a marker for esophageal candidiasis in the acquired immuno-deficiency syndrome, by A. Tavitian, et al. ANNALS OF INTERNAL MEDI-CINE 104(1):54-55, January 1986.

Oral candidiasis in high-risk patients as the initial manifestation of the acquired immunodeficiency syndrome, by R. S. Klein, et al. NEW ENGLAND JOUR-NAL OF MEDICINE 311(6):354-358, August 9, 1984.

Oral candidosis and AIDS [letter], by L. P. Samaranayake. BRITISH DENTAL JOURNAL 157(10):342-343, November 24, 1984.

Oral findings in people with or at high risk for AIDS: a study of 375 homosexual males, by S. Silverman, Jr., et al. JOURNAL OF THE AMERICAN DENTAL ASSOCIATION 112(2):187-192, February 1986.

Oral manifestation of disseminated Mycobacterium avium intracellulare in a patient with AIDS, by F. Volpe, et al. ORAL SURGERY, ORAL MEDICINE, ORAL PATHOLOLOGY 60(6):567-570, December 1985.

Oral viral lesion (hairy leukplakia) associated with acquired immunodeficiency syndrome. JAMA 254:1694, October 4, 1985; also in MMWR 34(36):549-550, September 13, 1985.

Oral viral leukoplakea—a new AIDS-associated condition, by J. S. Greenspan, et al. ADVANCES IN EXPERIMENTAL MEDICINE AND BIOLOGY 187:123-128, 1985.

Orbital Brukitt's lymphoma in a homosexual man with acquired immune deficiency, by H. L. Brooks, Jr., et al. ARCHIVES OF OPHTHALMOLOGY 102(10): 1533-1537, October 1984.

Organic brain syndrome in three cases of acquired immune deficiency syndrome, by E. Kermani, et al. COMPREHENSIVE PSYCHIATRY 25(3):294-297, May-June 1984.

Otolaryngologic and head and neck manifestations of acquired immunodificiency syndrome (AIDS), by D. C. Marcusen, et al. LARYNGOSCOPE 95(4):401-405, April 1985.

Overview of infectious diseases and other nonmalignant conditions in the ac-quired immune deficiency syndrome, by D. F. Busch. FRONTIERS OF RADIATION THERAPY AND ONCOLOGY 19:52-58, 1985.

Overwhelming mycobacteriosis in an immunodeficient homosexual, by J. S. Waxman, et al. MOUNT SINAI JOURNAL OF MEDICINE 50(1):19-21, January-February 1983.

Paraproteinemia in patients with acquired immunodeficiency syndrome (AIDS) or lymphadenopathy syndrome (LAS), by K. Heriot, et al. CLINICAL CHEMISTRY 31(7):1224-1226, July 1985.

Patient with opportunistic infections due to acquired immunodeficiency syndrome, by C. S. de Graaff, et al. NEDERLANDS TIJDSCHRIFT VOOR GENEESKUNDE 128(12):549-553, March 24, 1984.

Peripheral neuropathy of the inflammatory polyradiculoneuritis-type in immune disorders, evoking the acquired immunodeficiency syndrome [letter], by H. Dehen, et al. PRESSE MEDICALE 14(4):226, February 2, 1985.

Persistent generalized adenopathies in subjects at high risk of AIDS. Diagnostic and prognostic value of lymph node lesion syndromes. Apropos of 8 cases, by D. Canioni, et al. ARCHIVES D'ANATOMIE ET DE CYTOLOGIE PATHOLOGIQUES 33(3):129-139, 1985.

Phlegmonous gastritis associated with the acquired immunodeficiency syndrome/pre-acquired immunodeficiency syndrome, by R. E. Mittleman, et al. ARCHIVES OF PATHOLOGY AND LABORATORY MEDICINE 109(8):765-767, August 1985.

Plasmacytoma and the acquired immunodeficiency syndrome, by A. M. Israel, et al. ANNALS OF INTERNAL MEDICINE 99(5):635-636, November 1983.

Positive direct antiglobulin test associated with hyperglobulinemia in acquired immunodeficiency syndrome (AIDS), by P. T. Toy, et al. AMERICAN JOURNAL OF HEMATOLOGY 19(2):145-150, June 1985.

Precoccious thymic involution manifest by epithelial injury in the acquired immune deficiency syndrome, by T. A. Seemayer, et al. HUMAN PATHOLOGY 15(5): 469-474, May 1984.

Prevalence of neurologic abnormalities in AIDS patients. AMERICAN FAMILY PHYSICIAN 31:158, January 1985.

Primary Addison's disease in a patient with the acquired immunodeficiency syndrome by E E. Guenthner, et al. ANNALS OF INTERNAL MEDICINE 100(6): 847-848, June 1984.

Primary lymphoma of the brain associated with AIDS. A study of one case, by M. J. Payan, et al. ACTA NEUROPATHOLOGICA 64(1):78-80, 1984.

Primary lymphoma of the nervous system associated with acquired immune-deficiency syndrome [letter],by W. D. Snider, et al. NEW ENGLAND JOURNAL OF MEDICINE 308(1):45, January 6, 1983.

Primary malignant lymphoma of the brain in acquired immune deficiency syndrome [letter], by C. V. Reyes. ACTA CYTOLOGICA 29(1):85-86, January-February 1985.

Principal muco-cutaneous aspects encountered in AIDS, by O. Picard, et al. REVUE FRANCAISE DE TRANSFUSION ET IMMUNOHEMATOLOGIE 27(4):427-436, September 1984.

Problems raised by the treatment of Kaposi's sarcoma in subjects with AIDS, by H. Félix, et al. BULLETIN DE LA SOCIETE DE PATHOLOGIE EXOTIQUE ET DE SES FILLIALES 77(4, Part 2):592-598, 1984.

Progressive encephalopathy in children with acquired immune deficiency syndrome, by L. G. Epstein, et al. ANNALS OF NEUROLOGY 17(5):488-496, May 1985.

Pseudomembranous necrotizing bronchial aspergillosis. A variant of invasive aspergillosis in a patient with hemophilia and acquired immune deficiency syndrome, by N. K. Pervez, et al. AMERICAN REVIEW OF RESPIRATORY DISEASE 131(6):961-963, June 1985.

Psoriasis in acquired immunodeficiency syndrome—new aspects for an immuno-pathogenesis of psoriasis, by G. K. Steigleder, et al. ZEITSCHRIFT FUR HAUTKRANKHEITEN 60(24):1913-1914, December 15, 1985.

Pyogenic otorhinologic infections in acquired immune deficiency syndrome, by M. D. Poole, et al. ARCHIVES OF OTO-RHINO-LARYNGOLOGY 110(2):130-131, February 1984.

Pyrexia of undetermined origin, diarrhoea, and primary cerebral lymphoma associated with acquired immunodeficiency, by C. R. Shiach, et al. BRITISH MEDICAL JOURNAL 288(6415):449-450, February 11, 1984.

Recurrent infectious diseases and AIDS, by F. di Nola. MINERVA MEDICA 75(47-48):2847-2848, Decembr 15, 1984.

Recurrent Salmonella typhimurium bacteremia associated with the acquired immunodeficiency syndrome, by J. B. Glaser, et al. ANNALS OF INTERNAL MEDICINE 102(2):189-193, February 1985.

Renal disease and the acquired immunodeficiency syndrome [letter], by S. J. Bennett, et al. ANNALS OF INTERNAL MEDICINE 102(2):274-275, February 1985.

Renal disease in patients with AIDS: a clinicopathologic study, by M. H. Garden-swartz, et al. CLINICAL NEPHROLOGY 21(4):197-204, April 1984.

Replication of Epstein-Barr virus within the epithelial cells of oral "hairy" leuko-plakia, an AIDS-associated lesion, by J. S. Greenspan, et al. NEW ENGLAND JOURNAL OF MEDICINE 313(25):1564-1571, December 19, 1985.

Retroperitoneal nodal aplasia, asplenia, chylous effusion and lymphatic dysplasia: an acquired immunodeficiency syndrome?, by L. Carini, et al. LYMPHOLOGY 18(1):31-36, March 1985.

Ritodrine-responsive bullous pemphigoid in a patient with AIDS-related complex [letter],by P. M. Levy, et al. BRITISH JOURNAL OF DERMATOLOGY 114(5): 635-636, May 1986.

Salmonella infections in patients with acquired immunodeficiency syndrome, by S. Profeta, et al. ARCHIVES OF INTERNAL MEDICINE 145(4):670-672, April 1985.

—, by J. L. Jacobs, et al. ANNALS OF INTERNAL MEDICINE 102(2):186-188, February 1985.

Salmonella septicemia in acquired immunodeficiency syndrome [letter], by D. Fassin, et al. PRESSE MEDICALE 14(16):894, April 20, 1985.

Salmonella typhimurium aenteritis and bacteremia in the acquired immunodeficiency syndrome, by P. D. Smith, et al. ANNALS OF INTERNAL MEDICINE 102(2):207-209, February 1985.

Scrapie-associated fibrils and AIDS encephalopathy [letter],by P. H. Gibson. LANCET 2(8455):612-613, September 14, 1985.

—, by P. N. Goldwater, et al. LANCET 2(8467):1300, December 7, 1985.

Seborrheic dermatitis and acquired immunodeficiency syndrome [letter],by R. B. Skinner, Jr., et al. JOURNAL OF THE AMERICAN ACADEMY OF DERMA-TOLOGY 14(1):147-148, January 1986.

Seborrheic dermatitis and butterfly rash in AIDS [letter], by B. A. Eisenstat, et al. NEW ENGLAND JOURNAL OF MEDICINE 311(3):189, July 19, 1984.

Seborrheic dermatitis may signify AIDS in high-risk groups, by B. M. Mathes. AMERICAN FAMILY PHYSICIAN 33:263, March 1986.

Seborrheic-like dermatitis of acquired immunodeficiency syndrome. A clinico-pathologic study, by F. F. Soeprono, et al. JOURNAL OF THE AMERICAN ACADEMY OF DERMATOLOGY 14(2, Part 1):242-248, February 1986.

Secondary pulmonary alveolar proteinosis occurring in two patients with acquired immune deficiency syndrome, by F. L. Ruben, et al. AMERICAN JOURNAL OF MEDICINE 80(6):1187-1190, June 1986.

Severe hyponatremia after colonoscopy preparation in a patient with the acquired immune deficiency syndrome, by J. M. Salik, et al. AMERICAN JOURNAL OF GASTROENTEROLOGY 80(3):177-179, March 1985.

Shigella flexneri bacteraemia in a patient with acquired immune deficiency syndrome, by Y. Glupczynski, et al. ACTA CLINICA BELGICA 40(6):388-390, 1985.

Simultaneous occurrence of Pneumocystis carinii pneumonia, cytomegalovirus infection , Kaposi's sarcoma, and B-immunoblastic sarcoma in a homosexual man, by R. L. Brukes, et al. JAMA 253(23):3425-3428, June 21, 1985.

Sinusitis caused by Legionella pneumophila in a patient with the acquired immune deficiency syndrome, by G. Schlanger, et al. AMERICAN JOURNAL OF MEDICINE 77(5):957-960, November 1984.

Skin disease in homosexual patients with acquired immune deficiency syndrome (AIDS) and lesser forms of human T cell leukaemia virus (HTLV III) disease, by

C. F. Farthing, et al. CLINICAL AND EXPERIMENTAL DERMATOLOGY 10(1):3-12, January 1985.

Small bowel lymphoma associated with AIDS, by P. E. Collier. JOURNAL OF SURGERY AND ONCOLOGY 32(2):131-133, June 1986.

Small intestinal lymphoma in three patients with acquired immune deficiency syndrome, by J. J. Steinberg, et al. AMERICAN JOURNAL OF GASTROENTER-OLOGY 80(1):21026, January 1985.

Small noncleaved B cell Burkitt-like lymphoma with chromosome t(8;14) translocation and Epstein-Barr virus nuclear-associated antigen in a homosexual man with acquired immune deficiency syndrome, by J. M. Petersen, et al. AMERI-CAN JOURNAL OF MEDICINE 78(1):141-148, January 1985.

Specific gastrointestinal manifestations of a generalized cytomegalovirus infection in a patient with acquired immune deficiency syndrome, by A. Krämer, et al. DEUTSCHE MEDIZINISCHE WOCHENSCHRIFT 110(12):462-468, March 22, 1985.

Specific translocations characterize Burkitt's-like lymphoma of homosexual men with the aquired immunodeficiency syndrome, by R. S. Chaganti, et al. BLOOD 61(6):126-1268, June 1983.

Spectrum of central nervous system complications in homosexual men with acquired immune deficiency syndrome [letter], by S. D. Pitlik, et al. JOURNAL OF INFECTIOUS DISEASES 148(4):771-772, October 1983.

Spectrum of liver disease in the acquired immunodeficiency syndrome, by S. C. Gordon, et al. JOURNAL OF HEPATOLOGY 2(3):475-484, 1986.

Spectrum of morphologic changes of lymph nodes from patients with AIDS or AIDS-related complexes, by P. Rácz, et al. PROGRESS IN ALLERGY 37:81-181, 1986.

Spectrum of renal abnoramalities in acquired immune deficiency syndrome, by N. D. Vaziri, et al. JOURNAL OF THE NATIONAL MEDICAL ASSOCIATION 77(5):369-375, May 1985.

Spinal cord degeneration in AIDS, by L. Goldstick, et al. NEUROLOGY 35(1): 103-106, January 1985.

Spontaneous colonic perforation secondary to cytomegalovirus in a patient with acquired immune deficiency syndrome, by H. B. Kram, et al. CRITICAL CARE MEDICINE 12(5):469-471, May 1984.

Squamous cell carcinoma of the epiglottis in a homosexual man at risk for AIDS [letter], by M. M. Alhashimi, et al. JAMA 253(16):2366, April 26, 1985.

Streptococcus bovis bacteremia and acquired immunodeficiency syndrome [letter], by J. B. Glaser, et al. ANNALS OF INTERNAL MEDICINE 99(6):878, December 1983.

Structures resembling scrapie-associated fibrils in AIDS encephalopathy [letter],by P. N. Goldwater, et al. LANCET 2(8452):447-448, August 24, 1985.

535

Subacute encephalitis in acquired immune deficiency syndrome: a postmortem study, by S. L. Nielsen, et al. AMERICAN JOURNAL OF CLINICAL PATHOLOGY 82(6):678-682, December 1984.

Talcosis in AIDS victims? [letter] by D. Brauner, et al. AMERICAN JOURNAL OF CLINICAL PATHOLOGY 81(1):145, January 1984.

Testicular cancer in homosexual men with cellular immune deficiency: report of 2 cases, by C. J. Logothetis, et al. JOURNAL OF UROLOGY 133(3):484-486, March 1985.

Testicular toxoplasmosis in two men with the acquired immunodeficiency syndrome (AIDS), by M. Nistal, et al. ARCHIVES OF PATHOLOGY AND LABORATORY MEDICINE 110(8):744-746, August 1986.

Thirty-eight-year-old male with bilateral pulmonary infiltrates and the septic picture of fatal development [clinical conference]. REVISTA CLINICA ESPANOLA 177(9):459-467, December 1985.

Thirty-nine-year-old man with thrombocytopenia, cough, fever, and shaking chills [clinical conference]. NEW YORK STATE JOURNAL OF MEDICINE 85(1):27-33, January 1985.

Thoracic manifestations of the acquired immune deficiency syndrome, by H. I. Pass, et al. JOURNAL OF THORACIC AND CARDIOVASCULAR SURGERY 88(5, Part 1):654-658, November 1984.

Three fungal infections in an AIDS patient, by G. P. Holmes, et al. JOURNAL OF THE KENTUCKY MEDICAL ASSOCIATION 84(5):225-226, May 1986.

Thymic dysplasia in acquired immunodeficiency syndome [letter], by R. Elfie, et al. NEW ENGLAND JOURNAL OF MEDICINE 308(14):841-842, April 7, 1983.

Thymus fragment transplantation in the acquired immunodeficiency syndrome [letter], by N. Ciobanu, et al. ANNALS OF INTERNAL MEDICINE 103(3):479, September 1985.

Thymus in AIDS [letter], by K. Welch. AMERICAN JOURNAL OF CLINICAL PATHOLOGY 85(4):531, April 1986.

Thymus involution in the acquired immunodeficiency syndrome, by W. W. Grody, et al. AMERICAN JOURNAL OF CLINICAL PATHOLOGY 84(1):85-95, July 1985.

Tinea faciale mimicking seborrheic dermatitis in a patient with AIDS, by C. Perniciaro, et al. NEW ENGLAND JOURNAL OF MEDICINE 314:315-316, January 30, 1986.

Tumor infiltrates in acquired immunodeficiency syndrome [letter], by A. J. Cochran, et al. LANCET 1(8321):416, February 19, 1983.

Tumorlike proliferation of 'granular histiocytes' in a lymph node, by D. Dharkar, et al. ULTRASTRUCTURAL PATHOLOGY 7(4):339-343, 1984.

Two cases of AIDS with florid Mycobacterium avium-intracellalare infection in the T-cell areas of the spleen [letter], by B. Seshi. HUMAN PATHOLOGY 16(9): 964-965, September 1985.

Unilateral cytomegalovirus retinochoroiditis and bilateral immunodeficiency syndrome, by M. M. Rodrigues, et al. OPHTHALMOLOGY 90(12):1577-1582, December 1983.

Unusual and newly recognized patterns of nontuberculous mycobacterial infection with emphasis on the immunocompromised host, by A. C. Chester, et al. PATHOLOGY ANNUAL 21(Part 1):251-270, 1986.

Unusual CT presentation of cerebral toxoplasmosis, by W. Cohen, et al. JOURNAL OF COMPUTER ASSISTED TOMOFRAPHY 9(2):384-386, March-April 1985.

Unusual diseases in homosexual men. AMERICAN FAMILY PHYSICIAN 26:249, September 1982.

Vacuolar myelopathy in patients with the acquired immunodeficiency syndrome [letter], by R. D. Kimbrough. NEW ENGLAND JOURNAL OF MEDICINE 313(13):827, September 26, 1985.

Vacuolar myelopathy pathologically resembling subacute combined degeneration in patients with the acquired immunodeficiency syndrome, by C. K. Petito, et al. NEW ENGLAND JOURNAL OF MEDICINE 312(14):874-879, April 4, 1985.

Variably acid-fast bacteria in vivo in a case of reactive lymph node hyperplasia occurring in a young male homosexual, by A. R. Cantwell, Jr. GROWTH 46(4: 331-336, Winter 1982.

Vasculitis in a suspected AIDS patient, by R. A. Berg, et al. SOUTHERN MEDICAL JOURNAL 79(7):914-915, July 1986.

Whipple-like disease in AIDS [letter], by C. D. Kooijman, et al. HISTOPATHOLOGY 8(4):705-708, July 1984.

Widespread cytomegalovirus gastroenterocolitis in a patient with acquired immunodeficiency syndrome, by A. B. Knapp, et al. GASTROENTEROLOGY 85(6):1399-1402, December 1983.

AFRICA

Acquired immunodeficiency syndrome and homozygote sickle cell anemia. Apropos of a Zairian case, by K. W. Izzia, et al. ANNALES DE LA SOCIETE BELGE DE MEDECINE TROPICALE 64(4):391-396, 1984.

AIDS and cryptococcosis (Zaire, 1977) [letter], by J. Vandepitte, et al. LANCET 1(8330):925-926, April 23, 1983.

Hepatitis B and AIDS in Africa [letter], by J. F. Cook. MEDICAL JOURNAL OF AUSTRALIA 142(12):661, June 10, 1985.

Multiple opportunistic infection due to AIDS in a previously healthy black woman from Zaire [letter], by G. Offenstadt, et al. NEW ENGLAND JOURNAL OF MEDICINE 308(13):775, March 31, 1983.

Squamous-cell carcinoma, Kaposi's sarcoma and Burkitt's lymphoma are consequences of impaired immune surveillance of ubiquitous viruses in acquired immune deficiency syndrome, allograft recipients and tropical African patients, by D. T. Purtilo, et al. IARC SCIENTIFIC PUBLICATIONS 63:749-770, 1984.

AUSTRALIA
AIDS and related conditions. One year's experience in St. Vincent's Hospital, Sydney, by A. B. Hill, et al. MEDICAL JOURNAL OF AUSTRALIA 141(9): 573-578, October 27, 1984.

HAITI
Acquired immunodeficiency syndrome with severe gastrointestinal manifestation in Haiti, by R. Malebranche, et al. LANCET 2(8355):873-878, October 15, 1983.

14q+ abnormality with probable t(8;14)(q24;q32) in a young Haitian immigrant with acquired immunodeficiency syndrome and concomitant Burkitt's-like lymphoma, by M. Gyger, et al. CANCER GENETICS AND CYTOGENETICS 17(4):283-288, August 1985.

SECONDARY LESIONS—BACTERIAL PNEUMONIA
Life-threatening bacterial pneumonia in male homosexuals with laboratory features of the acquired immunodeficiency syndrome, by S. White, et al. CHEST 87(4):486-488, April 1985.

SECONDARY LESIONS—DIAGNOSIS
Bronchoalveolar lavage and transbronchial biopsy for the diagnosis of pulmonary infections in the acquired immunodeficiency syndrome, by c. Broaddus, et al. ANNALS OF INTERNAL MEDICINE 102(5)Ú747-752, June 1985.

Bronchoalveolar lavage as the exclusive diagnosic modality for Pneumocystis carinii pneumonia. A prospective study among patients with acquired immunodeficiency syndrome, by J. A. Golden, et al. CHEST 90(1):18-22, July 1986.

CT biopsy of cerebral toxoplasmosis in AIDS, by B. A. Rodan, et al. JOURNAL OF THE FLORIDA MEDICAL ASSOCIATION 71(3):158-160, March 1984.

Cytologic diagnosis of Pneumocystis carinii infection by bronchoalveolar lavage in acquired immune deficiency syndrome, by M. Orenstein, et al. ACTA CYTOLOGICA 29(5):727-731, September-October 1985.

Diagnosis for interstitial lung disease in patients with acquired immunodeficiency syndrome (AIDS): a prospective comparison of bronchial washing, alveolar lavage, transbronchial lung biopsy, and open-lung biopsy, by R. J. McKenna, Jr., et al. ANNALS OF THORACIC SURGERY 41(3):318-321, March 1986.

Diagnosis of intracranial lesions in AIDS [letter], by I. C. Denton, Jr., et al. JAMA 253(23):3398, June 21, 1985.

Diagnosis of Pneumocystis carinii pneumonia in patients with the acquired immunodeficiency syndrome using subsegmental bronchoalveolar lavage, by F. P. Ognibene, et al. AMERICAN REVIEW OF RESPIRATORY DISEASE 129(6):929-932, June 1984.

Diagnosis of pulmonary complications of the acquired immune deficiency syndrome, by M. J. Rosen, et al. THORAX 40(8):571-575, August 1985.

Diagnosis of pulmonary disease in acquired immune deficiency syndrome (AIDS) [letter], by R. Kern, et al. AMERICAN REVIEW OF RESPIRATORY DISEASE 131(5):802-803, May 1985.

Diagnosis of pulmonary disease in acquired immune deficiency syndrome (AIDS). Role of bronchoscopy and bronchoalveolar lavage, by D. E. Stover, et al. AMERICAN REVIEW OF RESPIRATORY DISEASE 130(4):659-662, October 1984.

Diagnosis of Toxoplasma encephalitis in absence of neurological signs by early computerised tomographic scanning in patients with AIDS [letter], by R. Roué, et al. LANCET 2(8417-8418):1472, December 22, 1984.

Diagnostic utility of fiberoptic bronchoscopy in patients with Pneumocystis carinii pneumonia and the acquired immune deficiency syndrome, by D. L. Coleman,et al. AMERICAN REVIEW OF RESPIRATORY DISEASE 128(5):795-799, November 1983.

Electron microscopic diagnosis of cerebral toxoplasmosis. Case report, by L. Cerezo, et al. JOURNAL OF NEUROSURGERY 63(3):470-472, September 1985.

Evaluation of patients with the acquired immunodeficiency syndrome (AIDS) by fiberoptic bronchoscopy, by C. Harcup, et al. ENDOSCOPY 17(6):217-220, November 1985.

Multiple infections by cytomegalovirus in patients with acquired immunodeficiency syndrome: documentation by Southern blot hybridizatin, by W. L. Drew, et al. JOURNAL OF INFECTIOUS DISEASES 150(6):952-953, December 1984.

Percutaneous needle lung aspiration for diagnosing pneumonitis in the patient with acquired immunodeficiency syndrome (AIDS), by J. M. Wallace, et al. AMERICAN REVIEW OF RESPIRATORY DISEASE 131(3):389-392, March 1985.

Respiratory cryptosporidiosis in the acquired immune deficiency syndrome. Use of modified cold Kinyoun and Hemacolor stains for rapid diagnoses, by P. Ma, et al. JAMA 252(10):1298-1301, September 14, 1984.

GREAT BRITAIN
Early experience and difficulties with bronchoalveolar lavage and transbronchial biopsy in the diagnosis of AIDS associated pneumonia in Britain, by c. R. Swinburn, et al. THORAX 40(3):166-170, March 1985.

SECONDARY LESIONS—HEMOPHILIACS
Natural history of the AIDS related complex in hemophilia—relationships to Epstein Barr virus, by F. Gervais, et al. AIDS RESEARCH 1(3):197-209, 1983-1984.

SECONDARY LESIONS—HETEROSEXUALS
Unilateral cytomegalovirus retinochoroiditis and bilateral cytoid bodies in a bisexual man with the acquired immunodeficiency syndrome, by M. M.

Rodrigues, et al. OPHTHALMOLOGY 9(Suppl. 1):1577-1582, January 1984.

SECONDARY LESIONS—INTERSTITIAL PNEUMONIA

Lymphocytic interstitial pneumonia associated with the acquired immune deficiency syndrome, by M. H. Grieco, et al. AMERICAN REVIEW OF RESPIRATORY DISEASE 131(6)952-955, June 1985.

Lymphoid interstitial pneumonitis in acquired immunodeficiency syndrome-related complex, by P. Solal-Celigny, et al. AMERICAN REVIEW OF RESPIRATORY DISEASE 131(6):956-960, June 1985.

SECONDARY LESIONS—KAPOSI'S SARCOMA

Absence of Kaposi's sarcoma in hemophiliacs with the acquired immunodeficiency syndrome [letter], by D. I. Cohn, et al. ANNALS OF INTERNAL MEDICINE 101(3): 401, September 1984.

Acquired immune deficiency syndrome (AIDS) and disseminated Kaposi's sarcoma. A new infectious disease?, by C. E. Orfanos. HAUTARZT 34(7):319-321, July 1983.

Acquired immune deficiency syndrome, leading to opportunistic infections, Kaposi's sarcoma, and other malignancies, by P. W. Mansell. CRITICAL REVIEWS IN CLINICAL LABORATORY SCIENCES 20(3):191-204, 1984.

Acquired immune deficiency syndrome, opportunistic infections and Kaposi's sarcoma: epidemic of a new disease, by P. Francioli, et al. SCHWEIZERISCHE MEDIZINISCHE WOCHENSCHRIFT 113(26):938-942, July 2, 1983.

Acquired immune deficiency syndrome presenting as oral pharyngeal and cutaneous Kaposi's sarcoma, by B. L. NaPier, et al. LARYNGOSCOPE 93(11, Part 1):1466-1469, November 1983.

Acquired immunodeficiency syndrome (AIDS) and Kaposi's sarcoma, by J. Martin. INTERNATIONAL JOURNAL OF DERMATOLOGY 23(7):482-486, September 1984.

Acquired immunodeficiency syndrome (AIDS) with Kaposi's sarcoma in homosexuals in Argentina [letter], by M. E. Estevez, et al. MEDICINA 43(4):477, 1983.

Acquired immunodeficiency syndrome and Kaposi's sarcoma, by M. F. Muhlemann, et al. JOURNAL OF THE ROYAL SOCIETY OF MEDICINE 78(20:158-189, February 1985.

Acquired immunodeficiency syndrome in a drug addict with Kaposi's sarcoma and chronic hepatitis B [letter], by A. García Díez, et al. MEDICINA CLINICA 83(12):518, October 20, 1984.

Acquired immunodeficiency syndrome is an opportunistic infection and Kaposi's sarcoma results from secondary immune stimulation, by J. A. Levy, et al. LANCET 2(8341):78-81, July , 1983.

Acquired immunodeficiency syndrome, Kaposi's disease and cerebral toxoplasmosis in a young man. Review of the literature apropos of a case, by M.

Janier, et al. ANNALES DE DERMATOLOGIE ET DE VENEREOLOGIE 111(1):11-23, 1984.

Acquired immunodeficiency syndrome with Kaposi's sarcoma in Ireland, by F. N. O'Keeffe, et al. IRISH JOURNAL OF MEDICAL SCIENCE 152(9):353-356, September 1983.

Adenovirus and acquired immunodeficiency syndrome/Kaposi sarcoma [letter], by D. Ingrand, et al. PRESSE MEDICALE 12(46):2949, December 17, 1983.

AIDS and Kaposi's sarcoma, by M. A. Conant. CURRENT PROBLEMS IN DERMATOLOGY 13:92-108, 1985.

AIDS in a Haitian woman with cardiac Kaposi's sarcoma and Whipple's disease [letter], by B. Autram, et al. LANCET 1(8327):767-768, April 2, 1983.

AIDS, Kaposi's sarcoma and the dermatologist [editorial], by N. P. Smith. JOURNAL OF THE ROYAL SOCIETY OF MEDICINE 78(2):97-99, February 1958.

Analysis of T cell subsets in different clinical subgroups of patients with the acquired immune deficiency syndrome. Comparison with the 'classic' form of Kaposi's sarcoma, by A. Mittelman, et al. AMERICAN JOURNAL OF MEDICINE 78(6, Part 1):951-956, June 1985.

Atypical infections and Kaposi's sarcoma in AIDS—radiographic findings, by M. P. Federle. FRONTIERS OF RADIATION THERAPY AND ONCOLOGY 19:117-122, 1985.

Atypical mycobacteria and Kaposi's sarcoma in the same biopsy speciments [letter], by T. S. Croxson, et al. NEW ENGLAND JOURNAL OF MEDICINE 308(24):1476, June 16, 1983.

Basement membrane and connective tissue proteins in early lesions of Kaposi's sarcoma associated with AIDS, by R. H. Kramer, et al. JOURNAL OF INVESTIGATIVE DERMATOLOGY 84(6):516-520, June 1985.

Biology and therapy of Kaposi's sarcoma, by R. T. Mitsuyasu, et al. SEMINARS IN ONCOLOGY 11(10;53-59, March 1984.

Cardiac involvement by Kaposi's sarcoma in acquired immune deficiency syndrome (AIDS), by M. A. Silver, et al. AMERICAN JOURNAL OF CARDIOLOGY 53(7):983-985, March 15, 1984.

Changing biclonal gammopathy due to different lymphocyte clones in acquired immunodeficiency syndrome with Kaposi's sarcoma, by H. Piechowiak, et al. KLINISCHE WOCHENSCHRIFT 63(20):1083-1086, October 15, 1985.

Clinical features of Kaposi's sarcoma/acquired immune deficiency syndrome and its management, by B. Safai. ANTIBIOTIC CHEMOTHERAPY 32:54-70, 1983.

Cutaneous and lymphadenopathic Kaposi's sarcoma in Africa and the USA with observations on persistent lymphadenopathy in homosexual men at risk for the acquired immunodeficiency syndrome, by R. F. Dorfman. FRONTIERS OF RADIATION THERAPY AND ONCOLOGY 19:105-116, 1985.

541

Cytomegalovirus meningoencephalitis in a homosexual man with Kaposi's sarcoma: isolatin of CMV from CSF cells, by R. H. Edwards, et al. NEUROLOGY 35(4):560-562, April 1985.

Disseminated Kaposi's sarcoma associated with cytomegalic infection and systemic candidiasis in a male homosexual patient (acquired immunodeficiency syndrome), by E. Simó-Camps. MEDICINA CLINICA 83(19):807-811, December 8, 1984.

Disseminated Kaposi's sarcoma in pregnancy: a manifestation of acquired immune deficiency syndrome, by K. F. Rawlinson, et al. OBSTETRICS AND GYNECOLOGY 63(Suppl. 3):2S-6S, March 1984.

Disseminated Kaposi's-sarcoma within the framework of acquired immunodeficiency syndrome, by H. Mensing, et al. IMMUNITAT UND INFEKTION 12(5):253-255, October 1984.

Endemic Kaposi's sarcoma vs. Kaposi's sarcoma in AIDS: a brief communication, by J. A. Malliwah, et al. HIROSHIMA JOURNAL OF MEDICIAL SCIENCES 34(3):201-296, September 1985.

Epidemic Kaposi's sarcoma and opportunistic infections, by D. A. Cooper. MEDICAL JOURNAL OF AUSTRALIA 1(12):564-566, June 11, 1983.

Epidemic Kaposi's sarcoma: a manifestation of the acquired immune deficiency syndrome, by A. E. Friedman-Kien. JOURNAL OF DERMATOLOGIC SURGERY AND ONCOLOGY 9(8):637-640, August 1983.

Epidemic of acquired immune deficiency syndrome (AIDS) and Kaposi's sarcoma. First workshop of the European Study Group on AIDS/KS, Naples, June 25, 1983. ANTIBIOTICS AND CHEMOTHERAPY 32:1-164, 1983.

Expression of endothelial cell surface antigens by AIDS-associated Kaposi's sarcoma. Evidence for a vascular endothelial cell origin, by J. L. Rutgers, et al. AMERICAN JOURNAL OF PATHOLOGY 122(3):493-499, March 1986.

Extracorporeal perfusion of plasma over immobilized protein A in a patient with Kaposi's sarcoma and acquired immunodeficiency, by D. D. Kiprov, et al. JOURNAL OF BIOLOGICAL RESPONSE MODIFIERS 3(3):341-346, 1984.

Frequency and anatomic distribution of lymphadenopathic Kaposi's sarcoma in the acquired immunodeficiency syndrome: an autopsy series, by L. B. Moskowitz, et al. HUMAN PATHOLOGY 16(5):447-456, May 1985.

Gastrointestinal Kaposi's sarcoma in AIDS: radiographic manifestations, by S. D. Wall, et al. JOURNAL OF CLINICAL GASTROENTEROLOGY 6(2):165-171, April 1984.

Gastrointestinal Kaposi's sarcoma in patients with acquired immunodeficiency syndrome. Endoscopic and autopsy findings, by S. L. Friedman, et al. GASTROENTEROLOGY 89(1):102-108, July 1985.

Hematologic manifestations in homosexual men with Kaposi's sarcoma, by D. I. Abrams, et al. AMERICAN JOURNAL OF CLINICAL PATHOLOGY 81(1):13-18, January 1984.

Heterogeneity of epidemic Kaposi's sarcoma. Implications for therapy, by R. T. Mitsuyasu, et al. CANCER 57(Suppl. 8):1657-1661, April 15, 1986.

HLA studies in acquired immune deficiency syndrome patients with Kaposi's sarcoma, by H. E. Prince, et al. JOURNAL OF CLINICAL IMMUNOLOGY 4(3):242-245, May 1984.

Hypervascular follicular hyperplasia and Kaposi's sarcoma in patients at risk for AIDS [letter], by N. L. Harris. NEW ENGLAND JOURNAL OF MEDICINE 10(7):462-463, February 16, 1984.

Immunological variablies as predictors of prognosis in patients with Kaposi's sarcoma and the acquired immunodeficiency syndrome, by S. Vadhan-Raj, et al. CANCER RESEARCH 46(1):417-425, January 1986.

Incidence of Kaposi's sarcoma and mycosis fungoides in the United States including Puerto Rico, 1973-81, by R. J. Biggar, et al. JOURNAL OF THE NATIONAL CANCER INSTITUTE 73(1):89-94, July 1984.

Involvement of cytomegalovirus in acquired immune deficiency syndrome and Kaposi's sarcoma, by g. Giraldo, et al. PROGRESS IN ALLERGY 37:319-331, 1986.

Kaposi sarcoma and lymphadenopathy syndrome: limitations of abnominal CT in acquired immunodeficiency syndrome, by K. L. Moon, Jr., et al. RADIOLOGY 150(2):479-483, February 1984.

Kaposi sarcoma in acquired immune deficiency syndrome (AIDS). I: Clinical findings and laboratory diagnosis], by H. Weidauer, et al. LARYNGOLOGIE, RHINOLOGIE, OTOLOGIE 64(8):418-422, August 1985.

Kaposi's sarcoma—alpha-fetoprotein in amniotic fluid, by K. Shibusawa. KANGO 37(6):98-99, May 1985.

Kaposi's sarcoma among four different AIDS risk groups [letter],by D. C. De Jarlais, et al. NEW ENGLAND JOURNAL OF MEDICINE 310(17):119, April 26, 1984.

Kaposi's sarcoma—an acquired immunodeficiency syndrome, by J. A. Price, et al. OHIO STATE MEDICAL JOURNAL 80(2):143-145, February 1984.

Kaposi's sarcoma and acquired immune deficiency syndrome—the British experience, by N. P. Smith. ANTIBIOTIC CHEMOTHERAPY 32:71-75, 1983.

Kaposi's sarcoma and the acquired immunodeficiency syndrome [letter],by R. R. Bailey. NEW ZEALAND MEDICAL JOURNAL 97(748):50, January 25, 1984.

Kaposi's sarcoma and acquired immunodeficiency syndrome (AIDS), by I. Frydecka, et al. POLSKI TYGODNIK LEKARSKI 40(39):1109-1111, September 30, 1985.

Kaposi's sarcoma and the diagnosis of acquired immunodeficiency syndrome. Case report and brief review, by M. A Kielhofner, et al. MISSOURI MEDICINE 81(10):662-666, October 1984.

Kaposi's sarcoma and AIDS. AMERICAN FAMILY PHYSICIAN 30:268, October 1984.

—, by F. M. Muggia, et al. MEDIAL CLINICS OF NORTH AMERICA 70(1): 139-154, January 1986.

—, by H. Reich, et al. KLINISCHE MONATSBLATTER FUR AUGENHEIL-KUNDE 187(1):1-8, July 1985.

—, by W. Rozenbaum. BULLETIN DE LA SOCIETE DE PATHOLOGIE EXOTIQUE ET DE SES FILIALES 77(4, Part 2):589-591, 1984.

Kaposi's sarcoma and community-acquired immune deficiency syndrome, by E. Abemayor, et al. ARCHIVES OF OTOLARYNGOLOGY 109(8):536-542, August 1983.

Kaposi's sarcoma and fatal opportunistic infections in a homosexual man with immunodeficiency, by M. F. Prummel, et al. NEDERLANDS TIJDSCHRIFT VOOR GENEESKUNDE 127(19):820-824, May 7, 1983.

Kaposi's sarcoma and HTLV-III infection. Virus-like particles in skin lesions: experimental observations, by P. Cuneo Crovari, et al. BOLLETTINO DELL I ISTITUTO SIEROTERAPICO MILANESE 64(5):353-362, 1985.

Kaposi's sarcoma and immunoblastic sarcoma in the acquired immune deficiency syndrome [letter], by R. A. Figlin, et al. JAMA 251(3):342-343, January 20, 1984.

Kaposi's sarcoma and malignant lymphoma in AIDS, by H. J. Leu, et al. VIRCHOWS ARCHIV. A. PATHOLOGICAL ANATOMY AND HISTOPATHOL-OGY 903(2):205-212, 1984.

Kaposi's sarcoma and variably acid-fast bacteria in vivo in two homosexual men, by A. R. Cantwell, Jr. CUTIS 32(1):58-61+, July 1983.

Kaposi's sarcoma, aplastic pancytopenia, and multiple infections in a homosexual [letter], by W. Sterry, et al. LANCET 1(8330):924-925, April 23, 1983.

Kaposi's sarcoma causing pulmonary infiltrates and respiratory failure in the acquired immunodeficiency syndrome, by F. P. Ognibene, et al. ANNALS OF INTERNAL MEDICINE 102(4):471-475, April 1985.

Kaposi's sarcoma, chronic ulcerative herpes simplex, and acquired immunodeficiency, by W. I. Dotz, et al. ARCHIVES OF DERMATOLOGY 119(1):93-94, January 1983.

Kaposi's sarcoma: a comparison of classical, endemic, and epidemic forms, by J. L. Ziegler, et al. SEMINARS IN ONCOLOGY 11(1):47-52, March 1984.

Kaposi's sarcoma: gastrointestinal manifestations, by D. F. Altman. FRONTIERS OF RADIATION THERAPY AND ONCOLOGY 19:123-125, 1985.

Kaposi's sarcoma in the acquired immune deficiency syndrome, by W. Leslie, et al. MEDICAL PEDIATRICS AND ONCOLOGY 12(4):336-342, 1984.

Kaposi's sarcoma in acquired immune deficiency syndrome (AIDS), by N. D. F rancis, et al. JOURNAL OF CLINICAL PATHOLOGY 39(5):469-474, May 1986.

Kaposi's sarcoma in AIDS, by J. H. Dobloug, et al. TIDSSKRIFT FOR DEN NORSKE LAEGEFORENING 105(28):1964-1968, October 10, 1985.

Kaposi's sarcoma in the light of epidemiologic and immunologic studies, by B. Toruniowa, et al. WIADOMOSCI LEKARSKIE 37(19):1537-1543, October 1, 1984.

Kaposi's sarcoma in a patient with acquired immune deficiency syndrome, by G. B. Nickles, et al. JOURNAL OF ORAL AND MAXILLOFACIAL SURGERY 42(1):56-60, January 1984.

Kaposi's sarcoma in transfusion-associated AIDS [letter], by E. Vélez-García, et al. NEW ENGLAND JOURNAL OF MEDICINE 312(10):648, March 7, 1985.

Kaposi's sarcoma in young male homosexuals. Report of 2 cases, by V. Petri, et al. AMB 30(7-8):161-164, July-August 1984.

Kaposi's sarcoma: a new staging classification, by R. L. Krigel, et al. CANCER TREATMENT REPORTS 67(6):531-534, June 1983.

Kaposi's sarcoma of the head and neck in the acquired immune deficiency syndrome, by C. A. Patow, et al. OTOLARYNGOLOGY—HEAD AND NECK SURGERY 2(3):255-260, June 1984.

Kaposi's sarcoma of the skin and its relation to AIDS, by W. Meigel, et al. OFFENTLICHE GESUNDHEITSWESEN 46(10);519-521, October 1984.

Kaposi's sarcoma: an oncologic looking glass, by J. E. Groopman, et al. NATURE 299:103-104, September 9, 1982.

Kaposi's sarcoma presenting as homogeneous pulmonary infiltrates in a patient with acquired immunodeficiency syndrome, by L. Rucker, et al. WESTERN JOURNAL OF MEDICINE 142(6):831-833, June 1985.

Kaposi's sarcoma presenting as pulmonary disease in the acquired immunodeficiency syndrome:diagnosis by lung biopsy, by G. Nash, et al. HUMAN PATHOLOGY 15(10):999-1001, October 1984.

Kaposi's sarcoma, tuberculosis and Hodgkin's lymphoma in a lymph node—possible acquired immunodeficiency syndrome. A case report, by M. M. Hayes, et al. SOUTH AFRICAN MEDICAL JOURNAL 66(6):226-229, August 11, 1984.

Lymphadenopathic and oropharyngeal Kaposi's sarcoma in a drug addict with acquired immunodeficiency syndrome. Immunological abnormalities in peripheral blood and lymphoid tissue, by F. Facchetti, et al. APPLIED PATHOLOGY 2(2):103-109, 1984.

Malignant lymphoma presenting as Kaposi's sarcoma in a homosexual man with the acquired immunodeficiency syndrome, by S. E. Lind, et al. ANNALS OF INTERNAL MEDICINE 102(3):338-340, March 1985.

Minute foci of Kaposi's sarcoma in a patient with acquired immunodeficiency syndrome [letter], by S. H. Swerdlow, et al. ARCHIVES OF PATHOLOGY AND LABORATORY MEDICINE 109(2):106-107, Feburary 1985.

Multicentric angiofollicular lymph node hyperplasia (Castleman's disease) followed by Kaposi's sarcoma in two homosexual males with the acquired immunodeficiency syndrome (AIDS), by N. A. Lachant, et al. AMERICAN JOURNAL OF CLINICAL PATHOLOGY 83(1):27-33, January 1985.

Multicentric Kaposi's sarcoma of the conjunctiva in a male homosexual with the acquired immunodeficiency syndrome, by A. M. Macher, et al. OPHTHAL MOLOGY 90(8):879-884, August 1983.

National case-control study of Kaposi's sarcoma and Pneumocystis carinii pneumonia in homosexual men: Part I. Epidemiologic results, by H. W. Jaffe, et al. ANNALS OF INTERNAL MEDICINE 99(2):145151, August 1983.

—: Part 2. Laboratory results, by M. F. Rogers, et al. ANNALS OF INTERNAL MEDICINE 99(2):151-158, August 1983.

Natural history of Kaposi's sarcoma in the acquired immunodeficiency syndrome, by B. Safai, et al. ANNALS OF INTERNAL MEDICINE 103(5):744-750, November 1985.

Opportunistic infections and Kaposi's sarcoma among Haitians: evidence of a new acquired immunodeficiency state, by A. E. Pitchenik, et al. ANNALS OF INTERNAL MEDICINE 98(3):377-384, March 1983.

Oral Kaposi's sarcoma associated with acquired immunodeficiency syndrome among homosexual males, by L. R. Eversole, et al. JOURNAL OF THE AMERICAN DENTAL ASSOCIATION 107(2):248-253, August 1983.

Oral manifestations of tumor and opportunistic infections in the acquired immunodeficiency syndrome (AIDS): findings in 53 homosexual men with Kaposi's sarcoma, by F. Lozada, et al. ORAL SURGERY 56(5):491-494, November 1983.

Outbreak of an acquired immunodeficiency syndrome associated with opportunistic infections and Kaposi's sarcoma in male homosexuals: an epidemic with forensic implications, by M. L. Taff, et al. AMERICAN JOURNAL OF FORENSIC MEDICINE AND PATHOLOGY 3(3):259-264, September 1982.

Pharyngeal obstruction by Kaposi's sarcoma in a homosexual male with acquired immune deficiency syndrome, by C. A. Patow, et al. OTOLARYNGOLOGY AND HEAD AND NECK SURGERY 92(6):713-716, December 1984.

Prevalence of Kaposi's sarcoma among patients with AIDS [letter], by H. W. Haverkos, et al. NEW ENGLAND JOURNAL OF MEDICINE 312(23):1518, June 6,1985.

Problem of Kaposi's sarcoma in AIDS, by P. A. Volberding. FRONTIERS OF RADIATION THERAPY AND ONCOLOGY 19:91-98, 1985.

Prodrome, Kaposi sarcoma, and infections associated with acquired immunodeficiency syndrome: radiologic findings in 39 patients, by C. A. Hill, et al. RADIOLOGY 149(2):383-399, November 1983.

Prognostically significant classification of immune changes in AIDS with Kaposi's sarcoma, by J. Taylor, et al. BLOOD 67(3):666-671, March 1986.

Pulmonary Kaposi's sarcoma in the acquired immune deficiency syndrome. Clinical, radiographic, and pathologic manifestations, by G. U. Meduri, et al. AMERICAN JOURNAL OF MEDICINE 81(1):11-18, July 1986.

Regression of Kaposi's sarcoma in AIDS after treatment with dapsone [letter], by A. Poulsen, et al. LANCET 1(8376):560, March 10, 1984.

Retroviruses in Kaposi-sarcoma cells in AIDS [letter], by F. Gyorkey, et al. NEW ENGLAND JOURNAL OF MEDICINE 311(18):1183-1184, November 1, 1984.

Spectrum of Kaposi's sarcoma in the epidemic of AIDS, by B. Safai, et al. CANCER RESEARCH 45(Suppl. 9):4646s-4648s, September 1985.

Spontaneous regression of Kaposi's sarcoma in patients with AIDS [letter], by F. X. Real, et al. NEW ENGLAND JOURNAL OF MEDICINE 313(26):1659, December 26, 1985.

Spontaneously healing Kaposi's sarcoma in AIDS [letter], by M. Janier, et al. NEW ENGLAND JOURNAL OF MEDICINE 312(25):1638-1639, June 20, 1985.

Sporadic, endemic and AIDS-related Kaposi's sarcoma. Different clinical course variants of the tumor demonstrated by 3 typical cases, by H. Rasokat, et al. ZEITSCHRIFT FUR HAUTKRANKHEITEN 60(1-2):109-115, January 1985.

Therapy of Kaposi's sarcoma in AIDS, by P. Volberding. SEMINARS IN ONCOLOGY 11(1):60-70, March 1984.

Tubuloreticular structures in peripheral blood cells from patients with AIDS-associated Kaposi's sarcoma, by P. Schenk, et al. ARCHIVES OF DERMATOLOGICAL RESEARCH 278(3):249-251, 1986.

Ultrastructural morphology and histogenesis of Kaposi sarcoma in AIDS, by H. J. Leu. VASA 13(2):107-113, 1984.

Ultrastructure of Kaposi's sarcoma in acquired immune deficiency syndrome (AIDS), by P. Schenk, et al. ARCHIVES OF OTORHINOLARYNGOLOGY 242(3):305-313, 1985.

Upper airway obstruction secondary to acquired immunodeficiency syndrome-related Kaposi's sarcoma, by J. E. Greenberg, et al. CHEST 88(4):638-640, October 1985.

Vincristine and Kaposi's sarcoma in the acquired immunodeficiency syndrome [letter], by E. Rieber, et al. ANNALS OF INTERNAL MEDICINE 101(6):876, December 1984.

Viral infections and cell-mediated immunity in immunodeficient homosexual men with Kaposi's sarcoma treated with human lymphoblastoid interferon, by W. R. Frederick, et al. JOURNAL OF INFECTIOUS DISEASES 152(1):162-170, July1 985.

547

What's new: acquired immunodeficiency syndrome (AIDS) and Kaposi's sarcoma, by H. L. Lucia. TEXAS MEDICINE 79(6):39-40, June 1983.

AFRICA
African 'eosinophilic bodies' in vivo in two American men with Kaposi's sarcoma and AIDS, by A. . Cantwell, Jr., et al. JOURNAL OF DERMATOLOGIC SURGERY AND ONCOLOGY 11(4):408-412, April 1985.

African Kaposi's sarcoma and AIDS, by R. G. Downing, et al. LANCET 1(8375):478-480, March 3, 1984.

AIDS associated Kaposi's sarcoma in Africa [letter], by K. H. Marquart. BRITISH MEDICAL JOURNAL 292(6518):484, February 15, 1986.

Is AIDS an epidemic form of African Kaposi's sarcoma? Discussion paper, by J. Weber. JOURNAL OF THE ROYAL SOCIETY OF MEDICINE 77(7): 572-576, July 1984.

Kaposi's sarcoma associated with AIDS in a woman from Uganda [letter], by D. Edwards, et al. LANCET 1(8377):631-632, March 17, 1984.

Kaposi's sarcoma in Burundi and the Central Arican Republic in the framework of acquired immunodeficiency syndrome (AIDS), by R. Laroche, et al. MEDECINE TROPICALE 46(2):121-129, April-June 1986.

GREAT BRITAIN
Kaposi's sarcoma/AIDS surveillance in the UK [letter], by B. H. O.Connor, et al. LANCET 1(8329):872, April 16, 1983.

UNITED STATES
African 'eosinophilic bodies' in vivo in two American men with Kaposi's sarcoma and AIDS, by A. . Cantwell, Jr., et al. JOURNAL OF DERMATOLOGIC SURGERY AND ONCOLOGY 11(4):408-412, April 1985.

Kaposi's sarcoma in Los Angeles, California, by R. K. Ross, et al. JOURNAL OF THE NATIONAL CANCER INSTITUTE 75(6):1011-1015, December 1985.

SECONDARY LESIONS—KAPOSI'S SARCOMA—DIAGNOSIS
Kaposi's sarcoma: immunoperoxidase staining for cytomegalovirus, by J. Civantos, et al. AIDS RESEARCH 1(2):121-125, 1983-1984.

SECONDARY LESIONS—KAPOSI'S SARCOMA—ETIOLOGY
Speculations on the viral etiology of acquired immune deficiency syndrome and Kaposi's sarcoma, by M. A. Conant. JOURNAL OF INVESTIGATIVE DERMATOLOGY 83(Supl. 1):57s-62s, July 1984.

SECONDARY LESIONS—KAPOSI'S SARCOMA—INFANTS
Kaposi sarcoma in two infants with acquired immune deficiency syndrome, by B. E. Buck, et al. JOURNAL OF PEDIATRICS 103(6):911-913, December 1983.

SECONDARY LESIONS—KAPOSI'S SARCOMA—TRANSMISSION
Polymicrobial cholangitis and Kaposi's sarcoma in blood product transfusion-related acquired immune deficiency syndrome, by f. R. Cockerill, 3d, et al. AMERICAN JOURNAL OF MEDICINE 80(6):1237-1241, June 1986.

Alpha interferon therapy of Kaposi's sarcoma in AIDS, by P. Volberding, et al. AN-NALS OF THE NEW YORK ACADEMY OF SCIENCES 437:439-446, 1984.

Dapsone for AIDS-associated Kaposi's sarcoma [letter], by G. J. Hruza, et al. LANCET 1(8429):642, March 16, 1985.

Initial observations of the effect of radiotherapy on epidemic Kaposi's sarcoma, by J. S. Cooper, et al. JAMA 252(7):934-935, August 17, 1984.

Interferon-induced 2'-5' oligoadenylate synthetase during interferon-alpha therapy in homosexual men with Kaposi's sarcoma: marked deficiency in biochemical response to interferon in patients with acquired imunodeficiency syndrome, by O. T. Preble, et al. JOURNAL OF INFECTIOUS DISEASES 152(3):457-465, September 1985.

Interferon may help some AIDS patients with Kaposi's sarcoma, researchers re-port. PUBLIC HEALTH REPORTS 98(3):228, May-June 1983.

Interferons and other biological response modifiers in the treatment of Kaposi's sarcoma, by S. E. Krown, et al. FRONTIERS OF RADIATION THERAPY AND ONCOLOGY 19:138-149, 1985.

Kaposi's sarcoma and the acquired immune deficiency syndrome. Treatment with recombinant interferon alpha and analysis of prognostic factors, by S. E. Krown, et al. CANCER 57(Suppl. 8):1662-1665, April 15, 1986.

Kaposi's sarcoma in AIDS: the role of radiation therapy, by J. W. Harris, et al. FRONTIERS OF RADIATION THERAPY AND ONCOLOGY 19:126-132, 1985.

Radiation therapy of Kaposi's sarcoma in AIDS. Memorial Sloan-Kettering experi-ence, by L. Z. Nisce, et al. FRONTIERS OF RADIATION THERAPY AND ON-COLOGY 19:133-137, 1985.

Radiotherapy for AIDS-related Kaposi's sarcoma. AMERICAN FAMILY PHYSI-CIAN 31:245-246, April 1985.

Recombinant alpha-2 interferon therapy for Kaposi's sarcoma associated with the acquired immunodeficiency syndrome, by J. E. Groopman, et al. ANNALS OF INTERNAL MEDICINE 100(5):671-676, May 1984.

Recombinant interferon alpha in the treatment of acquired immune deficiency syndrome-related Kaposi's sarcoma, by P. A. Volberding, et al. SEMINARS IN ONCOLOGY 12(4, Suppl. 5):2-6, December 1985.

Treatment of acquired immunodeficiency syndrome-related Kaposi's sarcoma with lymphoblastoid interferon, by A. Rios, et al. JOURNAL OF CLINICAL ONCOLOGY 3(4):506-512, April 1985.

Treatment of Kaposi's sarcoma and thrombocytopenia with vincristine in patients with the acquired immunodeficiency syndrome, by D. M. Mintzer, et al. ANNALS OF INTERNAL MEDICINE 102(2):200-202, February 1985.

Vinblastine therapy fo Kaposi's sarcoma in the acquired immunodeficiency syn-drome, by P. A. Volberding, et al. ANNALS OF INTERNAL MEDICINE 103(3):335-338, September 1985.

Kaposi's sarcoma and T-cell lymphoma in an immunodeficienct woman: a case report, by M. T. Sabatini, et al. AIDS RESEARCH 1(2):135-137, 1983-1984.

SECONDARY LESIONS—LEUKOENCEPHALOPATHY
Progressive multifocal leukoencephalopathy in acquired immune deficiency syndrome, by L. W. Blum, et al. ARCHIVES OF NEUROLOGY 42(2):137-139, February 1985.

Progressive multifocal leukoencephalopathy in a case of acquired immune deficiency syndrome, by J. D. Speelman, et al. CLINICAL NEUROLOGY AND NEUROSURGERY 87(1):27-33, 1985.

Progressive multifocal leukoencephalopathy in a patient with acquired immune deficiency syndrome, by C. Bernick, et al. ARCHIVES OF NEUROLOGY 41(7):780-   782, July 1984.

—, by M. Morente Gallego, et al. MEDICINA CLINICA 83(16):680-682, November 17, 1984.

Progressive multifocal leukoencephalopathy occurring with the acquired immune deficiency syndrome, by J. D. England, et al. SOUTHERN MEDICAL JOURNAL 77(8):1041-1043, August 1984.

SECONDARY LESIONS—PNEUMOCYSTIS CARINII PNEUMONIA
Bedside bronchoalveolar lavage for the diagnosis of Pneumocystis carinii pneumonia in patients with the acquired immunodeficiency syndrome, by G. R. Flick, et al. AIDS RESEARCH 2(1):31-41, February 1986.

Bronchoalveolar lavage as the exclusive diagnosic modality for Pneumocystis carinii pneumonia. A prospective study among patients with acquired immuno-deficiency syndrome, by J. A. Golden, et al. chest 90(1):18-22, July 1986.

Case of acquired immune deficiency syndrome (AIDS) with Pneumocystis carinii pneumonia, by A. B. Adams, et al. RESPIRATORY CARE 29(1):50-53, January 1984.

Gallium-67 scintigraphy in acquired immune deficiency syndrome complicated by Pneumocystis carinii pneumonia, by F. R. Graybeal, Jr., et al. CLINICAL NUCLEAR MEDICINE 10(9):669-670, September 1985.

Humoral responses to Pneumocystis carinii in patients with acquired immuno-deficiency syndrome and in immunocompromised homosexual men, by B. Hofmann, et al. JOURNAL OF INFECTIOUS DISEASES 152(4):838-840, October 1985.

National case-control study of Kaposi's sarcoma and Pneumocystis carinii pneumonia in homosexual men: Part I. Epidemiologic results, by H. W. Jaffe, et al. ANNALS OF INTERNAL MEDICINE 99(2):145151, August 1983.

—: Part 2. Laboratory results, by M. F. Rogers, et al. ANNALS OF INTERNAL MEDICINE 99(2):151-158, August 1983.

Persistence of Pneumocystis carinii in lung tissue of acquired immunodeficiency syndrome patients treated for pneumocystis pneumonia, by J. H. Shelhamer, et al. AMERICAN REVIEW OF RESPIRATORY DISEASE 130(6): 1161-1165, December 1984.

Persistence of Pneumosystis carinii pneumonia in the acquired immunodeficiency syndrome. Evaluation of therapy by follow-up transbronchial lung biopsy, by L. J. deLorenzo, et al. CHEST 88(1):79-83, July 1985.

Pneumocystis carinii infection in a homosexual adult subject with immunodeficiency : apropos of a case, by F. L. Goncales Júnior, et al. REVISTA PAULISTA DE MEDICINA 101(4):160-164, July-August 1983.

Pneumocystis carinii: a misunderstood opportunist, by L. L. Pifer. EUROPEAN JOURNAL OF CLINICAL MICROBIOLOGY 3(3):169-173, June 1984.

Pneumocystis carinii pneumonia, by C. B. Wofsy. FRONTIERS OF RADIATION THERAPY AND ONCOLOGY 19:74-81, 1985.

Pneumocystis carinii pneumonia and disseminated cytomegalovirus infection in previously healthy bisexual man, by G. F. Ragalie, et al. WISCONSIN MEDICAL JOURNAL 82(11):10-14, November 1983.

Pneumocystis carinii pneumonia: a comparison between patients with the acquired immunodeficiency syndrome and patients with other immunodeficiencies, by J. A. Kovacs, et al. ANNALS OF INTERNAL MEDICINE 100(5): 663-6672, May 1984.

Pneumocystis carinii pneumonia in the acquired immune deficiency syndrome: response to inadvertent steroid therapy, by d. K. MacFadden, et al. CANADIAN MEDICAL ASSOCIATION JOURNAL 132(10):1161-1163, May 15, 1985.

Pneumocystis carinii pneumonia in the acquired immunodeficiency syndrome (AIDS). Diagnosis with bronchial brushings, biopsy, and bronchoalveolar lavage, by B. Hartman, et al. CHEST 87(5):603-607, May 1985.

Pneumocystis carinii pneumonia in homosexual males with AIDS, by L. Bergmann, et al. PRAXIS UND KLINIK DER PNEUMOLOGIE 37(Suppl. 1):1035-1038, October 1983.

Pneumocystis carinii pneumonia in the patient with AIDS, by J. R. Catterall, et al. CHEST 88(5):758-762, November 1985.

Pneumocystis carinii pneumonia treated with alpha-difluoromethylornithine. A prospective study among patients with the acquired immunodeficiency syndrome, by J. A. Golden, et al. WESTERN JOURNAL OF MEDICINE 141(5): 613-623, November 1984.

Pneumocystis pneumonia and disseminated toxoplasmosis in a male homosexual, by W. R. Gransden, et al. BRITISH MEDICAL JOURNAL 286(6378): 1614, May 21, 1983.

Pneumocystis pneumonia as an expression of acquired immune deficiency (AIDS) in homosexual men, by P. Stark, et al. PRAXIS UND KLINIK DER PNEUMOLOGIE 38(1):26-28, January 1984.

Pneumonia due to Pneumocystis carinii in AIDS patients, by V. G. Pereira, et al. REVISTA DO HOSPITAL DAS CLINICAS; FACULDADE DE MEDICINA DA UNIVERSIDADE DE SAO PAULO 39(3):123-125, May-June 1984.

Prognosis of Pneumocystis carinii pneumonia in the acquired immunodeficiency syndrome [letter], by M. J. Rosen, et al. ANNALS OF INTERNAL MEDICINE 101(2);276, August 1984.

SECONDARY LESIONS—PNEUMOCYSTIS CARINII PNEUMONIA—DIAGNOSIS
Pneumocystis with normal chest X-ray film and arterial oxygen tension. Early diagnosis in a patient with the acquired immune deficiency syndrome, by J. L. Good- man, et al. ARCHIVES OF INTERNAL MEDICINE 143(10):1981-1982, October 1983.

Role of bronchial brush biopsy in AIDS with Pneumocystis carinii pneumonia [letter], by T. K. Sarkar, et al. CHEST 87(4):553-554, April 1985.

Serodiagnosis of Pneumocystis carinii [letter] by L. L. Pifer. CHEST 87(5):698-700, May 1985.

SECONDARY LESIONS—PNEUMOCYSTIS CARINII PNEUMONIA—TREATMENT
Complications of co-trimoxazole in treatment of AIDS-associated Pneumocystis carinii pneumonia in homosexual men, by H. S. Jaffe, et al. LANCET 2(8359):

Pentamidine treatment of Pneumocystis carinii pneumonia in the acquired immunodeficiency syndrome. Association with acute renal failure and myoglobinuria, by J. W. Sensakovic, et al. ARCHIVES OF INTERNAL MEDICINE 145(12):2247, December 1985.

Successful treatment of Pneumocystis carinii pneumonia with trimethoprim-sulfamethoxazole in hypersensitive AIDS patients, by R. B. Gibbons, et al. JAMA 253:1259-1260, March 1,1985.

Treatment of Pneumocystis carinii pneumonia in the acquired immunodeficiency syndrome, by C. B. Small, et al. ARCHIVES OF INTERNAL MEDICINE 145(5):837-840, May 1985.

SECONDARY LESIONS—PNEUMONIA
Management of AIDS pneumonia, by A. L. Pozniak, et al. BRITISH JOURNAL OF DISEASES OF THE CHEST 79(2):105-114, April 1985.

Management of opportunistic pneumonia in AIDS, by A. s. Teirstein, et al. ANNALS OF THE NEW YORK ACADEMY OF SCIENCES 437:461-465, 1984.

Pneumonia in the acquired immune deficiency syndrome [editorial], by N. M. Johnson. BRITISH MEDICAL JOURNAL 290(678):1299-1301, May 4, 1985.

Pneumonia in AIDS patients. AMERICAN FAMILY PHYSICIAN 33:266, January 1986.

Streptococcus pneumoniae infections and bacteremia in patients with acquired immune deficiency syndrome, with report of a pneumococcal vaccine failure, by M. S. Simberkoff, et al. AMERICAN REVIEW OF RESPIRATORY DISEASE 130(6):1174-1176, December 1984.

Pulmonary cell populations in the immunosuppressed patient. Bronchoalveolar lavage findings during episodes of pneumonitis, by D. A. White, et al. CHEST 88(3):352-359, September 1985.

SECONDARY LESIONS—PREVENTION
Tetanus prophylaxis in AIDS patients, by R. T. Chen, et al. JAMA 255:1061, February 28, 1986.

SECONDARY LESIONS—PULMONARY
Pulmonary complications of the acquired immunodeficiency syndrome: a clinico-pathologic study of 70 cases, by A. Marchevsky, et al. HUMAN PATHOLOGY 16(7):659-670 July 1985.

Pulmonary complications of AIDS. AMERICAN FAMILY PHYSICIAN 31:215, March 1985.

Pulmonary complications of AIDS [letter], by J. R. Masci, et al. NEW ENGLAND JOURNAL OF MEDICINE 311(18):1182-1183, November 1, 1984.

Pulmonary complications of AIDS. Evaluating the tests [editorial], by J. Glassroth. CHEST 87(5):562-563, May 1985.

Pulmonary complications of AIDS: radiologic features, by B. A. Cohen, et al. AJR 143(1):115-122, July 1984.

Pulmonary cryptosporidiosis in acquired immune deficiency syndrome, by E. M. Brady, et al. JAMA 252:89-90, July 6, 1984.

Pulmonary disease in the acquired immune deficiency syndrome, by M. S. Gottlieb. CHEST 86(Suppl 3):29S-31S, September 1984.

Pulmonary involvement in the acquired immunodeficiency syndrome, by P. C. Hopewell, et al. CHEST 87(1):104-112, January 1985.

Pulmonary involvement in AIDS. Postmortem study of 50 cases, by E. Lam-poureux, et al. ARCHIVES D'ANATOMIE ET DE CYTOLOGIE PATHOLO-GIQUES 34(1):12-16, 1986.

Pulmonary manifestations of the acquired immunodeficiency syndrome (AIDS), by C. M. Wollschlager, et al. CHEST 85(2):197-202, February 1984.

—, by H. C. Hu, et al. CHUNG-HUA CHIEH HO HO HU HSI HSI CHI PING TSA CHIH 8(6):364-366, December 1985.

Radiographic features in patients with pulmonary manifestations of the acquired immune deficiency syndrome, by C. W. Heron, et al. CLINICAL RADIOLOGY 36(6):583-588, November 1985.

Spectrum of pulmonary diseases associated with the acquired immune deficiency syndrome, by D. E. Stover, et al. AMERICAN JOURNAL OF MEDICINE 78(3): 429-437, March 1985.

Thirty-two-year-old AIDs patient with progressive pulmonary infiltrates [clinical conference], by A. White, et al. INDIANA MEDICINE 78(10):884-890, October 1985.

Unusual pulmonary infection in a puzzling presentation of AIDS [letter], by J. M. Tourani, et al. LANCET 1(8435):989, April 27, 1985.

SECONDARY LESIONS—PULMONARY—DIAGNOSIS
Use of the transbronchial biopsy for diagnosis of opportunistic pulmonary infections in acquired immunodeficiency syndrome (AIDS), by W. Blumfeld, et al. AMERICAN JOURNAL OF CLINICAL PATHOLOGY 8(1):1-5, January 1984.

SECONDARY LESIONS—TOXOPLASMOSIS
Toxoplasma encephalitis in acquired immunodeficiency syndrome by A. Vital, et al. ANNALS OF PATHOLOGY 4(1):80-82, January-March 1984.

Toxoplasma encephalitis in Haitian adults with acquired immunodeficiency syndrome: a clinical-pathologic-CT correlation, by M. J. Post, et al. AJR 140(5):861-868, May 1983.

Toxoplasmic encephalitis in patients with acquired immune deficiency syndrome, by B. J. Luft, et al. JAMA 252(7):913-917, August 17, 1984.

Toxoplasmosis. Immunohistochemical study of a case of acquired toxoplasmosis in a patient with AIDS and of a case of congenital toxoplasmosis, by C. Herbert, et al. REVUE MEDICALE DE LA SUISSE ROMANDE 105(1):89-100, January 1985.

Toxoplasmosis and AIDS. AMERICAN FAMILY PHYSICIAN 31:345, February 1985.

Toxoplasmosis diagnosis and immunodeficiency [editorial]. LANCET 1(8377): 605-606, March 17, 1984.

Toxoplasmosis encephalitis in patients with AIDS, by W. Enzensberger, et al. DEUTSCHE MEDIZINISCHE WOCHENSCHRIFT 110(3):83-87, January 18, 1985.

Toxoplasmosis in immunosuppression and AIDS, by B. Velimirovic. INFECTION 12(5):315-317, September-October 1984.

Toxoplasmosis presenting as panhypopituitarism in a patient with the acquired immune deficiency syndrome, by S. A. Milligan, et al. AMERICAN JOURNAL OF MEDICINE 77(4):760-764, October 1984.

SECONDARY LESIONS—TREATMENT
Care of pentamadine ulcers in AIDS patients, by J. R. Gottlieb, et al. PLASTIC AND RECONSTRUCTIVE SURGERY 76(4):630-632, October 1985.

Immunotherapy and therapy of complications of AIDS, by H. Masur. TOPICS IN CLINICAL NURSING 6(2):53-60, July 1984.

9-(1,3 Dinydroxy-2-propoxymethyl)quanine for cytomegalovirus infections in patients with the acquired immunodeficiency syndrome, by M. C. Bach, et al. ANNALS OF INTERNAL MEDICINE 103(3):381-382, September 1985.

Pentamidine isethionate approved for P. Carinii pneumonia. FDA DRUG BULLETIN 14(3):25-26, December 1984.

Problems in the therapy of AIDS-associated malignancies, by R. E. Wittes, et al. ANNALS OF THE NEW YORK ACADEMY OF SCIENCES 437:454-460, 1984.

Treatment of opportunistic infections in AIDS, by S. Staszewski, et al. MUENCH-ENER MEDIZINISCHE WOCHENSCHRIFT 125(39):841-844, September 30, 1983.

Treatment of serious cytomegalovirus infections with 9-(1,3-dihydroxy-2-propoxymethyl)guanine in patients with AIDS and other immunodeficiencies, by the Collaborative DHPG Treatment Study Group. NEW ENGLAND JOURNAL OF MEDICINE 314(13):801-805, March 27, 1986.

Update: treatment of cryptosporidiosis in patients with acquired immunodeficiency syndrome (AIDS). MMWR 33(9):117-119, March 9, 1984.

SECONDARY LESIONS—TUBERCULOSIS
Tuberculosis as a manifestation of the acquired immunodeficiency syndrome (AIDS), by G. Sunderam, et al. JAMA 256(3):362-366, July 18, 1986.

Tuberculosis—United States, 1985—and possible impact of human T-I Lymphotropic virus type III/lymphadenopathy-associated virus infection. JAMA 255:1010+, February 28, 1986.

Tuberculous brain abscess and Toxoplasma encephalitis in a patient with the acquired immunodeficiency syndrome, by M. A. Fischl, et al. JAMA 253(23):3428-3430, June 21, 1985.

SECONDARY LESIONS—TUBERCULOSIS—HAITIANS
Tuberculosis, atypical mycobacteriosis, and the acquired immunodeficiency syndrome among Haitian and non-Haitian patients in south Florida, by A. E. Pitchenik, et al. ANNALS OF INTERNAL MEDICINE 101(5):641-645, November 1984.

SEMEN
HTLV-III in cells cultured from semen of two patients with AIDS, by D. Zagury, et al. SCIENCE 226(4673):449-451, October 26, 1984.

HTLV/III in the semen and blood of a healthy homosexual man, by D. D. Ho, et al. SCIENCE 226(4673):451-453, October 26, 1984.

SEX
AIDS and promiscuity, by R. Royal. GAY COMMUNITY NEWS 11(5):6, August 13, 1983.

AIDS and prostitutes [letter], by D. A. Cooper, et al. MEDICAL JOURNAL OF AUSTRALIA 145(1):55, July 7, 1986.

AIDS and sexual behavior reported by gay men in San Francisco, by L. McKusick, et al. AMERICAN JOURNAL OF PUBLIC HEALTH 75(5):493-496, May 1985.

AIDS (and STD) prophylaxis: urgent need for an effective genital antiseptic [letter], by A. Comfort. JOURNAL OF THE ROYAL SOCIETY OF MEDICINE 79(5):311-312, May 1986.

AIDS, condoms, and gay abandon [letter], by C. J. Mitchell. MEDICAL JOURNAL OF AUSTRALIA 142(11):617, May 27, 1985.

AIDS epidemic: the price of promiscuity. HUMAN EVENTS 43:5+, June 18, 1983.

AIDS fear is leading to safer sex, expert says [views of Dr. L. Edwards]. JET 68:5, September 2, 1985.

AIDS found in female prostitute. RN 46:15, April 1983.

AIDS goes hetero, by M. Castleman. MEDICAL SELF CARE 30:18, September 1985.

AIDS goes straight, by N. Fain. VILLAGE VOICE 30:30-31, May 14, 1985.

AIDS hygiene: practices and precautions, by D. Bille. ADVOCATE 421:34, May 28, 1985.

AIDS: a nurse's responsibility. Safe sex guidelines for women. CALIFORNIA NURSE 82(4):8, May 1986.

AIDS: "safer sex" is the best solution so far, by M. Jay. NEW SOCIETY December 12, 1985, p. 12-13.

Are you ready to die for sexual lib, by C. Shively. FAG RAG 40:1, 1983.

Aspects of anal sexual practices, by J. Agnew. JOURNAL OF HOMOSEXUALITY 12(1):75, Fall 1985.

Can sex survive AIDS?, by Arthur Kretchmer. PLAYBOY 33:48+, February 1986.

CDC bans "explicit sex" from AIDS education, by K. Westheimer. GAY COM- MUNITY NEWS 13(26):1, January 18, 1986.

CDC: "Hands off safe sex," by J. Irving. GAY COMMUNITY NEWS 13(31):2, February 15, 1986.

Changes in sexual behaviour and fear of AIDS [letter], by M. T. Schechter, et al. LANCET 1(8389):1293, June 9, 1984.

Cluster of cases of the acquired immune deficiency syndrome. Patients linked by sexual contact, by D. M. Auerbach, et al. AMERICAN JOURNAL OF MEDI- CINE 76(3):487-492, March 1984.

Condom mania! Sex sensation sweeping the nation, by C. Wittke. GAY COM- MUNITY NEWS 13(37):6, April 1, 1986.

Condoms, by K. Orr. BODY POLITIC 109:31, December 1984.

Condoms help stop AIDS. BODY POLITIC 123:23, February 1986.

Condoms prevent transmission of AIDS-associated retrovirus [letter], by M. Conant, et al. JAMA 255(13):1706, April 4, 1986.

Decreased helper T lymphocytes in homosexual men. I. Sexual contact in high-incidence areas for the acquired immunodeficiency syndrome, by J. J. Goedert, et al. AMERICAN JOURNAL OF EPIDEMIOLOGY 121(5):629-636, May 1985.

—. II. Sexual practices, by J. J. Goedert, et al. AMERICAN JOURNAL OF EPIDEMIOLOGY 121(5):637-644, May 1985.

Eroticizing safe sex, "south-of-Market" style, by B. Beuse. ADVOCATE 452:30, August 5, 1986.

Farewell, sexual revolution. Hello, new Victorianism, by E. Cornish. THE FUTURIST 20:2+, January-February 1986.

Fear—loving in NYC—life after AIDS, by J. Fouralt. BODY POLITIC 1:37, January 1984.

Female prostitutes: a risk group for infection with human T-cell lymphotropic virus type III, by P. Van de Perre, et al. LANCET 2(8454):524-527, September 7, 1985.

Fever all through the night: is disease shaping a new sexual ethic? by N. Gallagher. MOTHER JONES 7:36-43, November 1982.

Gay erotic fantasies: don't let AIDS destroy, by E. Ingle. ADVOCATE 449:9, June 24, 1986.

Goodbye to promiscuity, by W. J. Weatherby. GUARDIAN August 30, 1985, p. 13.

Health Director closes Bay Area sex businesses, by C. Guilfoy. GAY COMMUNITY NEWS 12(14):1, October 20, 1984.

Health officials close baths and sex clubs. BODY POLITIC 1(8):17, November 1984.

Helquist report—is oral sex safe?, by M. Helquist. ADVOCATE 444:23, April 15, 1986.

Homosexual promiscuity and the fear of AIDS [letter],by R. Golubjatnikov, et al. LANCET 2(8351):681, September 17, 1983.

Homosexuality and sexually transmitted diseases, including the acquired immunologic deficiency syndrome, by C. H. Coester, et al. INTERNIST 24:334-345, June 1983.

If your partner contracts AIDS. RN 47:15, February 1984.

Inside a bathhouse [gay bathhouse in New York City], by P. Weiss. THE NEW REPUBLIC 193:12-13, December 2, 1985.

Is there death after sex?, by B. D. Colen. ROLLING STONE February 3, 1983, p. 17.

Is there gay life after AIDS?, by R. King. COSMOPOLITAN 199:198+, December 1985.

557

Is there life after sex?, by B. D. Colen. ROLLING STONE February 3, 1983, p. 17.

Is there safe sex?, by R. Bebout. BODY POLITIC 99:33, December 1983. SEX

Kiss is still a kiss?, by N. Fain. VILLAGE VOICE 29:11, October 9, 1984.

Lack of correlation between promiscuity and seropositivity to HTLV-III from a low-incidence area for AIDS, by L. H. Calabrese, et al. NEW ENGLAND JOURNAL OF MEDICINE 312:1256-1257, May 9, 1985.

LAV/HTLV-III infection after a one-time sexual contact with an AIDS patient, by P. Reiss, et al. NEDERLANDS TIJDSCHRIFT VOOR GENEESKUNDE 129(40): 1933-1934, October 5, 1985.

Life and love after AIDS, by R. Joyce. BODY POLITIC 126:13, May 1986.

New York bath owners to promote safe sex,by S. Hyde. GAY COMMUNITY NEWS 12(35):1, March 23, 1985.

New York: where intimacy is in, by G. Whitmore. ADVOCATE 3(73):22, August 4, 1983.

Next they'll tax it: sex diseases. ECONOMIST 285:29-30, October 2, 1982.

No sex for gays, High Court says. GUARDIAN 38(39):5, July 9, 1986.

Passive anal intercourse, by N. Fain. ADVOCATE 3(78):22, October 13, 1983.

Passive anal intercourse as a risk factor for AIDS in homosexual men [letter], by W. W. Darrow, et al. LANCET 2(8342):160, July 16, 1983.

Prime time for instant monogamy, by A. Duncan. TIMES December 1, 1986, p. 15.

Progress toward the 1990 objectives for sexually transmitted diseases: good news and bad, by W. C. Parra, et al. PUBLIC HEALTH REPORTS 100(3): 261-269, May-June 1985.

Prophylactic lover, by R. Bebout. BODY POLITIC 126:25, May 1986.

Relation between sexual practices and T-cell subsets in homosexually active men, by R. Detels, et al. LANCET 1(8325):609-611, March 19, 1983.

Reported changes in the sexual behavior of men at risk for AIDS, San Francisco, 1982-84—the AIDS Behavioral Research Project, by L. McKusick, et al. PUBLIC HEALTH REPORTS 100(6):622-629, November-December 1985.

Safe sex: guidelines that could save your life, by M. Helquist. ADVOCATE 426: 36, August 6, 1985.

Safe sex: warm, approaching hot, by K. Bowling. OUT 4(8):8, June 1986.

Sensible summer sex , by Bronski, et al. GAY COMMUNITY NEWS 12(40):4, April 27, 1985.

Serological markers as indicators of sexual orientation in AIDS virus-infected men [letter], by J. J. Potterat, et al. JAMA 256(6):712, August 8, 1986.

Sex and germs, by K. Hale-Wehmann. SCIENCE FOR THE PEOPLE 18(4):26, July 1986.

Sex for the second millennium, by M. Pye. OBSERVER October 29, 1985, p. 41.

Sex in the age of AIDS, by L. Giteck.. ADVOCATE 450:42, July 8, 1986.

—, Part 2, by L. Giteck. ADVOCATE 451:28, July 22, 1986.

Sex scolding ignores fact: gays have changed. OUT 3(12):4, October 1985.

Sexual slander, by D. Rist. ADVOCATE 446:42, May 13, 1986.

Sodomy and the Supreme Court, by D. Robinson, Jr. COMMENTARY 82:57-61, October 1986.

Some sex out of danger?, by K. Popert. BODY POLITIC 123:15, February 1986.

State plans to trace sex, needle partners. OUT 4(5):1, April 1986.

Taking a sexual history, by R. A. Gremminger. WISCONSIN MEDICAL JOURNAL 82(11):20-24, November 1983.

Zoo sex, by R. Emmett Tyrrell Jr. AMERICAN SPECTATOR 18:8, November 1985.

CANADA
   Vancouver AIDS study ranks risk of sex acts, by K. Popert. BODY POLITIC 113:8, April 1985.

HAITI
   AIDS in a Canadian woman who had helped prostitutes in Port-au-Prince [letter], by D. B. Rose, et al. LANCET 2(8351):680-681, September 17, 1983.

INDIA
   Acquired immune deficiency syndrome . . . impact of heredity and East Indian sexual practices, by S. Khanna. NURSING JOURNAL OF INDIA 76(4):91-93, April 1985.

SEX—COLLEGES
   Campus sex: new fears. AIDS is the latest STD to hit the nation's colleges, by M. Bruno, et al. NEWSWEEK 106(18):81-82, October 28, 1985.

SEX—LAWS AND LEGISLATION
   Sex ban in baths proposed in D.C., by J. Ryan. GAY COMMUNITY NEWS 12(346):3, March 30, 1985.

SEX—TRANSMISSION
   Sex transmits AIDS. THE ECONOMIST 300:14, July 5, 1986.

Acquired immunodeficiency syndrome (AIDS) in an economically disadvantaged population, by S. Maayan, et al. ARCHIVES OF INTERNAL MEDICINE 145(9):1607-1612, September 1985.

Age of AIDS: a great time for defensive living (editorial], by G. D. Lundberg. JAMA 253(23):3440-3441, June 21, 1985.

AIDS and social change, by D. A. Feldman. HUMAN ORGANIZATION 44:343-348, Winter 1985.

AIDS—the end of permissive society?, by J. Clements. NEW ZEALAND NURSING JOURNAL 78(7):12-13, July 1985.

AIDS: a legal, medical, and social problem, by C. J. Postell. TRIAL 22(8):76-78, August 1986.

AIDS: a link with poverty? [Belle Glade, Florida], by J. Conant. NEWSWEEK 105:37, June 24, 1985.

AIDS not a 'social disease' [letter]. NATURE 303(5916):371, June 2-8, 1983.

Change in gay life-style, by V. Coppola. NEWSWEEK 101:80, April 18, 193.

Coping with the threat of AIDS. An approach to psychosocial assessment, by J. G. Joseph, et al. AMERICAN PSYCHOLOGIST 39(11):1297-1302, November 1984.

Desperate living—analysis—gay health. RFD 36:21, Fall 1983.

Double life of an AIDS victim, by G. Clarke. TIME 126:106, October 14, 1985.

Draconian law or human decencies, by L. Gostin. NEW STATESMAN June 20, 1986, p. 17-18.

Effects of the acquired immune deficiency syndrome on gay lifestyle and the gay individual, by D. A. Hirsch, et al. ANNALS OF THE NEW YORK ACADEMY OF SCIENCES 437:273-282, 1984.

Etiquette for an epidemic: when someone has AIDS, by R. Boucheron. ADVOCATE 434:9, November 26, 1985.

Gay America in transition, by T. Morganthau. NEWSWEEK 102:30-36+, August 8, 1983.

Incognito in Colorado, by B. Maschinot. IN THESE TIMES 9(38):4, October 9, 1985.

Learning to live with AIDS, by J. Interrante. GAY COMMUNITY NEWS 12(32):6, March 2, 1985.

—, by P. Ungvarski. NURSING MIRROR 160(2):20-22, May 22, 1985.

Men with AIDS: dying of red tape, by S. Hyde. GAY COMMUNITY NEWS 11(5):1, August 13, 1983.

Moral, ethical, and legal aspects of infection control, by B. Parent. AMERICAN JOURNAL OF INFECTION CONTROL 13(6):278-280, December 1985.

"Morals", medicine, and the AIDS epidemic, by P. M. Kayal. JOURNAL OF RE-LIGION AND HEALTH 24:218-238, Fall 1985.

National AIDS candlelight vigil. ADVOCATE 3(78):17, October 13, 1983.

National AIDS vigil: at a low time, by J. Irvine. GAY COMMUNITY NEWS 11(12):1, October 7, 1983.

National AIDS vigil set for Oct. 8. GAY COMMUNITY NEWS 11(9):1, September 17, 1983.

Of AIDS, gays and repression. NEW STATESMAN 109:3, March 1, 1985.

Only a moral revolution can contain this scourge, by I. Jakobowits. TIMES December 27, 1986, p. 20.

People with AIDS honored at 70 vigils worldwide, by Bisticas-Cocoves. GAY COMMUNITY NEWS 13(45):1, June 7, 1986.

Pols, actors, art crowd help gays fight AIDS, by H. Hanson. CHICAGO 34:18, July 1985.

Poverty's harvest: AIDS, by J. Murphy. GUARDIAN 38(15):1, January 15, 1986.

Pro and con: should AIDS victims be isolated? [interview]. U.S. NEWS & WORLD REPORT 99(14):50, September 30, 1985.

Reaching out to someone with AIDS, by G. Whitmore. NEW YORK TIMES MAGA-ZINE May 19, 1985, p. 68-71+.

Review of a support group for patients with AIDS, by D. A. Newmark. TOPICS IN CLINICAL NURSING 6(2):38-44, July 1984.

Ride for wellness: positive radicalism, by T. Barrus. GAY COMMUNITY NEWS 13(16):6, November 2, 1985.

San Francisco AIDS vigil in 12th week, by S. Poggi. GAY COMMUNITY NEWS 13(27):1, January 25, 1986.

San Francisco AIDS vigilers stand firm in 8th month, by Bisticas-Cocoves. GAY COMMUNITY NEWS 13(48):1, June 28, 1986.

San Francisco vigil for AIDS funds enters fourth week, by K. Westheimer. GAY COMMUNITY NEWS 13(20):1, November 30, 1985.

Self-reported behavioral change among gay and bisexual men—San Francisco. MMWR 34(40):613-615, October 11, 1985.

Social aspects of the AIDS problem. The best possibility lies in reality-oriented ac-tions, by R. Osterwalder. KRANKENPFLEGE. SOINS INFIRMIERS 79(5):43-45, May 1986.

Social consequences of the acquired immunodeficiency syndrome, by B. J. Cassens. ANNALS OF INTERNAL MEDICINE 103(5):768-771, November 1985.

Social disease [editorial]. NATION 241(7):195, September 14, 1985.

Social meaning of AIDS, by P. Conrad. SOCIAL POLICY 17(1):51, Summer 1986.

Social networks and the spread of infectious diseases: the AIDS example, by A. S. Klovdahl. SOCIAL SCIENCE & MEDICINE 21(11):1203-1216, 1985.

Social work and AIDS, by A-L. Furstenberg, et al. SOCIAL WORK IN HEALTH CARE 9(4):45-62, 1984.

Ten thousand join AIDS vigil, by M. Cocoves. GAY COMMUNITY NEWS 12(26):1, June 8, 1985.

Vigil—a profile of gay courage, by M. Hippler. ADVOCATE 444:42, April 15, 1986.

SPORTS

AIDS, athletes, and fears about contact, by M. M. Gauthier. PHYSICIAN SPORTS-MEDICINE 14:41, January 1986.

STATISTICS

AIDS cases expected to triple. SCIENCE DIGEST 94:9, May 1986.

AIDS cases surpass 15,000. CHRISTIANITY TODAY 29(16):66, November 8, 1985.

AIDS cases top 7000; 5244 are gay men, by E. Guilfoy. GAY COMMUNITY NEWS 12(23):3, December 22, 1984.

AIDS numbers don't add up, by K. Hale. ARKANSAS TIMES 12:21-24, March 1986.

AIDS: statistics in Puerto Rico and useful references, by J. G. Rigau-Pérez, et al. BOLETIN—ASOCIACION MEDICA DE PUERTO RICO 76(3):120-122, March 1984.

AIDS statistics released. OUT 3(4):1, February 1985.

AIDS trends: projections from limited data, by C. Norman. SCIENCE 230:1018-1021, November 29, 1985.

AIDS will increase tenfold in the US. NEW SCIENTIST 110:26, June 19, 986.

CDC reports AIDS cases in U.S. top 15,000, by Bisticas-Cocoves. GAY COMMUNITY NEWS 13(22):3, December 14, 1985.

CDC reports 10,000 diagnosed with AIDS, by M. Cocoves. GAY COMMUNITY NEWS 12(45):1, June 1, 1985.

DNCB data released, by M. Helquist. ADVOCATE 443:21, April 1, 1986.

Domestic AIDS cases clear 4000 mark, by C. Guilfoy. GAY COMMUNITY NEWS 12(1):1, July 14, 1984.

Estimation of risk of outcomes of HTLV-III infection [letter], by D. J. Hunter, et al. LANCET 1(8482):677-678, March 22, 1986.

Figures don't lie, they tell half-truths, by E. Jackson. BODY POLITIC 116:14, July 1985.

Life table analysis of children with acquired immunodeficiency syndrome, by R. Lampert, et al. PEDIATRIC INFECTIOUS DISEASE 5(3):374-375, May-June 1986.

Some problems in the prediction of future numbers of cases of the acquired immunodeficiency syndrome in the UK, by M. McEvoy, et al. LANCET 2(8454):541-542, September 7, 1985.

UNITED STATES
Acquired immune deficiency syndrome (AIDS) trends in the United States, 1978-1982, by R. M. Selik, et al. AMERICAN JOURNAL OF MEDICINE 76(3):493-500, March 1984.

Acquired immune deficiency syndrome in the United States: the first 1,000 cases, by H. W. Jaffe, et al. JOURNAL OF INFECTIOUS DISEASES 286(6374):1354, April 23, 1983.

Massachusetts AIDS caseload rises to 296, by C. Guilfoy. GAY COMMUNITY NEWS 13(3):3, July 27, 1985.

United States AIDS cases pass the 20,000 mark, by Bisticas-Cocoves. GAY COMMUNITY NEWS 13(43):1, May 24, 1986.

SURGERY
Acquired immune deficiency syndrome. A surgical perspective, by J. M. Davis, et al. ARCHIVES OF SURGERY 119(1):90-95, January 1984.

Acquired immunodeficiency syndrome (AIDS)—apheresis and operative risks, by D. D. Kiprov, et al. JOURNAL OF CLINICAL APHERESIS 2(4):427-440, 1985.

AIDS after coronary bypass surgery [letter], by G. Delpre, et al. LANCET 1(8368): 103, January 14, 1984.

AIDS and the reluctant surgeon, by H. A. Dudley. MEDICAL JOURNAL OF AUS-TRALIA 142(12):651-652, June 10, 1985.

AIDS: a surgeon's responsibility, by M. T. Lotze. BULLETIN OF THE AMERICAN COLLEGE OF SURGEONS 70(9):6-12, September 1985.

AIDS and surgery [editorial], by J. Ludbrook. AUSTRALIA AND NEW ZEALAND JOURNAL OF SURGERY 56(2):97-98, February 1986.

— [letter], by E. Owen. MEDICAL JOURNAL OF AUSTRALIA 142(2):164, January 21, 1985.

563

Hematologic care of the surgical patient, by S. A. Berkman. HOSPITAL PRAC-TICE 21(2):124DD+, Feburary 15, 1986.

Performing safe phlebotomy on AIDS patients, by S. A. Diffley. MLO 15(11):75-76, November 1983.

Surgeon and HTLV-III infection [editorial], by C. D. Forbes. BRITISH JOURNAL OF SURGERY 73(3):168-169, March 1986.

Surgical perspective on AIDS. AMERICAN FAMILY PHYSICIAN 29:265, June 1984.

AFRICA
AIDS in a Danish surgeon (Zaire, 1976) [letter], by I. C. Bygbjerg. LANCET 1(8330):925, April 23, 1983.

TESTING
AIDS and accuracy: Is TV testing positive?, by Jim Fiske. EMMY 8:38+, May-June 1986.

AIDS antibody testing and counseling [letter], by G. H. Hall. BRITISH MEDICAL JOURNAL 29(6506):1424, November 16, 1985.

AIDS serology testing in low- and high-risk groups, by J. R. Carlson, et al. JAMA 253(23):3405-3408, June 21, 1985.

AIDS testing sought. BODY POLITIC 127:23, June 1986.

AIDS tests could trigger world blood shortage, by O. Sattaur. NEW SCIENTIST 106:6, May 16, 1985.

Blood banks give HTLV-III test positive appraisal at five months, by C. Marwick. JAMA 254:1681-1683, October 4, 1985.

California wants AIDS test on organs. NEW SCIENTIST 107:19, August 1, 1985.

CDC advises HTLV-3 test for all "at risk", by Bisticas-Cocoves. GAY COMMUNITY NEWS 13(37):1, April 1, 1986.

CDC issues HTLV-III screening guidelines, by C. Guilfoy. GAY COMMUNITY NEWS 12(27):1, January 26, 1985.

CDC sees no need to test health workers for AIDS; two SNA's launch campaigns "to reduce anxiety." AMERICAN JOURNAL OF NURSING 86:200-202, February 1986.

Consensus conference. The impact of routine HTLV-III antibody testing of blood and plasma donors on public health. JAMA 256(13):1778-1783, October 3, 1986.

DC insurers barred from testing for AIDS, by J. Firshein. HOSPITALS 60(13): 50+, July 5, 1986.

Drug test advances, civil rights abuses. BODY POLITIC 128:22, July 1986.

FDA advises blood centers on phase-in of AIDS test. MLO17(4):21-23, April 1985.

FDA approves blood screen for AIDS, by C. Foty. OFF OUR BACKS 15(4):2, April 1985.

Gay father ordered to take HTLV-3 test, by P. Freiberg. ADVOCATE 448:D15, June 10, 1986.

Gay/lesbian community statement on HTLV-III test. GAY COMMUNITY NEWS 12(33):9, March 9, 1985.

Gay men urged not to take AIDS-virus test,by D. Walter. ADVOCATE 414:12, February 19, 1985.

Health experts call for improved HIV testing , by D. Walter. ADVOCATE 453:22, August 19, 1986.

HTLV3 screening—a cautious perspective, by B. Andrews. GAY COMMUNITY NEWS 12(4):5, August 4, 1984.

HTLV-3 screening: problematic but available, by C. Guilfoy. GAY COMMUNITY NEWS 12(2):3, July 21, 1984.

HTLV-III: should testing ever be routine?,by D. Miller, et al. BRITISH MEDICAL JOURNAL 292(6525):941-943, April 5, 1986.

HTLV-3 test availability elicits mixed response, by C. Guilfoy. GAY COMMUNITY NEWS 12(40):3, April 27, 1985.

HTLV-III test sought as basis for insurance, by M. Cocoves. GAY COMMUNITY NEWS 13(10):1, September 21, 1985.

Large-scale AIDS testing program delayed, by L. Famiglietti. AIR FORCE TIMES 46:10, June 16, 1986.

Massachusetts sets sites for HTLV-3 test, by C. Guilfoy. GAY COMMUNITY NEWS 12(39):6, April 20, 1985.

Medical editor revises AIDS testing remark, by K. Westheimer. GAY COMMUNITY NEWS 13(40):1, April 26, 1986.

Medical expert views potential for abuse in AIDS screening, by R. L. Cohen. THE NATIONAL PRISON PROJECT JOURNAL 6:5-6, Winter 1985.

NIMH study: gay men shun AIDS test, by J. Folkenberg. ADAMHA NEWS 11(11): 2, November 1985.

PHS issues guidelines on AIDS testing and follow-up for positives. MLO 17(3): 25-27, March 1985.

Researchers discuss safety of AIDS testing, by L. Goldsmith. GAY COMMUNITY NEWS 12(3):3, July 28, 1984.

San Francisco AIDS antibody testing program, by M. Helquist. ADVOCATE 424: 14, July 9, 1985.

Screening for acquired immunodeficiency syndrome [letter],by N. M. Arnott. CANADIAN MEDICAL ASSOCIATION JOURNAL 129(5):412, September 1, 1983.

Screening for acquired immune deficiency syndrome with dinitrochlorobenzene [letter],by W. A. McLeod, et al. CANADIAN MEDICAL ASSOCIATION JOURNAL 130(2):100-101, January 15, 1984.

Screening for AIDS. MEDICAL LETTER ON DRUGS AND THERAPEUTICS 27(684):29-30, March 29, 1985.

Screening for AIDS or for gays?, by T. Ensign. GUARDIAN 37(44):5, September 11, 1985.

Screening for HIV antibodies, by N. P. Guarda, et al. NURSING 16(11):28-29, November 1986.

Screening for HTLV-III antibodies—a government blunder?, by C. S. Bryan. JOURNAL OF THE SOUTH CAROLINA MEDICAL ASSOCIATION 81(4):242-244, April 1985.

Screening for HTLV-III antibodies: the relation between prevalence and positive predictive value and its social consequences [letter]. JAMA 253(23):3395-3398, June 21, 1985.

Screening for risk of acquired immune-deficiency syndrome [letter],by F. Greenberg, et al. NEW ENGLAND JOURNAL OF MEDICINE 307(24):1521-1522, December 9, 1982.

Screening test for HTLV-III (AIDS agent) antibodies. Specificity, sensitivity, and applications, by S. H. Weiss, et al. JAMA 253(2):221-225, January 11, 1985.

Should actors take AIDS test before filming a kiss? JET 68:60-61, September 9, 1985.

Should I take the test? OUT 4(1):3, November 1985.

Special report: AIDS testing. CITIZEN AIRMAN 37:8, Winter 1985-1986.

State seeking sites for antibody testing. OUT 3(6):3, April 1985.

Status report on the acquired immunodeficiency syndrome: human T-cell lymphotropic virus type III testing, by AMA Council on Scientific Affairs. CONNECTICUT MEDICINE 49(10):667-670, October 1985; also in JAMA 254(10):1342-1345, September 13, 1985.

Take the test!, by B. Voeller. ADVOCATE 419:5, April 30, 1985.

Test shows AIDS bug well established here. BODY POLITIC 111:14, February 1985.

Tuberculin testing for persons with positive serologic studies for HTLV-III, by A. E. Pitchenik, et al. NEW ENGLAND JOURNAL OF MEDICINE 314:447, February 13, 1986.

United States cities fight HTLV-3 test plan, by M. Cocoves. GAY COMMUNITY NEWS 12(40):1, April 27, 1985.

United States prepares for AIDS blood test. NEW SCIENTIST 105:3, January 17, 1985.

Use of AIDS antibody test may provide more answers , by C. Marwick. JAMA 253(12):1694-1695+, March 22-29, 1985.

CANADA
AIDS: testing program launched in Vancouver, by M. Rekart. RNABC NEWS 17(6):23, November-December 1985.

FRANCE
French claim on AIDS testing, by R. Rhein, et al. CHEMICAL WEEK 137:11, October 16, 1985.

GERMANY
Scholars face AIDS test [West Germany]. THE TIMES HIGHER EDUCATION SUPPLEMENT 684:8, December 13, 1985.

GREAT BRITAIN
Lytic infection by British AIDS virus and development of rapid cell test for anti-viral antibodies, by A. Karpas, et al. LANCET 2(8457):695-697, September 28, 1985.

SPAIN
HTLV-III antibody testing in Spain [letter], by R. Nájera, et al. LANCET 2(8458):783, October 5, 1985.

SRI LANKA
Seroepidemiologic screening for antibodies to LAV/HTLV-III in Sri Lanka, 1908-1982, by R. A. Miller, et al. NEW ENGLAND JOURNAL OF MEDICINE 313:1352-1353, November 21, 1985.

TESTING—ECONOMICS
Test centers: shifting funds, by D. Walter. ADVOCATE 420:13, May 14, 1985.

TESTING—INSURANCE
Test insurance applicants for signs of AIDS? [interviews with S. Rish and J. Corcoran]. US NEWS & WORLD REPORT 99:71, November 25, 1985.

TESTS
AIDS antibody screening test: controversy surrounds a new ELISA assay designed to prevent the spread of AIDS through blood transfusions. ANALYTICAL CHEMISTRY 57:773A-4A+, June 1985.

AIDS: the antibody test, by S. Anderson. PROFESSIONAL MEDICAL ASSISTANT 19(2):22-25, March-April 1986.

AIDS antibody tests effectively screen blood supply. AMERICAN FAMILY PHYSICIAN 32:274-275, October 1985.

AIDS control: problems of new blood test [news],by S. Budiansky. NATURE 309(5964):106, May 10-16, 1984.

AIDS diagnostic tests. CHEMICAL MARKETING REPORTER 228:5, August 5, 1985.

AIDS research funding stalled; diagnostic test advances. AMERICAN FAMILY PHYSICIAN 30:18, August 1984.

AIDS screening test now available to everyone, by D. Bradford. AUSTRALIAN FAMILY PHYSICIAN 14(5):463, May 1985.

AIDS-test ambiguities raise concert. BODY POLITIC 107:17, October 1984.

AIDS: test companies chosen [news], by S. Budiansky. NATURE 310(5972):6, July 5-11, 1984.

"AIDS test" guidelines issued, by N. Fain. ADVOCATE 417:26, April 2, 1985.

"AIDS" test a misnomer [letter], by A. J. Pinching. BRITISH MEDICAL JOURNAL 291(6498):821, September 21, 1985.

AIDS test: no comfort to many, by B. Bower, et al. SCIENCE NEWS 128:2, September 7, 1985.

AIDS tests alarm blood banks, by S. Budiansky. NATURE 313:87, January 10, 1985.

AIDS tests and cures [news]. AMERICAN FAMILY PHYSICIAN 28(6):250, December 1983.

AIDS tests that could offer proof positive, by J. O. Hamilton. BUSINESS WEEK April 28, 1986, p. 27-28.

Amid the debate over AIDS tests, some progress. DISCOVER 6:12, March 1985.

Antibody Test Amendment passes, by M. Martinek. OUT 3(9):3, July 1985.

Antibody-test debate ranges in Atlanta, by D. Walter. ADVOCATE 420:9, May 14, 1985.

Bad blood? [screening tests for AIDS virus inconclusive]. SCIENTIFIC AMERICAN 253:78, December 1985.

Close to FDA's finish line: five AIDS-linked tests, by R. Rhein, et al. CHEMICAL WEEK 136:25-26, March 6, 1985.

Coombs' test and the acquired immunodeficiency syndrome [letter], by S. Gupta, et al. ANNALS OF INTERNAL MEDICINE 100(3):462, March 984.

Crash development of AIDS test nears goal, by B. J. Culliton. SCIENCE 225 (4667):1128+, September 14, 1984.

Dubious test approved; funding cuts loom. BODY POLITIC 113:21, April 1985.

Evaluation of commercial AIDS screening test kits [letter], by J. R. Carlson, et al. LANCET 1(8442):1388, June 15, 1985.

568

FDA approves Pasteur's AIDS test kit, by C. Norman. SCIENCE 231:1063, March 7, 1986.

FDA postpones licensing of HTLV-III test, by C. Guilfoy. GAY COMMUNITY NEWS 12(32):1, March 2, 1985.

Great AIDS race: testing the test, by J. Silberner. SCIENCE NEWS 127:36, January 19, 1985.

High-stakes race is on to develop blood test to detect AIDS virus, by A. Cooper. NATIONAL JOURNAL 16:1470-1472, August 4, 1984.

HTLV-III antibody test is licensed, by Freiberg, et al. ADVOCATE 417:11, April 2, 1985.

HTLV-III antibody test: what it can and cannot do. CHART 83(5):5, May-June 1986.

Immunity syndrome: new test, new ideas, by J. A. Miller. SCIENCE NEWS 123: 197, March 26, 1983.

Leveraging AIDS [race to develop reliable blood test], by R. Teitelman. FORBES 135:115, April 8, 1985.

Looking for an answer: the AIDS test. NEW YORK 18:31, October 7, 1985.

New AIDS test? THE ECONOMIST 298:82, February 22, 1986.

—. US NEWS & WORLD REPORT 98(6):48, February 18, 1985.

No trend yet in test for HTLV-III antibody. OUT 4(2):1, December 1985.

Oncor to offer test to detect AIDS virus. CHEMICAL AND ENGINEERING NEWS 64:6, October 6, 1986.

Plans underway for blood test, by C. Guilfoy. GAY COMMUNITY NEWS 12(36):7, March 30, 1985.

Sharper tests for AIDS, by O. Sattaur. NEW SCIENTIST 106:23, May 2, 1985.

Struggle looms over AIDS tests, by L. J. Lyons. THE NATIONAL UNDERWRITER 90:1+, March 1, 1986.

Sure fire blood test for AIDS sought, by N. Fain. ADVOCATE 8(78):23, October 13, 1983.

Test with no right answers, by S. Burke. OUT 3(5):1, March 1985.

Transamerica Occidental using controversial blood test to detect the presence of AIDS virus, by L. Kocolowski. THE NATIONAL UNDERWRITER 89:6, October 19, 1985.

United States licenses blood test for AIDS, by C. Joyce, et al. NEW SCIENTIST 105:3-4, March 7, 1985.

GERMANY
West Germany moves to register HTLV-3 positive test, by E. Gill. ADVOCATE 432:25, October 29, 1985.

GREAT BRITAIN
AIDS: two British blood tests launched, by M. Clarke. AIDS NATURE 316: 474, August 8, 1985.

New British test for AIDS is quicker and cheaper, by O. Sattaur. NEW SCIENTIST 108:20-21, October 3, 1985.

Two British blood tests launched [news], by M. Clarke. NATURE 316(6028): 474, August 8-14, 1985.

JAPAN
Japan buys British 'litmus test' for AIDS, by S. Connor. NEW SCIENTIST 111: 16, August 28, 1986.

New AIDS test comes to light in Japan, by B. Johnstone. NEW SCIENTIST 106:8, April 18, 1985.

TESTS—ATTITUDES
Opposition to antibody test grows, by N. Fain. ADVOCATE 418:22, April 16, 1985.

TESTS—BLOOD
Racing to sell an AIDS test to blood banks, by E. t. Smith, et al. BUSINESS WEEK February 18, 1985, p. 136.

Results of human T-lymphotropic virus type III test kits reported from blood collection centers—United States, April 22 to May 19, 1985. JAMA 254:741, August 9, 1985.

United States blood-bank tests established [news], by T. Beardsley. NATURE 316(6028):474, August 8-14, 1985.

TRANSMISSION
Acquired immune deficiency syndrome (AIDS) HTLV-III/LAV; the causal agent and modes of transmission, by A. Smithies. HEALTH BULLETIN 44(4):234-238, July 1986.

Acquired immune deficiency syndrome in low-risk patient. Evidence for possible transmission by an asymptomatic carrier, by A. E. Pitchenik, et al. JAMA 250(10):1310-1312, September 9, 1983.

Acquired immunodeficiency syndrome possibly arthropod-borne [letter], by M. J. Blaser. ANNALS OF INTERNAL MEDICINE 99(6):877, December 1983.

Acquired immunodeficiency syndrome: rules for pestilential contagion revisited, by L. L. Rosendorf, et al. AMERICAN JOURNAL OF INFECTION CONTROL 12(1):31-33, February 1984.

AIDS and artificial insemination by donor [editorial], by a. Galvao-Teles. ACTA MEDICA PORTUGUESA 7(1):3-4, January-February 1986.

AIDS and the baths, by Freiberg, et al. ADVOCATE 3(75):20, September 1, 1983.

AIDS and the needle. NEW SCIENTIST 112:15, October 2, 1986.

AIDS: casual contact exonerated, by J. Silberner. SCIENCE NEWS 128:213, October 5, 1985.

AIDS: epidemiology and potential for nosocomial transmission, by D. K. Henderson. TOPICS IN CLINICAL NURSING 6(2):1-11, July 1984.

AIDS: an imported disease?, by B. Somaini. SCHWEIZERISCHE MEDIZINISCHE WOCHENSCHRIFT 116(24):818-821, June 14, 1986.

AIDS in the bathhouse, by T. Allen-Mills. SPECTATOR March 9, 1985, p. 7-8.

AIDS is less transmissible than hepatitis, say guidelines. AMERICAN JOURNAL OF NURSING 86:201, February 1986.

AIDS—the transmissible immunologic deficiency disease, by U. A. Baumann, et al. VASA 13(2):94-98, 1984.

AIDS transmission. AMERICAN FAMILY PHYSICIAN 29:388+, March 1984.

AIDS transmission [letter], by J. M. Campbell. WESTERN JOURNAL OF MEDICINE 144(1):92, January 1986.

AIDS transmission: what about the hepatitis B vaccine? [news], by C. Macek. JAMA 249(6):685-686, February 11, 1983

Anderson closes bathhouse, cites AIDS, by Brooke, et al. ADVOCATE 424:16, July 9, 1985.

Bathhouses reopen, but must clean up act. BODY POLITIC 110:19, January 1985.

Bathhouses—scapegoats for AIDS fear, by R. Oloughlin. ADVOCATE 3(90):16, March 20, 1984.

Casual contact theories incite AIDS, by B. Nelson. GAY COMMUNITY NEWS 10(47):3, June 18, 1983.

Communicable disease report. April to June 1983. COMMUNITY MEDICINE 5(4): 330-332, November 1983.

—. October to December 1984. COMMUNITY MEDICINE 7(2):136-144, May 1985.

Community-acquired opportunistic infections and defective cellular immunity in heterosexual drug abusers and homosexual men, by C. B. Small, et al. AMERICAN JOURNAL OF MEDICINE 74(3):433-441, March 1983.

Contact tracing in the acquired immune deficiency syndrome (AIDS). Evidence for transmission of virus and disease by an asymptomatic carrier, by D. A. Cooper, et al. MEDICAL JOURNAL OF AUSTRALIA 141(9):579-582, October 27, 1984.

Current AIDS epidemiology and potential for nosocomial transmission, by D. K. Henderson. TOPICS IN CLINICAL NURSING 6(2):1-22, July 1984.

Deadly spread of AIDS, by C. Wallis. TIME 120:55, September 6, 1982.

Everybody out of the pool. THE PROGRESSIVE 47:11-12, September 1983.

How do you get AIDS, by N. Fain. ADVOCATE 3(79):20, October 27, 1983.

How a virus that is very hard to catch crossed the world; AIDS and public health, by J. Meldrum. NEW STATESMAN 110:14-15, September 27, 1985.

HTLV-III transmission [editorial], by L. D. Grouse. JAMA 254(15):2130-2131, October 18, 1985.

Inhalation-induced immunosuppression: sniffing out the volatile nitrite-AIDS connection [editorial], by K. H. Mayer. PHARMACOTHERAPY 4(5):235-236, September-October 1984.

Is nobody safe from AIDS? ECONOMIST 298:79-81, February 1, 1986.

Is there unwarranted risk in cohorting AIDS patients? [letter], by C. B. Burrus. INFECTION CONTROL 6(10):389, October 1985.

Lack of effect of hepatitis B vaccine on T-cell phenotypes, by I. M. Jacobson, et al. NEW ENGLAND JOURNAL OF MEDICINE 311:1030-1032, October 18, 1984.

Lack of transmission of HTLV-III/LAV infection to household contacts of patients with AIDS or AIDS-related complex with oral candidiasis, by G. H. Friedland, et al. NEW ENGLAND JOURNAL OF MEDICINE 314:344-349, February 6, 1986.

New directions in AIDS transmission, by J. Silberner. SCIENCE NEWS 129:101, February 15, 1986.

"Not an easy disease to come by", by G. J. Church. TIME 126(12):27, September 23, 1985.

One man connected to forty cases of AIDS in 10 cities across nation. JET 66:37, April 23, 1984.

Possible AIDS transmission is concern to nurses. AMERICAN FAMILY PHYSICIAN 28:17, July 1983.

Precautions prevent transmission of HTLV-III virus, by J. Prescott. TEXAS HOSPITALS 41(11):16-17, April 1986.

Risk of AIDS with artificial insemination, by J. Morgan, et al. NEW ENGLAND JOURNAL OF MEDICINE 314:386, February 6, 1986.

Spread of AIDS sparks new health concern, by J. L. Marx. SCIENCE 219:42-43, January 7, 1983.

Transmission of AIDS [letter], by G. A. Ahronheim. NATURE 313(6003):534, February 14-20, 1985.

572

Transmission of AIDS: the case against casual contagion, by M. A. Sande. NEW ENGLAND JOURNAL OF MEDICINE 314:380-382, February 6, 1986.

Transmission of AIDS virus at renal transplantation [letter], by C. A. Prompt, et al. LANCET 2(8456):672, September 21, 1985.

Transmission of hepatitis B and AIDS, by R. A. Garibaldi. INFECTION CONTROL 7(2 Supl):132-134, February 1986.

Transmission of HTLV-III [letter], by H. S. Kant. JAMA 254(14):1901, October 11, 1985.

Transplacental transmission of HTLV-III virus [letter], by N. Lapointe, et al. NEW ENGLAND JOURNAL OF MEDICINE 312(20):1125-1126, May 16, 1985.

Transplacental transmission of human immunodeficiency virus [letter], by H. di Maria, et al. LANCET 2(8500):215-216, July 26, 1986.

When is AIDS communicable? [letter], by H. H. Neumann. JAMA 251(12):1553, March 23-30, 1984.

TRANSMISSION—ANIMALS
NIH scientists report transmission of clinical AIDS infection from humans to chimpanzees, by J. Murphy. NEWS & FEATURES FROM NIH November 1984, p. 12-13.

TRANSMISSION—BLOOD TRANSFUSION
Abnormal T-lymphocyte subpopulations associated with transfusion of blood-derived products [letter], by C. M. Kessler, et al. LANCET 1(8331):991-992, April 30, 1983.

Acquired immune deficiency syndrome in the Middle East from imported blood, by M. E. Kingston, et al. TRANSFUSION 25(4):317-318, July-August 1985.

Acquired immune deficiency syndrome possibly related to transfusion in an adult without known disease-risk factors, by S. M. Gordon, et al. JOURNAL OF IN-FECTIOUS DISEASES 149(6):1030-1032, June 1984.

Acquired immunodeficiency and the "one donor-one patient" principle, by A. I. Vorob'ev, et al. TERAPEVTICHESKII ARKHIV 57(7):3-6, 1985.

Acquired immunodeficiency in an infant: possible transmission by means of blood products, by A. J. Ammann, et al. LANCET 1(8331):956-958, April 30, 1983.

Acquired immunodeficiency syndrome (AIDS) and blood products, by R. D. Miller, et al. ANESTHESIOLOGY 58(6):493-494, June 1983.

Acquired immunodeficiency syndrome (AIDS) associated with transfusions by J. W. Curran, et al. NEW ENGLAND JOURNAL OF MEDICINE 310(2):69-75, January 12, 1984.

Acquired immunodeficiency syndrome and the transfusion service, by M. Hrubisko. VNITRNI LEKARSTVI 30(2):147-151, February 1984.

Acquired immunodeficiency syndrome—another blood-transmitted disease?, by H. Seyfriedowa. ACTA HAEMATOLOGICA POLONICA 15(1-2):79-82, January-June 1984.

Acquired immunodeficiency syndrome associated with blood-product transfusions, by J. R. Jett,e t al. ANNALS OF INTERNAL MEDICINE 99(5):621-624, November 1983.

Acquired immunodeficiency syndrome associated with transfusions: the evolving perspective, by J. W. Curran, et al. ANNALS OF INTERNAL MEDICINE 100(2):298-300, February 1984.

AIDS and the blood bank, by H. F. Polesky. CLINICAL ENGINEERING INFORMATION SERVICE 7(5):152-153, September-October 1983.

AIDS and the blood bankers, by R. D. Eckert. REGULATION 10:15-24+, September-October 1986.

AIDS and blood donors [editorial], by A. I. Adams. MEDICAL JOURNAL OF AUSTRALIA 141(9):558, October 27, 1984.

AIDS and blood donors in Brazil [letter], by S. N. Wendel, et al. LANCET 2(8453): 506, August 31, 1985.

AIDS and blood products, by G. F. Rolland. BULLETIN DE LA SOCIETE DES SCIENCES MEDICALES DU GRAND-DUCHE DE LUXEMBOURG 121(2):7-12, 1984.

AIDS and the blood supply. KANSAS MEDICINE 87(3):76, March 1986.

AIDS and the blood supply, by R. D. Eckert. CONSUMERS' RESEARCH MAGAZINE 68:20-25, October 1985.

AIDS and blood transfusion in New Zealand [letter], by S. G. Whyte, et al. NEW ZEALAND MEDICAL JOURNAL 97(770):905, December 26, 1984.

AIDS and blood transfusions. NORTH CAROLINA MEDICAL JOURNAL 45(2): 109-110, February 1984.

AIDS and homologous blood transfusion [letter], by S. Flecknoe-Brown. MEDICAL JOURNAL OF AUSTRALIA 143(2):89, July 22, 1985.

AIDS and the importance of donated blood, by L. K. Altman. THE NEW YORK TIMES MAGAZINE November 18, 1984, p. 136-137+.

AIDS and the paid donor [letter], by D. J. Gury. LANCET 2(8349):575, September 3, 1983.

AIDS: the blood-bank scare, by M. Clark, et al. NEWSWEEK 105(4):62, January 28, 1985.

AIDS contaminates world's blood, by S. Connor. NEW SCIENTIST 104:5, November 22, 1984.

AIDS, ethics, and the blood supply. A report of a conference of the American Blood Commission and the Hastings Center, Institute of Society, Ethics and

the Life Sciences, January 29 and 30, 1985, by W. V. Miller, et al. TRANSFU-
SION 25(2):174-175, March-April 1985.

AIDS fear prompts recall of blood products, by S. Connor. NEW SCIENTIST
111:19, July 17, 1986.

AIDS, hepatitis, and the national blood policy. REGULATION 9(4):5-7, July-
August 1985.

AIDS in a child 5 1/2 years after a transfusion [letter], by M. J. Maloney, et al. NEW
ENGLAND JOURNAL OF MEDICINE 312(19):1256, May 9, 1985.

AIDS—a new concern for blood transfusion services, by J. Leikola. KRANKEN-
PFLEGE 76(10):60-61, October 1983.

AIDS panic disrupts American blood banks, by I. Anderson. NEW SCIENTIST 98:
927, June 30, 1983.

AIDS-related complex in a heterosexual man seven weeks after a transfusion, by
R. M. E. Fincher, et al. NEW ENGLAND JOURNAL OF MEDICINE 313:1226-
1227, November 7, 1985.

AIDS tests alarm blood banks, by S. Budiansky. NATURE 313:87, January 10,
1985.

AIDS: the trail of tainted blood, by M. Clark. NEWSWEEK 108(8):55, August 24,
1986.

AIDS, transfusion and hemophilia, still a mysterious relationship. Comments and
hypotheses, by J. F. Bach. REVUE FRANCAISE DE TRANSFUSION ET
IMMUNOHEMATOLOGIE 27(4):455-458, September 1984.

AIDS: transfusion patients may be at risk, by O. Sattaur. NEW SCIENTIST 97:
289, February 3, 1983.

AIDS transmission via transfusion therapy [letter], by S. C. Dereinski, et al.
LANCET 1(8368):102, January 14, 1984.

AIDS: US blood-bank test established, by T. Beardsley. NATURE 316:474,
August 8, 1985.

As AIDS scare hits nation's blood supply, by J. Mann. U.S. NEWS & WORLD RE-
PORT 95:71-72, July 25, 1983.

Autologous blood transfusion [letter], by R. Yomtovian. JAMA 253(17):2491,
May 3, 1985.

Bad blood: "gift of life" may be also an agent of death in some AIDS [acquired
immunodeficiency syndrome] cases, by M. Chase. WALL STREET JOUR-
NAL 203:1+, March 12, 1984.

Blood bank now accepts lesbian, by B. Brown. WOMEN'S PRESS 13(4):2,
November 1983.

Blood bankers send out AIDS alert, by A. Weller. PATHOLOGIST 37(6):431-432,
June 1983.

Blood bankers set the AIDS record straight. COLORADO MEDICINE 80(11):318, November 1983.

Blood banking—public or private, isologous or autologous?, by R. Beal. MEDICAL JOURNAL OF AUSTRALIA 1444(8):393-394, April 14, 1986.

Blood banks and AIDS [editorial], by A. Krosnick. JOURNAL OF THE MEDICAL SOCIETY OF NEW JERSEY 81(2):105, February 1984.

Blood banks still cope with AIDS fears and myths, by J. Riffer. HOSPITALS 60(1):74, January 5, 1986.

Blood-borne agent in immune deficiency and rare infection implicated. SCIENCE NEWS 123:8, January 1, 1983.

Blood brotherhood: a risk factor for AIDS? [letter], by L. Morfeldt-Manson, et al. LANCET 2(8415):1346, December 8, 1984.

Blood donation by persons at high risk of AIDS [letter], by J. J. Goedert. NEW ENGLAND JOURNAL OF MEDICINE 312(18):1190, May 2, 1985.

Blood donor services and liability issues relating to acquired immune deficiency syndrome, by K. S. Lipton. JOURNAL OF LEGAL MEDICINE 7(2):131-186, June 1986.

Blood donors at high risk of transmitting the acquired immune deficiency syndrome, by M. Contreras, et al. BRITISH MEDICAL JOURNAL 290(6470):749-750, March 9, 1985.

Blood drive unsettling Providence, by C. Guilfoy. GAY COMMUNITY NEWS 11(21):3, December 10, 1983.

Blood groups act to cut AIDS transmission risk. HOSPITALS 57(9):61-62, May 1, 1983.

Blood groups 'look back' for AIDS, by B. McCormick. HOSPITALS 60(16):72, August 20, 1986.

Blood-handling precautions and the human T-leukemia virus [letter], by T. R. Franson, et al. ANNALS OF INTERNAL MEDICINE 100():765, May 1984.

Blood product immunosuppression and the acquired immunodeficiency syndrome [letter], by R. J. Ablin, et al. ANNALS OF INTERNAL MEDICINE 104(1):130, January 1986.

Blood shortage fails to materialize, by J. E. Fox. US MEDICINE 19(17):3+, September 1, 1983.

Blood story. Part II. AIDS—current concepts and implications for blood transfusion services and nursing staff, by C. J. Burrell, et al. AUSTRALIAN NURSES JOURNAL 14(7):45-47, February 1985.

Blood supply safety: NIH panel sees reduced AIDS risk. CHEMICAL AND ENGINEERING NEWS 64:4, July 14, 1986.

Blood transfusion and acquired immunodeficiency syndrome (AIDS), by B. Habibi, et al. REVUE FRANCAISE DE TRANSFUSION ET IMMUNO-HEMATOLOGIE 26(5):447-465, Novemebr 1983.

Blood transfusion and susceptibility to AIDS [letter], by G. M. Shearer, et al. NEW ENGLAND JOURNAL OF MEDICINE 310(24):1601, June 14, 1984.

Blood transfusion, blood donation, and AIDS [editorial], by A. J. Grindon,e t al. JOURNAL OF THE MEDICAL ASSOCIATION OF GEORGIA 72(9):641-642, September 193.

Blood transfusion, haemophilia, and AIDS [editorial]. LANCET 2(8417-8418): 1433-1435, December 22, 1984.

Blood transfusions and the acquired immunodeficiency syndrome [letter], by J. Herman. ANNALS OF INTERNAL MEDICINE 100(3):461, March 1984.

Blood transfusions and AIDS: the facts, by P. Gadsby GOOD HOUSEKEEPING 200:222, June 1985.

Blood treatment may not kill AIDS virus, by S. Connor. NEW SCIENTIST 109:13-14, February 20, 1986.

Blood, virus: new links to AIDS, by D. Franklin. SCIENCE NEWS 125:21, January 14, 1984.

Blood will tell—but only with difficulty, by A. Veitch. GUARDIAN May 9, 1985, p. 19.

Care study—HTLV-III: spread of infection via blood, by C. Emery. NURSING 3(4): 147-148, April 1986.

Case 46—1984: AIDS associated with transfusion of blood products [letter], by G. F. Leparc. NEW ENGLAND JOURNAL OF MEDICINE 312(10):648, March 7, 1985.

Civilian blood banks to help monitor AIDS, by P. Smith. AIR FORCE TIMES 46: 24, August 26, 1985.

Continued risk of transfusion-transmitted AIDS, by J. Kolins. PATHOLOGIST 40(6):9-10, June 1986.

Cost of transfusion in AIDS. Experience at the Claude-Bernard Hospital apropos of 28 cases, by M. Simonneau, et al. REVUE FRANCAISE DE TRANSFU-SION ET IMMUNO-HEMATOLOGIE 27(4):557-560, September 1984.

Directed blood program to prevent AIDS contamination? AMERICAN FAMILY PHYSICIAN 33:253, February 1986.

Dr. Alfred Katz says fear, not AIDS, is causing a Red Cross blood loss, by M. Ryan. PEOPLE 20:32-33, July 11, 1983.

Effect of the acquired immune deficiency syndrome (AIDS) on blood transfusion and donation patterns in the state of Minnesota, by E. P. Scott, et al. MINNESOTA MEDICINE 68(9):665-669, September 1985.

Effects of AIDS on various aspects of blood banking, by M. Kuriyan, et al. JOURNAL OF THE MEDICAL SOCIETY OF NEW JERSEY 81(10):875--877, October 1984.

Effects of exposure to factor concentrates containing donations from identified AIDS patients. A matched cohort study, by J. Jason, et al. JAMA 256(13): 1758-1762, October 3, 1986.

Gays and the stigma of bad blood, by R. Bayer. HASTINGS CENTER REPORT 13(2):5-7, April 1983.

How blood traders could have launched AIDS. NEW SCIENTIST 105:7, March 28, 1985.

How to prevent spreading AIDS via blood transfusions. RN 46:11-12, April 1983.

Immunodeficiency syndrome, acquired post-transfusionally in a non-hemophilac (letter), by M. F. Legrand, et al. PRESSE MEDICALE 14(30):1609-1610, September 14, 1985.

Impact of AIDS on blood services in the United States, by S. G. Sandler, et al. VOX SANGUINIS 46(1):1-7, 1984.

Impact of AIDS on the voluntary blood donor system: a preliminary analysis, by A. J. Katz, et al. ANNALS OF THE NEW YORK ACADEMY OF SCIENCES 437: 487-492, 1984.

Infection, immunity, and blood transfusion [editorial], by L. J. Bruce-Chwatt. BRITISH MEDICAL JOURNAL 288(6433):1782-1783, June 16, 1984.

Infection, immunity, and blood transfusion. Proceedings of the XVIth Annual Scientific Symposium of the American Red Cross. Washington, DC, May 9-11, 1984. PROGRESS IN CLINICAL AND BIOLOGICAL RESEARCH 182:1-464, 1985.

Infection with HTLV-III/LAV and transfusion-associated acquired immunodeficiency syndrome. Serologic evidence of an association, by H. W. Jaffe, et al. JAMA 254(6):770-773, August 9, 1985.

Infectious complications of blood transfusions, by S. A. Berkman. SEMINARS IN ONCOLOGY 11(1):68-76, March 1984.

Intravenous gammaglobulin, thrombocytopenia, and the acquired immunodeficiency syndrome [letter], by J. F. Delfraissy, et al. ANNALS OF INTERNAL MEDICINE 103(3):478-479, September 1985.

Is our blood supply safe?, by R. D. Fritz, et al. WISCONSIN MEDICAL JOURNAL 82(11):26-27, November 1983.

Joint statement on acquired immune deficiency syndrome (AIDS) related to transfusion. TRANSFUSION 23(2):87-88, March-April 1983.

Keeping the AIDS virus out of blood supply, by D. M. Barnes. SCIENCE 233: 514-515, August 1, 1986.

Keeping the blood supply safe. WISCONSIN MEDICAL JOURNAL 82(11):26, November 1983.

Latency period in transfusion-related AIDS may exceed five years. AMERICAN FAMILY PHYSICIAN 32:144, July 1985.

May a blood bank refuse donations to prevent the spread of AIDS?, by L. G. Smith, et al. JOURNAL OF THE MEDICAL SOCIETY OF NEW JERSEY 81(2):125-129, February 1984.

Measures to decrease the risk of acquired immunodeficiency syndrome transmission by blood transfusion. Evidence of volunteer blood donor cooperation, by J. Pindyck, et al. TRANSFUSION 25(1):3-9, January-February 1985.

More on AIDS from blood. DISCOVER 6:13, July 1985.

More on blood transfusion and AIDS [letter], by R. S. Gordon, Jr. NEW ENGLAND JOURNAL OF MEDICINE 310(26):1742, June 28, 1984.

Natural history of primary infection with LAV in multitranfused patients, by the AIDS-Hemophilia French Study Group. BLOOD 68(1):89-94, July 1986.

Oat-cell carcinoma in transfusion-associated acquired immunodeficiency syndrome [letter], by R. J.\ Moser, 3d, et al. ANNALS OF INTERNAL MEDICINE 103(3):478, September 1985.

Of AIDS and the national blood supply. EMERGENCY MEDICINE 18(8):130+, April 30, 1986.

Pilot study of surrogate tests to prevent transmission of acquired immune deficiency syndrome by transfusion, by T. L. Simon, et al. TRANSFUSION 24(5):373-378, September-October 1984.

Plasma products withdrawn after donor dies of AIDS. AMERICAN FAMILY PHYSICIAN 28:18, December 1983.

Possible transfusion-associated acquired immune deficiency syndrome (AIDS)—California. MMWR 31(48):652-654, December 10, 1982.

Post-transfusion AIDS outside of hemophilia: facts, questions and commentary, by B. Habibi. REVUE FRANCAISE DE TRANSFUSION ET IMMUNOHEMATOLOGIE 27(4):497-507, September 1984.

Potential liability for transfusion-associated AIDS, by P. J. Miller, et al. JAMA 253(23):3419-3424, June 21, 1985.

Reactions and counter-reactions to transfusion-associated-AIDS [news], by M. F. Goldsmith. JAMA 251(2):177-179, January 13, 1984.

Red blood's not good enough. BODY POLITIC 119:25, October 1985.

Red Cross backs off donor policy, by E. Jackson. BODY POLITIC 93:11, May 1983.

Risk of transferring AIDS or hepatitis via immune globulin, by M. A. Kane, et al. JAMA 252:1057, August 24, 1984.

Safe blood for transfusion. MEDICAL LETTER ON DRUGS AND THERA-PEUTICS 25(646):93-95, October 14, 1983.

Significance of non-A, non-B hepatitis, cytomegalovirus and the acquired im-mune deficiency syndrome in transfusion practice, by W. L. Bayer, et al. CLINICS IN HAEMATOLOGY 13(1):253-269, February 1984.

Transfusion-associated acquired immunodeficiency syndrome: evidence for persistent infection in blood donors, by P. M. Feorino, et al. NEW ENGLAND JOURNAL OF MEDICINE 312:1293-1296, May 16, 1985.

Transfusion-associated acquired immunodeficiency syndrome in the United States, by T. A. Peterman, et al. JAMA 254:2913-2917, November 22-29, 1985.

Transfusion associated AIDS, by J. E. Menitove. JOURNAL OF CLINICAL APHERESIS 2(4):423-426, 1985.

—, by H. A. Perkins. AMERICAN JOURNAL OF HEMATOLOGY 19(3):307-313, July 1985; also in FRONTIERS OF RADIATION THERAPY AND ONCOLOGY 19:23-25, 1985.

— [editorial], by S. Bar-Shani. HAREFUAH 108(5):264-266, March 1, 1985.

Transfusion-associated AIDS—a cause for concern [editorial], by J. R. Bove. NEW ENGLAND JOURNAL OF MEDICINE 310(2):115-116, January 12, 1984.

Transfusion-associated AIDS: serologic evidence of human T-cell leukemia virus infection of donors, by H. W. Jaffe, et al. SCIENCE 223(4642):1309-1312, March 23, 1984.

Transmission of AIDS, and blood donors, by D. G. Penington. MEDICAL JOUR-NAL OF AUSTRALIA 142(3):213, February 4, 1985.

Transmission of lymphotropic retroviruses (HTLV-I and LAV/HTLV-III) by blood transfusion and blood products, by C. J. Melief, et al. VOX SANGUINIS 50(1):1-11, 1986.

Virologic studies in a case of transfusion-associated AIDS [letter], by D. J. Salberg. NEW ENGLAND JOURNAL OF MEDICINE 312(13):857-858, March 28, 1985.

—, by J. E. Groopman, et al. NEW ENGLAND JOURNAL OF MEDICINE 311(22): 1419-1422, November 29, 1984.

Whose blood can now be safe?, by T. Beardsley. NATURE 303(5913):102, May 12-18, 1983.

CANADA
AIDS and the safety and adequacy of the Canadian blood supply [editorial], by J. B. Derrick. CANADIAN ANAESTHETISTS SOCIETY JOURNAL 33(2):117-122, March 1986.

FRANCE
French doctors ban American blood imports. NEW SCIENTIST 98:529, May 26, 1983.

GERMANY
Interview with Dr. W. Stille, Frankfurt. Will AIDS-suspected blood donors soon be identifiable?, by W. Stille. MUENCHENER MEDIZINISCHE WOCHENSCHRIFT 125(48):Suppl. 2, December 2, 1983.

GREAT BRITAIN
British AIDS; whose blood can now be safe? by T. Beardsley. NATURE 303: 102, May 12, 1983.

British blood is almost clean. NEW SCIENTIST 109:15, February 13, 1986.

ISRAEL
Blood bank policy in Israel in relation to AIDS, by D. Michaeli. ANNALS OF THE NEW YORK ACADEMY OF SCIENCES 437:485-486, 1984.

ITALY
Rapid spread of HTLV-III infection among drug addicts in Italy [letter], by G. Angarano, et al. LANCET 2(8467):1302, December 7, 1985.

JAPAN
AIDS: Japan screens donated blood, by D. Swinbanks. NATURE 319:610, February 20, 1986.

How adult T-cell leukaemia spread in Japan, by J. Bell. NEW SCIENTIST 105: 22, March 7, 1985.

Japan blames US blood for AIDS cases, by B. Johnstone. NEW SCIENTIST 106:22, July 4, 1985.

Japan screens donated blood, by D. Swinbanks. NATURE 319(6055):610, February 20-26, 1986.

MIDDLE EAST
Acquired immune deficiency syndrome in the Middle East from imported blood, by M. E. Kingston, et al. TRANSFUSION 25(4):317-318, July-August 1985.

AIDS tests could trigger world blood shortage, by O. Sattaur. NEW SCIENTIST 106: 6, May 16, 1985.

TRANSMISSION—FAMILY
Apparent transmission of human T-lymphotrophic virus type III/lymphadenopathy-associated virus from a child to a mother providing health care. MMWR 35(5): 76-79, February 7, 1986; also in JAMA 255:1005+, February 28, 1986.

CDC reports first AIDS transmission from child to parent. AMERICAN FAMILY PHYSICIAN 33:17-18, March 1986.

Maternal transmission of acquired immune deficiency syndrome, by M. J. Cowan, et al. PEDIATRICS 73(3):382-386, March 1984.

Maternal transmission of AIDS studied. RESEARCH RESOURCES REPORTER 9(2):11-12, February 1985.

Risk of HTLV-III/LAV transmission to household contacts [letter]. NEW ENGLAND JOURNAL OF MEDICINE 315(4):257-259, July 24, 1986.

FRANCE
AIDS: France to screen blood donors, by R. Walgate. NATURE 315:705, June 27, 1985.

TRANSMISSION—HEALTH CARE WORKERS
Hospital waste: states confront task of disposal, by L. Lehrer. PROFESSIONAL SANITATION MANAGEMENT 17(3):39, October0November 1985.

You're not likely to get AIDS from patients. RN 48:12-13, June 1985.

TRANSMISSION—HETEROSEXUALS
Apparent transmission of human T-cell leukemia virus type III to a heterosexual woman with the acquired immunodeficiency syndrome, by J. E. Groopman, et al. ANNALS OF INTERNAL MEDICINE 102(1):63-66, January 1985.

Potential check on heterosexual transmission of AIDS [letter], by A. Comfort. JOURNAL OF THE ROYAL SOCIETY OF MEDICINE 78(11):969-970, November 1985.

Transmission of the acquired immunodeficiency syndrome through heterosexual activity, by M. M. Lederman. ANNALS OF INTERNAL MEDICINE 104(1):115-117, January 1986.

TRANSMISSION—HOSPITALS
AIDS: a time bomb at hospitals' door, by D. Burda, et al. HOSPITALS 60(1):54-61, January 5, 1986.

Nosocomial acquired immunodeficiency syndrome and human T-cell leukaemia lymphoma virus associated disease, by D. C. Shanson. JOURNAL OF HOSPITAL INFECTION 5(1):3-6, March 1984.

Risk of nosocomial infection with human T-cell lymphotropic virus III (HTLV-III), by M. S. Hirsch, et al. NEW ENGLAND JOURNAL OF MEDICINE 312(1):1-4, January 3, 1985.

Risks of transmission of the HTLV-III and hepatitis B virus in the hospital, by D. Shanson. INFECTION CONTROL 7(2):128-132, February 1986.

GREAT BRITAIN
Incidence and risk of transmission of HTLV III infections to staff at a London hospital, 1982-85, by D. C. Shanson, et al. JOURNAL OF HOSPITAL INFECTION 6(Suppl. C):15-22, December 1985.

TRANSMISSION—INSECTS
Can hepatitis B virus and AIDS-associated retrovirus (LAV/HTLV-III) be transmitted by insects?, by T. G. Jaenson. LAKARTIDNINGEN 82(47):4133-4136, November 20, 1985.

Insect-borne transmission of AIDS?, by D. P. Drotman. JAMA 254:1085, August 23-30, 1985.

Survival of HIV in the common bedbug [letter],by S. F. Lyons, et al. LANCET 2(8497):45, July 5, 1986.

TRANSMISSION—NEEDLE PRICK
HIV infection with seroconversion after a superficial needlestick injury to the finger, by E. Oksenhendler, et al. NEW ENGLAND JOURNAL OF MEDICINE 315(9):582, August 28, 1986.

HTLV-III infection among health care workers. Association with needle-stick injuries, by S. H. Weiss, et al. JAMA 254(15):2089-2093, October 18, 1985.

In-hospital needlesticks and other significant blood exposures to blood from patients with acquired immunodeficiency syndrome and lymphadenopathy syndrome, by F. S. Rhame. AMERICAN JOURNAL OF INFECTION CONTROL 12(20:69-75, April 1984.

Needle-prick injury and AIDS. NEW ZEALAND NURSING FORUM 14(2):3, August 1986.

Needle-stick injuries during the care of patients with AIDS [letter], by G. P. Wormser, et al. NEW ENGLAND JOURNAL OF MEDICINE 310(22):1461-1462, May 31, 1984.

Risk of transmission of HTLV-III by needle stick [letter], by C. E. DuBeau. NEW ENGLAND JOURNAL OF MEDICINE 312(17):1128-1129, April 25, 1985.

Transmission of hepatitis B without transmission of AIDS by accidental needle-stick [letter], by J. L. Gerberding, et al. NEW ENGLAND JOURNAL OF MEDICINE 312(1):56-57, January 3, 1985.

AFRICA
Needlestick transmission of AIDS and Africa [letter], by J. Desmyter. LANCET 1(8422):217, January 26, 1985.

Needlestick transmission of HTLV-III from a patient infected in Africa [editorial]. LANCET 2(8416):1376-1377, December 15, 1984.

TRANSMISSION—PREGNANCY
Fetal transmission of AIDS through the mother's womb, by A. Rubinstein. COMPREHENSIVE THERAPY 11(5):6-11, May 1985.

TRANSMISSION—RESEARCH
Transmission experiments with human T-lymphotropic retroviruses and human AIDS tissue [letter], by D. C. Gajdusek, et al. LANCET 1(8391):1415-1416, June 23, 1984.

TRANSMISSION—SALIVA
AIDS: saliva is safe. NEW SCIENTIST 105:7, February 28, 1985.

AIDS saliva link is questioned. NEW SCIENTIST 105:5, February 14, 1985.

AIDS: the saliva scare, by J. Seligmann, et al. NEWSWEEK 104(17):103, October 22, 1984.

AIDS spitting case dismissed. CRIME CONTROL DIGEST 20(33):8, August 18, 1986.

AIDS virus rarely in saliva, researchers say. CORRECTIONS DIGEST 17(3):10, January 29, 1986.

Infrequency of isolation of HTLV-III virus from saliva in AIDS [letter], by D. D. Ho, et al. NEW ENGLAND JOURNAL OF MEDICINE 313(24):1606, December 19, 1985.

Much ado about HTLV-III saliva study, by C. Guilfoy. GAY COMMUNITY NEWS 12(14):1, October 20, 1984.

No AIDS from saliva. NEWSWEEK 106:69, December 30, 1985.

No AIDS test to be required in biting of police officer. CORRECTIONS DIGEST 16(17):10, August 14, 1985; also in CRIME CONTROL DIGEST 19(33):2-3, August 19, 1985.

TRANSMISSION—SEMEN

Semen and AIDS [letter],by G. M. Shearer, et al. NATURE 308(5956):230, March 15-21, 1984.

—, by R. E. Rewell. NATURE 309(5967):394, May 31-June 6, 1984.

Semen polyamines in AIDS pathogenesis [letter], by J. D. Williamson. NATURE 310(5973):103, July 12-18, 1984.

Seminal lymphocytes, plasma and AIDS, by G. P. Olsen, et al. NATURE 309:116-117, May 10, 1984.

Transmission of human T-cell lymphotropic virus type III (HTLV-III) by artificial insemination by donor, by G. J. Stewart, et al. LANCET 2(8455):581-585, September 14, 1985.

TRANSMISSION—SEX

Additional recommendations to reduce sexual and drug abuse-related transmission of human T-lymphotropic virus type III/lymphadenopathy-associated virus. JAMA 255(14):1843-1844+, April 11, 1986; also in: MMWR 35(10): 152-155, March 14, 1986.

AIDS as a sexually transmissible disease, by B. Donovan, et al. AUSTRALIAN FAMILY PHYSICIAN 15(5):620-633, May 1986.

AIDS—discounting promiscuity theory, by B. Lewis. BODY POLITIC 92:11, April 1983.

AIDS epidemic and gay bathhouses: a constitutional analysis, by J. A. Rabin. JOURNAL OF HEALTH POLITICS, POLICY AND LAW 10(4):729-747, Winter 1986.

Can AIDS transmission by prevented by use of a condom? by D. T. Purtilo. JAMA 252:826, August 10, 1984.

Minimal risk of transmission of AIDS-associated retrovirus infection by oral-genital contact [letter], by D. Lyman, et al. JAMA 255(13):1703, April 4, 1986.

Prostitutes taking the heat for the AIDS, by A. Phibbs. GAY COMMUNITY NEWS 13(36):3, March 29, 1986.

Potential for transmission of AIDS-associated retrovirus from bisexual men in San Francisco to their female sexual contacts, by W. Winkelstein, Jr., et al. JAMA 255:901, February 21, 1986.

TRANSMISSION—SPERM
AIDS—status 1985. Implications for sperm banks, by J. O. Nielsen. INTERNA-TIONAL JOURNAL OF ANDROLOGY 8(2):97-100, April 1985.

Spermatozoa and immune dysregulation in homosexual men [letter]. JAMA 252(9):1130, September 7, 1984.

CANADA
Sperm wary: Aussie AIDS puts Calgary insemination on hold, by K. Diotte, et al. ALBERTA REPORT 12:35, August 12, 1985.

TRANSMISSION—TEARS
AIDS virus not transmitted through tears, experts say. OHIO NURSES REVIEW 61(1):3, January 1986.

TRANSMISSION—TEARS—PREVENTION
Recommendations for preventing possible HTLV-III/LAV virus from tears. JAMA 254(11):1429, September 20, 1985.

Recommendations for preventing possible transmission of human T-lymphotropic virus type III/lymphadenopathy-associated virus from tears. MMWR 34(34):533-534, August 30, 1985.

TRANSMISSION—VACCINATION
AIDS, hepatitis, and the national blood policy. REGULATION 9(4):5-7, July-August 1985.

TRANSMISSION—VACCINATION—HEPATITIS B
Laboratory and serological studies argue against possible transmission of AIDS by hepatitis B vaccine [letter], by F. Barré-Sinoussi, et al. LANCET 2(8449): 274, August 1985.

No AIDS from HB vaccine. AMERICAN JOURNAL OF NURSING 85:1268, November 1985.

No HTLV-III antibodies after HBV vaccination, by L. Muylie, et al. NEW ENGLAND JOURNAL OF MEDICINE 314:581, February 27, 1986.

No increased incidence of AIDS in recipients of hepatitis B vaccine [letter], by J. A. Golden. NEW ENGLAND JOURNAL OF MEDICINE 308(19):1163-1164, May 12, 1983.

Question of possible relationship between hepatitis B vaccine and AIDS [letter], by L. B. Taubman,e t al. AMERICAN JOURNAL OF MEDICINE 76(4):A59, April 1984.

Risk of AIDS after hepatitis vaccination [letter]. JAMA 253(20):296-2961, May 24-31, 1985.

Risk of AIDS in recipients of hepatitis B vaccine [letter], by G. Papaevangelou, et al. NEW ENGLAND JOURNAL OF MEDICINE 312(6):376-377, February 7, 1985.

Should the risk of acquired immunodeficiency syndrome deter hepatitis B vaccination? A decision analysis, by H. S. Sacks, et al. JAMA 252(24):3375-3377, December 28, 1984.

Virologists discount fear of AIDS in hepatitis B vaccine. NEW SCIENTIST 108:21, November 7, 1985.

You won't get AIDS from hepatitis vaccine. RN 48:11, April 1985.

TREATMENT

Acquired immunodeficiency syndrome and a trimethoprim-sulfamethoxazole adverse reaction [letter], by D. L. Cohn, et al. ANNALS OF INTERNAL MEDICINE 100(2):311, February 1984.

Acquired immunodeficiency syndrome, chronic coccidiosis and Salmonella typhimurium septicemia in a couple from Zaire. Immunological functions and attempt at immunostimulation by thymopentin, by R. C. Martin-Du Pan, et al. SCHWEIZERISCHE MEDIZINISCHE WOCHENSCHRIFT 114(46):1645-1650, November 17, 1984.

Acquired immunodeficiency syndrome: guidelines for the control of infections in the ambulatory patient and in the hospitalized patient, by C. H. Ramírez-Ronda. BOLETIN—ASOCIACION MEDICA DE PUERTO RICO 77(4):143-150, April 1985.

Administration of 3'-azido-3'-deoxythymidine, an inhibitor of HTLV-III/LAV replication, to patients with AIDS or AIDS-related complex, by R. Yarchoan, et al. LANCET 1(8481):575-580, March 15, 1986.

Adverse effects of interferon in virus infections, autoimmune diseases, and acquired immunodeficiency, by J. Vilcek. PROGRESS IN MEDICAL VIROLOGY 30:62-77, 1984.

Adverse reactions associated wih pyrimethamine-sulfadoxine prophylaxis for Pneumocystis carinii infections in AIDS [letter], by T. R. Navin, et al. LANCET 1(8441):1332, June 8, 1985.

Adverse reactions to pyrimethamine-sulfadoxine in context of AIDS [letter], by M. S. Gottlieb, et al. LANCET 1(8442):1389, June 15, 1985.

Adverse reactions to trimethoprim-sulfamethoxazole in patients with the acquired immunodeficiency syndrome, by F. M. Gordin, et al. ANNALS OF INTERNAL MEDICINE 100(4):495-499, April 1984.

AIDS and AIDS-related diseases—clinical manifestations and therapy, by A. Sönnerborg, et al. LAKARTIDNINGEN 82(20):1877-1880, May 15, 1985.

AIDS and taurolin [letter], by P. Bayardelle. CANADIAN MEDICAL ASSOCIATION JOURNAL 134(5):476, March 1, 1986.

AIDS, associated disorders pose complex therapeutic challenges [news], by H. Cole. JAMA 252(15):1987-1988, October 19, 1984.

AIDS drug shows promise in preliminary clinical trial [news], by J. L. Marx. SCIENCE 231(4745):1504-1505, March 28, 1986.

AIDS drugs: some relief, but adverse side effects, by S. Siwolop. DISCOVER
6:38-42+, December 1985.

AIDS exorcism—suck toes, by J. McNiel. FAG RAG 40:1, 1983.

AIDS: new victims but maybe a treatment, by J. Arehart-Treichel. SCIENCE
NEWS 124:54, July 23, 1983.

AIDS pill that offers hope, by J. Carey. US NEWS & WORLD REPORT 101(13):
69-70, September 29, 1986.

AIDS prevention and treatment, by A. Ranki. DUODECIM 102(7):429-438, 1986.

AIDS: the promise of alternative treatments, by C. Reuben. EAST WEST JOUR-
NAL 16(9):52, September 1986.

AIDS research: promising drug forces reassessment. CHEMICAL AND ENGI-
NEERING NEWS 64:6-7, September 29, 1986.

AIDS research stirs bitter fight over use of experimental drugs, by M. Chase.
WALL STREET JOURNAL 207:29, June 18, 1986.

AIDS: a suitable place for treatment?, by N. Heneson, et al. NEW SCIENTIST
109:24, March 13, 1986.

AIDS therapy by blocking CD4+ cells [letter], by A. Singer, et al. NATURE
320(6058):113, March 13-19, 1986.

AIDS therapy: new push for clinical trials [news], by C. Norman. SCIENCE
230(4732):1355-1358, December 20, 1985.

AIDS therapy: a step closer?, by M. Clark. NEWSWEEK 107(8):60, February 24,
1986.

AIDS: what is now known: part 4, psychosocial aspects, treatment prospects, by
P. A. Selwyn. HOSPITAL PRACTICE 21(10):125-128+, October 15, 1986.

Alternative therapies: hope for people w/AIDS?, by M. Helquist. ADVOCATE
435:43, Decemebr 10, 1985.

AMI hopes to convert Houston hospital into AIDS research and treatment center.
REVIEW OF THE FEDERATION OF AMERICAN HEALTH SYSTEMS 19(2):
108-109, March-April 1986.

Amprolium for coccidiosis in AIDS [letter], by S. J. Veldhuyze van Zanten, et al.
LANCET 2(8398):345-346, August 1984.

Another AIDS treatment , by J. Rogers. MACLEAN'S 98:61, November 11,
1985.

Antimoniotungstate (GPA 23) treatment of three patients with AIDS and one with
prodrome [letter], by W. Rozenbaum, et al. LANCET 1(8426):450-451,
February 23, 1985.

Antiviral agents join fight against AIDS. CHEMICAL AND ENGINEERING NEWS
64:6, August 11, 1986.

Antiviral chemotherapy against HTLV-III/LAV infections, by B. Oberg. JOURNAL OF ANTIMICROBIAL CHEMOTHERAPY 17(5):549-552, May 1986.

Antiviral drugs for AIDS. Current status and future prospects, by E. Sandström. DRUGS 31(6):463-466, June 1986.

Approaches to AIDS therapy, by D. Klatzmann, et al. NATURE 319:10-11, January 2, 1986.

Aseptic techniques for AIDS [letter], by B. E. Evans. JOURNAL OF THE AMERICAN DENTAL ASSOCIATION 107(5):706+, November 1983.

At last, hope for AIDS victims: while no cure, a new drug may prolong life,by M. Clark, et al. NEWSWEEK 108(13):57-58, September 29, 1986.

Attempted treatment of acquired immunodeficiency syndrome (AIDS) with thymic humoral factor, by Y. Berner, et al. ISRAEL JOURNAL OF MEDICAL SCIENCES 20(12):1195-1196, December 1984.

Black market forces legalisation of AIDS drug, by I. Anderson. NEW SCIENTIST 106:6, May 16, 1985.

Bone marrow transplantation in AIDS [letter, by J. M. Hassett, et al. NEW ENGLAND JOURNAL OF MEDICINE 309(11):665, September 15, 1983.

Breakthrough of cytomegalovirus infection despite 9-(1,3-dihydroxy-2-propoxy-methyl)guanine therapy [letter],by M. C. Bach. ANNALS OF INTERNAL MEDICINE 104(4):587, April 1986.

Chemotherapeutic approaches to the treatment of the acquired immune deficiency syndrome (AIDS), by E. De Clercq. JOURNAL OF MEDICINAL CHEMISTRY 29(9):1561-1569, September 1986.

Cincinnati prepares for treatment of AIDS, by J. Zeh. GAY COMMUNITY NEWS 10(26):3, January 22, 1983.

Clinical. A new approach to combat viruses, by S. Hopkins. NURSING MIRROR 160(18):28-29, May 1, 1985.

Clinical pharmacokinetics of suramin in patients with HTLV-III/LAV infection, by J. M. Collins, et al. JOURNAL OF CLINICAL PHARMACOLOGY 26(1):22-26, January 1986.

Clinical trials of interleukin-2 in the acquired immune deficiency syndrome: warning to autopsy prosectors and other health care professionals [letter], by W. M. Mitchell. HUMAN PATHOLOGY 16(1):97-98, January 1985.

Cryptosporidiosis: assessment of chemotherapy of males with acquired immune deficiency syndrome (AIDS). MMWR 31(44):589-592, November 12, 1982.

Cutaneous reaction to trimethoprim-sulfamethoxazole in patients with AIDS and Kaposi's sarcoma, by R. Mituyasu, et al. NEW ENGLAND JOURNAL OF MEDICINE 308(25):1535-1537, June 2, 1983.

Debate continues over treatment of workers with AIDS. SAVINGS INSTITUTIONS 107:76-77, January 1986.

Desperate American AIDS victims journey to Paris, hoping that a new drug can stave off death, by J. Jarvis, et al. PEOPLE 24(7):42-43, August 12, 1985.

Disabling fear of AIDS responsive to imipramine, by M. A. Jenike, et al. PSYCHO-SOMATICS 27(2):143-144, February 1986.

Drug therapy for the opportunistic diseases associated with AIDS, by D. Glickman, et al. AMERICAN PHARMACY NS23(10):23-28, October 1983.

Drug trials: four stages of testing, by M. Helquist. ADVOCATE 450:23, July 8, 1986.

Early results show drug helps patients to fight AIDS. NEW SCIENTIST 109:23, March 20, 1986.

Effective rehabilitation of immune deficiency, by R. Miles. RFD 45:36, Winter 1985.

Effects of intravenous recombinant gamma-interferon on the respiratory burst of blood monocytes from patients with AIDS, by J. e. Pennington, et al. JOURNAL OF INFECTIOUS DISEASES 153(3):609-612, March 1986.

Effects of suramin on HTLV-III/LAV infection presenting as Kaposi's sarcoma or AIDS-related complex: clinical pharmacology and suppression of virus replication in vivo, by S. Broder, et al. LANCET 2(8456):627-630, September 21, 1985.

Etoposide in AIDS therapy. AMERICAN FAMILY PHYSICIAN 31:276, March 1985.

Failure (and danger) of mitozantrone in AIDS-related Kaposi's sarcoma [letter], by L. Kaplan, et al. LANCET 2(8451):396, August 17, 1985.

Feds to rush AIDS drugs, by K. Popert. BODY POLITIC 129:15, August 1986.

Gallo testing new drug. BODY POLITIC 121:25, December 1985.

Gamma interferon and AIDS [letter], by J. L. Moore, et al. NEW ENGLAND JOURNAL OF MEDICINE 312(7):442-443, February 14, 1985.

General strategy for the use of allogeneic lymphocyte infusions in the treatment of disorders characterized by impaired helper or suppressor T cell function: autoimmune diseases and the acquired immunodeficiency syndrome (AIDS), by M. F. McCarty. MEDICAL HYPOTHESES 16(3):189-206, March 1985.

Guide to the investigation and treatment of patients with AIDS and AIDS-related disorders, by F. A. Shepherd, et al. CANADIAN MEDICAL ASSOCIATION JOURNAL 134(9):999-1008, May 1, 1986.

Helquist report—round two for cyclosporin, by M. Helquist. ADVOCATE 449:21, June 24, 1986.

Hepatitis B immune globulin as treatment of CMV infections in patients with AIDS, by W. C. Jordan. JOURNAL OF THE NATIONAL MEDICAL ASSOCIATION 78(1):61-62, January 1986.

Hepatitis B immunization and AIDS, by R. Thomssen, et al. DEUTSCHE MEDIZIN-ISCHE WOCHENSCHRIFT 108(36):1373-1374, September 9, 1983.

Holistic aid for AIDS, by C. McPartland. NEW AGE 9(4):17, November 1983.

Holistic antidote to the epidemic of fear, by C. Hall. RFD 45:46, Winter 1985.

Hope for therapies in 1986, by M. Helquist. ADVOCATE 437:21, January 7, 1986.

Human alpha- and beta-interferon but not gamma- suppress the in vitro replication of LAV, HTLV-III, and ARV-2, by J. K. Yamamoto, et al. JOURNAL OF INTER-FERON RESEARCH 6(2):143-152, April 1986.

Human interferon-alpha production in homosexual men with the acquired immune deficiency syndrome [letter], by J. Abb, et al. JOURNAL OF INFEC-TIOUS DISEASES 150(1):158-189, July 1984.

Hypoglycemic coma from pentamadine in an AIDS patient [letter], by M. P. S Spadafora, et al. AMERICAN JOURNAL OF EMERGENCY MEDICINE 4(4): 384, July 1986.

Immunotoxins to combat AIDS [letter],by A. Surolia, et al. NATURE 322(6075): 119-120, July 10-16, 1986.

In-vivo immunomodulation by isoprinosine in patients with the acquired immuno-deficiency syndrome and related complexes, by M. H. Grieco,e t al. ANNALS OF INTERNAL MEDICINE 101(2):206-207, August 1984.

Inactivation of human T-cell lymphotropic retrovirus (HTLV-III) by LDtm, by P. S. Sarin, et al. NEW ENGLAND JOURNAL OF MEDICINE 313:1416, November 28, 1985.

Inhibitors of retroviral DNA polymerase: their implication in the treatment of AIDS, by P. Chandra, et al. CANCER RESEARCH 45(Suppl. 9):4677s-4684s, September 1985.

Interferon and interferon inactivators in patients with acquired immune deficiency syndrome and Kaposi's sarcoma. A preliminary report, by M. G. Ikossi-O'Connor, et al. RESEARCH COMMUNICATIONS IN CHEMICAL PATHOL-OGY AND PHARMACOLOGY 45(2):271-277, August 1984.

Interferon helps AIDS victims. NEW SCIENTIST 98:681, June 9, 1983.

Interferon may help AIDS victims. NEW SCIENTIST 100:324, November 3, 1983.

Interleukin 2 therapy in infectious diseases: ratinale and prospects, by J. P. Siegel, et al. INFECTION 12(4):298-302, July-August 1984.

Interleukin 2 trial will try to spark flagging immunity of AIDS patients [news], by C. Marwick. JAMA 250(9):1125, September 2, 1983.

Interventions to minimize AIDS [letter], by M. W. Ross. MEDICAL JOURNAL OF AUSTRALIA 142(4):279-280, February 18, 1985.

Isoprinosine and Imuthiol, two potentially active compounds in patients with AIDS-related complex symptoms, by a. Pompidou, et al. CANCER RESEARCH 45(Suppl. 9):4671s-4673s, Setpember 1985.

Isoprinosine unproven. FDA CONSUMER 19:37-38, September 1985.

Ketoconazole therapy for AIDS patients with disseminated histoplasmosis [letter], by P. R. Gustafson, et al. ARCHIVES OF INTERNAL MEDICINE 145(12): 2272, December 1985.

Lymphocyte transfusion in case of acquired immunodeficiency syndrome [letter],by K. C. Davis, et al. LANCET 1(8324):599-600, March 12, 1983.

Miracle cure; holism or hokum?, by K. Schneider. NEW AGE September 1985, p. 14.

Modulation of T- and B-lymphocyte functions by isoprinosine in homosexual subjects with prodromata and in patients with acquired immune deficiency syndrome (AIDS), by P. H. Tsang, et al. JOURNAL OF CLINICAL IMMUNOLOGY 4(6):469-478, November 1984.

Modulation of virus-specific immunity in vitro by the addition of interleukin-1 and interleukin-2 in patients with the acquired immune deficiency syndrome, by J. F. Sheridan, et al. ANNALS OF THE NEW YORK ACADEMY OF SCIENCES 437:53-534, 1984.

Neutralization of HTLV-III/LAV replication by antiserum to thymosin a_1, by P. S. Sarin, et al. SCIENCE 232:1135-1137, May 30, 1986.

Neutralization of human T-lymphotropic virus type III by sera of AIDS and AIDS-risk patients, by R. A. Weiss, et al. NATURE 316(6023):69-72, July 4, 1985.

New developments in the acquired immunodeficiency syndrome: are treatment, prevention, and control possible?, by J. M. Luce. RESPIRATORY CARE 31(2):113-116, February 1986.

New drug boost for AIDS research. THE TIMES HIGHER EDUCATION SUPPLEMENT 675:11, October 11, 1985.

New drug joins front line against AIDS, by C. Joyce. NEW SCIENTIST 111:16, September 25, 1986.

New hope from old drug, by M. Helquist. ADVOCATE 428:30, September 3, 1985.

New strategies for AIDS therapy and prophylaxis [letter], by E. C. M. Mariman, et al. NATURE 318(6045):414, December 5-11, 1985.

New treatment helps AIDS victims. CHEMICAL INDUSTRY 11:349, June 3, 1985.

No new ways of treating AIDS, by J. Maddox. NATURE 308(5955):107, March 8-14, 1984.

Old cure fights AIDS, by N. Underwood. MACLEAN'S 99:52, April 28, 1986.

One against the plague . . . AIDS treatment team, by P. Goldman, et al. NEWS-
WEEK 108(3):38-45+, July 21, 1986.

Partial restoration of impaired interleukin-2 production and Tac antigen (putative
interleukin-2 receptor) expression in patients with acquired immune deficiency syndrome by isoprinosine treatment in vitro, by K. Y. Tsang, et al.
JOURNAL OF CLINICAL INVESTIGATION 75(5):1538-1544, May 1985.

Pentamidine-induced hypoglycemia in patients with the acquired immune deficiency syndrome, by C. M. Stahl-Bayliss, et al. CLINICAL PHARMACOLOGY
AND THERAPEUTICS 39(3):271-275, March 1986.

Pentamidine methanesulfonate to be distributed by CDC. JAMA 251(20):2641,
May 25, 1985; also in MMWR 33(17):225-226, May 4, 1984.

Perspectives on the immunotherapy of AIDS, by J. W. Hadden. ANNALS OF
THE NEW YORK ACADEMY OF SCIENCES 437:76-87, 1984.

Possible AIDS cure, by K. Scanlon. MACLEAN'S 99:46, March 24, 1986.

Possible AIDS remedy tested, by L. Goldsmith. GAY COMMUNITY NEWS
11(3):1, July 30, 1983.

Possible cure for crytosporidiosis . . . spiramycin. EMERGENCY MEDICINE
16(14):115-116, August 15, 1984.

Possible risk of steroid administration in patients at risk for AIDS [letter], by R. W.
Shafer, et al. LANCET 1(8434):934-935, April 20, 1985.

Pre-AIDS patients will get experimental drug, by S. Burke. OUT 3(4):2, February
1985.

Preferences of homosexual men with AIDS for life-sustaining treatment, by R.
Steinbrook, et al. NEW ENGLAND JOURNAL OF MEDICINE 314:457-460,
February 13, 1986.

Preliminary clinical observations with recombinant interleukin-2 in patients with
AIDS or LAS, by P. Kern, et al. BLUT 50(1):1-6, 1985.

Preliminary results on clinical and immunological effects of thymopentin in AIDS,
by N. Clumeck, et al. INTERNATIONAL JOURNAL OF CLINICAL PHARMA-
COLOGICAL RESEARCH 4(6):459-463, 1984.

Promising results halt trial of anti-AIDS drug, by D. M. Barnes. SCIENCE 234:15-
16, October 3, 1986.

Promising treatment, by N. Underwood. MACLEAN'S 99:58, October 13, 1986.

Prophylaxis of Pneumocystis carinii infection in AIDS with pyrimethamine-
sulfadoxine [letter], by M. S. Gottlieb, et al. LANCET 2(8399):398-399,
August 18, 1984.

Prospects for treatment of human retrovirus-associated diseases, by D. P.
Bolognesi, et al. CANCER RESEARCH 45(Suppl. 9):4700s-4705s, September 1985.

Prospects of therapy for infections with human T-lymphotropic virus type III, by M. S. Hirsch, et al. ANNALS OF INTERNAL MEDICINE 103(5):750-755, November 1985.

Ray of hope in the fight against AIDS . . . an experimental drug called AZT prolongs the life of patients, by J. Levine, et al. TIME 128(13):60-61, September 29, 1986.

Recommendations for providing dialysis treatment to patients infected with human T-lymphotropic virus type III/lymphadenopathy-associated virus. ANNALS OF INTERNAL MEDICINE 105(4):558-559, October 1986; also in MMWR 35(23):376-378+, June 13, 1986.

Recommended precautions for patients undergoing hemodialysis who have AIDS or non-A, non-B hepatitis, by M. S. Favero. INFECTION CONTROL 6(8):301-305, August 1985.

Remission without drugs/drugs without remission, by M. Helquist. ADVOCATE 431:21, October 15, 1985.

Repairing the T-cell defect in AIDS [letter], by D. Zagury, et al. LANCET 2(8452): 449, August 24, 1985.

Risks with danazol in the acquired immunodeficiency syndrome [letter], by . E Metroka, et al. ANNALS OF INTERNAL MEDICINE 101(4)564-565, October 1984.

Role of interferon in AIDS, by O. T. Preble, et al. ANNALS OF THE NEW YORK ACADEMY OF SCIENCES 437:65-75, 1984.

Senate votes to expand anti-AIDS drug trials, by D. M. Barnes. SCIENCE 233: 1382, September 26, 1986.

Serotherapy for AIDS and pre-AIDS syndrome [letter], by H. F. Sewell, et al. NATURE 320(6058):113-114, March 13-19, 1986.

Severe neutropenia during pentamidine treatment of immunodeficiency syndrome—New York City. JAMA 251(10):1253-1254, March 9, 1984; also in MMWR 33(6):65-67, February 17, 1984.

Short-term results with suramin for AIDS-related conditions [letter], by D. Rouvoy, et al. LANCET 1(8433):878-879, April 13, 1985.

Side effects of substitution therapy, by L. M. Aledort. SCANDINAVIAN JOURNAL OF HAEMATOLOGY. SUPPLEMENTUM 40:331-333, 1984.

Stimulation of cellular function by thymopentin (TP-5) in three AIDS patients [letter], by F. Mascart-Lemone, et al. LANCET 2(8352):735-736, September 24, 1983.

Successful treatment of lethal protozoal infections with the ornithine decarboxylase inhibitor, alpha-difluoromethylornithine, by A. Sjoerdsma, et al. TRANSACTIONS OF THE ASSOCIATION OF AMERICAN PHYSICIANS 97:70-79, 1984.

Sulphadiazine desensitisation in AIDS patients [letter], by E. T. Bell, et al. LANCET 1(8421):163, January 19, 1985.

Suramin drug is disappointing in AIDS. NEW SCIENTIST 107:30, September 26, 1985.

Suramin protection of T cells in vitro against infectivity and cytopathic effect of HTLV-III, by H. Mitsuya, et al. SCIENCE 226:172-174, October 12, 1984.

Suramin therapy in patients with LAS/AIDS (letter), by W. Busch, et al. DEUTSCHE MEDIZINISCHE WOCHENSCHRIFT 110(40)1552, October 4, 1985.

Suramin treatment for AIDS [letter], by w. Busch, et al. LANCET 2(8466):1247, November 30, 1985.

Theater as therapy: "AIDS/US" creates drama, by S. McDonald. ADVOCATE 450:39, July 8, 1986.

Therapeutic approaches to patients with AIDS, by H. C. Lane, et al. CANCER RESEARCH 45(Suppl. 9):4674s-4676s, September 1985.

Thymopentin treatment in AIDS and pre-AIDS patients, by N. Clumeck, et al. SURVEY OF IMMUNOLOGICAL RESEARCH 4(Suppl. 1):58-62, 1985.

Toughers virus of all: can a drug or vaccine be found to vanquish AIDS? TIME 128(18):76-77, November 3, 1986.

Treatment of the acquired immune deficiency syndrome, by S. Gupta, et al. JOURNAL OF CLINICAL IMMUNOLOGY 6(3):183-193, May 1986.

Treatment of immunodeficiency with interleukin-2: initial exploration, by R. Mertelsmann, et al. JOURNAL OF BIOLOGICAL RESPONSE MODIFIERS 3(5):483-490, October 1984.

Treatment of infections in patients with the acquired immunodeficiency syndrome, by D. Armstrong, et al. ANNALS OF INTERNAL MEDICINE 103(): 738-743, November 1985.

Treatment of infectious complications of acquired immunodeficiency syndrome, by M. M. Furio, et al. CLINICAL PHARMACY 4(5):539-554, September-October 1985.

Uncertainty surrounds anti-viral drug plan, by K. Westheimer. GAY COMMUNITY NEWS 14(11):1, September 28, 1986.

Use of interleukin-2 in patients with acquired immunodeficiency syndrome, by H. C. Lane, et al. JOURNAL OF BIOLOGICAL RESPONSE MODIFIERS 3(5): 512-516, October 1984.

Vitamin C in the treatment of acquired immune deficiency syndrome (AIDS), by R. F. Cathcart, 3d. MEDICAL HYPOTHESES 14(4):423-433, August 1984.

Volatile nitrites. Use and adverse effects related to the current epidemic of the acquired immune deficiency syndrome, by G. R. Newell, et al. AMERICAN JOURNAL OF MEDICINE 78(5):811-816, May 1985.

GREAT BRITAIN
British drug set to better AZT. NEW SCIENTIST 111:17, September 25, 1986.

HAITI
Cutaneous reactions to trimethoprim-sulfamethoxazole in Haitians [letter], by J. A. DeHovitz, et al. ANNALS OF INTERNAL MEDICINE 103(3):479-480, September1985.

TREATMENT—HEMOPHILIACS
AIDS and the treatment of hemophilia. MICHIGAN MEDICINE 84(1):62-63, January 1985.

AIDS retrovirus antibodies in hemophiliacs treated with factor VIII or factor IX concentrates, cryorecipitate, or fresh frozen plasma: prevalence, seroconversion rate, and clinical correlations, by M. V. Ragni, et al. BLOOD 67(3):592-595, March 1986.

Immunologic dysfunction in patients with classic hemophilia receiving lyophilized factor VIII concentrates and cryoprecipitate, by C. Tsoukas, et al. CANADIAN MEDICAL ASSOCIATION JOURNAL 129(7):713-717, October 1, 1983.

VACCINATION
Disseminated Mycobacterium bovis infection from BCG vaccination of a patient with acquired immunodeficiency syndrome. MMWR 34(16):227-228, April 26, 1985.

VACCINATION—HEPATITIS B
Absence of antibodies to HTLV-III in health workers after hepatitis B vaccination, by J. L. Dienstag, et al. JAMA 254:1064-1066, August 23-30, 1985.

Acquired immunodeficiency syndrome (AIDS): is vaccination against hepatitis B a prevention for the risk?, by D. Vuitton, et al. GASTROENTEROLOGIE CLINIQUE ET BIOLOGIQUE 8(1):37-41, January 1984.

Hepatitis B vaccination and AIDS [letter], by S. Kato, et al. JAMA 254(1):53, July 5, 1985.

Hepatitis B vaccination: the danger of AIDS transmission, by R. Scheier. ZEITSCHRIFT FUR HAUTKRANKHEITEN 59(8):502-506, April 15, 1984.

Hepatitis "B" vaccine. MEDICAL BULLETIN OF THE U.S. ARMY, EUROPE 41(2):14, February 1984.

Hepatitis B vaccine and AIDS. AMERICAN FAMILY PHYSICIAN 33:312, March 1986.

— [letter], by J. B. Epstein. CANADIAN DENTAL ASSOCIATION JOURNAL 5(2):115, February 1986.

Hepatitis B vaccine does not transmit AIDS. AMERICAN JOURNAL OF NURSING 83:1196, August 1983.

—. Pasteur Institute in AIDS fracas, by R. Walgate. NATURE 304(5922):104, July 14-20, 1983.

Hepatitis B vaccine: evidence confirming lack of AIDS transmission, by B. Poiesz, et al. JAMA 253:21-22, January 4, 1985; also in MMWR 33(49):685-687, December 1, 1984.

Hepatitis vaccine and the acquired immunodeficiency syndrome [letter], by A. M. Schwartz, et al. ANNALS OF INTERNAL MEDICINE 99(4):567-568, October 1983.

Safety of hepatitis B vaccine confirmed. FDA DRUG BULLETIN 15(2):14-15, August 1985.

VACCINE

AIDS controversies: scientists bicker while their search for a vaccine continues, by S. Gilbert. SCIENCE DIGEST 93:28, September 1985.

AIDS fears spark row over vaccine [news], by D. Dickson. SCIENCE 221(4609): 437, July 29, 1983.

AIDS progress. Synthetic vaccine only a distant prospect [news], by T. Beardsley. NATURE 314(6013):659, April 25-May 1, 1985.

AIDS vaccine: a glimmer of hope. THE ECONOMIST 298:90, March 22, 1986.

AIDS vaccine research: promising protein, by L. Davis. SCIENCE NEWS 129: 151, March 8, 1986.

AIDS victims still await vaccine, by O. Sattaur. NEW SCIENTIST 105:20, January 24, 1985.

Ambivalent support for AIDS vaccine, by N. Fain. ADVOCATE 419:22, April 30, 1985.

Answer to AIDS/ a herpes vaccine? SCIENCE DIGEST 92:42, January 1984.

Closer to an AIDS vaccine?, by C. Wallis, et al. TIME 127(14):44, April 7, 1986.

Gallo cautious about vaccine, by C. Guilfoy. GAY COMMUNITY NEWS 13(17):3, November 9, 1985.

Glimmer of hope; AIDS vaccine. THE ECONOMIST 298:90, March 22, 1986.

HB vaccine study. AMERICAN FAMILY PHYSICIAN 31:274, March 1985.

Hopes for an AIDS vaccine are fading fast, by S. Connor. NEW SCIENTIST 111:28-29, July 3, 1986.

Long shots: the race to develop vaccine against AIDS mobilizes researchers, by M. Chase. WALL STREET JOURNAL 204:1+ September 4, 1984.

Mutant virus worries vaccine researchers. NEW SCIENTIST 110:26, June 26, 1986.

New research leads to AIDS vaccine. NEW SCIENTIST 110:17, April 17, 1986.

596

Old cure points to an AIDS vaccine . . . vaccinia virus—or cowpox, by M. Clark, et al. NEWSWEEK 107(16):71, April 21, 1986.

PHS invites industry collaboration on AIDS vaccine, by D. M. Barnes. SCIENCE 233:1034-1035, September 5, 1986.

Prospects for and pathways toward a vaccine for AIDS, by D. P. Francis, et al. NEW ENGLAND JOURNAL OF MEDICINE 313(25):1586-1590, December 19, 1985.

Retrovaccine. SCIENTIFIC AMERICAN 253:62, August 1985.

Search for an AIDS vaccine, by W. Dowdle. PUBLIC HEALTH REPORTS 101(3): 232-233, May-June 1986.

Slow progress on AIDS vaccines. NEW SCIENTIST 111:17, September 11, 1986.

Strategies for an AIDS vaccine, by D. M. Barnes. SCIENCE 233:1149-1150+, September 12, 1986.

Subunit vaccines against exogenous retroviruses: overview and perspectives, by G. Hunsmann. CANCER RESEARCH 45(Suppl. 9):4691s-4693s, September 1985.

Thymus protein offers a clue to AIDS vaccine. NEW SCIENTIST 110:20, May 29, 1986.

Toughers virus of all: can a drug or vaccine be found to vanquish AIDS? TIME 128(18):76-77, November 3, 1986.

Unconventional vaccines: immunization with anti-idiotype antibody against viral diseases, by H. Koprowski. CANCER RESEARCH 45(Suppl. 9):4689s-4690s, September 1985.

Vaccine against AIDS is on the way. US NEWS & WORLD REPORT 96:12, May 7, 1984.

Vaccine for simian AIDS developed. CHEMICAL AND ENGINEERING NEWS 64:5, September 8, 1986.

When will we have an AIDS vaccine?, by N. Heneson. NEW SCIENTIST 109:20, March 27, 1986.

Why an AIDS vaccine is a long time coming. NEW SCIENTIST 109:39, January 2, 1986.

Will an AIDS vaccine bankrupt the company that makes it?, by D. M. Barnes. SCIENCE 233:1035, September 5, 1986.

VENEREAL DISEASE
ABC of sexually transmitted diseases. Acquired immune deficiency syndrome, by I. Weller. BRITISH MEDICAL JOURNAL 288(6411):136-137, January 14, 1984.

Acquired immune deficiency syndrome: a venereal disease? by P. A. Poulsen, et al. UGESKRIFT FOR LAEGER 146(5):355-356, January 30, 1984.

Acquired immunodeficiency syndrome (AIDS) manifested as severe genital herpes. Apropos of 2 cases, by J. De Maubeuge, et al. DERMATOLOGICA 168(3):105-111, 1984.

AIDS and herpes carry weighty policy implications for your Board, by K. McCormick. AMERICAN SCHOOL BOARD JOURNAL 172(10):37-38, October 1985.

AIDS-induced decline of the incidence of syphilis in Denmark, by A. Poulsen, et al. ACTA DERMATO-VENEREOLOGICA 65(6):567-569, 1985.

Gonorrhoea in homosexual men and media coverage of the acquired immune deficiency syndrome in London 1982-3, by I. V. Weller, et al. BRITISH MEDICAL JOURNAL 289(6451):1041, October 20, 1984.

Herpes may be a factor in getting AIDS: study. JET 66:35, July 30, 1984.

Herpes virus infections in the acquired immune deficiency syndrome, by G. V. Quinnan, Jr., et al. JAMA 252(1):72-77, July 6, 1984.

Herpes virus may have role in AIDS. AMERICAN FAMILY PHYSICIAN 27:268-269, April 1983.

Herpes without vesicles: limited, recurrent genital lesions in an immunodebili-tated host, by H. Schneiderman, et al. SOUTHERN MEDICAL JOURNAL 79(3):368-370, March 1986.

Herpes zoster and the acquired immunodeficienty syndrome [letter],by L. A. Cone, et al. ANNALS OF INTERNAL MEDICINE 100(3):462, March 1984.

Herpes zoster ophthalmicus and acquired immune deficiency syndrome, by E. L. Cole, et al. ARCHIVES OF OPHTHALMOLOGY 102(7):1027-1029, July 1984.

Herpes zoster ophthalmicus in patients at risk for AIDS [letter], by W. Sandor, et al. NEW ENGLAND JOURNAL OF MEDICINE 310(17):1118-1119, April 26, 1984.

Herpes zoster: a possible early clinical sign for development of acquired immuno-deficiency syndrome in high-risk individuals, by A. E. Friedman-Kien, et al. JOURNAL OF THE AMERICAN ACADEMY OF DERMATOLOGY 14(6):1023-1028, June 1986.

How to turn a disease into VD, by J. Seale. NEW SCIENTIST 106:38-41, June 20, 1985.

Immunogen for herpes, AIDS? by C. Wenz. NATURE 311(5985):404, October 4, 1984.

Secondary syphilis masquerading as AIDS in a young gay male, by R. A. Smego, Jr., et al. NORTH CAROLINA MEDICAL JOURNAL 45(4):253-254, April 1984.

Speaking VD, by P. Masters. GAY INFORMATION JOURNAL OF GAY STUDIES 12:19, Summer 1982.

VIROLOGY

Acquired immune deficiency syndrome (AIDS) manifesting as anogenital herpes zoster eruption: demonstration of virus-like particles in lymphosytes, by P. Thune, et al. ACTA DERMATO-VENEREOLOGICA. SUPPLEMENTUM 63(6):540-543, 1983.

Acquired immune deficiency syndrome: viral infections and etiology, by D. Armstrong. PROGRESS IN MEDICAL VIROLOGY 30:1-13, 1984.

Acquired immunodeficiency syndrome: epidemiology, virology, and immunology, by A. Weiss, et al. ANNUAL REVIEW OF MEDICINE 36:545-562, 1985.

Activation of a novel KpnI transcript by downstream integration of a human T-lymphotropic virus type I provirus, by T. Okamoto, et al. JOURNAL OF BIOLOGICAL CHEMISTRY 261:4615-4619, April 5, 1986.

Acute AIDS retrovirus infection. Definition of a clinical illness associated with seroconversion, by D. A. Cooper, et al. LANCET 1(8428):537-540, March 9, 1985.

Adenovirus isolates from urine of patients with acquired immunodeficiency syndrome, by P. J. deJong, et al. LANCET 1(8337):1293-1296, June 11, 1983.

Advances in the isolation of HTLV-III from patients with AIDS and AIDS-related complex and from donors at risk, by P. D. Markham, et al. CANCER RESEARCH 45(Suppl. 9):4588s-4591s, September 1985.

AIDS, acquired immunodeficiency syndrome and its possible link to human T-cell leukemia-lymphoma virus, the retrovirus inducer of T-cell leukemia in the adult, by C. Dosne Pasqualini, et al. MEDICINA 43(4):472-474, 1983.

AIDS and HTLV-III infection, by H. M. Glenister. NURSING 3(6):229-231, June 1986.

AIDS and its association with human tumors and viruses. A viral and/or immunogenetic cause?, by G. Mathé. BIOMEDICINE AND PHARMACOTHERAPY 37(4):153-159, 1983.

AIDS and its relation to a virus infection, by H. Bauer. DEUTSCHE MEDIZINISCHE WOCHENSCHRIFT 110(12):443-444, March 22, 1985.

AIDS and 'slow viruses,' by R. W. Smith. ANNALS OF THE NEW YORK ACADEMY OF SCIENCES 437:576-607, 1984.

AIDS and the spectrum of HTLV-III/LAV infection, by A. J. Pinching, et al. INTERNATIONAL REVIEW OF EXPERIMENTAL PATHOLOGY 28:1-44, 1986.

AIDS-associated retroviruses (ARV) can productively infect other cells besides human T helper cells, by J. A. Levy, et al. VIROLOGY 147:442-448, December 1985.

AIDS-associated virus yields data to intensifying scientific study, by C. Marwick. JAMA 254:2865-2868+, November 22-29, 1985.

AIDS development: NIH to license HTLV [news],by S. Budiansky. NATURE 309(5969):577, June 14-20, 1984.

AIDS investigators identify second retrovirus [news], by J. Maurice. JAMA 2 250(8):1010-1011+, August 26, 1983.

AIDS related virus found. BODY POLITIC 126:23, May 1986.

AIDS research. Is there really a virus? [news], by G. Linnebank. NATURE 305(5932):264, September 22-28, 1983.

AIDS research, virus both advance, J. Silberner. SCIENCE NEWS 127:7, January 5, 1985.

AIDS retrovirus (ARV-2) clone replicates in transfected human and animal fibro-blasts, by J. A. Levy, et al. SCIENCE 232:998-1001, May 23, 1986.

AIDS virology: a battle on many fronts [news], by C. Norman. SCIENCE 230 (4725):518-521, November 1, 1985.

AIDS virus, by T. Kitamura. NIPPON RINSHO43(8):1783-1789, August 1985.

AIDS virus and HTLV-I differ in codon choices [letter], by P. Grantham, et al. NATURE 319(6056):727-728, February 27-March 5, 1986.

AIDS: virus clones multiply, by T. Beardsley. NATURE 311:195, September 20, 1984.

AIDS virus entry pinpointed in brain [news], by R. Lewin. SCIENCE 233(4760): 160, July 11, 1986.

AIDS virus genome sequenced, by R. Baum. CHEMICAL AND ENGINEERING NEWS 63:32-34, February 18, 1985.

AIDS virus genomes [news], by J. L. Marx. SCIENCE 227(4686):503, February 1, 1985.

AIDS virus has new name—perhaps, by J. L. Marx. SCIENCE 232:699-700, May 9, 1986.

AIDS virus: how many kinds? SCIENCE 6:8, November 1985.

AIDS virus in the brain. NEW SCIENTIST 108:29, December 5, 1985.

AIDS virus infection: prognosis and transmission [letter]. JOURNAL OF THE ROYAL SOCIETY OF MEDICINE 79(2):121-123, February 1986.

AIDS virus infection: prognosis and transmission [editorial], by J. Seale. JOUR-NAL OF THE ROYAL SOCIETY OF MEDICINE 78(8):613-615, August 1985.

AIDS virus: infection up? SCIENCE NEWS 128:325, November 23, 1985.

AIDS: the virus is not immune, by J. Weber. NEW SCIENTIST 109:37-39, January 2, 1986.

AIDS virus is spreading and mutating, by C. Joyce. NEW SCIENTIST 104:9, October 18, 1984.

AIDS virus might cause brain disease, by O. Sattaur. NEW SCIENTIST 106:21, April 25, 1985.

AIDS virus presents moving target, by C. Norman. SCIENCE 230:1357, December 20, 1985.

AIDS virus shows a chink in its armour. THE ECONOMIST 297:105, November 16, 1985.

AIDS virus structure and disease transmission analyzed. AMERICAN FAMILY PHYSICIAN 31:275-276+, April 1985.

AIDS: what is now known: part 1, history and immunovirology, by P. A. Selwyn. HOSPITAL PRACTICE 21(5):67-76, May 15, 1986.

AIDS— a virus infection?, by J. Abb, et al. HAUTARZT 35(12):615-616, December 1984.

Alteration of T-cell functions by infection with HTLV-I or HTLV-II, by M. Popovic, et al. SCIENCE 226:459-462, October 26, 1984.

Another cell victim of AIDS virus? SCIENCE NEWS 129:24, January 11, 1986.

Antigens on HTLV-infected cells recognized by leukemia and AIDS sera are related to HTLV viral glycoprotein, by J. Schüpbach, et al. SCIENCE 224 (4649):607-610, May 11, 1984.

Antiserum to a synthetic peptide recognizes the HTLV-III envelope glycoprotein, by R. C. Kennedy, et al. SCIENCE 231:1556-1559, March 28, 1986.

Binding of HTLV-III/LAV to T4+ cells by a complex of the 110K viral protein and the T4 molecule, by J. S. McDougal, et al. SCIENCE 231:382-385, January 24, 1986.

Biological nature of AIDS virus, by D. Bardell. AMERICAN BIOLOGY TEACHER 48:75-77, February 1986.

Body composition studies in patients with the acquired immunodeficiency syndrome, by D. P. Kotler, et al. AMERICAN JOURNAL OF CLINICAL NUTRITION 42(6):1255-1265, December 1985.

Boston PWAs included in anti-viral drug study, by K. Westheimer. GAY COMMUNITY NEWS 13(50):3, July 6, 1986.

Caution on AIDS viruses [letter],by J. A. Sonnabend. NATURE 310(5973):103, July 12-18, 1984.

CD4 (T4) antigen is an essential component of the receptor for the AIDS retrovirus, by A. G. Dalgleish, et al. NATURE 312(5996):763-767, December 20, 1984-January 2, 1985.

Characterization of a continuous T-cell line susceptible to the cytopathic effects of the acquired immunodeficiency syndrome (AIDS)-associated retrovirus, by T. Folks, et al. PROCEEDINGS OF THE NATIONAL ACADEMY OF SCIENCES USA 82(13):4539-4543, July 1985.

Characterization of the acquired immune deficiency syndrome at the cellular and molecular level, by D. J. Barrett. MOLECULAR AND CELLULAR BIOCHEMISTRY 63(1):3-11, August 1984.

Characterization of adenovirus isolates from AIDS patients, by M. S. Horwitz, et al. ANNALS OF THE NEW YORK ACADEMY OF SCIENCES 437:161-174, 1984.

Characterization of the AIDS-associated retrovirus reverse transcriptase and optimal conditions for its detection in virions, by A. D. Hoffman, et al. VIROLOGY 147:326-235, December 1985.

Characterization of long terminal repeat sequences of HTLV-III, by B. Starcich, et al. SCIENCE 227:538-540, February 1, 1985.

Classification of HTLV-III infection based on 75 cases seen in a suburban community, by M. H. Kaplan, et al. CANCER RESEARCH 45(Suppl. 9):4655s-4658s, September 1985.

Classification of HTLV-III/LAV-related diseases [letter],by H. W. Haverkos, et al. JOURNAL OF INFECTIOUS DISEASES 152(5):1095, November 1985.

Classification system for human T-lymphotropic virus type III/lymphadenopathy-associated virus infections, by Centers for Disease Control, U.S. Department of Health and Human Services. ANNALS OF INTERNAL MEDICINE 105(2): 234-237, August 1986.

Clinical work-load of HTLV-III infection [letter], by B. A. Evans, et al. LANCET 1(8442):1388, June 15, 1985.

Clonal selection of T lymphocytes infected by cell-free human T-cell leukemia/ lymphoma virus type I: parameters of virus integration and expression, by A. DeRossi, et al. VIROLOGY 143:640-645, June 1985.

Coming of AIDS: a viral update, by J. F. Grutsch, et al. AMERICAN SPECTATOR 19:18-20, September 1986.

Common disinfectants kill AIDS virus. RN 49:81, January 1986.

Complete nucleotide sequence of the AIDS virus, HTLV-III, by L. Ratner, et al. NATURE 313(6000):277-284, January 24-30, 1985.

Consultation 7—here everything turns around the AIDS virus, by I. Lernevall. VARD-FACKET 9(22):10-12, December 12, 1985.

Correlation between exposure to human T-cell leukemia-lymphoma virus-III and the development of AIDS, by P. D. Markham, et al. ANNALS OF THE NEW YORK ACADEMY OF SCIENCES 437:106-109, 1984.

Cytomegalovirus and carcinogenesis, by F. Rapp. JOURNAL OF THE NATIONAL CANCER INSTITUTE 72(4):783-787, April 1984.

Cytomegalovirus- and Cryptosporidium-associated acalculous gangrenous cholecystitis, by R. S. Blumberg, et al. AMERICAN JOURNAL OF MEDICINE 76(6):1118-1123, June 1984.

Detection, isolation, and continuous production of cytopathic retroviruses (HTLV-III) from patients with AIDS and pre-AIDS, by M. Popovic, et al. SCIENCE 224:497-500, May 4, 1984.

Detection of AIDS virus in macrophages in brain tissue from AIDS patients with encephalopathy, by S. Koenig, et al. SCIENCE 233:1089-1093, September 5, 1986.

Detection of infectious HTLV-III/LAV virus in cell-free plasma from AIDS patients [letter], by D. Zagury, et al. LANCET 2(8453):505-506, August 31, 1985.

Detection of two human T cell leukemia/lymphotropic viruses in cultured lymphocytes of a hemophiliac with acquired immunodeficiency syndrome, by E. L. Palmer, et al. JOURNAL OF INFECTIOUS DISEASES 151(3):559-563, March 1985.

Disinfection in LAV/HTLV-III infections. KRANKENPFLEGE. SOINS INFIRMIERS 79(5):40-42+, May 1986.

Diversity of clinical spectrum of HTLV-III infection, by S. L. Valle, et al. LANCET 1(8424):301-304, February 9, 1985.

Does prostaglandin aid the AIDS virus?, by B. Johnstone. NEW SCIENTIST 110:28, April 10, 1986.

Does quinine facilitate AIDS?, by V. Ruocco,e t al. ANTIBIOTIC CHEMO-THERAPY 32:159-160, 1983.

Effect of Cohn fractionation conditions on infectivity of the AIDS virus, by A. M. Prince, et al. NEW ENGLAND JOURNAL OF MEDICINE 314:386, February 6, 1986.

Electron microscopic evidence of non-A, non-B hepatitis markers and virus-like particles in immunocompromised humans, by S. Watanabe, et al. HEPA-TOLOGY 4(4):628-632, July-August 1984.

Evidence of a virus in multiple sclerosis. NEW SCIENTIST 108:30, November 21, 1985.

Expression of human immunodeficiency virus antigen (HIV-Ag) in serum and cerebrospinal fluid during acute and chronic infection, by J. Goudsmit, et al. LANCET 2(8500):177--180, July 26, 1986.

Expression of the 3' terminal region of human T-cell leukemia viruses, by W. Wachsman, et al. SCIENCE 226:177-179, October 12, 1984.

French, US viral isolates compared in search for cause of AIDS [news], by C. Marwick, et al. JAMA 251(22):2901-2903+, June 8, 1984.

Frequent detection and isolation of cytopathic retroviruses (HTLV-III) from patients with AIDS and at risk for AIDS, by R. C. Gallo, et al. SCIENCE 224 (4648):500-503, May 4, 1984.

Functional properties of antigen-specific T cells infected by human T-cell leukemia-lymphoma virus (HTLV-I), by H. Mitsuya, et al. SCIENCE 225:1484-1486, September 28, 1984.

Functional relation between HTLV-III *x* and adenovirus EIA proteins in transcriptional activation, by I.S. Y. Chen, et al. SCIENCE 230:570-573, November 1, 1985.

Hepatitis B surface antigen could harbour the infective agent of AIDS, by M. I. McDonald, et al. LANCET 2(8355):882-884, October 15, 1983.

Hepatitis B virus and the prevention of primary cancer of the liver, by B. S. Blumberg, et al. JOURNAL OF THE NATIONAL CANCER INSTITUTE 74(2):267-273, February 1985.

Hepatitis B virus DNA sequences in lymphoid cells from patients with AIDS and AIDS-related complex, by F. Laure, et al. SCIENCE 229(4713):561-563, August 9, 1985.

Hepatitis B virus (HBV) DNA in leucocytes in acquired immune deficiency syndrome (AIDS), by L. E. Lie-Injo, et al. CYTOBIOS 44(176):119-128, 1985.

Hepatitis B virus in AIDS [letter],by L. E. Lie-Injo. LANCET 1(8367):54, January 7, 1984.

Hepatitis B virus infection in the acquired immunodeficiency syndrome, by V. K. Rustgi, et al. ANNALS OF INTERNAL MEDICINE 101(6):795-797, December 1984.

How HTLV causes leukaemia, by O. Sattaur. NEW SCIENTIST 103:35, August 2, 1984.

HTLV and AIDS. AMERICAN FAMILY PHYSICIAN 28:255, July 1983.

— [editorial]. LANCET 1(8335):1200, May 28, 1983.

HTLV exposure and AIDS. AMERICAN FAMILY PHYSICIAN 33:358, March 1986.

HTLV/III, AIDS, and the brain [editorial], by P. H. Black. NEW ENGLAND JOURNAL OF MEDICINE 313(2):1538-1540, December 12, 1985.

HTLV-III AIDS link, by J. A. Bennett. AMERICAN JOURNAL OF NURSING 85(10): 1086-1089, October 1985.

HTLV-III and LAV: similar, or identical? by C. Norman. SCIENCE 230:643, November 8, 1985.

HTLV-III gag protein is processed in yeast cells by the virus *pol*-protease, by R. A. Kramer, et al. SCIENCE 231:1580-1584, March 28, 1986.

HTLV-III infection in kidney transplant recipients [letter], by J. L'age-Stehr, et al. LANCET 2(8468):1361-1362, December 14, 1985.

HTLV-III infections and AIDS—current epidemiology and serology, by G. Biberfeld, et al. LAKARTIDNINGEN 82(20):1867-1870, May 15, 1985.

HTLV-III, LAV, ARV are variants of same AIDS virus [letter], by L. Ratner, et al. NA-
TURE 313(6004):636-637, February 21-27, 1985.

HTLV-III/LAV-like retrovirus particles in the brains of patients with AIDS encephalopathy, by L. G. Epstein, et al. AIDS RESEARCH 1(6):447-454, 1984-
1985.

HTLV-III seroconversion associated with heat-treated factor VIII concentrate
[letter], by G. C. White, 2d, et al. LANCET 1(8481):611-612, March 15, 1986.

HTLV-III seropositivity in AIDS [letter],by W. M. Behan, et al. LANCET 1(8389):
1292, June 9, 1984.

Human T-cell leukemia (lymphotropic) retroviruses and their causative role in T-
cell malignancies and acquired immune deficiency syndrome, by R. C. Gallo.
CANCER 55(10):2317-2323, May 15, 1985.

Human T-cell leukemia/lymphotropic retroviruses (HTLV) family: past, present,
and future, by R. C. Gallo. CANCER RESEARCH 45(Suppl. 9):4524s-4533s,
September 1985.

Human T-cell leukemia virus and AIDS [letter],by P. H. Black, et al. NEW
ENGLAND JOURNAL OF MEDICINE 309(14):856, October 6, 1983.

Human T-cell leukemia virus family, adult T cell leukemia, and AIDS, by R. C. Gallo,
et al. HAMATOLOGIE UND BLUTTRANSFUSION 29:317-325, 1985.

Human T-cell leukemia virus in acquired immune deficiency syndrome: preliminary
observation. JAMA 249(21)L2878-2879, June 3, 1983.

Human T-cell leukemia virus infection in patients with acquired immune deficiency
syndrome: preliminary observations. MMWR 32(18):233-234, May 13, 1983.

Human T-cell leukemia virus linked to AIDS, by J. L. Marx. SCIENCE 220(4599):
806-809, May 20, 1983.

Human T-cell leukemia virus type II: primary structure analysis of the major internal
protein, p24 and the nucleic acid binding protein, p15, by S. G. Devare, et al.
VIROLOGY 142:206-210, April 15, 1985.

Human T-cell leukemia viruses (HTLV): a unique family of pathogenic retroviruses, by S. Broder, et al. ANNUAL REVIEW OF IMMUNOLOGY 3:321-
336, 1985.

Human 'T' leukemia virus still suspected in AIDS [interview by John Maurice], by
R. C. Gallo. JAMA 250(8):1015+, August 26, 1983.

Human T-lymphotropic retrovirus and AIDS. HTLV-III is probably the cause of acquired immunodeficiency syndrome, by J. H. Dobloug. TIDSSKRIFT FOR
DEN NORSKE LAEGEFORENING 105(1):50-52, January 10, 1985.

Human T-lymphotropic retroviruses, by F. Wong-Staal, et al. NATURE 317:395-
403, October 3, 1985.

Human T lymphotropic virus type III infection of human alveolar macrophages, by
S. Z. Salahuddin, et al. BLOOD 68(1):281-284, July 1986.

Identification and antigenicity of the major envelope glycoprotein of lymphadeno-pathy-associated virus, by L. Montagnier, et al. VIROLOGY 144:283-239, July 15, 1985.

Identification of the putative transforming protein of the human T-cell leukemia viruses HTLV-I and HTLV-II, by D. J. Slamon, et al. SCIENCE 226:61-65, October 5, 1984.

Implications of the discovery of HTLV-III for the treatment of AIDS, by R. Yarchoan, et al. CANCER RESARCH 45(Suppl. 9):4685s-4688s, September 1985.

Inactivation of AIDS virus in clothing, by I. H. Linden, et al. JAMA 253:2580, May 3, 1985.

Indications of a new virus in MS patients, by J. L. Marx. SCIENCE 230:1028, November 29, 1985.

Induction of HTLV-III/LAV from a nonvirus-producing T-cell lime: implications for latency, by T. Folks, et al. SCIENCE231:600-602, February 7, 1986.

Infection by the LAV virus and the acquired immunodeficiency syndrome, by J. C. Gluckman, et al. PRESSE MEDICALE 14(27):1451-1453, July 6, 1985.

Infection by the retrovirus associated with the acquired immunodeficiency syn-drome. Clinical, biological, and molecular features, by J. A. Levy, et al. ANNALS OF INTERNAL MEDICINE 103(5):694-699, November 1985.

Infection of HTLV-III/LAV in HTLV-I-carrying cells MT-2 and MT-4 and application in plaque assay, by S. Harada, et al. SCIENCE 229:563-566, August 9, 1985.

Infection of human T-lymphotropic virus type I (HTLV-I)-bearing MT-4 cells with HTLV-III (AIDS virus): chronological studies of early events, by S. Harada, et al. VIROLOGY 146:272-281, October 30, 1985.

Is the AIDS virus recombinant?, by H. Toh, et al. NATURE 316(6023):21-22, July 4-10, 1985.

Isolation and identification of a novel virus from patients with AIDS, by S. C. Lo. AMERICAN JOURNAL OF TROPICAL MEDICINE AND HYGIENE 35(4):675-676, July 1986.

Isolation of AIDS-associated retrovirus from genital secretions of women with antibodies to the virus, by C. B. Wofsy, et al. LANCET 1(8480):527-529, March 8, 1986.

Isolation of AIDS-associated retroviruses from cerebrospinal fluid and brain of pa-tients with neurological symptoms, by J. a. Levy, et al. LANCET 2(8455):586-588, September 14, 1985.

Isolation of AIDS virus from cell-free breast milk of three healthy virus carriers [letter], by L. Thiry, et al. LANCET 2(8460):891-892, October 19, 1985.

Isolation of HTLV-III from cerebrospinal fluid and neural tissues of patients with neurologic syndromes related to the acquired immunodeficiency syndrome, by D. D. Ho, et al. NEW ENGLAND JOURNAL OF MEDICINE 313(24):1493-1497, December 12, 1985.

Isolation of HTLV-III/LAV from cervical secretions of women at risk for AIDS, by M. W. Vogt, et al. LANCET 1(8480):525-527, March 8, 1986.

Isolation of human T-cell leukemia virus in acquired immune deficiency syndrome (AIDS), by R. C. Gallo, et al. SCIENCE 220(4599):865-867, May 20, 1983.

Isolation of human T-lymphotropic virus type III from the tears of a patient with the acquired immunodeficiency syndrome, by L. S. Fujikawa, et al. LANCET 2(8454):529-530, September 7, 1985.

Isolation of infectious human T-cell leukemia/lymphotropic virus type III (HTLV-III) from patients with acquired immunodeficiency syndrome (AIDS) or AIDS-related complex (ARC) and from healthy carriers: a study of risk groups and tissue sources, by S. Z. Salahuddin, et al. PROCEEDINGS OF THE NATIONAL ACADEMY OF SCIENCES USA82(16):5530-5534, August 1985.

Isolation of LAV/HTLV-III from a patient with amyotrophic lateral sclerosis [letter], by P. M. Hoffman, et al. NEW ENGLAND JOURNAL OF MEDICINE 313(5): 324-325, August 1, 1985.

Isolation of a lymphadenopathy-associated virus from a patient with the acquired immune deficiency syndrome, by M. L. Bechker, et al. SOUTH AFRICAN MEDICAL JOURNAL 68(3):144-147, August 3, 1985.

Isolation of a new retrovirus in a patient at risk for acquired immunodeficiency syndrome, by J. C. Chermann, et al. ANTIBIOTIC CHEMOTHERAPY 32:48-53, 1983.

Isolation of a T-lymphotropic retrovirus from a patient at risk for acquired immune deficiency syndrome (AIDS), by F. Barré-Sinoussi, et al. SCIENCE 220 (4599):868-871, May 20, 1983.

Kaplan memorial lecture. The family of human lymphotropic retroviruses called HTLV: HTLV-I in adult T-cell leukemia (ATL), HTLV-II in hairy cell leukemias, and HTLV-III in AIDS, by R. C. Gallo. INTERNATIONAL SYMPOSIUM OF THE PRINCESS TAKAMATSU CANCER RESEARCH FUND 15:13-38, 1984.

LAV/HTLV-III—new discoveries on its properties, isolation, vaccination and therapy, by B. Asjö, et al. LAKARTIDNINGEN 82(20):1870-1875, May 15, 1985.

Laying the groundwork for neturalizing AIDS-linked virus, by J. E. Groopman. NATURE 316:12, July 4, 1985.

Leu 3a/TQ 1 and leu 2a/leu 15 double marker studies of AIDS and ARC patients [letter], by M. J. Warzynski, et al. AIDS RESEARCH 1(6):vi-ix, 1984-1985.

Leukemia virus linked to AIDS. NEW SCIENTIST 98:439, May 19, 1983.

Like sheep virus, AIDS virus infects brain, by D. D. Bennett. SCIENCE NEWS 127:22, January 12, 1985.

Location of the *trans*-activating region on the genome of human T-cell lympho-tropic virus type III, by J. Sodroski, et al. SCIENCE 229:74-77, July 5, 1985.

Looking for the virus overlooking other causes, by K. Kelley. GUARDIAN 37(39): 7, July 10, 1985.

Low prevalence in the UK of HTLV-I and HTLV-II infection in subjects with AIDS, with extended lymphadenopathy, and at risk of AIDS, by R. S. Tedder, et al. LANCET 2(8395):125-128, July 21, 1984.

Lymphotropic virus type III, by D. P. Francis, et al. ANNALS OF INTERNAL MEDI-CINE 103(5):719-722, November 1985.

Mixed results found in Boston HTLV-III project, by S. Hyde. GAY COMMUNITY NEWS 12(35):6, March 23, 1985.

Molecular biology of human T-lymphotropic retroviruses, by F. Wong-Staal, et al. CANCER RESEARCH 45(Suppl. 9):4539s-4544s, September 1985.

Molecular biology of human T-lymphotropic retroviruses (HTLV), by F. Dorner, et al. WIENER MEDIZINISCHE WOCHENSCHRIFT 36(708):181-188, April 30, 1986.

Molecular biology of viruses associated with AIDS and current attempts to prevent its spread, by J. Holy. CASOPIS LEKARU CESKYCH 125(16):496-498, April 18, 1986.

Molecular characterization of human T-cell leukemia (lymphotropic) virus III in the acquired immune deficiency syndrome, by G. M. Shaw, et al. SCIENCE 226: 1165-1171, December 7, 1984.

Molecular comparison of retroviruses associated with human and simian AIDS, by M. L. Bryant, et al. HEMATOLOGICAL ONCOLOGY 3(3):187-197, July-September 1985.

Molecular studies of human T cell leukemia/lymphotropic retroviruses, by F. Wong-Staal. HAMATOLOGIE UND BLUTTRANSFUSION 29:326-330, 1985.

More about the HTLV's and how they act, by J. L. Marx. SCIENCE 229:37-38, July 5, 1985.

More progress on the HTLV family, by J. L. Marx. SCIENCE 227:156-157, January 11, 1985.

Morphology of the retroviruses associated with AIDS and SAIDS, by G. Lecatsas, et al. PROCEEDINGS OF THE SOCIETY FOR EXPERIMENTAL BIOLOGY AND MEDICINE 177(3):495-498, December 1984.

Mystery of AIDS could be solved [T-cell leukaemia virus type III (HTLV III)]. NEW SCIENTIST 102:3, April 19, 1984.

Name for AIDS virus [letter], by F. Wong-Staal. NATURE 314(6012):574, April 18-24, 1985.

Natural history of HTLV-III infection is studied, by S. H. Weiss. AMERICAN FAMILY PHYSICIAN 32:176, August 1985.

Natural history of human T lymphotropic virus-III infection: the cause of AIDS, by M. Melbye. BRITISH MEDICAL JOURNAL 292(6512):5-12, January 4, 1986.

Natural history of infection with the lymphadenopathy-associated virus/human T-lymphotropic virus type III, by D. P. Francis, et al. ANNALS OF INTERNAL MEDICINE 103(5):719-722, November 1985.

New AIDS viruses spark more rivalry. NEW SCIENTIST 110:20, April 3, 1986.

New clues link leukemia virus to AIDS, by P. Taulbee. SCIENCE NEWS 123:324, May 21, 1983.

New HTLV-III/LAV encoded antigen detected by antibodies from AIDS patients, by J. S. Allan, et al. SCIENCE 230:810-813, November 15, 1985.

New human retrovirus associated with acquired immunodeficiency syndrome (AIDS) or AIDS-related complex, by J. C. Chermann, et al. PROGRESS IN CLINICAL AND BIOLOGICAL RESEARCH 182:329-342, 1985.

New relatives of AIDS virus found [news],by J. L. Marx. SCIENCE 232(4747): 157, April 11, 1986.

New viral infections and the acquired immunodeficiency syndrome, by V. M. Zhdanov, et al. SOVIET MEDICINE 10:41-46, 1985.

Nucleic acid structure and expression of the human AIDS/lymphadenopathy retrovirus, by M. A. Muesing, et al. NATURE 313(6002):450-458, February 7-13, 1985.

Nucleotide sequence and expression of an AIDS-associated retrovirus (ARV-2), by R. Sanchez-Pescador, et al. SCIENCE 227(4686):484-492, February 1, 1985.

Nucleotide sequence evidence for relationship of AIDS retrovirus to lentiviruses, by I. M. Chiu, et al. NATURE 317(6035):366-368, October 26, 1985.

Nucleotide sequence of the AIDS virus, LAV, by S. Wain-Hobson, et al. CELL

On HTLV-III's trail. ALBERTA REPORT 12:50, November 25, 1985.

Parvovirus infection and the acquired immunodeficiency syndrome [letter], by M. J. Anderson, et al. ANNALS OF INTERNAL MEDICINE 102(2):275, February 1985.

Parvovirus infections: features reminiscent of AIDS, by M. E. Bloom. ANNALS OF THE NEW YORK ACADEMY OF SCIENCES 437:110-120, 1984.

Pathogenic retrovirus—current facts and hypotheses, by E. Kazimierska. POLSKI TYGODNIK LEKARSKI 41(3):86-87, January 21, 1986.

Pathogenic retrovirus (HTLV-III) linked to AIDS, by S. Broder, et al. NEW ENGLAND JOURNAL OF MEDICINE 311(20):1292-1297, November 15, 1984.

Persistent infection with human T-lymphotropic virus type III/lymphadenopathy-associated virus in apparently healthy homosexual men, by H. W. Jaffe, et al. ANNALS OF INTERNAL MEDICINE 102(5):627-628, May 1985.

Persistent noncytopathic infection of normal human T lymphocytes with AIDS-associated retrovirus, by J. A. Hoxie, et al. SCIENCE 229:1400-1402, September 27, 1985.

Possible role of a new lymphotropic retrovirus (LAV) in the pathogeny of AIDS and AIDS-related diseases, by F. Brun-Vezinet, et al. PROGRESS IN MEDICAL VIROLOGY 32:189-194, 1985.

Possible viral interactions in the acquired immunodeficiency syndrome (AIDS), by M. S. Hirsch, et al. REVIEWS OF INFECTIOUS DISEASES 6(5):726-731, September-October 1984.

Possible viral link to AIDS, by L. Goldsmith. GAY COMMUNITY NEWS 11(9):1, September 17, 1983.

Post-transcriptional regulation accounts for the transactivation of the human T-lymphotrophic virus type III, by C. A. Rosen, et al. NATURE 319:555-559, February 13, 1986.

Prevalence of AIDS-associated retrovirus and antibodies among male homosexuals at risk for AIDS in Greenwich Village, by D. Casareale, et al. AIDS RESEARCH 1(5):407-421, 1984-1985.

Proliferation of accessory cells in LAS and AIDS [letter], by H. Müller, et al. DEUTSCHE MEDIZINISCHE WOCHENSCHRIFT 111(7):278, February 14, 1986.

Proviral DNA of a retrovirus, human T-cell leukemia virus, in two patients with AIDS, by E. P. Gelmann, et al. SCIENCE 220(4599):862-865, May 20, 1983.

PX protein of HTLV-I is a transcriptional activator of its long terminal repeats, by B. K. Felber, et al. SCIENCE 229:675-679, August 16, 1985.

Quantitative analysis of AIDS-related virus-carrying cells by plaque-forming assay using an HTLV-I-positive MT-4 cell line, by S. Harada, et al. GANN 76(6):432-435, June 1985.

Recovery of AIDS-associated retroviruses from patients with AIDS or AIDS-related conditions and from clinically healthy individuals, by J. A. Levy, et al. JOURNAL OF INFECTIOUS DISEASES 152(4):734-738, October 1985.

Recovery of herpes viruses from cerebrospinal fluid of immunodeficient homosexual men, by R. D. Dix, et al. ANNALS OF NEUROLOGY 18(5):611-614, November 1985.

Relationship of AIDS to other retroviruses [letter], by S. Wain-Hobson, et al. NATURE 313(6005):743, February 28-March 6, 1985.

Retrovirus and malignant lymphoma in homosexual men, by A. M. Levine, et al. JAMA 254:1921-1925, October 11, 1985.

Retrovirus associated with AIDS. AMERICAN FAMILY PHYSICIAN 31:249, March 1985.

Retrovirus-induced acquired immunodeficiencies, by M. Bendinelli, et al. AD-
VANCES IN CANCER RESEARACH 45:125-181, 1985.

Retrovirus-like particles in salivary glands, prostate and testes of AIDS patients, by
G. Lecatsas, et al. PROCEEDINGS OF THE SOCIETY FOR EXPERIMENTAL
BIOLOGY AND MEDICINE 178(4):653-655, April 1985.

Retrovirus resembling HTLV in macrophages of patients with AIDS [letter], by F.
Gyorkey, et al. LANCET 1(8420):106, January 12, 1985.

Retroviruses, AIDS and systemic lupus erythematosus [editorial],by A. Schattner.
HAREFUAH 109(9):251-253, November 1985.

Retroviruses and acquired immunodeficiency syndrome (AIDS), by J. C.
Chermann, et al. BULLETIN DE L'ACADEMIE NATIONALE DE MEDECINE
168(1-2):288-295, January-February 1984.

Retroviruses and human disease [editorial], by R. A. Weinberg. HOSPITAL
PRACTICE 18(7):13+, July 1983.

Retroviruses linked with AIDS, by R. Weiss. NATURE 309(5963):12-13, May 3,
1984.

Role of Epstein-Barr virus in acquired immune deficiency syndrome, by D. T.
Purtilo, et al. ADVANCES IN EXPERIMENTAL MEDICINE AND BIOLOGY
187:53-65, 1985.

Role of hepatitis B virus in acquired immunodeficiency syndrome, y R. T. Ravenholt. LANCET 2(8355):885-886, October 15, 1983.

Second virus linked to AIDS cancer, by O. Sattaur, et al. NEW SCIENTIST 106:8,
April 11, 1985.

Selective cytotoxicity of AIDS virus infection towards HTLV-I-transformed cell
lines, by Y. Koyanagi, et al. INTERNATIONAL JOURNAL OF CANCER 36(4):
445-451, October 15, 1985.

Sequence homology and morphologic similarity of HTLV-III and visna virus, a
pathogenic lentivirus, by M. A. Gonda, et al. SCIENCE 227:173-177, January
11,   1985.

Seroepidemiological studies of human T-lymphotropic retrovirus type III in
acquired immunodeficiency syndrome, by B. Safai, et al. LANCET 1(8392):
1438-1440, June 30, 1984.

Seroepidemiology of human T-lymphotropic virus type III among homosexual
men with the acquired immunodeficiency syndrome or generalized lymphadenopathy and among asymptomatic controls in Boston, by J. E. Groopman,
et al. ANNALS OF INTERNAL MEDICINE 102(3):334-337, March 1985.

Serum interferon and clinical manifestations of infection with human T-lymphotropic virus type III, by J. Abb. MEDICAL MICROBIOLOGY AND IMMUNOLO-
GY 174(4):205-210, 1985.

Slow, insidious natures of the HTLV's, by J. L. Marx. SCIENCE 231:50-51, January 31, 1986.

611

Structural analysis of p19 and p24 core polypeptides of primate lymphotropic retroviruses (PLRV), by E. Jurkiewicz, et al. VIROLOGY 150:291-298, April 15, 1986.

Structure and function of human leukemia and AIDS viruses, by W. A. Haseltine, et al. INTERNATIONAL SYMPOSIUM OF THE PRINCESS TAKAMATSU CANCER RESEARCH FUND 15:187-196, 1984.

Studies of the putative transforming protein of the type I human T-cell leukemia virus, by D. J. Slamon, et al. SCIENCE 228:1427-1430, June 21, 1985.

Subcellular localization of the product of the long open reading frame of human T-cell leukemia virus type, by I. W. C. Goh, et al. SCIENCE 227:1227-1228, March 8, 1985.

Supergerms: the new health menace, by J. Mann. US NEWS AND WORLD REPORT 94:35-36, February 28, 1983.

Surprising action for the AIDS virus, by J. L. Marx. SCIENCE 231:798, February 21, 1986.

Trans-acting transcriptional regulation of human T-cell leukemia virus type III long terminal repeat, by J. Sodroski, et al. SCIENCE 227:171-173, January 11, 1985.

Trans-activator gene of HTLV-II induces IL-2 receptor and IL-2 cellular gene expression, by W. C. Greene, et al. SCIENCE 232:877-880, May 16, 1986.

Trans-activator gene of human T-lymphotropic virus type III (HTLV-III), by S. K. Arva, et al. SCIENCE 229:69-73, July 5, 1985.

Transactivation induced by human T-lymphotropic virus type III (HTLV-III) maps to a viral sequence encoding 58 amino acids and lacks tissue specificity, by L. J. Seigel, et al. VIROLOGY 148:226-231, January 15, 1986.

Transcription of novel open reading frames of AIDS retrovirus during infection of lymphocytes, by A. B. Rabson, et al. SCIENCE 229(4720):1388-1390, September 27, 1985.

Transcriptional activator protein encoded by the *x-lor* region of the human T-cell leukemia virus, by J. Sodroski, et al. SCIENCE 228:1430-1434, June 21, 1985.

Type D retrovirus in prodromal AIDS? [letter], by T. F. Warner, et al. LANCET 1(8381):860, April 14, 1984.

Viral AIDS suspect stripped of alibi, by D. Franklin. SCIENCE NEWS 126:6, July 7, 1984.

Viral cancers: AIDS virus at the centre, by J. Palca. NATURE 319:170, January 16, 1986.

Virologic, immunologic, and epidemiologic associations with AIDS among gay males in a low incidence area, by C. Rinaldo, et al. ANNALS OF THE NEW YORK ACADEMY OF SCIENCES 437:544-548, 1984.

Virology of AIDS: taxonomy, molecular biology, and pathogenicity, by J. T. Griffith. JOURNAL OF MEDICAL TECHNOLOGY 3(3):149-151+, March 1986.

Virus by any other name . . . would still cause AIDS, by J. L. Marx. SCIENCE 227(4693): 1449-1451, March 22, 1985.

Virus clones multiply [news], by T. Beardsley. NATURE 311(5983):195, September 20-26, 1984.

Virus envelope protein of HTLV-III represents major target antigen for antibodies in AIDS patients, by F. Barin, et al. SCIENCE 228(4703):1094-1096, May 31, 1985.

'Virus-like particles' in lymphocytes in AIDS are normal organelles, not viruses [letter], by T. Gardiner, et al. LANCET 2(8356):963-964, October 22,1 983.

Virus linked to AIDS: variant of cancer virus may be cause. CHEMICAL AND ENGINEERING NEWS 62:4, April 23, 1984.

Virus-neutralizing activity, serologic heterogeneity, and retrovirus isolation from homosexual men in the Los Angeles area, by S. Rasheed, et al. VIROLOGY 150(1):1-9, April 15, 1986.

Viruses linked to AIDS. FDA CONSUMER 18:5-6, October 1984.

What is the role of cytomegalovirus in AIDS?, by W. L. Drew, et al. ANNALS OF THE NEW YORK ACADEMY OF SCIENCES 437:320-324, 1984.

What proportion of HTLV-III antibody positives will proceed to AIDS? [letter], by A. R. Moss. LANCET 2(8448):223-224, July 27, 1985.

Where is the AIDS virus harbored? SCIENCE 232:1197, June 6, 1986.

Why the AIDS virus is not like HTLVs-I or II. NEW SCIENTIST 105:4, February 7, 1985.

AFRICA
Acquired immune deficiency syndrome and related complex. A report of 2 confirmed cases in Cape Town with comments on human T-cell lymphotropic virus type III infections, by F. H. Spracklen, et al. SOUTH AFRICAN MEDICAL JOURNAL 68(3):139-143, August 3, 1985.

Isolation of human T-lyphotropic retrovirus (LAV) from Zairian married couple, one with AIDS, one with prodromes, by A. Ellrodt, et al. LANCET 1(8391):1383-1385, June 23, 1984.

Isolation of a new human retrovirus from West African patients with AIDS, by F. Clavel, et al. SCIENCE 233(4761):343-346, July 18, 1986.

LAV type II: a second retrovirus associated with AIDS in West Africa, by F. Clavel, et al. COMPTES RENDUS DE L'ACADEMIE DES SCIENCES. SERIE III, SCIENCES DE LA VIE 302(13):485-488, 1986.

Tests show virus common, long-established/Africa. BODY POLITIC 114:21, May 1985.

AFRICA
Virus-like particles in lymphocytes of seven cases of AIDS in Black Africans [letter], by W. Feremans, et al. LANCET 2(8340):52-53, July 2, 1983.

BAHAMAS
Isolation of HTLV-III/LAV from samples of serum proteins given to cancer patients—Bahamas. JAMA 254:1139, September 6, 1985.

FRANCE
HTLV and AIDS in France [letter], by D. Mathez, et al. LANCET 1(8380):799, April 7, 1984.

United States French studies link leukemia virus to AIDS [news]. HOSPITAL PRACTICE 18(7):33+, July 1983.

GERMANY
HTLV and AIDS in West Germany [letter],by M. Born, et al. LANCET 1(8370): 222, January 28, 1984.

HAITI
Characteristics of the acquired immunodeficiency syndrome (AIDS) in Haiti, by J. W. Pape, et al. NEW ENGLAND JOURNAL OF MEDICINE 309(16): 945-950, October 20, 1983.

ISRAEL
Human T-cell lymphotropic virus type-I antibodies in Falashas and other ethnic groups in Israel, by Z. Ben-Ishai, et al. NATURE 315:665-666, June 20, 1985.

JAPAN
ATLV in Japanese patient with AIDS [letter],by I. Miyoshi, et al. LANCET 2(8344):275, July 30, 1983.

Viruses and cancer: the Japanese connection [adult T-cell leukemia and HTLV-I], by G. Vines. NEW SCIENTIST 107:36-37+, July 11, 1985.

THE NETHERLANDS
Acquired immune deficiency syndrome, altered T cell subset ratios, and cytomegalo-virus infections among male homosexuals in The Netherlands, by J. Goudsmit, et al. ANTIOBIOTIC CHEMOTHERAPY 32:138-146, 1983.

TRINIDAD
Racial and other characteristics of human T cell leukemia/lymphoma (HTLV-I) and AIDS (HTLV-III) in Trinidad, by C. Bartholomew, et al. BRITISH MEDI-CAL JOURNAL 290(6477):1243-1246, April 27, 1985.

UNITED STATES
Isolation of lymphadenopathy-associated virus (LAV) and detection of LAV antibodies from US patients with AIDS, by F. Barré-Sinoussi, et al. JAMA 253(12):1737-1739, March 22-29, 1985.

Isolation of lymphocytopahic retroviruses from San Francisco patients with AIDS, by J. A. Levy, et al. SCIENCE 225(4664):840-842, August 24, 1984.

UNITED STATES
United States French studies link leukemia virus to AIDS [news]. HOSPITAL PRACTICE 18(7):33+, July 1983.

VIROLOGY—CHILDREN
HTLV-I antibodies in childhood leukemia, by D. L. Williams, et al. JAMA 253: 2496, May 3, 1985.

Role of mononuclear phagocytes in HTLV-III/LAV infection, by S. Gartner, et al. SCIENCE 233(4760):215-219, July 11, 1986.

WOMEN
Acquired immunodeficiency syndrome and opportunistic infections in a female, by E. Thornston, et al. SCHWEIZERISCHE MEDIZINISCHE WOCHEN-SCHRIFT 113(1):28-30, January 8, 1983.

AIDS and women, by E. Cameron. CHATELAINE 59:56+, February 1986.

AIDS from women to men. NEW SCIENTIST 108:27, November 7, 1985.

AIDS: how real is the risk for women? GLAMOUR 83:308+, November 1985.

AIDS in an apparently risk-free woman [letter], by J. Cabane, et al. LANCET 2(8394):105, July 14, 1984.

AIDS in the female, by W. Stille, et al. ARCHIVES OF GYNECOLOGY 238(1-4):825-832, 1985.

AIDS is not for men only, by C. Norwood. MADEMOISELLE 91:198-199+, September 1985.

AIDS: the risk for women, by Farrell, et al. COMMUNIQU'ELLES 12(2):20, March 1986.

AIDS risk groups include some women, by P. Turner. OUT 4(4):7, February 1986.

AIDS: what women must know now!, by D. R. Zimmerman, et al. GOOD HOUSE-KEEPING 201:245-246, November 1985.

AIDS—women get, more rarely give, by A. Henry. OFF OUR BACKS 15:12-13, November 1985.

Boston women meet, discuss AIDS, by S. Hyde. GAY COMMUNITY NEWS 11(11):1, October 1, 1983.

Case records of the Massachusetts General Hospital. Case 2-1986 [a 58-year-old woman with fever and nodular pulmonary infiltrates], by R. E. Scully, et al. NEW ENGLAND JOURNAL OF MEDICINE 314:167-174, January 16, 1986.

Mothers on the front lines, by M. Helquist. ADVOCATE 438:22, January 21, 1986.

Taking control—women, sex and AIDS, by C. Patton. GAY COMMUNITY NEWS 11(9):5, September 17, 1983.

Women and AIDS, by A. G. Fettner. HEALTH 18(11):61-66, November 1986.

—, by M. Clark, et al. NEWSWEEK 108(2):60-61, July 14, 1986.

Women of the year, by L. Van Gelder. MS. 14:31-34+, January 1986.

Women susceptible to AIDS, too? AMERICAN JOURNAL OF NURSING 83: 1199, August 1983.

617

620

625

Goudot, P. 196
Goudsmit, J. 12, 127, 133, 165, 195
Goulden, T. 34
Gracie, J. A. 14
Grady, D. 65, 197
Graf, T. M. 276
Graham, B. S. 5
Gransden, W. R. 227
Grant, I. H. 195
Grantham, P. 76
Gravell, M. 272
Gray, R. H. 257
Graybeal, F. R., Jr. 141
Greaves, W. 62
Greco, R. S. 146
Greco, S. 94
Green, D. 36
Green, J. 53, 82
Greenberg, F. 252
Greenberg, J. E. 278
Greenberg, M. L. 99
Greene, E. R., Jr. 25
Greene, L. W. 28
Greene, W. C. 270
Greenspan, J. S. 218, 244
Gregg, M. B. 229
Gremminger, R. A. 266
Grenville, D. 89
Grieco, M. H. 127, 170
Griese, O. N. 46
Griffin, J. P. 14
Griffith, J. T. 282
Griffiths, C. 50
Grimley, P. M. 175
Grimm, I. 112
Grindon, A. J. 91
Grodin, M. A. 131
Grody, W. w. 269
Groocock, V. 250
Groopman, J. E. 8, 9, 46, 78, 83, 84,
    98, 105, 128, 158, 184, 187, 221,
    241, 254, 255, 281
Gross, L. 220
Grossi, C. E. 265
Grouse, L. D. 159
Grubb, R. 203
Grutsch, J. F. 107
Gu, C. H. 28
Guarda, L. A. 15
Guarda, N. P. 11, 252, 253
Guards, L. A. 160
Gubernick, L. 235
Guenot, O. 187
Guenthner, E. E. 233
Guerin, J. M. 15, 256, 285
Guilfoy, C. 31, 32, 43, 48, 49, 50, 63,
    64, 68, 89, 91, 92, 98, 117, 124,
    135, 136, 138, 141, 142, 146,

148, 155, 159, 195, 196, 197,
    202, 208, 209, 212, 213, 226,
    239, 250, 261, 269, 276
Guilfoy, E. 42
Guinan, M. E. 151
Gunderson, C. 215
Gupta, S. 87, 103, 110, 133, 193,
    200, 273
Gurevich, I. 97
Gury, D. J. 37
Gustafson, P. R. 171, 184, 232
Gyger, M. 139
Gyorkey, F. 246
Haber, S. L. 284
Habermehl, K. O. 31
Habibi, B. 91, 229
Hachem, S. 71
Hacket, D. 285
Hadden, J. W. 224
Hadden, L. 203
Hager, T. 284
Hagerty, A. D. 187
Hagerty, P. J. 51
Haggerty, C. M. 141
Hahn, B. H. 144, 199
Haire, W. D. 20
Halak, G. 75, 266
Halcrow, A. 44, 56
Hale, K. 62
Hale, W. K. 99,
Hale-Wehmann, K. 58, 256
Hall, C. 153
Hall, G. H. 39
Hall, J. 188
Hall, R. 108
Haller, S. 54, 81, 137, 187
Halper, H. R. 44
Hamilton, J. O. 73
Hamilton, M. 72
Hammar, S. P. 201
Hammarström, L. 166
Hammond, A. 39
Hampton Sides, W. 250
Hancock, L. 135
Hanczyk, B. 30
Handler, M. 177
Handsfield, H. H. 16
Handy, W. 124, 286
Handzel, Z. T. 164
Hanks, C. 287
Hannon, G. 125
Hanrahan, J. P. 234
Hansen, R. S. 8
Hanson, H. 228
Harada, S. 173, 239
Harbeck, W. 144
Harcup, C. 132
Hardie, J. 36, 212

626

627

Johnson, N. M. 227
Johnson, T. 109
Johnson, T. M. 47
Johnstone, B. 124, 181, 208
Johson, J. A. 31
Johson, M. E. 97
Johson, R. E. 20
Johson, T. 37
Joller-Jemelka, H. I. 166
Jonas, C. 113, 256
Joncas, J. H. 13, 247
Jonckheer, T. 106
Jonderko, K. 49
Jones, J. 170, 220
Jones, K. A. 26
Jones, M. 229
Jones, N. L. 125
Jones, P. 22, 32, 35, 157
Jones, P. G. 122
Jonsen, A. 131
Jonsen, A. R. 34
Jordan, B. D. 207
Jordan, W. C. 150
Joseph, J. G. 110
Joshi, V. V. 221, 222
Jothy, S. 66, 116
Joy, M. 218
Joyce, C. 49, 77, 156, 209, 279
Joyce, R. 188, 261
Jörgensen, G. 156
Judson, F. N. 135
Jurgens, N. N. 67
Jurkiewicz, E. 262
Kabbash, L. 57
Kadzielski, M. A. 28, 70, 187
Kal Bo Zanon, R. 138
Kalden, J. R. 166
Kalish, R. S. 265
Kalish, S. B. 24
Kalter, D. C. 194
Kalter, S. 13
Kalyanaraman, V. S. 82
Kan, N. C. 163
Kandel, W. L. 56
Kane, M. A. 248
Kanki, P. J. 83, 180, 254
Kant, H. S. 272
Kantrowitz, A. 140
Kantrowitz, B. 145
Kaplan, H. S. 41
Kaplan, J. 199
Kaplan, J. E. 132, 159
Kaplan, L. 134
Kaplan, M. H. 104
Karam, D. B. 34
Karg, O. 120
Karlovac, M. 47
Karpas, A. 185, 194, 277

Karpatkin, S. 163
Kaslow, R. A. 68
Katlama, C. 18
Kato, S. 150
Katz, A. J. 169
Katz, B. Z. 173
Katz, J. C. 52
Katzman, M. 200
Kawai, T. 214
Kawala, K. S. 230
Kawata, P. 261
Kay, N. E. 103
Kayal, P. M. 200
Kaye, J. A. 111
Kaye, R. 61, 142, 228
Kazimierska, E. 7, 221
Kearns, M. 142
Keeling, R. P. 63
Keen, L. M. 224
Keenan, G. 55
Keerdoja, E. 154
Keikola, J. 61
Kekow, J. 265
Kelinberg, S. 142
Kelley, K. 49, 191, 228, 253
Kellner, A. 36
Kelly, T. A. 10
Kelly, W. M. 25
Kenkelen, B. 58, 121, 206
Kenkelsen, B. 171
Kennedy, R. C. 84
Kenny, P. 278
Kenny, P. M. 215
Kermani, E. 219
Kern, P. 118, 167, 230, 240
Kern, R. 119
Kernoff, P. B. 57
Kerr, P. 37
Kerrison, R. 60
Kerschner, P. 263
Kesselring, J. 87, 206
Kessler, C. M. 4
Kestelyn, P. 223, 235
Kestens, L. 5
Khadem, M. 217
Khaitov, R. M. 8
Khan, F. A. 8
Khanna, S. 12, 15
Khojasteh, A. 194, 195
Khurana, M. 49
Kiel, R. A. 30, 78
Kielhofner, M. A. 182
Kiely, J. 95, 148, 225, 279
Kikukawa, R. 120
Kim, B. S. 172
Kimble, V. 225
Kimbrough, R. D. 280
King, N. W. 257

629

632

639

641

Wilson, G. 128
Wilson, J. 187
Wilson, J. D. 10
Wing, D. L. 50, 59
Wingerter, R. 111
Winkelstein, A. 116
Winkelstein, W., Jr. 229
Winkler, W. P. 138
Winter, S. M. 162
Winters, P. 48
Winterton, S. J. 274
Wisecarver, J. 107
Witek, T. J., Jr. 11
Witkin, S. S. 162, 172
Witte, M. H. 55
Wittees, R. E. 233
Witti, F. P. 205
Wittke, C. 108
Wittner, M. 134
Wofford, D. T. 11
Wofsy, C. B. 179, 226
Wolcott, D. L. 10
Wolff, P. H. 50
Wolke, A. 203
Wollschlager, C. M. 238
Wong, B. 100, 110
Wong-Staal, F. 134, 144, 162, 199,
    204
Wood, G. S. 165, 170
Wood, G. S. 170
Wood, R. 102
Woodfield, D. G. 146
Wormser, G. P. 24, 203, 206
Wright, K. 67
Wright, P. M. 37
Wu, J. M. 120
Wykoff, R. F. 166, 232
Wynne, P. 170
Yales, G. 43
Yamamoto, J. K. 159
Yancey, P. 181
Yanchinski, S. 45, 94
Yankauer, A. 224
Yarbrough, J. 248
Yarchoan, R. 28, 170
Yomtovian, R. 87
Yonay, E. 212
Young, F. E. 188
Young, K. R., Jr. 94
Young, S. B. 50, 64, 223
Zack, R. 243
Zagury, D. 118, 132, 158, 190, 244
Zakowski, P. 122
Zaloga, G. P. 162
Zar, F. 86
Zeffren, B. 97
Zegerius, L. 112
Zeh, J. 33, 88, 103

Zeithuber, U. 149
Zhdanov, V. M. 211
Ziegler, J. B. 229
Ziegler, J. L. 37, 152, 183, 213
Zielinski, C. C. 271
Zimmerman, D. R. 78, 89
Ziza, J. M. 68, 192
Zolla-Pazner, S. 239, 279
Zuck, T. F. 145
Zucker-Franklin, D. 191
Zumbrunnen, R. 236